PRINCIPLES OF
PHARMACOLOGY
for MEDICAL ASSISTING

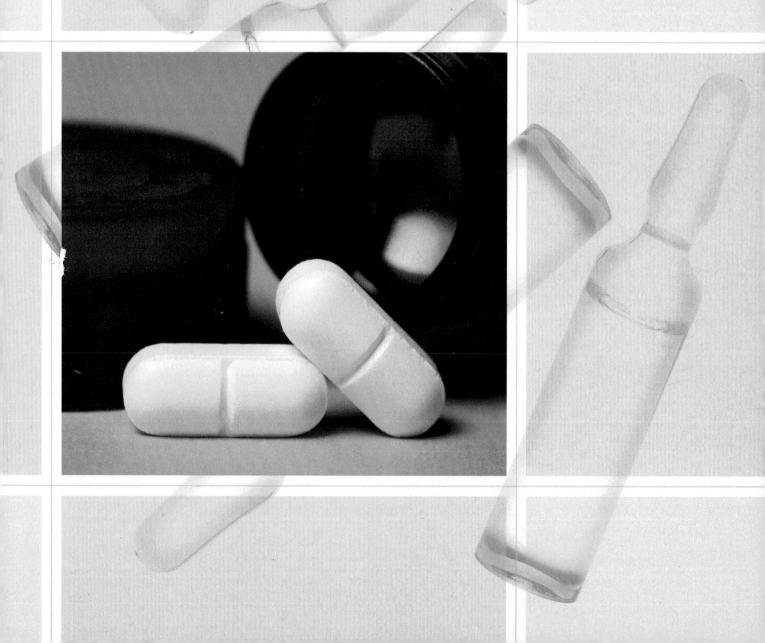

PRINCIPLES OF
PHARMACOLOGY
for MEDICAL ASSISTING

Jane Rice, RN, CMA-C

Fifth Edition

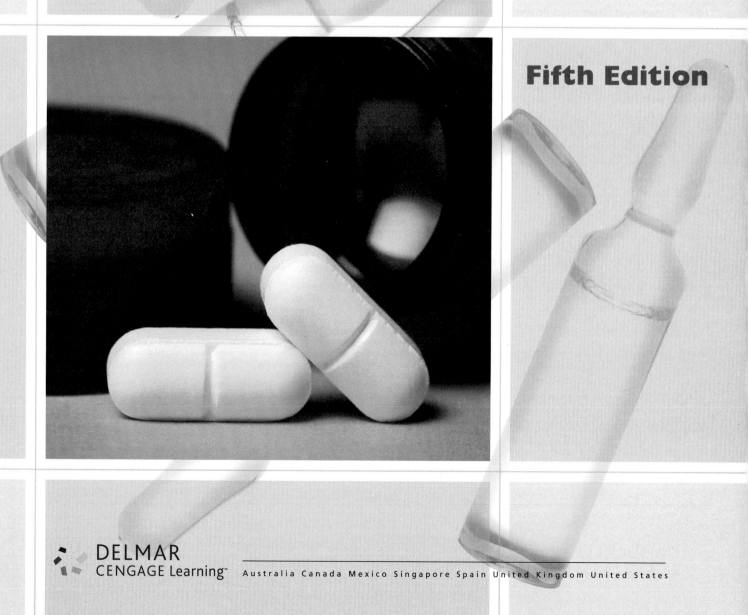

DELMAR
CENGAGE Learning™

Australia Canada Mexico Singapore Spain United Kingdom United States

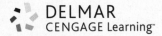

Principles of Pharmacology for Medical Assisting, Fifth Edition
Jane Rice

Vice President, Career and Professional Editorial: Dave Garza

Director of Learning Solutions: Matthew Kane

Senior Acquisitions Editor: Rhonda Dearborn

Managing Editor: Marah Bellegarde

Senior Product Manager: Sarah Prime

Editorial Assistant: Lauren Whalen

Vice President, Career and Professional Marketing: Jennifer Baker

Marketing Director: Wendy E. Mapstone

Senior Marketing Manager: Nancy Bradshaw

Marketing Coordinator: Erica Ropitzky

Production Director: Carolyn Miller

Content Project Manager: Thomas Heffernan

Senior Art Director: Jack Pendleton

Technology Project Manager: Patti Allen

For product information and technology assistance, contact us at
Cengage Learning Customer & Sales Support, 1-800-354-9706
For permission to use material from this text or product,
submit all requests online at **cengage.com/permissions**
Further permissions questions can be emailed to
permissionrequest@cengage.com

Library of Congress Control Number: 2010927188

ISBN-13: 978-1-1111-3182-1

ISBN-10: 1-1111-3182-1

Delmar
5 Maxwell Drive
Clifton Park, NY 12065-2919
USA

Cengage Learning is a leading provider of customized learning solutions with office locations around the globe, including Singapore, the United Kingdom, Australia, Mexico, Brazil, and Japan. Locate your local office at:
international.cengage.com/region

Cengage Learning products are represented in Canada by Nelson Education, Ltd.

To learn more about Delmar, visit **www.cengage.com/delmar**

Purchase any of our products at your local college store or at our preferred online store **www.cengagebrain.com**

Printed in the United States of America
2 3 4 5 6 7 14 13 12 11

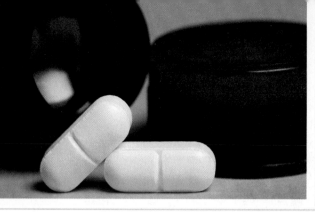

Contents

SECTION 4

Effects of Medications on Body Systems   351

Preface

Principles of Pharmacology for Medical Assisting, Fifth Edition is designed for the medical assistant. Although directed at the medical assistant, any health care professional who needs essential information about mathematics and pharmacology can use this text.

The text reflects current and commonly used practices, procedures, medications, and drug preparations. The content is explained in a clear and easy-to-understand language. At all times, safety is emphasized for the health care professional administering medications and for the patient receiving medications.

Graphic icons pinpoint information that relates to legal implications, safety, warnings and cautions, documentation, ethical considerations, patient teaching, spotlights, special considerations: older adults, special considerations: children, critical thinking questions and activities, and spot checks.

SECTION 1

Section 1—Mathematics and Dosage Calculations explains how to work each mathematical process, with emphasis placed on accuracy. Practice problems follow the mathematical presentation for immediate reinforcement. This section builds the mathematical skills necessary for the safe preparation and administration of medications to adult and pediatric patients. Each mathematical process is presented in a clear, concise, step-by-step format with numerous solved problems as examples. Practice problems are based upon actual clinical situations and involve the use of current drugs and dosages. Self-Assessment exercises at the end of each unit allow students to assess their understanding of each unit's content.

Key Features

- Extensive practice in working with metric units of measurement is provided.
- Guidelines are presented for administering medications to a pediatric patient. Calculations of pediatric dosages is based on the method and kilogram of body weight method.
- The presentation of each mathematical concept is clear and concise, with a step-by-step format and numerous solved examples.
- Practice problems follow each step-by-step explanation for immediate reinforcement.
- Review problems and Self-Assessment exercises are presented at the end of the unit to allow students to assess their understanding of each unit's content.

SECTION 2

Section 2—Introduction to Pharmacology presents a detailed explanation of topics essential to a thorough understanding of drug sources, herbs and supplements, legislation relating to drugs, drug references, forms of drugs, drug classifications and actions, the medication order, basic principles for the administration of medications, universal precautions, standard precautions, nonparenteral medications, parenteral equipment and supplies, preventing needlestick injuries in health care settings, Needlestick Safety and Prevention Act, and administration of parenteral medications.

Key Features

- Stresses the seven rights of proper drug administration:
  — The Right Patient
  — The Right Drug
  — The Right Dose
  — The Right Route
  — The Right Time
  — The Right Technique
  — The Right Documentation
- Drugs cited are current and commonly used.
- Numerous photographs, drawings, tables, and examples of drugs and equipment are provided.
- Basic principles for the administration of medications are presented.
- Drug administration procedures include standard precautions, purpose, equipment and supplies, procedure steps, and performance checklist.
- An overview of allergy therapy includes diagnosis, treatment, and administration of allergenic extracts. Latex allergy is also included.
- Multiple choice and matching review questions are provided for each unit.

SECTION 3

Section 3—Medications, Supplements, and Drug Abuse provides quality information about antibiotics, antiseptics, disinfectants, antifungal, antiviral, immunizing agents, antineoplastics, vitamins, minerals, and herbals, and psychotropic agents, and substance abuse.

Key Features

- New tables summarize currently used drugs.
- Each major drug classification includes:
  — description   — action
  — uses   — adverse reactions
  — contraindications   — warnings, when indicated
  — dosage and route   — implications for patient care
  — patient teaching   — special considerations
- Multiple choice and matching review questions are provided for each unit.
- Among the features are:
  — spotlights   — special considerations: older adult
  — special considerations: children   — critical thinking questions and activities
  — spot checks

SECTION 4

Section 4—Effects of Medications on Body Systems provides students with an explanation of the effects of specific medications on the musculoskeletal, gastrointestinal, cardiovascular, respiratory, urinary, endocrine, nervous, and reproductive systems.

Key Features

- New tables summarizing currently used drugs
- Each major drug classification includes:
  - description
  - uses
  - contraindications
  - dosage and route
  - patient teaching
  - action
  - adverse reactions
  - warnings, when indicated
  - implications for patient care
  - special considerations
- Multiple choice and matching review questions are provided for each unit
- Among the features are:
  - spotlights
  - special considerations: children
  - spot checks
  - special considerations: older adults
  - critical thinking questions and activities

INDEX

Two indexes are provided for ready reference to learners. A drug reference allow individuals to be able to locate any of the drugs described in the text and a general index covers all other topics for ready reference.

SPECIAL FEATURES

- Competency-based objectives guide students in their study of each unit.
- Each unit contains a vocabulary list in which important terms are identified, defined, and their pronunciation indicated.
- Emphasis throughout the text is placed on the legal implications of drug therapy, safety, and accuracy in calculating and administering medications.
- An excellent table is provided listing the classifications of drugs and giving examples of commonly used drugs.
- Needlestick Safety and Prevention Act included.
- National Institute for Occupation Safety and Health's (NIOSH) recommendations presented on preventing needlestick injuries in health care settings.
- Use of safety syringe-needle units discussed.
- Information on MedWatch and reporting drug errors included.
- Numerous implications for patient care and patient teaching are included.
- Important information about infectious diseases, including AIDS (with drug therapy), and guidelines for the safe handling of infectious materials are provided.
- Included is current information about immunization based on materials from the U.S. Department of Health and Human Services, Public Health Service, and Centers for Disease Control and Prevention in Atlanta, Georgia.

- Answers to practice problems, learning exercises, review questions, and critical thinking questions and activities are found on this book's online student companion website and in the Instructor's Manual.

- Self-assessment exercises in the math and calculations units allow students to assess their understanding of the content. Answers to self-assessment exercises are found on this book's online student companion website and in the Instructor's Manual.

- Spotlights present current findings in pharmacology and medicine along with interesting facts about the subject highlighted.

- Special Considerations: Older Adults presents important information as related to aging, drugs, and diseases and conditions.

- Special Considerations: Children presents important information as related to growth and development, drugs, and diseases and conditions.

- Critical thinking questions and answers provide students with the opportunity to enhance their learning concepts.

- Spot Checks provide students with a quick refresher of selected material from the unit.

New To This Edition

- Appendix A: *A Color Photo Quick Reference Guide* provides rapid identification of 101 most commonly prescribed drugs. Actual-sized tablets and capsules, with their strength, are organized alphabetically by generic name and include appropriate trade name and manufacturer.

- The author used www.Drugs@FDA.gov to check each drug entry in the text and to update the content, thereby reflecting the current status of the drug. Many trade or brand names were removed from the text due to withdrawal of that specific name from the market. If the generic equivalent of the drug was found to be on the market, then it is still included in the text.

- The author used FDA MedWatch, Center for Drug Evaluation and Research (CDER), and (Center for Drug Evaluation and Research) and Drugs@FDA for new cautions, alerts, and black-box warnings for NSAIDS; fluoroquinolones; zanamivir (Relenza); benzodiazepines; antipsychotic agents; SSRIs, SNRAs, and triptans; Enbrel, Remicade, Humira and Cimzia; bisphosphonates; Epogen; Avandia; proton pump inhibitors (PPIs); Singulair; multisymptoms cold medicines, and others.

- The previous editions of Unit 5 (Household Measures) and Unit 6 (Temperature Equivalents) were removed from the text. The household abbreviations, equivalent tables, and relationship between household measures are included in Appendix B. Also included in Appendix B is the relationship of differences between Celsius and Fahrenheit temperature scales.

- *Unit 6* includes the "seven rights" of medication administration and new dosage forms of medications as they relate to children, and the author has removed material on calculating children's dosages by body surfaces area.

- *Unit 7* includes new material and a table on biologics. Material on herbals and supplements was removed from Unit 7 (Drug Sources, Schedules, and Dosages) and was placed in Unit 18 (Vitamins, Minerals, and Herbals), in response to reviewer recommendations.

- *Unit 8* includes new material on fast-dissolving drug delivery systems (FDDS).

- *Unit 9* includes new material and screen shots on electronic medical records (EMRs) and e-prescribing, and the Institute For Safe Medication Practices's (ISMP's) List of Error-Prone Abbreviations, Symbols, and Dose Designations.

- *Unit 10* includes new material on "the right technique" (one of the "seven rights"), a new figure for standard precautions from the CDC, and documentation examples both in a paper chart and in an electronic medical record.

- *Unit 11 to 14* include new figures of medicine cups with approximate equivalent measures, and updated "cc" to "mL" measurements. Performance checklists have been moved to Appendix C.

- *Unit 15* includes new material on methicilin-resistant *Staphylococcus aureus* (MRSA), *Clostridium difficile*-associated diarrhea (CDAD), dangers of antibiotic resistance, carbapenems, and a warning box about fluoroquinolones.

- *Unit 16* includes new material on H1N1 influenza, vaccines/immunizations, including H1N1 and live attenuated influenza vaccine, and a warning box about zanamivir (Relenza).

- *Unit 17* includes new material on cancer treatment, distinguishing local and systemic therapy; how chemotherapy works; additional types of cancer drugs; and new and expected advances in chemotherapy.

- *Unit 19* includes a new caution box on the combined use of SSRIs, SNRIs, and triptan medications.

- *Unit 21* includes a new warning box on NSAIDs; new material and a warning box on Enbrel, Remicade, Humira, and Cimzia; new material and a table on agents used to treat osteoporosis; and other antiresorptive medications.

- *Unit 22* includes a new caution box on the combined use of Plavix and Prilosec.

- *Unit 23* includes new material and a warning box on Epogen.

- *Unit 24* includes new material on pertussis (whooping cough) and the vaccine DTaP, and new figures for airborne and droplet precautions from the CDC.

- *Unit 26* includes new safety information on the use of insulin pens and insulin cartridges; information on dipeptidyl peptidase-4 (DPP-4) inhibitor, a new class of oral hypoglycemic agent; and a warning box on congestive heart failure and myocardial ischemia.

- *Unit 28* includes new material on estrogen and hormone replacement therapy.

SUPPLEMENTS

- **StudyWARE CD-ROM.** The StudyWARE™ CD-ROM includes a basic math pretest, math tutorials and animations, interactive syringe activities, and Audio Library of drug names and medical terminology. ISBN-13: 978-1-1115-3815-6

- **Premium Website.** The Premium website includes an online version of StudyWARE™, along with printable procedure checklists and additional review quizzes. Follow the directions on the Printed Access Card to log in at www.CengageBrain.com. ISBN-13: 978-1-1115-4149-1

- **Instructor's Manual.** The Instructor's Manual includes course outlines, suggestions for instructors using this book, lecture outlines and class notes, post-tests with answers, and an answer key for textbook review questions. ISBN-13: 978-1-1111-3183-8

- **Instructor Resources.** This CD-ROM includes instructor slides in Microsoft PowerPoint® for each chapter; computerized Test Bank in ExamView®; and electronic Instructor's Manual files in Microsoft Word®, for instructor customization. ISBN-13: 978-1-1111-3184-5

- **Instructor Companion Site.** The instructor companion site includes customizable procedure checklists, answer keys, electronic Instructor's Manual files, and instructor slides in Microsoft PowerPoint®. Log in at login.cengage.com/sso with your Cengage instructor account. If you are a first-time user, click Create a new Faculty Account and follow the prompts.

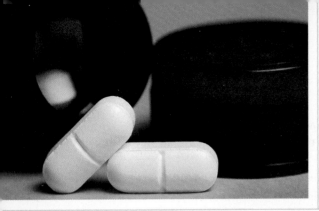

Acknowledgments

I wish to express my deepest appreciation to those individuals who assisted me in this revision of *Principles of Pharmacology for Medical Assisting*. Thank you for your time, knowledge, encouragement, expertise, and your valuable input.

- Husband and partner, Charles Larry Rice
- Rhonda Dearborn, Sarah Prime, Tom Heffernan, Jack Pendleton, Ben Knapp, and Patti Allen

REVIEWERS

The author and publisher would like to thank the following individuals for their many suggestions for improvement in the manuscript. Their constructive evaluation contributed to an outstanding edition of the text.

Connie Allen, MAED/CI-AE, CMA (AAMA)
Medical Assistant Clinical Coordinator
    and Instructor
Wallace State Community College
Hanceville, AL

Cherika DeJesus, CMA (AAMA)
Minnesota School of Business
Plymouth, MN

Linda Demain, LPN, BS, MA, EDS
Medical Curriculum Development
Wichita Technical Institute
Wichita, KS

Patricia Dudek, RN, RMA (AMT), CHI
Program Director, Medical Assisting
McCann School of Business
    and Technology

Rhonda Epps, CMA (AAMA), AS
Director of Healthcare Education
National College
Knoxville, TN

Pamela Fleming, RN, MPA, CMA (AAMA)
Quinsigamond Community College
Worcester, MA

Dr. Henry Gomez
Assistant Chair, Clinical Disciplines
ASA Institute
Brooklyn, NY

Helen Houser, RN, MSHA, RMA (AMT)
Director, Medical Assisting and Patient
    Care Technician Programs
Phoenix College
Phoenix, AZ

Diana Kendrick, RN, RMA (AMT)
Medical Assisting Instructor
Griffin Technical College
Griffin, GA

Donna Otis, LPN
Medical Program Director
Metro Business College
Rolla, MO

Agnes Pucillo, LPN, BSN, ACI, RHE, CMBCS
Medical Billing and Coding Instructor
Prism Career Institute
Cherry Hill, NJ

Lynn G. Slack, BS, CMA (AAMA)
Medical Programs Director
Kaplan Career Institute—ICM Campus
Pittsburgh, PA

Sherry Stanfield, RN, BSN, MSHPE
Assistant Program Director—Medical Assisting
Miller-Motte Technical College
North Charleston, SC

Tammy Summerson, BSN, RMA (AMT)
Faculty/Program Director
Westwood College, Chicago River Oaks Campus
Calumet, IL

Marilyn Turner, RN, CMA (AAMA)
Program Director
Ogeechee Technical College
Statesboro, GA

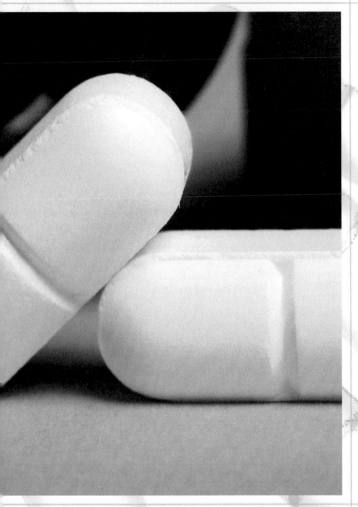

SECTION ONE

Mathematics and Dosage Calculations

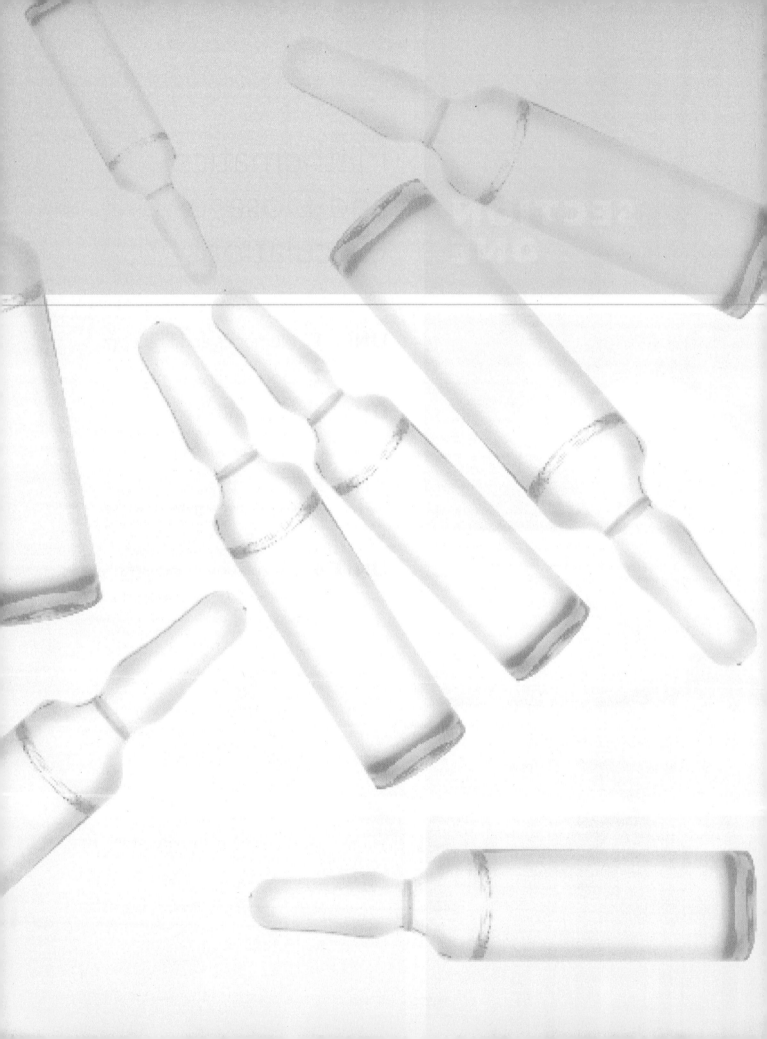

UNIT I
Numerals and Fractions

OBJECTIVES

Upon completing this unit, you should be able to:

- Define the terms listed in the vocabulary.
- Express Arabic numerals as Roman numerals.
- Express Roman numerals as Arabic numerals.
- Express a fraction as a simple, compound, complex, proper, or improper fraction.
- Express fractions as equivalents.
- Determine the relative values of fractions.
- Express improper fractions as mixed numbers.
- Add, subtract, multiply, and divide fractions and mixed numbers.
- Work the practice problems and review problems correctly.
- Successfully complete the Self-Assessment.

VOCABULARY

denominator (dee-nom"a-na'ter). The number *below* the line in a fraction. It indicates the number of equal parts into which the whole is divided. It is also known as the *divisor*.

Example: $\frac{1}{2}\underline{\text{ denominator}}$

2 divided into 1 or 1 divided by 2

dividend (div'a-dend). The number that is *divided*. It is also known as the *numerator*.

divisor (di-vy'-zer). The number that is divided into another number or the number by which another can be divided. It is also known as the *denominator*.

fraction (frak'shun). The result of dividing or breaking a whole number into parts.

lowest common denominator (LCD). The least number into which all the denominators will go evenly.

lowest terms. The process of reducing the fraction to the *least* number possible.

minuend (min'yoo-end). The top number from which the lower number is to be subtracted.

Example: 765 (minuend)
− 432

mixed number. A whole number plus a fraction.

Example: $2\frac{1}{2}$

numerator (nu'me-ra"ter). The number *above* the line in a fraction. It is the number of parts into which a unit or number may be divided. It is also known as the *dividend*.

Example: $\frac{1}{2}\overline{\text{ numerator}}$

1 of 2 parts or 1 divided by 2 or 2 divided into 1

product (prod'ukt). The number found by multiplying two or more numbers.

quotient (kwo'shant). The number found when one number is divided by another number.

subtrahend (sub'tra-hend). The lower number that is to be subtracted from the top number.

Example: 765
− 432 (subtrahend)

sum (sum). The total amount.

unit (u'nit). The smallest whole number; one.

3

ARABIC AND ROMAN NUMERALS

Arabic numerals are those we use in our everyday calculations. They include the figures 0 through 9 or any combination of these figures.

Roman numerals make use of letters to represent numeric values. They are a part of the apothecaries' system of measurement. On occasion, you may see Roman numerals being used on prescriptions or medication orders. Table 1-1 shows some Arabic numbers and their Roman numeral equivalents.

TABLE 1-1 Arabic and Roman Numerals

ARABIC NUMERALS	ROMAN NUMERALS	ARABIC NUMERALS	ROMAN NUMERALS	ARABIC NUMERALS	ROMAN NUMERALS
1	I	8	VIII	60	LX
2	II	9	IX	70	LXX
3	III	10	X	80	LXXX
4	IV	20	XX	90	XC
5	V	30	XXX	100	C
6	VI	40	XL	500	D
7	VII	50	L	1000	M

Reading and Writing Roman Numerals

The following steps will guide you as you learn to read and write Roman numerals:

1. When using two Roman numerals of the same value that are repeated in sequence, you add their values. A Roman numeral may not be repeated more than three times.

   EXAMPLE

   XXX = 30

2. When a Roman numeral of a larger value is followed by one of a lesser value, you add the values.

   EXAMPLE

   XI = (10 + 1) = 11

3. When a Roman numeral of a lesser value is followed by one of a larger value, you subtract the values.

   EXAMPLE

   IV = (5 − 1) = 4

4. When a Roman numeral is placed between two numerals of a larger value, you subtract the lesser value from the following numeral.

   EXAMPLE

   XIV = (10 + 5 − 1) = 14

5. Roman numerals over 100 are seldom used in medicine. The following are the basic Roman numerals and their Arabic equivalents:

ROMAN NUMERALS	ARABIC NUMERALS	ROMAN NUMERALS	ARABIC NUMERALS
I	1	C	100
V	5	D	500
X	10	M	1000
L	50		

PRACTICE PROBLEMS

1. Arabic and Roman numerals. Express the following as Arabic or Roman numerals:

    a. 3 _____ f. 7 _____ k. XVI _____

    b. 5 _____ g. 50 _____ l. XIX _____

    c. 8 _____ h. 60 _____ m. IX _____

    d. 10 _____ i. XXIV _____ n. VIII _____

    e. 100 _____ j. IV _____ o. XX _____

FRACTIONS

The *word* **fraction** literally means the result of breaking, dividing. It is used to indicate a small part that is broken off; a small amount, degree, or fragment. In mathematics, a fraction is a quantity that is less than a whole. It may be written in either of the following ways and still have the same value: 0.2 (decimal fraction); $\frac{2}{10}$ (common fraction).

 A *common fraction* is a part of a whole number. It is obtained by dividing a number into a **numerator** separated from the **denominator** by a *horizontal* line ($\frac{2}{10}$) or by a *diagonal* line (2/10). In the fraction $\frac{2}{10}$, the 2 is the numerator, and the 10 is the denominator. The line separating the numerator from the denominator expresses the process of division: the numerator is divided by the denominator.

EXAMPLE

$$\text{denominator } 10\overline{)2.0}^{\,0.2}\text{ numerator}$$
$$2.0$$

Types of Common Fractions

Simple fractions are fractions that contain only one numerator and one denominator, such as $\frac{1}{3}$, $\frac{1}{4}$, and $\frac{2}{10}$.

 Compound fractions are those in which an arithmetical process is necessary in either the numerator or denominator, as in $\frac{2 \times 4}{12} = \frac{8}{12}$ or $\frac{10}{6-4} = \frac{10}{2} = 5$.

 Complex fractions may have simple fractions in either the numerator or the denominator, or both, as in

$$\frac{1\frac{1}{2}}{6}\text{ numerator}\qquad\qquad \frac{6}{1\frac{1}{2}}\text{ denominator}\qquad\qquad \frac{1\frac{1}{2}}{6\frac{1}{2}}\text{ both}$$

 Proper fractions have a numerator that is smaller than the denominator, as in $\frac{6}{8}$ or $\frac{4}{5}$.

 Improper fractions have a numerator that is larger than the denominator, as in $\frac{16}{4}$ or $\frac{15}{3}$.

 A **mixed number** contains a whole number and a fraction, as in $3\frac{1}{3}$ or $2\frac{1}{2}$.

 Equivalent fractions are those that have the same value, as in $\frac{4}{8} = \frac{1}{2}$ or $\frac{5}{10} = \frac{1}{2}$.

Expressing Fractions as Equivalents

To express fractions as equivalents, one must find the largest whole number that will divide evenly into both the numerator and the denominator. This is called reducing the fraction to **lowest terms**. It is easier and safer to work with smaller numbers than with larger numbers.

EXAMPLE

Reduce $\frac{27}{81}$ to lowest terms.

Divide the numerator and the denominator by 27: $\frac{27}{81} = \frac{1}{3}$

PRACTICE PROBLEMS

2. Reduce the following fractions to lowest terms:

   a. $\dfrac{75}{100}$ = _____

   b. $\dfrac{34}{102}$ = _____

   c. $\dfrac{14}{56}$ = _____

   d. $\dfrac{33}{66}$ = _____

   e. $\dfrac{60}{1200}$ = _____

   f. $\dfrac{21}{105}$ = _____

Expressing Improper Fractions as Mixed Numbers

To express improper fractions as mixed numbers, follow these steps:

1. Divide the numerator by the denominator.
2. Place the remainder as a fraction and reduce to lowest terms.

   EXAMPLE

   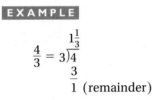

PRACTICE PROBLEMS

3. Express the following improper fractions as mixed numbers, reducing to lowest terms:

   a. $\dfrac{16}{12}$ = _____

   b. $\dfrac{24}{18}$ = _____

   c. $\dfrac{9}{6}$ = _____

   d. $\dfrac{8}{5}$ = _____

   e. $\dfrac{10}{9}$ = _____

   f. $\dfrac{15}{13}$ = _____

Expressing Mixed Numbers as Improper Fractions

To express mixed numbers as improper fractions, follow these steps:

1. Multiply the whole number by the denominator.
2. Add the numerator to the product of Step 1.
3. Place the **sum** over the denominator.

   EXAMPLE

   $$2\dfrac{1}{2} = \dfrac{(2 \times 2) = 4 + 1}{2} = \dfrac{5}{2} = 2\dfrac{1}{2}$$

PRACTICE PROBLEMS

4. Express the following mixed numbers as improper fractions, checking your work by changing the fractions back into mixed numbers:

   a. $3\dfrac{1}{3}$ = _____

   b. $4\dfrac{1}{4}$ = _____

   c. $5\dfrac{2}{3}$ = _____

   d. $6\dfrac{7}{10}$ = _____

   e. $7\dfrac{1}{7}$ = _____

   f. $9\dfrac{1}{9}$ = _____

RELATIVE VALUES OF FRACTIONS

To determine the relative values of a series of fractions, you need to determine which fraction is the largest. Which is the largest, $\frac{1}{4}$, $\frac{1}{15}$, or $\frac{1}{3}$? To assist you in determining which fraction is the largest, follow these steps:

1. Make each fraction a whole number. The fraction that takes fewer parts to make a whole number is the largest.

$$\frac{1}{3} + \frac{2}{3} = \frac{3}{3} = 1$$

$$\frac{1}{4} + \frac{3}{4} = \frac{4}{4} = 1$$

$$\frac{1}{15} + \frac{14}{15} = \frac{15}{15} = 1$$

EXAMPLE

$\frac{1}{3}$ is the largest fraction in this series, because it takes 2 additional parts to make a whole.

$\frac{1}{4}$ is the next largest fraction, because it takes 3 additional parts to make a whole.

$\frac{1}{15}$ is the smallest fraction in this series, because it takes 14 additional parts to make a whole.

2. When the fractions have the same denominators, the fraction with the largest numerator is the largest, because it takes fewer parts to make a whole. Which is the largest, $\frac{2}{8}$, $\frac{4}{8}$, or $\frac{7}{8}$?

$$\frac{7}{8} + \frac{1}{8} = \frac{8}{8} = 1$$

$$\frac{4}{8} + \frac{4}{8} = \frac{8}{8} = 1$$

$$\frac{2}{8} + \frac{6}{8} = \frac{8}{8} = 1$$

EXAMPLE

$\frac{7}{8}$ is the largest fraction in this series, because it takes 1 additional part to make a whole.

$\frac{4}{8}$ is the next largest fraction, because it takes 4 additional parts to make a whole.

$\frac{2}{8}$ is the smallest fraction, because it takes 6 additional parts to make a whole.

PRACTICE PROBLEMS

5. To determine the relative values of fractions, analyze each series of fractions that follows, and give the largest value on the first line and the smallest value on the second line.

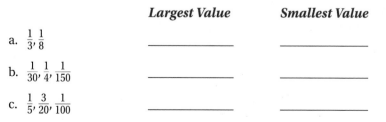

		Largest Value	*Smallest Value*
a.	$\frac{1}{3}, \frac{1}{8}$	_____	_____
b.	$\frac{1}{30}, \frac{1}{4}, \frac{1}{150}$	_____	_____
c.	$\frac{1}{5}, \frac{3}{20}, \frac{1}{100}$	_____	_____

	Largest Value	*Smallest Value*
d. $\frac{2}{5}, \frac{4}{5}, \frac{3}{5}$	_____	_____
e. $\frac{2}{40}, \frac{8}{40}, \frac{10}{40}$	_____	_____
f. $\frac{1}{150}, \frac{1}{125}, \frac{1}{100}$	_____	_____
g. $\frac{1}{4}, \frac{3}{8}, \frac{3}{4}$	_____	_____
h. $\frac{1}{3}, \frac{1}{2}, \frac{1}{5}$	_____	_____
i. $\frac{25}{100}, \frac{75}{100}, \frac{50}{100}$	_____	_____
j. $\frac{3}{10}, \frac{5}{10}, \frac{8}{10}$	_____	_____

ADDITION OF FRACTIONS

Adding Common Fractions

When adding common fractions, the denominators must be the same figure. The following fractions can be added because their denominators are the same:

$$\frac{1}{4} + \frac{3}{4} = \frac{4}{4} = 1$$

To add fractions that have unlike denominators, follow these steps:

1. Express the fractions as equivalent fractions by finding the lowest common denominator (LCD).
2. Add the numerators and place the sum over the lowest common denominator.

EXAMPLE

$$\frac{1}{4} + \frac{1}{2} = ?$$

4 is the LCD

$$\frac{1}{4} = \frac{1}{4}$$

$$\frac{1}{2} = \frac{2}{4}$$

$$\frac{1}{4} + \frac{2}{4} = \frac{3}{4}$$

Adding Mixed Numbers

When adding fractions and whole numbers, the denominators must be the same figure. When the denominators are the same, add the fractions, and then add the results to the whole numbers.

EXAMPLE

$$
\begin{array}{r}
7\frac{1}{8} \\
+\, 6\frac{2}{8} \\
\hline
13\frac{3}{8}
\end{array}
$$

To add fractions and whole numbers that have unlike denominators, follow these steps:

1. Express the fractions as equivalent fractions by finding the LCD.
2. Add the fractions and then add the whole numbers.

EXAMPLE

$$1\frac{1}{4} + 2\frac{5}{8} + 3\frac{1}{2} = ?$$

Step 1.   8 is the LCD

$$\frac{1}{4} = \frac{2}{8}$$

$$\frac{5}{8} = \frac{5}{8}$$

$$\frac{1}{2} = \frac{4}{8}$$

Step 2.
$$
\begin{array}{r}
1\frac{2}{8} \\
+\ 2\frac{5}{8} \\
+\ 3\frac{4}{8} \\
\hline
6\frac{11}{8}
\end{array}
$$

3. When adding the fractions results in a numerator that is larger than the denominator, divide the numerator by the denominator and then add the results to the whole number.

EXAMPLE

$$6\frac{11}{8}$$

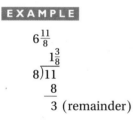

$$
\begin{array}{r}
1\frac{3}{8} \\
8\overline{)11} \\
\underline{8} \\
3 \text{ (remainder)}
\end{array}
$$

Step 3.
$$
\begin{array}{r}
6 \\
+\ 1\frac{3}{8} \\
\hline
7\frac{3}{8}
\end{array}
$$

■ ■ PRACTICE PROBLEMS

6. Addition of fractions. Correctly add the following fractions:

a. $\frac{1}{6}$ c. $\frac{6}{16}$ e. $22\frac{3}{4}$ g. $9\frac{1}{3}$ i. $13\frac{2}{5}$ k. $\frac{1}{5}$

$+\frac{3}{4}$ $\frac{7}{8}$ $+76\frac{1}{4}$ $+33\frac{2}{3}$ $16\frac{4}{10}$ $\frac{14}{25}$

              $+\frac{1}{4}$ $+7\frac{5}{30}$ $+\frac{11}{50}$

b. $\frac{4}{7}$ d. $\frac{2}{5}$ f. $49\frac{1}{7}$ h. $18\frac{14}{12}$ j. $24\frac{3}{9}$ l. $\frac{1}{4}$

$+\frac{1}{3}$ $\frac{6}{10}$ $+106\frac{5}{7}$ $+9\frac{20}{12}$ $8\frac{16}{18}$ $+\frac{3}{4}$

              $+\frac{8}{20}$ $+3\frac{40}{36}$

SUBTRACTION OF FRACTIONS

Subtracting Common Fractions

When subtracting common fractions, the denominators must be the same figure. The following fractions can be subtracted because their denominators are the same:

$$\frac{3}{4} - \frac{1}{4} = \frac{2}{4} = \frac{1}{2}$$

To subtract fractions that have unlike denominators, follow these steps:

1. Express the fractions as equivalent fractions by finding the LCD.
2. Subtract the numerators and place your answer over the lowest common denominator.

EXAMPLE

$$\frac{1}{2} - \frac{1}{4} = ?$$

4 is the LCD

$$\frac{1}{2} = \frac{2}{4}$$

$$\frac{1}{4} = \frac{1}{4}$$

$$\frac{2}{4} - \frac{1}{4} = \frac{1}{4}$$

Subtracting Mixed Numbers

When subtracting fractions and whole numbers, the denominators must be the same figure. When the denominators are the same, subtract the fractions, and then subtract the whole numbers.

EXAMPLE

$$\begin{array}{r} 7\frac{9}{10} \\ -2\frac{6}{10} \\ \hline 5\frac{3}{10} \end{array}$$

To subtract fractions and whole numbers that have unlike denominators, follow these steps:

1. Express the fractions as equivalent fractions by finding the LCD.
2. Subtract the fractions and then subtract the whole numbers.
3. When subtracting fractions in which the **subtrahend** (bottom number) is larger than the **minuend** (top number):
   a. borrow one whole unit from the whole number,
   b. add the borrowed unit (1) to the fraction of the minuend,
   c. subtract the fractions and then subtract the whole numbers.

EXAMPLE

$$\begin{array}{r} 10\frac{1}{5} \\ -8\frac{3}{5} \\ \hline \end{array}$$
$$\text{borrow} \quad \begin{array}{r} 10\frac{1}{5} \\ -\frac{5}{5} \ (1) \\ \hline 9\frac{6}{5} \end{array} \qquad \frac{5}{5} + \frac{1}{5} = \frac{6}{5}$$

$$10\frac{1}{5} \text{ becomes} \quad \begin{array}{r} 9\frac{6}{5} \\ \text{now subtract} \quad -8\frac{3}{5} \\ \hline 1\frac{3}{5} \end{array}$$

4. Check the accuracy of your work by adding the answer and the subtrahend together. The sum will equal the minuend.

$$8\tfrac{3}{5} \text{ (subtrahend)}$$
$$+ \ 1\tfrac{3}{5} \text{ (answer)}$$
$$9\tfrac{6}{5} = 10\tfrac{1}{5} \text{ (minuend)}$$

■ ■ PRACTICE PROBLEMS

7. Subtraction of fractions. Correctly subtract the following fractions:

a. $\dfrac{7}{8}$
  $-\dfrac{2}{16}$

c. $\dfrac{16}{32}$
  $-\dfrac{9}{32}$

e. $21\tfrac{3}{9}$
  $- \ 5\tfrac{5}{9}$

g. $17\tfrac{9}{10}$
  $- \ 9\tfrac{12}{10}$

i. $91\tfrac{45}{25}$
  $-42\tfrac{7}{25}$

k. $\dfrac{11}{12}$
  $-\dfrac{5}{6}$

b. $\dfrac{4}{15}$
  $-\dfrac{1}{45}$

d. $66\tfrac{2}{3}$
  $-33\tfrac{1}{3}$

f. $14\tfrac{3}{15}$
  $- \ 5\tfrac{6}{30}$

h. $106\tfrac{7}{8}$
  $- \ 23\tfrac{3}{8}$

j. $\dfrac{25}{75}$
  $-\dfrac{16}{150}$

l. $16\tfrac{5}{6}$
  $-14\tfrac{3}{8}$

THE PROCESS OF CANCELLATION

When multiplying or dividing fractions, it is easier and more accurate to work with smaller numbers. To arrive at a smaller number, use the process of cancellation.

Steps to Cancel

1. Divide any numerator and any denominator by the largest number contained in each.

2. After canceling, continue with the mathematical process of the problem.

> **EXAMPLE**
>
> *Multiplication:*

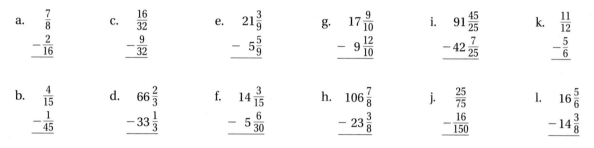

$$16 \times \frac{3}{8} = \frac{16}{1} \times \frac{3}{8}$$
$$= 16 \div 8 = 2$$
$$= 8 \div 8 = 1$$
$$= \frac{\overset{2}{16}}{1} \times \frac{3}{\underset{1}{8}} \quad \frac{2 \times 3}{1 \times 1} = \frac{6}{1}$$
$$= 6$$

MULTIPLICATION OF FRACTIONS

Multiplying Common Fractions

To multiply common fractions, multiply the numerator by the numerator and the denominator by the denominator. Reduce to lowest terms when possible.

> **EXAMPLE**

$$\frac{3}{7} \times \frac{4}{5} = \frac{12}{35} \quad \frac{(3 \times 4)}{(7 \times 5)}$$

EXAMPLE

Reduce to lowest terms:

$$\frac{1}{6} \times \frac{3}{4} = \frac{3}{24} \frac{(3 \times 1)}{(6 \times 4)}$$

$$= \frac{3}{24} \frac{(3 \div 3)}{(24 \div 3)} = \frac{1}{8}$$

Multiplying a Fraction and a Whole Number

To multiply a fraction and a whole number, follow these steps:

1. Change the whole number to a fraction by placing the whole number over one (1).
2. Then multiply the numerator by the numerator and the denominator by the denominator.
3. Reduce the **product** to lowest terms when possible.

EXAMPLE

$$16 \times \frac{3}{8} =$$

$$\frac{16}{1} \times \frac{3}{8} = \frac{48 \,(16 \times 3)}{8 \,(1 \times 8)}$$

$$= 48 \div 8 = 6$$

Multiplying Mixed Numbers

To multiply mixed numbers, follow these steps:

1. Change the mixed numbers to improper fractions.
2. Then multiply the numerator by the numerator and the denominator by the denominator.
3. Reduce to lowest terms when possible.

EXAMPLE

$$2\frac{7}{8} \times \frac{3}{5}$$

$$8 \times 2 = 16 + 7 = \frac{23}{8} \times \frac{3}{5} = \frac{69 \,(23 \times 3)}{40 \,(8 \times 5)} = 69 \div 40 = 1\frac{29}{40}$$

■ ■ PRACTICE PROBLEMS

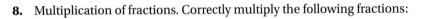

8. Multiplication of fractions. Correctly multiply the following fractions:

a. $\frac{23}{9} \times \frac{7}{16}$ = _____

b. $\frac{2}{5} \times \frac{1}{3}$ = _____

c. $\frac{14}{8} \times \frac{2}{4}$ = _____

d. $6\frac{10}{12} \times \frac{15}{3}$ = _____

e. $91\frac{2}{3} \times \frac{4}{6}$ = _____

f. $\frac{18}{24} \times 5\frac{1}{10}$ = _____

g. $42 \times \frac{1}{2}$ = _____

h. $56 \times \frac{9}{20}$ = _____

i. $365 \times \frac{12}{30}$ = _____

j. $18 \times \frac{2}{3}$ = _____

k. $\frac{2}{3} \times \frac{3}{4}$ = _____

l. $\frac{4}{5} \times \frac{1}{8}$ = _____

m. $\frac{4}{9} \times \frac{3}{8}$ = _____

n. $\frac{5}{7} \times 5\frac{1}{4}$ = _____

o. $\frac{5}{12} \times 4\frac{3}{4}$ = _____

DIVISION OF FRACTIONS

Dividing Common Fractions

To divide common fractions, invert the divisor. *Inverting* a fraction means turning it upside down. It is most important that you invert the **divisor** and not the dividend. When $\frac{3}{4}$ is inverted, it becomes $\frac{4}{3}$.

To divide common fractions, follow these steps:

1. Invert the *divisor*.
2. Then multiply the numerator by the numerator and the denominator by the denominator.
3. Reduce the **quotient** to lowest terms when possible.

> **EXAMPLE**
>
> $$\frac{1}{6} \div \frac{3}{4} \,(\text{divisor})$$
>
> $$\frac{1}{6} \times \frac{4}{3} = \frac{4(4 \times 1)}{18(6 \times 3)}$$
>
> $$= \frac{4}{18} = \frac{2}{9}$$

Dividing a Fraction and a Whole Number

To divide a fraction and a whole number, follow these steps:

1. Change the whole number to a fraction by placing the whole number over one (1).
2. Invert the *divisor*.
3. Then multiply the numerator by the numerator and the denominator by the denominator.
4. Reduce to lowest terms when possible.

> **EXAMPLE**
>
> $$16 \div \frac{3}{8} = \frac{16}{1} \div \frac{3}{8}$$
>
> $$= \frac{16}{1} \times \frac{8}{3} = \frac{128(16 \times 8)}{3(1 \times 3)} = 128 \div 3 = 42\frac{2}{3}$$

Dividing Mixed Numbers

To divide mixed numbers, follow these steps:

1. Change the mixed number to an improper fraction.
2. Invert the *divisor*.

3. Then multiply the numerator by the numerator and the denominator by the denominator.
4. Reduce to lowest terms when possible.

EXAMPLE

$$2\frac{7}{8} \div \frac{3}{5}$$

$$8 \times 2 = 16 + 7 = \frac{23}{8}$$

$$\frac{23}{8} \div \frac{3}{5}$$

$$\frac{23}{8} \times \frac{5}{3} = \frac{115(23 \times 5)}{24(8 \times 3)} = 115 \div 24 = 4\frac{19}{24}$$

■■ PRACTICE PROBLEMS

9. Division of fractions. Correctly divide the following fractions:

a. $\frac{23}{9} \div \frac{7}{16}$ = _____   i. $\frac{7}{8} \div \frac{3}{4}$ = _____

b. $\frac{2}{5} \div \frac{1}{3}$ = _____   j. $\frac{2}{3} \div \frac{1}{3}$ = _____

c. $\frac{14}{8} \div \frac{2}{4}$ = _____   k. $\frac{1}{5} \div \frac{1}{10}$ = _____

d. $6\frac{10}{12} \div \frac{15}{3}$ = _____   l. $\frac{1}{150} \div \frac{1}{100}$ = _____

e. $91\frac{2}{3} \div \frac{4}{6}$ = _____   m. $\frac{2}{5} \div \frac{10}{15}$ = _____

f. $\frac{18}{24} \div 5\frac{1}{10}$ = _____   n. $3 \div \frac{5}{3}$ = _____

g. $42 \div \frac{1}{2}$ = _____   o. $\frac{2}{3} \div 5\frac{1}{2}$ = _____

h. $56 \div \frac{9}{20}$ = _____   p. $\frac{3}{4} \div \frac{8}{9}$ = _____

■■ REVIEW PROBLEMS

1. Reduce the following fractions to lowest terms:

a. $\frac{6}{42}$ = _____   c. $\frac{18}{45}$ = _____   e. $\frac{24}{30}$ = _____   g. $\frac{9}{45}$ = _____   i. $\frac{100}{1000}$ = _____

b. $\frac{35}{50}$ = _____   d. $\frac{36}{48}$ = _____   f. $\frac{48}{60}$ = _____   h. $\frac{10}{100}$ = _____   j. $\frac{22}{88}$ = _____

2. Express the following improper fractions as mixed number, reducing to lowest terms:

a. $\frac{5}{2}$ = _____   c. $\frac{9}{8}$ = _____   e. $\frac{18}{3}$ = _____   g. $\frac{22}{4}$ = _____   i. $\frac{25}{5}$ = _____

b. $\frac{11}{10}$ = _____   d. $\frac{48}{12}$ = _____   f. $\frac{32}{6}$ = _____   h. $\frac{17}{5}$ = _____   j. $\frac{15}{3}$ = _____

3. Express the following mixed numbers as improper fractions, checking your work by changing the fractions back into mixed numbers:

a. $2\frac{1}{2}$ = _____   c. $8\frac{1}{4}$ = _____   e. $1\frac{1}{3}$ = _____   g. $9\frac{1}{7}$ = _____   i. $3\frac{9}{10}$ = _____

b. $5\frac{5}{6}$ = _____   d. $11\frac{1}{6}$ = _____   f. $3\frac{2}{3}$ = _____   h. $4\frac{4}{5}$ = _____   j. $4\frac{1}{6}$ = _____

4. In the following series of fractions, identify the *largest* value in each group, and place your answer on the appropriate line:

a. $\frac{5}{9}, \frac{2}{3}, \frac{11}{8}$ _____

b. $\frac{3}{4}, \frac{1}{2}, \frac{3}{5}$ _____

c. $\frac{2}{5}, \frac{9}{20}, \frac{3}{10}$ _____

d. $\frac{5}{24}, \frac{1}{4}, \frac{5}{12}$ _____

e. $\frac{6}{10}, \frac{10}{100}, \frac{2}{100}$ _____

f. $\frac{2}{10}, \frac{4}{10}, \frac{8}{10}$ _____

g. $\frac{25}{100}, \frac{50}{100}, \frac{75}{100}$ _____

h. $\frac{1}{100}, \frac{1}{125}, \frac{1}{150}$ _____

i. $\frac{2}{5}, \frac{4}{20}, \frac{2}{100}$ _____

j. $\frac{3}{4}, \frac{1}{4}, \frac{3}{8}$ _____

5. Correctly add the following fractions:

a. $6\frac{3}{4}$
$+\, 8\frac{3}{4}$

b. $8\frac{15}{18}$
$+\, 2\frac{1}{18}$

c. $26\frac{1}{3}$
$+\, 33\frac{2}{3}$

d. $\frac{6}{10}$
$\frac{5}{10}$
$+\, \frac{2}{10}$

e. $\frac{1}{100}$
$\frac{10}{100}$
$+\, \frac{50}{100}$

f. $4\frac{3}{10}$
$+\, 6\frac{9}{10}$

g. $5\frac{13}{40}$
$+\, 7\frac{10}{40}$

h. $4\frac{6}{32}$
$+\, 5\frac{7}{32}$

6. Correctly subtract the following fractions:

a. $7\frac{17}{21}$
$-\, 5\frac{12}{21}$

b. $10\frac{19}{25}$
$-\, 2\frac{4}{25}$

c. $\frac{5}{6}$
$-\, \frac{3}{6}$

d. $6\frac{1}{2}$
$-\, 3\frac{1}{4}$

e. $\frac{10}{12}$
$-\, \frac{5}{6}$

f. $13\frac{3}{15}$
$-\, 6\frac{6}{30}$

g. $9\frac{3}{10}$
$-\, 6\frac{9}{10}$

h. $5\frac{1}{8}$
$-\, 2\frac{7}{8}$

i. $104\frac{7}{8}$
$-\, 26\frac{3}{8}$

j. $66\frac{3}{4}$
$-\, 33\frac{1}{3}$

7. Correctly multiply the following fractions:

a. $\frac{3}{8} \times \frac{4}{9}$ = _____

b. $4\frac{3}{4} \times \frac{5}{12}$ = _____

c. $\frac{2}{3} \times \frac{1}{5}$ = _____

d. $\frac{3}{5} \times \frac{3}{8}$ = _____

e. $10 \times \frac{4}{5}$ = _____

f. $4 \times \frac{7}{8}$ = _____

g. $\frac{3}{7} \times \frac{2}{5}$ = _____

h. $\frac{8}{9} \times \frac{1}{3}$ = _____

i. $\frac{7}{10} \times \frac{3}{4}$ = _____

j. $3\frac{3}{4} \times \frac{8}{9}$ = _____

8. Correctly divide the following fractions:

a. $\frac{9}{10} \div \frac{3}{4}$ = _____

b. $\frac{3}{20} \div \frac{9}{16}$ = _____

c. $\frac{3}{5} \div \frac{6}{7}$ = _____

d. $3\frac{1}{2} \div \frac{3}{8}$ = _____

e. $1\frac{2}{3} \div \frac{5}{6}$ = _____

f. $7 \div \frac{7}{10}$ = _____

g. $10 \div \frac{5}{6}$ = _____

h. $1\frac{3}{4} \div \frac{1}{2}$ = _____

i. $3\frac{1}{3} \div \frac{4}{9}$ = _____

j. $\frac{15}{16} \div 2\frac{1}{4}$ = _____

■ ■ SELF-ASSESSMENT

This exercise is designed to assess your understanding of numerals and fractions. Follow the directions for each question. To verify your answers, you may check with your instructor or go to the student companion website:

1. Express the following as Arabic or Roman numerals:

   a. 15 _____   d. IV _____

   b. 25 _____   e. XIX _____

   c. 50 _____   f. XVI _____

2. Express the following mixed numbers as improper fractions:

   a. $5\frac{1}{2}$ _____   d. $6\frac{7}{8}$ _____

   b. $3\frac{1}{3}$ _____   e. $4\frac{2}{3}$ _____

   c. $8\frac{1}{6}$ _____   f. $2\frac{1}{2}$ _____

3. Express the following improper fractions as mixed numbers:

   a. $\frac{9}{6}$ _____   d. $\frac{15}{2}$ _____

   b. $\frac{7}{5}$ _____   e. $\frac{8}{6}$ _____

   c. $\frac{6}{4}$ _____   f. $\frac{3}{2}$ _____

4. Reduce the following fractions to lowest terms:

   a. $\frac{48}{96}$ _____   d. $\frac{60}{100}$ _____

   b. $\frac{75}{100}$ _____   e. $\frac{14}{56}$ _____

   c. $\frac{33}{66}$ _____   f. $\frac{3}{15}$ _____

5. Add the following fractions:

   a. $\frac{1}{8} + \frac{3}{4}$ _____   d. $9\frac{1}{3} + 31\frac{2}{3}$ _____

   b. $22\frac{14}{12} + 2\frac{1}{6}$ _____   e. $\frac{1}{3} + \frac{1}{9}$ _____

   c. $\frac{1}{7} + \frac{3}{21}$ _____   f. $102\frac{5}{6} + 98\frac{1}{3}$ _____

6. Subtract the following fractions:

   a. $\frac{3}{4} - \frac{1}{8}$ _____   d. $31\frac{2}{3} - 9\frac{1}{3}$ _____

   b. $21\frac{3}{9} - 5\frac{5}{9}$ _____   e. $\frac{25}{75} - \frac{16}{150}$ _____

   c. $\frac{11}{12} - \frac{5}{6}$ _____   f. $14\frac{3}{5} - 5\frac{6}{10}$ _____

7. Multiply the following fractions:

   a. $\frac{4}{9} \times \frac{1}{8}$ _____   c. $45 \times \frac{1}{5}$ _____

   b. $365 \times \frac{12}{30}$ _____   d. $6\frac{11}{12} \times \frac{7}{3}$ _____

8. Divide the following fractions:

   a. $\frac{1}{150} \div \frac{1}{100}$ _____   c. $\frac{2}{3} \div 5\frac{1}{2}$ _____

   b. $\frac{3}{4} \div \frac{8}{9}$ _____   d. $56 \div \frac{9}{20}$ _____

UNIT 2
Decimal Fractions

OBJECTIVES

Upon completing this unit, you should be able to:

- Define the terms listed in the vocabulary.
- Read and write decimals correctly.
- Define and use the powers of 10.
- Express a common fraction as a decimal fraction.
- Express a decimal fraction as a common fraction.
- Add, subtract, multiply, and divide decimals.
- Express common fractions and decimal fractions as percentages, and percentages as common fractions and decimal fractions.
- Answer the questions in the learning exercise correctly.
- Work the practice problems and review problems correctly.
- Successfully complete the Self-Assessment.

VOCABULARY

continuing number. A number that does not come out evenly but continues indefinitely. It is good practice to carry a continuing number to three decimal places and place a line over the last number.

Example:
$$
\begin{array}{r}
0.33\overline{3} \\
3\overline{)1.000} \\
\underline{9} \\
10 \\
\underline{9} \\
10 \\
\underline{9} \\
1
\end{array}
$$

decimal (dess'a-ml). A linear array of numbers based upon 10 or any multiple of 10.

decimal fraction (dess'a-ml frak'shun). A fraction with an unwritten denominator of 10 or a power of 10. It is expressed by placing a decimal point before the numerator.

decimal place (dess'a-ml plās). The position of a number to the right of a decimal point.

decimal point (dess'a-ml point). The period placed to the left of a decimal fraction.

decimal system (dess'a-ml sis'tem). A number system based upon the number 10 or multiples of 10.

multiplied (mul"ta-plide'). The process of finding the product of numbers by multiplication.

multiplier (mul"ta-ply'er). The number by which another number is multiplied. It is also known as the *multiplicand*.

UNDERSTANDING DECIMAL FRACTIONS

A decimal is a mathematical form that represents a straight line of units described as a fraction. The **decimal point** is in the center of the line. All the numbers to the left of the decimal point are *whole* numbers. All the numbers to the right of the decimal point are **decimals** or **decimal fractions**. The position of the number to the left or right of the decimal point is its *place value*. The value of each place *left* of the decimal point is *10* times that of the place to its right. The value of each place *right* of the decimal point is *one-tenth* the value of the place to its left (see Figure 2-1).

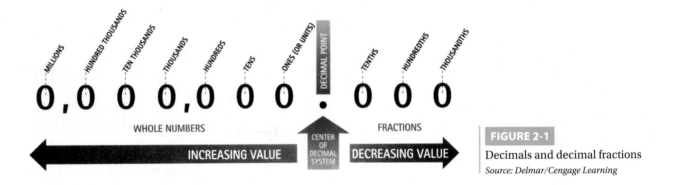

FIGURE 2-1

Decimals and decimal fractions

Source: Delmar/Cengage Learning

READING AND WRITING DECIMAL FRACTIONS

The following steps will guide you as you learn to read and write decimal fractions:

1. Note the place value of the decimal point.
2. Read the number to the right of the decimal point.
3. Use the name that applies to the decimal place of the last number.
4. Read using *th* or *ths* on the end of the denominator.
5. To read a whole number and a decimal fraction, the decimal point is read as *and* or *point*.
6. It is good practice to place a zero (0) before the decimal point. This is a safety measure that ensures the reading of the number as a decimal and not as a whole number.
7. Study the following chart and the examples given.

Reading Decimals	
0.1	Read as one-tenth
0.01	Read as one-hundredth
0.001	Read as one-thousandth
0.0001	Read as one ten-thousandth
0.00001	Read as one hundred-thousandth
0.000001	Read as one-millionth

EXAMPLE

1. Note that the number is directly to the right of the decimal point in 0.1 (read as one-tenth).
2. Note that the number is two places to the right of the decimal point in 0.01 (read as one-hundredth).

3. Note that the number is three places to the right of the decimal point in 0.001 (read as one-thousandth).

4. Note that the number is four places to the right of the decimal point in 0.0001 (read as one ten-thousandth).

5. Note that the number is five places to the right of the decimal point in 0.00001 (read as one hundred-thousandth).

6. Note that the number is six places to the right of the decimal point in 0.000001 (read as one-millionth).

7. The number 10.1 is a whole number and a decimal fraction (read as ten and one-tenth or ten point one).

Powers of 10

Finding the *power of 10* is the process of multiplying 10s together. The number of 10s multiplied determines the power. Remember that a decimal fraction is a fraction with an unwritten denominator of 10 or any power of 10. Study the following chart for an understanding of the powers of 10.

Power	Number	Name or Value
1st	10	ten
2nd	100	hundred
3rd	1,000	thousand
4th	10,000	ten thousand
5th	100,000	hundred thousand
6th	1,000,000	million
7th	10,000,000	ten million
8th	100,000,000	hundred million
9th	1,000,000,000	billion
10th	10,000,000,000	ten billion

■ ■ LEARNING EXERCISE

Mastering decimals. Answer the following questions that involve the use of decimals:

1. A _____ is a mathematical form that represents a straight line of units described as a fraction.

2. State the usage of a decimal.

3. All the numbers to the left of the decimal point are _____ numbers.

4. All the numbers to the right of the decimal point are _____ or _____.

5. The position of the number to the left or right of the decimal point is its _____.

6. The value of each place left of the decimal point is _____ times that of the place to its right.

7. The value of each place right of the decimal point is _____ of the value of the place to its left.

8. A _____ _____ is a fraction with an unwritten denominator of 10 or a power of 10.

9. Why is it important to place a 0 before the decimal point?

10. Finding the _____ _____ _____ is the process of multiplying 10s together.

11. Write out the following fractions in the spaces provided:

   a. $\frac{1}{10,000}$ _____

   b. $\frac{2}{10}$ _____

   c. $\frac{6}{100}$ _____

d. $\dfrac{10}{100,000}$ _____

e. $\dfrac{25}{1000}$ _____

12. Write out the following decimal fractions in the spaces provided:

a. 0.25 _____

b. 0.7 _____

c. 0.150 _____

d. 0.4200 _____

e. 0.00006 _____

13. Write out the following whole numbers and decimal fractions in the spaces provided:

a. 2.5 _____

b. 9.25 _____

c. 125.040 _____

d. 15.0150 _____

e. 4.00005 _____

EXPRESSING A COMMON FRACTION AS A DECIMAL FRACTION

A *common fraction* is part of a whole number. It is the process of dividing a number into a numerator separated from the denominator by either a horizontal or diagonal line ($\frac{1}{2}$ or $^1\!/_2$).

A *decimal fraction* is a fraction with an unwritten denominator of 10 or a power of 10 ($0.5 = \frac{5}{10}$).

To express a common fraction as a decimal fraction, follow these steps:

1. Divide the denominator of the fraction into the numerator.

$$\text{denominator } 2\overline{)1} \text{ numerator}$$

2. Place a decimal point after the numerator.

$$2\overline{)1.} \text{ numerator}$$

3. Place a decimal point in the *quotient* (answer) directly over the decimal point of the numerator.

$$\begin{array}{r} . \text{ quotient} \\ 2\overline{)1.} \text{ numerator} \end{array}$$

4. Place a 0 after the decimal point of the numerator.

$$\begin{array}{r} . \\ 2\overline{)1.0} \text{ numerator} \end{array}$$

5. Now divide.

$$\begin{array}{r} .5 \\ 2\overline{)1.0} \\ \underline{1\,0} \end{array}$$

6. Place a 0 before the decimal point of the quotient.

$$\begin{array}{r} 0.5 \text{ quotient} \\ 2\overline{)1.0} \\ \underline{1\,0} \end{array}$$

The common fraction $\frac{1}{2}$ is equal to the decimal fraction 0.5 ($\frac{5}{10}$). The number 0.5 is read as five-tenths and can be reduced to $\dfrac{\overset{1}{5}}{\underset{2}{10}} = \dfrac{1}{2}$.

7. To check the accuracy of your work, multiply the quotient by the denominator (divisor). This will give you the same number as the numerator (dividend).

$$
\begin{array}{ll}
0.5 & \text{quotient} \\
\underline{\times 2} & \text{denominator (divisor)} \\
1.0 & \text{numerator (dividend)}
\end{array}
$$

EXPRESSING A DECIMAL FRACTION AS A COMMON FRACTION

To express a decimal fraction as a common fraction, follow these steps:

1. Read the decimal fraction.
2. The numerator is the number you get when you move the decimal point to the right past the last number.
3. The denominator is the number of spaces you moved the decimal point.
4. Remember that each space is represented by a factor of 10.
5. Reduce to lowest terms.

> **EXAMPLE**   0.25   Read as twenty-five-hundredths.
>
> 0.25   Move the decimal point to the right of the last number; 0.25 becomes 25.
>
> You moved two spaces to the right, which is hundredths.
>
> $0.25 = \dfrac{25}{100}\ \dfrac{\text{numerator}}{\text{denominator}}$
>
> Reduce to lowest terms. $\dfrac{\overset{1}{25}}{\underset{4}{100}} = \dfrac{1}{4}$

▪▪ PRACTICE PROBLEMS

1. Mastering decimals. Express the following common fractions as decimal fractions:

    a. $\dfrac{2}{3} =$ _____

    b. $\dfrac{1}{4} =$ _____

    c. $\dfrac{3}{4} =$ _____

    d. $\dfrac{1}{5} =$ _____

    e. $\dfrac{7}{8} =$ _____

2. Express the following decimal fractions as common fractions:

    a. 0.4 _____

    b. 0.05 _____

    c. 0.010 _____

    d. 0.0006 _____

    e. 0.000002 _____

ADDITION OF DECIMALS

To add decimals, follow these steps:

1. To add decimals, arrange the numbers in a column.
2. Line up the decimal points.
3. Make sure you form a straight line with the decimal point, one under the other.
4. Add the numbers as in addition of whole numbers.
5. Now place the decimal point in your answer directly under the decimal points of the problem.

EXAMPLE

$$
\begin{array}{r}
0.5 \\
+\ 0.10 \\
\hline
0.60
\end{array}
\qquad
\begin{array}{r}
0.75 \\
0.125 \\
+\ 0.1000 \\
\hline
0.9750
\end{array}
$$

PRACTICE PROBLEMS

3. Mastering decimals. Correctly add the following decimals:

   a. $0.6 + 0.4 =$ _____

   b. $0.1 + 0.6 + 0.3 =$ _____

   c. $0.89 + 0.26 + 0.2 =$ _____

   d. $0.25 + 0.001 + 0.100 =$ _____

   e. $10.5 + 123.75 + 0.010 =$ _____

SUBTRACTION OF DECIMALS

To subtract decimals, follow these steps:

1. To subtract decimals, arrange the numbers in a column.
2. Line up the decimal points.
3. Make sure you form a straight line with the decimal point, one under the other.
4. Subtract the numbers as in subtraction of whole numbers.
5. Now place the decimal point in your answer directly under the decimal points of the problem.

   EXAMPLE

   $$
   \begin{array}{r}
   104.32 \\
   -\ 76.21 \\
   \hline
   28.11
   \end{array}
   \qquad
   \begin{array}{r}
   0.098 \\
   -\ 0.010 \\
   \hline
   0.088
   \end{array}
   $$

6. To subtract a smaller number from a larger number, place a 0 after the larger number. A 0 placed after the number will not alter or change the decimal place or the decimal value.

   EXAMPLE

   $$
   \begin{array}{r}
   0.1 \\
   -\ 0.03 \\
   \hline
   \end{array}
   \qquad
   \begin{array}{r}
   0.10 \\
   -\ 0.03 \\
   \hline
   0.07
   \end{array}
   $$

7. Check the accuracy of your work by adding the answer and the lower numbers (subtrahend) together. The sum will equal the upper numbers (minuend).

   EXAMPLE

   $$
   \begin{array}{rl}
   0.098 & \text{minuend} \\
   -\ 0.010 & \text{subtrahend} \\
   +\ 0.088 & \text{answer} \\
   \hline
   0.098 & \text{minuend}
   \end{array}
   \qquad
   \begin{array}{rl}
   0.10 & \text{minuend} \\
   -\ 0.03 & \text{subtrahend} \\
   +\ 0.07 & \text{answer} \\
   \hline
   0.10 & \text{minuend}
   \end{array}
   $$

PRACTICE PROBLEMS

4. Mastering decimals. Correctly subtract the following decimals:

   a. $0.1 - 0.04 =$ _____

   b. $2.25 - 1.75 =$ _____

   c. $304.65 - 264.26 =$ _____

   d. $9.123 - 6.055 =$ _____

   e. $1.000 - 0.556 =$ _____

   f. $0.2 - 0.07 =$ _____

   g. $0.1 - 0.04 =$ _____

   h. $0.3 - 0.09 =$ _____

   i. $0.6 - 0.08 =$ _____

   j. $0.5 - 0.06 =$ _____

MULTIPLICATION OF DECIMALS

To multiply decimals, follow these steps:

1. Multiply decimals just as you multiply whole numbers.
2. Count the number of decimal places in the **multiplier** and in the number to be **multiplied**. Total this number.
3. Start on the right of your *product* and count off the number of decimal places you counted in the previous step.
4. Remember that you count off decimal places in the product from right to left.

EXAMPLE		
	2.14	(two decimal places)
	× 0.76	(two decimal places)
	12 84	
	149 8	
	000	
Product	1.6264	(count off four decimal places from right to left)

Multiplying Decimals by 10 or Any Power of 10

To multiply decimals by 10 or any power of 10, follow these steps:

1. When you multiply by 10, you move the decimal point one place to the right.

$$0.6 \times 10 =$$
$$0.6. = 6$$

2. When you multiply by 100, you move the decimal point two places to the right.

$$0.6 \times 100 =$$
$$0.60. = 60$$

3. When you multiply by 1,000, you move the decimal point three places to the right.

$$0.6 \times 1{,}000 =$$
$$0.600. = 600$$

4. When you multiply by 10,000, you move the decimal point four places to the right.

$$0.6 \times 10{,}000 =$$
$$0.6000. = 6000$$

5. When you multiply by 100,000, you move the decimal point five places to the right.

$$0.6 \times 100{,}000 =$$
$$0.60000. = 60{,}000$$

6. *RULE:* When you multiply decimals by 10 or any multiple of 10, you move the decimal point to the right in the product as many places as there are 0s in the multiplier.

$$3.6 \times 10 = 36$$
$$(1)$$
$$3.6 \times 100 = 360$$
$$(2)$$
$$3.6 \times 1000 = 3{,}600$$
$$(3)$$
$$3.6 \times 10{,}000 = 36{,}000$$
$$(4)$$
$$3.6 \times 100{,}000 = 360{,}000$$
$$(5)$$

PRACTICE PROBLEMS

5. Mastering decimals. Correctly multiply the following decimals:

a. $4.25 \times 3.10 =$ _____

b. $3.75 \times 7.35 =$ _____

c. $83.126 \times 8.12 =$ _____

d. $66.66 \times 3.33 =$ _____

e. $0.0044 \times 72.16 =$ _____

f. $2.5 \times 100,000 =$ _____

g. $10.4 \times 10,000 =$ _____

h. $5.2 \times 1,000 =$ _____

i. $1.1 \times 100 =$ _____

j. $0.3 \times 10 =$ _____

DIVISION OF DECIMALS

The following methods of dividing decimals are designed to guide you step by step through dividing decimals by whole numbers, The following methods of dividing decimals, dividing decimals by decimals, and dividing decimals by 10 or any factor of 10. Master one step at a time and you will acquire a working understanding of dividing decimals.

Dividing Decimals by Whole Numbers

To divide decimals by whole numbers, follow these steps:

1. To divide a decimal by a whole number, set up the division process as follows:

$$12.6 \div 2$$
$$2\overline{)12.6}$$

2. Place a decimal point on the answer line directly over the decimal point of the dividend.

$$\overline{.} \quad \text{answer line}$$
$$2\overline{)12.6} \quad \text{dividend}$$

3. Now you divide the dividend by the *divisor*.

$$\begin{array}{r} 6.3 \quad \text{quotient} \\ \text{divisor} \quad 2\overline{)12.6} \quad \text{dividend} \\ \underline{12} \\ 6 \\ \underline{6} \end{array}$$

4. To check the accuracy of your work, multiply the quotient by the divisor. This will give you the same number as the dividend.

$$\begin{array}{r} 6.3 \quad \text{quotient} \\ \times \quad 2 \quad \text{divisor} \\ \hline 12.6 \quad \text{dividend} \end{array}$$

5. When you have a whole number (divisor) that will not go into the decimal (dividend), follow these steps:

a. $0.016 \div 4 =$

$$4\overline{)0.016}$$

b. Place a decimal point on the answer line directly over the decimal point of the dividend. To ensure accuracy, place a 0 before the decimal point.

$$\begin{array}{r} 0. \quad \text{answer line} \\ 4\overline{)0.016} \quad \text{dividend} \end{array}$$

c. Because 4 will not go into 0, you place a 0 on the answer line directly over the 0 of the dividend.

$$\begin{array}{r} 0.0 \quad \text{answer line} \\ 4\overline{)0.016} \quad \text{dividend} \end{array}$$

d. Because 4 will not go into 1, you place a 0 on the answer line directly over the 1 of the dividend.

$$\begin{array}{r} 0.00 \quad \text{answer line} \\ 4\overline{)0.016} \quad \text{dividend} \end{array}$$

e. Now 4 will go into 16, so divide.

$$\begin{array}{r} 0.004 \\ 4\overline{)0.016} \\ \underline{16} \end{array}$$

f. To check the accuracy of your work, multiply the quotient by the divisor. This will give you the same number as the dividend.

$$\begin{array}{r} 0.004 \quad \text{quotient} \\ \underline{\times 4} \quad \text{divisor} \\ 0.016 \quad \text{dividend} \end{array}$$

■ ■ PRACTICE PROBLEMS

6. Mastering decimals. Correctly divide the following decimals by whole numbers:

   a. $28.8 \div 4 =$ _____   f. $0.018 \div 9 =$ _____

   b. $36.12 \div 6 =$ _____   g. $0.025 \div 5 =$ _____

   c. $100.40 \div 20 =$ _____   h. $0.035 \div 7 =$ _____

   d. $56.14 \div 7 =$ _____   i. $0.04 \div 10 =$ _____

   e. $86.86 \div 43 =$ _____   j. $10.33 \div 3 =$ _____

Dividing Whole Numbers by Decimals

To divide a whole number by a decimal, make the decimal (divisor) a whole number. You can use the following two methods to make a decimal a whole number:

1. You can move the decimal point to the right as many places as necessary to make a whole number, or
2. You can multiply the decimal by the place value of the decimal point.

Moving the Decimal Point to the Right.

To move the decimal point to the right, follow these steps:

1. Place a decimal point at the end of the whole number of the dividend (for example, $100 \div 0.1 =$).

$$0.1\overline{)100.} \quad \text{dividend}$$

2. Place a 0 after the marked-off decimal point.

$$0.1\overline{)100.0}$$

3. Move the decimal point one place to the right in the divisor, and one place to the right in the dividend.

$$\text{divisor} \quad 0.1. \quad 100.0. \quad \text{dividend}$$

4. You have made the decimal (divisor) and the dividend whole numbers. Now you can divide.

$$\begin{array}{r} 1000 \\ 1\overline{)1000} \\ \underline{1} \\ 0 \\ \underline{0} \\ 0 \\ \underline{0} \\ 0 \\ \underline{0} \end{array}$$

5. To check the accuracy of your work, change the whole number and the decimal to fractions and then divide.

$$100 \div 0.1 = \frac{100}{1} \div \frac{1}{10} =$$

$$\frac{100}{1} \times \frac{10}{1} = \frac{1000}{1} = 1000$$

Multiplying the Decimal by the Place Value of the Decimal Point.

To multiply the decimal by the place value, follow these steps:

1. Multiply the decimal (divisor) and the dividend by the same value of the decimal point.

$$100 \div 0.1 = ?$$
0.1 (decimal, divisor) has a place value of 10.
$$0.1 \times 10 = 1$$
$$100 \times 10 = 1000$$

2. You have made the decimal (divisor) and the dividend whole numbers. Now you can divide.

$$\begin{array}{r} 1000 \\ 1\overline{)1000} \\ \underline{1} \\ 0 \\ \underline{0} \\ 0 \\ \underline{0} \\ 0 \\ \underline{0} \end{array}$$

Moving the decimal point to the right as many places as necessary to make a whole number and multiplying the decimal by the place value of the decimal point to make a whole number are two processes that will give you the same result.

0.1. = 1	Moving the decimal one place to the right
	is the same as multiplying by the place
$0.1 \times 10 = 1$	value of 10.
0.01. = 1	Moving the decimal two places to the right
	is the same as multiplying by the place
$0.01 \times 100 = 1$	value of 100.

0.001. = 1   Moving the decimal three places to the right

0.001 × 1,000 = 1   is the same as multiplying by the place
value of 1,000.

0.0001. = 1   Moving the decimal four places to the right

0.0001 × 10,000 = 1   is the same as multiplying by the place
value of 10,000.

0.00001. = 1   Moving the decimal five places to the right

0.00001 × 100,000 = 1   is the same as multiplying by the place
value of 100,000.

▪ ▪ PRACTICE PROBLEMS

7. Mastering decimals. Correctly divide the following whole numbers by decimals:

a. $20 \div 0.2 =$ _____

b. $60 \div 0.03 =$ _____

c. $150 \div 0.75 =$ _____

d. $100 \div 0.10 =$ _____

e. $1000 \div 0.01 =$ _____

f. $72 \div 0.009 =$ _____

g. $500 \div 0.0005 =$ _____

h. $86 \div 0.43 =$ _____

i. $60 \div 0.012 =$ _____

j. $36 \div 0.4 =$ _____

Dividing Decimals by Decimals

To divide decimals by decimals, follow these steps:

1. To divide a decimal by a decimal, make the divisor a whole number by moving the decimal point to the right as many places as necessary or by multiplying the decimal by the place value of the decimal point.

$$0.0016 \div 0.02 = \text{divisor} \qquad 0.02 \overline{)0.0016}$$

Moving the decimal 0.02. or multiplying 0.02 by the place value of 100 = 2.

$$
\begin{array}{r}
0.02 \\
\times\ 100 \\
\hline
0\ 00 \\
00\ 0 \\
002\ \\
\hline
002.00
\end{array}
$$

2. Now you must do the same thing to the dividend that you did to the divisor.

$$0.0016 \div 0.02 = \qquad 0.02 \overline{)0.0016} \qquad \text{dividend}$$

Moving the decimal 0.00.16 or multiplying by the place value of 100 = 0.16.

$$
\begin{array}{r}
0.0016 \\
\times\ \ \ \ \ 100 \\
\hline
0\ 0000 \\
00\ 0000 \\
000\ 16\ \ \\
\hline
000.1600
\end{array}
$$

3. Now set up the problem as follows:

$$2\overline{)\,.16}$$

To ensure accuracy, place a 0 before the decimal point of the dividend.

$$2\overline{)0.16} \quad \text{dividend}$$

Place a decimal point on the answer line directly over the new decimal place of the dividend.

$$\begin{array}{r} . \quad \text{answer line} \\ 2\overline{)0.16} \quad \text{dividend} \end{array}$$

Place a 0 before the marked-off decimal point.

$$\begin{array}{r} 0. \\ 2\overline{)0.16} \end{array}$$

4. Now you have $0.16 \div 2$. Divide.

$$\begin{array}{r} 0. \quad \text{answer line} \\ 2\overline{)0.16} \quad \text{dividend} \end{array}$$

5. But, 2 will not go into 1, so you place a 0 on the answer line directly over the 1 of the dividend.

$$\begin{array}{r} 0.0 \quad \text{answer line} \\ 2\overline{)0.16} \quad \text{dividend} \end{array}$$

6. Now 2 will go into 16.

$$\begin{array}{r} 0.08 \\ 2\overline{)0.16} \\ \underline{16} \end{array}$$

7. To check the accuracy of your work, multiply the quotient (answer) by the divisor. This will give you the same number as the dividend.

$$\begin{array}{r} 0.08 \quad \text{quotient (answer)} \\ \underline{\times 2} \quad \text{divisor} \\ 0.16 \quad \text{dividend} \end{array}$$

■ ■ PRACTICE PROBLEMS

8. Mastering decimals. Correctly divide the following decimals:

   a. $0.0024 \div 0.03 =$ _____   f. $7.5 \div 2.5 =$ _____

   b. $0.054 \div 0.18 =$ _____   g. $0.49 \div 0.007 =$ _____

   c. $0.02 \div 0.2 =$ _____   h. $0.81 \div 0.9 =$ _____

   d. $0.86 \div 0.43 =$ _____   i. $0.0138 \div 0.46 =$ _____

   e. $0.2 \div 0.002 =$ _____   j. $0.06 \div 0.6 =$ _____

Dividing Decimals by 10 or Any Power of 10

To divide decimals by 10 or any power of 10, follow these steps:

1. When you divide by 10, you move the decimal point one place to the left.

$$0.6 \div 10 =$$
$$.0.6 = 0.06$$

2. When you divide by 100, you move the decimal point two places to the left.

$$0.6 \div 100 =$$
$$.00.6 = 0.006$$

3. When you divide by 1000, you move the decimal point three places to the left.

$$0.6 \div 1000 =$$
$$.000.6 = 0.0006$$

4. When you divide by 10,000, you move the decimal point four places to the left.

$$0.6 \div 10,000 =$$
$$.0000.6 = 0.00006$$

5. When you divide by 100,000, you move the decimal point five places to the left.

$$0.6 \div 100,000 =$$
$$.00000.6 = 0.000006$$

6. *RULE:* When you divide by 10 or any multiple of 10, you move the decimal point to the left in the dividend as many places as there are 0s in the divisor.

$$3.6 \div 10 = 0.36$$
$$(1)$$
$$3.6 \div 100 = 0.036$$
$$(2)$$
$$3.6 \div 1000 = 0.0036$$
$$(3)$$
$$3.6 \div 10,000 = 0.00036$$
$$(4)$$
$$3.6 \div 100,000 = 0.000036$$
$$(5)$$

■ ■ PRACTICE PROBLEMS

9. Mastering decimals. Correctly divide the following decimals by the indicated power of 10:

a. $2.5 \div 100,000 =$ _____

b. $10.4 \div 10,000 =$ _____

c. $5.2 \div 1,000 =$ _____

d. $1.1 \div 100 =$ _____

e. $0.3 \div 10 =$ _____

f. $88.8 \div 10 =$ _____

g. $0.150 \div 100 =$ _____

h. $0.66 \div 100,000 =$ _____

i. $0.7 \div 10,000 =$ _____

j. $0.100 \div 1,000 =$ _____

In Review

Always remember that a *decimal fraction* is a fraction with an unwritten denominator of 10 or any power of 10. The *product* is the number found by multiplying two or more numbers. The *multiplier* is the number by which another number is multiplied. The *dividend* is the number that is divided. The *divisor* is the number that is divided into another number.

To multiply decimals by 10 or any power of 10, move the decimal point to the RIGHT in the *product* as many places as there are 0s in the *multiplier*.

$$3.6 \times 10 = 36$$
$$(1)$$

To divide decimals by 10 or any power of 10, move the decimal point to the LEFT in the *dividend* as many places as there are 0s in the *divisor*.

$$3.6 \div 10 = 0.36$$
$$(1)$$

PERCENTAGE

Percent means per hundred. Its symbol, %, indicates that the preceding number is a percentage. The whole is expressed as 100 percent. Therefore, a certain percent indicates parts of 100. For example, 34% means 34/100 or 0.34, or 340% means 340/100 or 3.4 or 3 2/5. Because the strength of solutions is expressed in percentage, it is necessary for you to be able to express percents as decimal fractions and common fractions. This is done by considering the percent sign as a denominator of 100, and then dividing the number by this 100.

- To express a percent as a fraction, remove the percent sign and write the percent as the numerator of a fraction. Write 100 as the denominator of the fraction and express in lowest terms.

  EXAMPLE $$50\% = \frac{50}{100} = \frac{1}{2}$$

- If the percent is a mixed number or a fraction, the numerator of the complex fraction is divided by the denominator (100). The process may be simplified by merely multiplying the percent by 1/100.

  EXAMPLE

  a. $$5.5\% = 5\frac{1}{2}\% = \frac{5\frac{1}{2}}{100} = \frac{11}{2} \div 100 = \frac{11}{2} \times \frac{1}{100} = \frac{11}{200}$$

  b. $$\frac{1}{4}\% = \frac{\frac{1}{4}}{100} = \frac{1}{4} \div 100 = \frac{1}{4} \times \frac{1}{100} = \frac{1}{400}$$

- To express a fraction as a percent, multiply by 100 and add the percent sign.

  EXAMPLE

  a. $$\frac{3}{4} = \frac{3}{4} \times \frac{\overset{25}{100}}{\underset{1}{1}} = 75\%$$

  b. $$\frac{29}{400} = \frac{29}{400} \times \frac{100}{1} = \frac{2900}{400} = 7\frac{1}{4}\%$$

- To express a percent as a decimal, simply remove the percent sign and move the decimal point two places to the left. This is the same as dividing by 100. If the percent has a fraction, the fraction must be expressed in decimal form before the decimal point may be moved.

  EXAMPLE 50% = 0.5   5.5% = 0.055   1/4% = 0.25% = 0.0025

- To express a decimal as a percent, move the decimal point two places to the right and add the percent sign. You are actually multiplying by 100.

  EXAMPLE 0.3 = 30%   0.35 = 35%   0.355 = 35.5%   0.0355 = 3.55%z

▪ ▪ PRACTICE PROBLEMS

10. Express the following common fractions as percentages:

a. $\frac{1}{4} =$ _____

b. $\frac{1}{3} =$ _____

c. $\frac{2}{5} =$ _____

d. $\frac{2}{3} =$ _____

e. $\frac{3}{25} =$ _____

11. Express the largest decimal in each of the following series as a percentage:

  a. 0.001   1.25   1.09   _____

  b. 0.7   0.69   0.349   _____

  c. 0.08   0.8   0.185   _____

  d. 0.495   4.95   0.049   _____

  e. 0.125   0.005   0.025   _____

12. Change each of the following percentages to a fraction *and* a decimal:

  a. 2%   _____ and _____

  b. $4\frac{3}{4}$ _____ and _____

  c. 40%   _____ and _____

  d. 19.3%   _____ and _____

  e. 64%   _____ and _____

DETERMINING QUANTITY IF A PERCENTAGE IS GIVEN

To find the percentage of a given number, express the percentage as a decimal or fraction; multiply the whole number by the decimal or fraction.

> **EXAMPLE**   How much is 5% of 48?
>
> **Conversion to decimal**   **Conversion to fraction**
>
> $5\% = 0.05$ $5\% = \frac{5}{100}$ or $\frac{1}{20}$
>
> $48 \times 0.05 = 2.4$ $48 \times \frac{1}{20} = \frac{48}{20}$ or $2\frac{2}{5}$
>
> *Note:* $2.4 = 2\frac{2}{5}$

▍▍ PRACTICE PROBLEMS

13. Solve each of the following problems and give the answer as a decimal and as a fraction:

Problem	*Decimal*	*Fraction*
a. How much is 20% of 36?	_____	_____
b. How much is 8% of 60?	_____	_____
c. How much is 1/2% of 750?	_____	_____
d. How much is 350% of 15?	_____	_____
e. How much is 2% of 10?	_____	_____

▍▍ REVIEW PROBLEMS

1. Express the following common fractions as decimal fractions:

  a. $\frac{1}{8} =$ _____   c. $\frac{1}{2} =$ _____   e. $\frac{1}{3} =$ _____   g. $\frac{3}{10} =$ _____   i. $\frac{2}{5} =$ _____

  b. $\frac{1}{16} =$ _____   d. $\frac{3}{25} =$ _____   f. $\frac{1}{4} =$ _____   h. $\frac{5}{6} =$ _____   j. $\frac{9}{16} =$ _____

2. Express the following decimal fractions as common fractions:

   a. 0.1 = _____

   b. 0.01 = _____

   c. 0.001 = _____

   d. 0.5 = _____

   e. 0.035 = _____

   f. 0.25 = _____

   g. 0.75 = _____

   h. 0.3 = _____

   i. 0.625 = _____

   j. 0.82 = _____

3. Correctly add the following decimals:

   a. 0.27 + 0.3 + 0.72 = _____

   b. 3.25 + 0.6 + 2.22 = _____

   c. 0.8 + 1.6 + 9.27 = _____

   d. 0.5 + 10.5 + 100.7 = _____

   e. 0.27 + 0.94 + 0.08 = _____

   f. 0.964 + 0.0086 + 0.05 = _____

   g. 246.1 + 56.7 + 11.9 = _____

   h. 6.7 + 72.5 + 21.4 = _____

   i. 1.76 + 2.86 + 7.52 = _____

   j. 2.24 + 2.20 + 3.33 = _____

4. Correctly subtract the following decimals:

   a. 0.36 − 0.09 = _____

   b. 0.3 − 0.26 = _____

   c. 3.8 − 2.96 = _____

   d. 9.7 − 2.82 = _____

   e. 0.63 − 0.402 = _____

   f. 0.15 − 0.07 = _____

   g. 3.25 − 1.12 = _____

   h. 5.8 − 0.299 = _____

   i. 0.7 − 0.462 = _____

   j. 6.75 − 3.33 = _____

5. Correctly multiply the following decimals:

   a. 5.1 × 2.6 = _____

   b. 0.8 × 0.09 = _____

   c. 0.6 × 9.1 = _____

   d. 0.4 × 82.6 = _____

   e. 0.36 × 0.526 = _____

   f. 3.8 × 0.526 = _____

   g. 0.065 × 0.4 = _____

   h. 1.29 × 26.2 = _____

   i. 0.02 × 0.10 = _____

   j. 0.24 × 10.6 = _____

6. Correctly divide the following decimals by whole numbers:

   a. 2.4 ÷ 12 = _____

   b. 6.6 ÷ 6 = _____

   c. 0.36 ÷ 18 = _____

   d. 0.75 ÷ 3 = _____

   e. 22.4 ÷ 2 = _____

   f. 4.8 ÷ 8 = _____

   g. 2.7 ÷ 9 = _____

   h. 16.2 ÷ 4 = _____

   i. 3.4 ÷ 5 = _____

   j. 7.6 ÷ 2 = _____

7. Correctly divide the following whole numbers by decimals:

   a. 168 ÷ 2.4 = _____

   b. 32 ÷ 0.64 = _____

   c. 9 ÷ 2.50 = _____

   d. 24 ÷ 0.4 = _____

   e. 66 ÷ 0.12 = _____

   f. 54 ÷ 4.5 = _____

   g. 3 ÷ 0.25 = _____

   h. 18 ÷ 0.36 = _____

   i. 48 ÷ 2.4 = _____

   j. 76 ÷ 0.38 = _____

8. Correctly divide the following decimals:

   a. $0.506 \div 0.1 =$ _____

   b. $22.8 \div 0.4 =$ _____

   c. $11.88 \div 0.18 =$ _____

   d. $0.333 \div 3.6 =$ _____

   e. $0.48 \div 0.008 =$ _____

   f. $7.5 \div 2.5 =$ _____

   g. $0.02 \div 0.2 =$ _____

   h. $40.42 \div 0.86 =$ _____

   i. $10.01 \div 0.02 =$ _____

   j. $0.001 \div 0.1 =$ _____

9. Correctly divide the following decimals by the powers of 10:

   a. $3.6 \div 100,000 =$ _____

   b. $10.5 \div 10,000 =$ _____

   c. $6.7 \div 1,000 =$ _____

   d. $2.2 \div 100 =$ _____

   e. $0.6 \div 10 =$ _____

   f. $99.9 \div 100 =$ _____

   g. $0.125 \div 1,000 =$ _____

   h. $0.7 \div 100 =$ _____

   i. $48.2 \div 100,000 =$ _____

   j. $3.33 \div 10 =$ _____

■ ■ SELF-ASSESSMENT

This exercise is designed to assess your understanding of decimal fractions and percentages. Answer the questions and follow the directions as provided. To verify your answers, you may check with your instructor or go to the student companion website.

1. All the numbers to the left of the decimal point are _____ numbers.

2. All the numbers to the right of the decimal point are _____ or _____ _____.

3. The value of each place left of the decimal point is _____ times that of the place to its right.

4. The value of each place right of the decimal point is _____ of the value of the place to its left.

5. Read the following fractions, decimal fractions, whole numbers, and decimal fractions. Write your answers in the following spaces:

   a. $\frac{5}{10}$ _____

   b. $\frac{10}{1000}$ _____

   c. 0.50 _____

   d. 0.00005 _____

   e. 2.25 _____

   f. 8.75 _____

6. Express the following as decimal fractions:

   a. $\frac{1}{3}$ _____

   b. $\frac{1}{4}$ _____

7. Express the following as common fractions:

   a. 0.5 _____

   b. 0.00005 _____

8. Add the following:

   a. $0.5 + 0.5$ _____

   b. $0.98 + 0.76$ _____

9. Subtract the following:

   a. $0.6 - 0.08$ _____

   b. $9.123 - 6.055$ _____

10. Multiply the following:

    a. 66.66×3.33 _____

    b. 1.1×100 _____

11. Divide the following:

    a. $0.018 \div 9$ _____

    b. $0.04 \div 10$ _____

    c. $86 \div 0.43$ _____

    d. $60 \div 0.012$ _____

    e. $0.06 \div 0.6$ _____

    f. $0.49 \div 0.007$ _____

12. Express the following as percentages:

    a. $\frac{1}{3}$ _____

    b. $\frac{1}{4}$ _____

    c. $\frac{2}{3}$ _____

UNIT 3
Ratio and Proportion

OBJECTIVES

Upon completing this unit, you should be able to:

- Define the terms listed in the vocabulary.
- Express a ratio as a quotient, as a fraction, and as a decimal.
- Name the four terms of a proportion.
- Solve for *x* and prove your answers.
- Work the practice problems and review problems correctly.
- Successfully complete the Self-Assessment.

VOCABULARY

extremes (eks-treemz'). The outer numbers or the first and fourth terms of the proportion.

means (meenz). The inner numbers or the second and third terms of the proportion.

negative (neg'a-tiv). A quantity less than 0; minus.

positive (poz'i-tiv). A quantity greater than 0; plus.

proof (proof). The stages in resolving the accuracy of your work.

proportion (pro-poor'shun). A way of expressing comparative relationships of a part, share, or portion with regard to size, amount, or number.

ratio (ra'shee-o). A way of expressing the relationship of a number, quantity, substance, or degree between two similar components.

UNDERSTANDING RATIO

Ratio is a way of expressing the relationship of a number, quantity, substance, or degree between two similar components. For example, the relationship of one to five is written 1 : 5. Note that the numbers are side by side and separated by a colon.

In mathematics, a ratio may be expressed as a quotient, a fraction, or a decimal.

Ratio Expressed as a Quotient

Remember that a quotient is the number found when one number is divided by another number. The ratio of one to five written as a quotient is $1 \div 5$.

Ratio Expressed as a Fraction

Remember that a fraction is the result of dividing or breaking a whole number into parts. The ratio of one to five written as a fraction is $\frac{1}{5}$.

Ratio Expressed as a Decimal

Remember that a decimal is a linear array of numbers based upon 10 or any multiple of 10. To express one to five as a decimal, you divide the denominator (5) into the numerator (1).

$$\text{denominator} \quad 5)\overline{1.0}^{\,0.2} \quad \text{numerator}$$

The RATIO 1 : 5 may be expressed as a:

	Quotient	Fraction	Decimal
	$1 \div 5$	$\frac{1}{5}$	0.2

PRACTICE PROBLEMS

Mastering ratios. Express the following numbers as a ratio, a quotient, a fraction, or a decimal, and reduce to lowest terms when possible:

1. Express as a Ratio   Reduce to Lowest Terms

   a. $\frac{1}{25}$ _____   _____

   b. $\frac{2}{100}$ _____   _____

   c. $\frac{10}{40}$ _____   _____

   d. $\frac{25}{75}$ _____   _____

   e. $\frac{8}{64}$ _____   _____

2. Express as a Quotient

   a. 24 : 48 _____   _____

   b. 12 : 6 _____   _____

   c. 76 : 304 _____   _____

   d. 5 : 25 _____   _____

   e. 2 : 92 _____   _____

3. Express as a Fraction   Reduce to Lowest Terms

    a. 55 : 66   _____   _____

    b. 4 : 10   _____   _____

    c. 75 : 100   _____   _____

    d. 22 : 88   _____   _____

    e. 43 : 86   _____   _____

4. Express as a Decimal

    a. 1 : 50   _____   _____

    b. 8 : 100   _____   _____

    c. 6 : 1000   _____   _____

    d. 5 : 4   _____   _____

    e. 1 : 500   _____   _____

UNDERSTANDING PROPORTION

Proportion is a way of expressing the comparative relationship between a part, share, or portion with regard to size, amount, or number. In mathematics, a proportion expresses the relationship between two ratios. In setting up a proportion, the ratios are separated by colons (: :) or an equal sign (=). In this text, the equal sign (=) is used to separate ratios.

> **EXAMPLE** $3 : 4 = 1 : 2$

Read: three is to four equals one is to two.

The four terms of a proportion are given special names. The means are the inner numbers or the second and third terms of the proportion.

> **EXAMPLE** $3 : 4 = 1 : 2$
>   (4) (1)
>
> *means*

The **extremes** are the outer numbers or the first and fourth terms of the proportion.

> **EXAMPLE** $3 : 4 = 1 : 2$
>   (3)   (2)
>
> *extremes*

In a *true* proportion, the product of the means equals the product of the extremes.

> **EXAMPLE** $8 : 16 = 1 : 2$
> $16 \times 1 = 16$ (*product of the means*)
> $8 \times 2 = 16$ (*product of the extremes*)

Solving for *x*

The proportion is a very useful mathematical tool. When a part, share, or portion of the problem is unknown, then *x* represents the unknown factor. You can determine the unknown by solving for *x*. The unknown factor *x* may appear any place in the proportion.

    Now solve for *x* in the problem $3 : 4 = x : 12$.

1. Multiply the terms that contain the *x* and place the *product* to the *left* of the equal sign (4x).

2. Multiply the other terms and place the product to the *right* of the equal sign (36).

3. To find x, divide the number in the product that contains x into the product of the other terms ($36 \div 4$).

4. Your answer will be equal to x (9).

EXAMPLE $3:4 = x:12$

$$4x = 36$$
$$x = 36 \div 4 = 9$$
$$x = 9$$

After finding the unknown factor, check your mathematical skills by determining if you have a *true* proportion. This technique is called constructing a **proof** or *proving* your answer. To prove your answer, follow these steps:

1. Place the answer you found for x back into the formula where you once had x.

2. Now multiply to find the *means* and the *extremes*.

3. The results will equal each other.

EXAMPLE   *Formula:* $3:4 = x:12$
          Proof: $3:4 = 9:12$
                $36 = 36$

■ ■ PRACTICE PROBLEMS

5. Solve for x and prove your answers for the following:

   a. $4:5 = x:10$ _____

   b. $25:x = 5:10$ _____

   c. $50:x = 25:1000$ _____

   d. $8:10 = x:30$ _____

   e. $4:8 = x:16$ _____

Now solve for x when a fraction of x is used in the formula: $\frac{1}{2}x:1000 = 1:500$

1. Multiply the fraction times x by the appropriate term and place the product to the *left* of the equal sign.

2. Multiply the other terms and place the product to the *right* of the equal sign.

3. To find x, divide the number in the product that contains x into the product of the other terms.

4. Your answer will be equal to x.

5. Prove your answer.

EXAMPLE $\frac{1}{2}x:1000 = 1:500$

$$\frac{1}{2} \times \frac{500}{1} = 250 \qquad \text{Steps 1, 2}$$
$$250x = 1000$$
$$x = 1000 \div 250 = 4 \qquad \text{Step 3}$$
$$x = 4 \qquad \text{Step 4}$$

Proof: $\frac{1}{2}\left(\frac{4}{1}\right) = 2$ Step 5

$2:1000 = 1:500$

$1000 = 1000$

PRACTICE PROBLEMS

6. Solve for x and prove your answers for the following:

   a. $\frac{1}{2}:x = 1:8$ _____

   b. $\frac{1}{4}:x = 20:4000$ _____

   c. $\frac{1}{6}:\frac{5}{6} = 4:x$ _____

   d. $\frac{1}{2}:1000 = x:500$ _____

   e. $\frac{3}{4}:x = \frac{9}{10}:\frac{2}{3}$ _____

   Now solve for x when decimals are used in the formula: $0.6:0.4 = 9:x$.

1. Multiply the terms containing the x and place the product to the *left* of the equal sign. Remember your steps in multiplying decimals.

2. Multiply the other terms and place the product to the *right* of the equal sign.

3. To find x, divide the number in the product that contains x into the product of the other terms. Remember your steps in how to divide decimals.

4. Your answer will be equal to x.

5. Prove your answer.

   EXAMPLE $0.6:0.4 = 9:x$

   $0.6x = 3.6$ Steps 1, 2

   $x = 3.6 \div 0.6$ Step 3

   $x = 6$

   $$0.6\overline{)3.6} \quad \begin{array}{r} 6 \\ \hline 3.6 \\ 3\,6 \end{array}$$

   Proof: $0.6:0.4 = 9:6$

   $3.6 = 3.6$

PRACTICE PROBLEMS

7. Solve for x and prove your answers for the following:

   a. $0.4:0.2 = 6:x$ _____

   b. $0.2:4 = 25:x$ _____

   c. $0.7:x = 70:500$ _____

   d. $0.5:15 = x:60$ _____

   e. $0.3:30 = 10:x$ _____

UNIT 4
The Metric System

OBJECTIVES

Upon completing this unit, you should be able to:

- Define the terms listed in the vocabulary.
- List 10 guidelines you will use as you work with the metric system.
- Name the seven common prefixes used in the metric system.
- Name the fundamental units of the metric system.
- State why you place a zero before the decimal point.
- Write the metric equivalents for length, volume, mass, and weight.
- Write the abbreviations for the metric equivalents of length, volume, mass, and weight.
- Name the metric equivalents that are most frequently used in the medical field.
- Use the proportional method to convert from one metric unit to another.
- Use the moving the decimal method to convert from one metric unit to another.
- Calculate dosage according to kilogram of body weight.
- Answer the questions in the learning exercise correctly.
- Work the practice problems and review problems correctly.
- Successfully complete the Self-Assessment.

VOCABULARY

centigram (sen'ti-gram). One hundredth of a gram.

centiliter (sen'ti-lee"ter). One hundredth of a liter.

centimeter (sen'ti-mee"ter). One hundredth of a meter.

decigram (des'i-gram). One tenth of a gram.

deciliter (des'ilee"ter). One tenth of a liter.

decimeter (des'i-mee"ter). One tenth of a meter.

dekagram (dek'ah-gram). Ten grams.

dekaliter (dek'ah-lee"ter). Ten liters.

dekameter (dek'ah-mee"ter). Ten meters.

gram (gram). The metric unit of mass or weight.

hectogram (hek'to-gram). One hundred grams.

hectoliter (hek'to-lee"ter). One hundred liters.

hectometer (hek'to-mee"ter). One hundred meters.

kilogram (kil'o-gram). One thousand grams. A kilogram is equal to 2.2 pounds.

kiloliter (kil'o-lee"ter). One thousand liters.

kilometer (kil'o-mee"ter). One thousand meters.

liter (lee'ter). The metric unit of volume.

meter (mee'ter). The fundamental unit of length in the metric system. It is derived from the Greek *metron*, which means to measure.

microgram (my'kro'gram). One thousandth of a milligram and one millionth of a gram.

milligram (mil'i-gram). One thousandth of a gram.

milliliter (mil'i-lee"ter). One thousandth of a liter.

millimeter (mil'i-mee"ter). One thousandth of a meter.

SI The International System of Units, derived from the French name Le Système International d'Unités.

INTRODUCTION

The *metric system* was first proposed in 1670 by Gabriel Mouton, a French clergyman. Adopted in 1801 by the French National Assembly, this system has become the official standard for scientific and industrial measurement in 92 percent of the world's developed countries. Known as the Système International d'Unités and abbreviated as SI, the modern metric system is used as the primary system of measurement in the field of medicine.

In the medical field, dosage of medications may be in micrograms, milligrams, grams, and per kilogram of body weight. The volume of the medication may be in milliliters or cubic centimeters. Blood pressure is measured in millimeters of mercury (mm Hg). The size and length of a wound, mole, tumor, or incision are measured in centimeters. Laboratory chemistry results may be measured in micrograms, milligrams, or grams per deciliter or as units per liter.

An average adult man's heart weighs 300 grams, and an individual who weighs 70 kg (154 pounds) has a blood volume of 5 liters (about 5 quarts). The normal body temperature is 37° Celsius (98.6° Fahrenheit).

The metric system provides a simple, flexible, and very accurate way to measure length, volume, and weight. It utilizes the concept of the decimal point, and measurements are in units of 10 or multiples of 10.

METRIC SYSTEM GUIDELINES

The following guidelines will help you as you learn basic facts about the metric system:

1. Arabic numbers are used to designate whole numbers: 1, 250, 500, 1000, and so forth.
2. Decimal fractions are used for quantities less than one: 0.1, 0.01, 0.001, 0.0001, and so forth.
3. To ensure accuracy, place a zero before the decimal point: 0.1, 0.001, 0.0001, and so forth.
4. The Arabic number precedes the metric unit of measurement: 10 grams, 2 milliliters, 5 liters, and so forth.
5. The abbreviation for gram may be written as gm or g. The preferred abbreviation is g.
6. The abbreviation for liter is capitalized (L).
7. Prefixes are written in lowercase letters: milli, centi, deci, deka, and so forth.
8. Capitalize the measurement and symbol when it is named after a person: Celsius (C).
9. Periods are no longer used with most abbreviations or symbols.
10. Abbreviations for units are the same for singular and plural. An "s" is not added to indicate a plural.

THE LANGUAGE OF THE METRIC SYSTEM

In the metric system, 14 prefixes are used to denote the size of a metric unit. Each prefix is based upon a multiple or submultiple of 10. These prefixes are tera-, giga-, mega-, kilo-, hecto-, deka-, deci-, centi-, milli-, micro-, nano-, pico-, femto-, and atto-. You will not have to learn all 14 prefixes for this course; however, you will need to know the seven common metric prefixes that are used in the medical field.

The Seven Common Metric Prefixes

Study the following list of prefixes. Once you know these prefixes, you will have a solid foundation for determining metric equivalents. When you combine a metric prefix with a root of physical quantity, you will know the multiples or submultiples of the metric system.

> **EXAMPLE** milli- (prefix) means one thousandth of a unit
> meter (root) a measure of length
> millimeter is one thousandth of a meter
>
> kilo- (prefix) means one thousand units
> liter (root) is a measure of volume
> kiloliter is one thousand liters

micro- (prefix) is one millionth of a unit
gram (root) is a measure of mass and/or weight
microgram is one millionth of a gram

EXAMPLE

micro- (mi'kro)	=	one millionth of a unit written as 0.000001
milli- (mil'i)	=	one thousandth of a unit written as 0.001
centi- (sen'ti)	=	one hundredth of a unit written as 0.01
deci- (des'i)	=	one tenth of a unit written as 0.1
deka- (dek'a)	=	ten units written as 10
hecto- (hek'to)	=	one hundred units written as 100
kilo- (kil'o)	=	one thousand units written as 1000

FUNDAMENTAL UNITS

The following are the fundamental units of the metric system:

meter (m)—length
liter (L)—volume
gram (g)—mass and/or weight

The **meter** is the fundamental unit of length in the metric system and originally formed the foundation for the entire system. A meter is equal to 39.37 inches, which is slightly more than a yard, or 3.28 feet.

Meter (m)	=	Length
1 millimeter (mm)	=	0.001 of a meter
1 centimeter (cm)	=	0.01 of a meter
1 decimeter (dm)	=	0.1 of a meter
1 meter (m)	=	1 meter
1 dekameter (dam)	=	10 meters
1 hectometer (hm)	=	100 meters
1 kilometer (km)	=	1000 meters

A millimeter is about the width of the head of a pin. It takes approximately $2\frac{1}{2}$ centimeters to make an inch; a decimeter is approximately 4 inches.

The **liter** is the liquid metric unit of volume. A liter is equal to 1.056 quarts, which is 0.26 of a gallon, or 2.1 pints.

Liter (L)	=	Volume
1 milliliter (mL)	=	0.001 of a liter
1 centiliter (cL)	=	0.01 of a liter
1 deciliter (dL)	=	0.1 of a liter
1 liter (L)	=	1 liter
1 dekaliter (daL)	=	10 liters
1 hectoliter (hL)	=	100 liters
1 kiloliter (kL)	=	1000 liters

A milliliter is equivalent to one cubic centimeter (cc), because the amount of space occupied by a milliliter is equal to one cubic centimeter. The weight of one milliliter of water equals approximately one gram. It takes approximately 15 milliliters to make one tablespoon.

The **gram** is the metric unit of solids, for mass and/or weight. It equals approximately the weight of one cubic centimeter or one milliliter of water. A gram is equal to approximately 15 grains, or 0.035 of an ounce.

Gram (g)	=	Mass and/or Weight
1 microgram (mcg, μg)	=	0.000001 gram
1 milligram (mg)	=	0.001 of a gram
1 centigram (cg)	=	0.01 of a gram
1 decigram (dg)	=	0.1 of a gram
1 gram (g)	=	1 gram
1 dekagram (dag)	=	10 grams
1 hectogram (hg)	=	100 grams
1 kilogram (kg)	=	1000 grams

Metric Equivalents Most Frequently Used in the Medical Field

Length		Volume	
$2\frac{1}{2}$ centimeters (cm) = 1 inch (in)		1000 milliliters (mL) or 1000 cubic centimeters (cc)	= 1 liter
Weight			
1000 micrograms (mcg)	=	1 milligram (mg)	
1000 milligrams (mg)	=	1 gram (g)	
1000 grams (g)	=	1 kilogram (kg)	
1 kilogram	=	2.2 pounds (lb)	

■ ■ LEARNING EXERCISE

Mastering the metric system. Place the correct answer in the space provided:

1. The fundamental units of the metric system are:

   a. _____ for length   b. _____ for volume   c. _____ for weight

2. Write the name of the prefix for each of the following:

   a. _____ one thousand units   e. _____ one thousandth of a unit

   b. _____ one tenth of a unit   f. _____ ten units

   c. _____ one millionth of a unit   g. _____ one hundredth of a unit

   d. _____ one hundred units

3. _____ are used for quantities less than one.

4. To ensure accuracy, place a _____ before the decimal point.

5. A meter is equal to _____ inches.

6. Write in the correct equivalent for each of the following:

   a. 1 mm = _____ meter   e. 1 dam = _____ meters

   b. 1 cm = _____ meter   f. 1 hm = _____ meters

   c. 1 dm = _____ meter   g. 1 km = _____ meters

   d. 1 m = _____ meter

7. It takes approximately _____ centimeters to make an inch.

8. A liter is equal to _____ quarts.

9. A milliliter is equivalent to _____ cubic centimeters.

10. A gram equals approximately the weight of _____ _____ _____ or _____ _____
    of water.

11. Write in the correct equivalent for each of the following:

    a. 1 mL = _____ liter   e. 1 daL = _____ liters

    b. 1 cL = _____ liter   f. 1 hL = _____ liters

    c. 1 dL = _____ liter   g. 1 kL = _____ liters

    d. 1 L = _____ liter

12. A gram is equal to approximately _____ grains or _____ of an ounce.

13. Write in the correct equivalent for each of the following:

    a. 1 mcg, μg = _____ gram   e. 1 g = _____ gram

    b. 1 mg = _____ gram   f. 1 dag = _____ grams

    c. 1 cg = _____ gram   g. 1 hg = _____ grams

    d. 1 dg = _____ gram   h. 1 kg = _____ grams

14. Name the metric equivalents that are most frequently used in the medical field. Start with the smallest and
    go to the largest:

Volume	*Weight*
a. _____	a. _____
b. _____	b. _____
	c. _____
	d. _____

15. Write the correct abbreviation and unit of measurement for each of the following:

   a. one gram _____

   b. one-fourth liter _____

   c. two hundred milligrams _____

   d. two-tenths of a milliliter _____

   e. twelve kilograms _____

16. Write in the abbreviation for the unit that makes the equivalent correct:

   a. 1000 mL = 1 _____   d. 2 kg = 4.4 _____

   b. 2000 mg = 2 _____   e. 0.5 g = 500 _____

   c. 1000 mcg, μg = 1 _____

CONVERSION

The process of changing into another form, state, substance, or product is known as *conversion*. In the metric system, changing from one unit to another involves multiplying or dividing by 10, 100, 1000, and so forth. This can be done by the proportional method or by moving the decimal in the correct direction.

Proportional Method for Converting Metric Equivalents

The proportional method has six basic steps , plus an additional step to prove your answer. The following example will serve as a model for future applications of the proportional method of converting metric equivalents. Study this example and then proceed to the practice problems.

> **EXAMPLE** Converting 1500 milligrams to grams. 1500 mg = _____ g

Step 1. Because the unknown factor in the given formula is the number of grams contained in 1500 milligrams, you will substitute the symbol x for grams in the equation.

Step 2. Setting up the proportion requires that you know your metric equivalents. For example, in this problem, you have to know that 1000 milligrams (mg) = 1 gram (g).

Step 3. Because you know that 1000 mg is equal to 1 g, you can create one-half of the equation. Write the equivalent that you know and place it on the *left* of the equal sign.

$$1000 \text{ mg}: 1 \text{ g} =$$

Step 4. Now that you have the *left* side of the equation, set up the right side by using the designated metric value 1500 mg : x g. Always write the smallest equivalent as to the largest equivalent— mg : g. By being consistent, you will be less likely to make errors.

$$1000 \text{ mg}: 1 \text{ g} = 1500 \text{ mg}: x \text{ g}$$

Step 5. Note that you have an equation—mg : g 5 mg : g. The *first* values on either side of the equal sign are *milligrams*, and the second values on either side are grams.

Step 6. Now solve for the unknown (x) by multiplication and division. Remember, multiply to get the means and the extremes. *Note:* Once you have the proportion correctly set up, you may simply use the numbers as you multiply and divide.

$$1000:1 = 1500:x$$

$$1000x = 1500$$
$$x = 1500 \div 1000$$
$$x = 1.5$$

$$\begin{array}{r} 1.5 \\ 1000\overline{)1500.0} \\ \underline{1000} \\ 500\,0 \\ \underline{500\,0} \end{array}$$

Step 7. To make sure that you have a correct answer, *prove* your work. Place your answer 1.5 g into the formula where you once had *x*. Now multiply. Note that the product of the means and the product of the extremes are the same.

$$1000 \text{ mg} : 1 \text{ g} = 1500 \text{ mg} : 1.5 \text{ g}$$
$$1500 = 1500$$

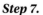 PRACTICE PROBLEMS

1. Conversion. Using the proportional method, convert each of the following metric equivalents:

   a. 250 mL = _____ L   f. 0.05 mg = _____ g

   b. 0.5 L = _____ mL   g. 1 mcg, μg = _____ mg

   c. 2 g = _____ mg   h. 2 mL = _____ cc

   d. 500 mg = _____ g   i. 1000 g = _____ kg

   e. 0.0300 g = _____ mg   j. 2 kg = _____ lb

Moving the Decimal Method for Converting Metric Equivalents

Four basic steps are used to move the decimal in the correct direction. It is essential that you understand the following concepts. Study this example and then proceed to the practice problems.

   EXAMPLE Converting 2.5 grams to milligrams. 2.5 g = _____ mg

Step 1. Establish the placement of the decimal in the unit that is to be converted to another unit.

convert 2.5 g to mg

Step 2. Determine if you are converting a larger unit to a smaller unit or a smaller unit to a larger unit.

convert g (larger) unit to mg (smaller) unit

Step 3. When converting from a larger unit to a smaller unit, you multiply by 1000, which is the same as moving the decimal point three places to the *right*.

Larger unit	$\dfrac{\times}{\text{multiply}}$	*to smaller unit*
milligram		microgram
gram		milligram
liter		milliliter
kilogram		gram

Convert: 2.5 g to _____ mg

Multiply	*Moving the decimal point*
2.5	2.500.
× 1000	
2500.0	1, 2, 3 places

Step 4. When converting a smaller unit to a larger unit, you divide by 1000, which is the same as moving the decimal point three places to the left.

Smaller unit	$\dfrac{\div}{\text{divide}}$	*to larger unit*
microgram		milligram
milligram		gram
milliliter		liter
gram		kilogram

Convert: 2500 mg to _____ g

Divide

$$\begin{array}{r} 2.5 \\ 1000\overline{)2500.0} \\ \underline{2000} \\ 500\,0 \\ \underline{500\,0} \end{array}$$

Moving the decimal point

2500.   2.500.

3, 2, 1

PRACTICE PROBLEMS

2. Conversion. Using the moving the decimal method, convert each of the following metric equivalents:

a. 60 mg   = _____ g   f.   3.5 mL   = _____ L

b. 0.005 L   = _____ mL   g.   4 kg   = _____ g

c. 200 mL   = _____ L   h.   1 mL   = _____ L

d. 1 g   = _____ kg   i.   0.1 L   = _____ mL

e. 0.0065 g   = _____ mg   j.   0.05 mg   = _____ g

CALCULATING DOSAGE ACCORDING TO KILOGRAM OF BODY WEIGHT

You may be responsibe for calculating the amount of dosage ordered by the physician according to the patient's body weight. The following example will guide you step by step through the mathematical process of calculating dosage according to kilogram of body weight.

EXAMPLE   The physician ordered an antiepileptic agent, Depakene (valproic acid) 15 mg/kg/day capsules, for Clark McGee, who weighs 110 pounds. The medication is to be given in three divided doses.

Step 1.   To express pounds in kilograms, divide the weight in pounds by 2.2. There are 2.2 pounds in one kilogram.

Convert patient's weight to kilograms:

$$110 \div 2.2 = 50 \text{ kilograms}$$

Step 2.   Now, calculate the prescribed dosage by placing 50 in the appropriate place.

$$15 \text{ mg/50/day}$$
$$15 \times 50 = 750 \text{ mg/day}$$

Step 3.   To determine the amount of each dose, divide 750 by 3 (divided doses).

$$750 \div 3 = 250 \text{ mg per dose}$$

Depakene is available in 250 mg capsules and 250 mg/5 mL syrup. The physician ordered the medication in capsules, so Clark will receive a 250 mg capsule every 8 hours.

PRACTICE PROBLEMS

3. Calculate the following dosages according to kilogram of body weight:
   a. The physician ordered a medication of 20 mg/kg/day in divided doses every 8 hours for a child who weighs 66 pounds. Convert pounds to kilograms and then calculate the prescribed dosage.
   b. The physician ordered a medication of 25 mg/kg/day in three equal doses every 8 hours for a child who weighs 50 pounds. Convert pounds to kilograms and then calculate the prescribed dosage.
   c. The physician ordered a medication of 50 mg/kg/day in equally divided doses four times a day for a child who weighs 40 pounds. Convert pounds to kilograms and then calculate the prescribed dosage.
   d. The physician ordered a medication of 50 mg/kg in equally divided doses at 6-hour intervals for a child who weighs 23 pounds. Convert pounds to kilograms and then calculate the prescribed dosage.

REVIEW PROBLEMS

1. Using the proportional method, convert each of the following metric equivalents:
   a. 1 mL = _____ L   f. 0.005 L = _____ mL
   b. 1500 mg = _____ g   g. 150.0 mg = _____ g
   c. 25,000 mL = _____ L   h. 0.25 g = _____ mg
   d. 0.006 g = _____ mg   i. 2 mcg = _____ mg
   e. 0.4 mg = _____ g   j. 2 kg = _____ lb

2. Using the moving the decimal method, convert each of the following metric equivalents:
   a. 0.0065 g = _____ mg   f. 0.5 L = _____ mL
   b. 100 mL = _____ L   g. 2 g = _____ kg
   c. 300 mL = _____ L   h. 1 mcg = _____ mg
   d. 0.04 mg = _____ g   i. 0.004 kg = _____ g
   e. 1 cc = _____ L   j. 0.06 mg = _____ g

3. Calculate the following dosages according to kilogram of body weight:

   a. The physician ordered Zovirax capsules 5 mg/kg every 8 hours for 7 days for a patient who has a diagnosis of herpes zoster. The patient weighs 132 pounds. Convert pounds to kilograms and then calculate the prescribed dosage.
   b. The physician ordered aminophylline 7.5 mg/kg for a child who weighs 66 pounds. Convert pounds to kilograms and then calculate the prescribed dosage.
   c. The physician ordered Rocephin 50 mg/kg in two divided doses for a child who weighs 44 pounds. Convert pounds to kilograms and then calculate the prescribed dosage.
   d. The physician ordered chloral hydrate 25 mg/kg for a child who weighs 55 pounds. Convert pounds to kilograms and then calculate the prescribed dosage.
   e. The physician ordered a medication of 50 mg/kg/day in divided doses at 8-hour intervals. The patient weighs 110 pounds. Convert pounds to kilograms and then calculate the prescribed dosage.

■ ■ SELF-ASSESSMENT

This exercise is designed to assess your understanding of the metric system. Place the correct answer in the space provided. To verify your answers, you may check with your instructor or go to the student companion website.

1. The fundamental units of the metric system are:

   a. _____ for length   b. _____ for volume   c. _____ for weight

2. Write the prefix for each of the following:

   a. _____ one thousand units   e. _____ one thousandth of a unit

   b. _____ one tenth of a unit   f. _____ ten units

   c. _____ one millionth of a unit   g. _____ one hundredth of a unit

   d. _____ one hundred units

3. It takes approximately _____ centimeters to make an inch.

4. A liter is equal to _____ quarts.

5. A milliliter is equivalent to _____ cubic centimeters.

6. Write in the abbreviation for the unit that makes the equivalency correct:

   a. 1000 mL = 1 _____   d. 2 kg = 4.4 _____

   b. 2000 mg = 2 _____   e. 0.5 g = 500 _____

   c. 1000 mcg = 1 _____

7. Correctly convert each of the following metric equivalents:

   a. 1 mcg = _____ mg   d. 0.2 L = _____ mL

   b. 4 g = _____ kg   e. 1 mL = _____ L

   c. 5 kg = _____ g   f. 3.5 mg = _____ g

8. Correctly convert the following pounds to kilograms:

   a. 176 lb = _____ kg   c. 64 lb = _____ kg

   b. 100 lb = _____ kg

UNIT 5
Calculating Adult Dosages: Oral and Parenteral Forms

OBJECTIVES

Upon completing this unit, you should be able to:

- Define the terms listed in the vocabulary.
- Describe the oral and parenteral routes of drug administration.
- Name two measures used to determine the amount of medication to be administered and give an example of each measure.
- List six medications that are measured in units.
- Calculate adult dosages by the proportional or formula method.
- Work the practice problems and review problems correctly.
- Successfully complete the Self-Assessment.

VOCABULARY

ampule (am'pyool). A small, sterile, prefilled glass container that holds a hypodermic solution.

cartridge-needle unit. A disposable unit containing a premeasured amount of medication. This unit is designed for use in a nondisposable cartridge-holder syringe, such as the Tubex and Carpuject.

hypodermic (hie"po-der 'mik). Pertaining to below the skin.

multiple dose. More than one dose per container.

oral (or'al). Pertaining to the mouth.

parenteral (par-en'ter-al). Pertaining to the injection of a liquid substance into the body via a route other than the alimentary canal. Parenteral means beside the intestine.

unit dose. A premeasured amount of medication that is individually packaged on a per-dose basis.

vial (vy'al). A small, sterile, prefilled glass bottle containing a hypodermic solution or a powder for reconstitution.

INTRODUCTION

As a medical assistant, you may be responsible for administering medications to adult patients. A bit of information worth knowing is that the "average" adult dose of medication is based upon the age and weight of an "average" patient who is between 20 and 60 years old, with a weight of 150 pounds.

THE ORAL AND PARENTERAL ROUTES OF ADMINISTRATION

The **oral** *route* of drug administration (by mouth) is the route most commonly used. It provides the safest, most convenient, and most economical means of giving a medication. Drugs administered by mouth may be in a solid or a liquid form. Solid forms include tablets, capsules, caplets, powders, and lozenges. Liquid preparations include solutions, elixirs, and syrups.

The term *parenteral* is used to describe the injection of a liquid substance into the body via a route other than the alimentary canal. The most frequently used parenteral routes are the following:

Subcutaneous—Just below the surface of the skin. A subcutaneous injection is usually given at a 45° angle.

Intramuscular—Within the muscle. An intramuscular injection is given at a 90° angle, passing through the skin and subcutaneous tissue, and penetrating deep into the muscle tissue.

Intradermal—Within the epidermal layer of the skin. An intradermal injection is given at an angle between 10° and 15°.

Intravenous—Within a vein. An intravenous injection is inserted (at less than a 15° angle) into the patient's vein.

Medications that have been prepared for use by injection are available in **multiple-dose** form (vials) and in **unit-dose** form (ampules and cartridge-needle units).

Vial—A small, sterile, prefilled glass bottle containing a **hypodermic** solution or a powder for reconstitution (see Figure 5-1).

Ampule—A small, sterile, prefilled container that usually holds a single dose of a hypodermic solution. (see Figure 5-1).

Cartridge-needle unit—A disposable unit containing a premeasured amount of medication. This unit is designed for use in a nondisposable cartridge-holder syringe such as the Tubex or the Carpuject (see Figure 5-1).

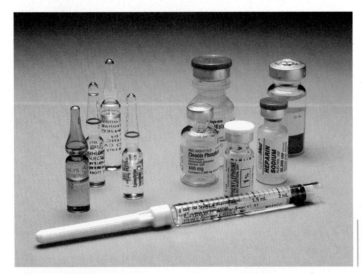

FIGURE 5-1

Ampules, vials, and a prefilled cartridge-needle unit

Source: Delmar/Cengage Learning

WEIGHT AND VOLUME

Two measures are used to determine the amount of medication to be administered: by weight and by volume. The weight of a medication may be expressed as any of the following: milliequivalents (mEq), micrograms (mcg, μg), milligrams (mg), grams (g), grains (gr), and units (U). The volume of a medication may be expressed in milliliters (mL), cubic centimeters (cc), or ounces (oz), and by a variety of household measures, such as the teaspoon (tsp).

CALCULATING ADULT DOSAGE

When a physician orders a medication and the dosage ordered is not the same as what is available, you may use two methods to determine the correct dosage. First is the proportional method, which may be used to solve almost any type of dosage problem, and second is the formula method. Both of these methods are described for you. Study each example carefully and then proceed to the practice problems.

As a medical assistant, remember that your physician and patients rely upon you. If you have any difficulty in calculating adult dosages, seek the assistance of someone who can help you. Always make sure that you administer the correct dosage of medication to your patient. You can, and do, make a difference in the quality of health care that is delivered to each patient. Your knowledge and ability to assist the physician and carry out orders precisely may make all the difference in a patient's life.

Calculating Adult Dosages Using the Proportional Method

EXAMPLE   The physician orders 0.2 g of meprobamate tabs. The dose on hand is 400 mg tabs.

Step 1.   Determine whether the medication ordered and the medication on hand are available in the same unit of measure.

Step 2.   If the medication ordered and the medication on hand *are not* in the same unit of measure, *convert* so that both measures are expressed using the same unit of measure.

Conversion: To change 0.2 g to mg
$$1000 \text{ mg} : 1 \text{ g} = x \text{ mg} : 0.2 \text{ g}$$
$$x = 200 \text{ mg}$$
or
multiply $0.2 \times 1000 = 200$

Step 3.   Now use the following proportion to calculate the dosage. Remember, you converted 0.2 g to 200 mg.

$$\frac{\text{Known unit}}{\text{on hand}} : \frac{\text{Known dosage}}{\text{form}} = \frac{\text{Dose}}{\text{ordered}} : \frac{\text{Unknown amount}}{\text{to be given}}$$

$$400 \text{ mg} : 1 \text{ tab} = 200 \text{ mg} : x \text{ tab}$$

$$400x = 200$$

$$x = \frac{\overset{1}{200}}{\underset{2}{400}} \quad (\text{Reduce fraction to lowest terms})$$

$$x = \frac{1}{2} \text{ tab}$$

Step 4.   Prove your answer. Remember to place your answer in the original formula in the x position.

$$400 \text{ mg} : 1 \text{ tab} = 200 \text{ mg} : \frac{1}{2} \text{ tab}$$

$$200 = 200$$

Calculating Adult Dosages Using the Formula Method

EXAMPLE The physician orders 0.2 g of meprobamate tabs. The dose on hand is 400 mg tabs.

Step 1. Determine whether the medication ordered and the medication on hand are available in the same unit of measure.

Step 2. If the medication ordered and the medication on hand *are not* in the same unit of measure, *convert* so that both measures are expressed using the same unit of measure.

$$\text{Conversion: To change } 0.2 \text{ } g \text{ to mg}$$
$$1000 \text{ mg} : 1 \text{ g} = x \text{ mg} : 0.2 \text{ g}$$
$$x = 200 \text{ mg}$$
$$\text{or}$$
$$\text{multiply } 0.2 \times 1000 = 200$$

Step 3. Now use the following formula to calculate the dosage.

$$\frac{\text{Dose ordered (desired)}}{\text{Dose on hand}} \times \text{Quantity (Q)} = \text{Amount to give (form of drug)}$$

$$\text{or } \frac{D}{H} \times Q = \text{Amount to give}$$

The physician ordered 0.2 g of meprobamate tabs (0.2 g converts to 200 mg). The dose on hand is 400 mg tabs.

$$\frac{200 \text{ mg}}{400 \text{ mg}} \times 1 \text{ tab} = \frac{\overset{1}{200}}{\underset{2}{400}} \text{ or } \frac{1}{2} \text{ tab}$$

▪ ▪ PRACTICE PROBLEMS

1. Using the proportional or formula method, calculate the following adult dosages:

   a. The physician orders 500 mcg (0.5 mg) of Lanoxin (digoxin). On hand you have 250 mcg (0.25 mg). How many tablets will you give? _____

   b. The physician orders 1000 mg of amoxicillin to be taken stat and then 500 mg every 8 hours for seven days. On hand you have 500 mg capsules. How many capsules will you give stat? _____

   c. The physician orders 100 mg of chlorpromazine HCl. On hand you have 100 mg tablets. How many tablets will you give? _____

   d. The physician orders 10 mg of Aricept (donepezil HCl). On hand you have 5 mg tablets. How many tablets will you give? _____

   e. The physician orders 100 mg of a medication IM (intramuscular). On hand you have 50 mg/mL. How many milliliters will you give? _____

   f. The physician orders 50 mg of chlorpromazine HCl IM. On hand you have 25 mg/mL. How many milliliters will you give? _____

   g. The physician orders 12.5 mg of meperidine IM. On hand you have 25 mg/mL. How many milliliters will you give? _____

   h. The physician orders 500 mg of Cipro (ciprofloxacin HCl). On hand you have 250 mg tablets. See Figure 5-2. How many tablets will you give? _____

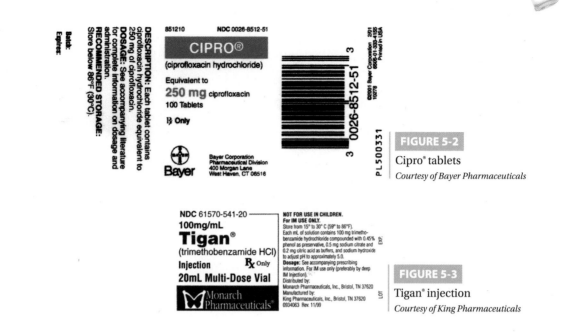

i. The physician orders 10 mg of Procardia (nifedipine). On hand you have 10 mg capsules. How many capsules will you give? _____

j. The physician orders 50 mg of Tigan (trimethobenzamide HCl) IM. On hand you have 100 mg/mL. See Figure 5-3. How many milliliters will you give? _____

MEDICATIONS MEASURED IN UNITS

Medications such as insulin, heparin, some antibiotics, hormones, vitamins, and vaccines are measured in units. These medications are standardized in units based on their strengths. The strength varies from one medicine to another, depending upon their sources, their conditions, and the methods by which they are obtained.

HOW TO CALCULATE UNIT DOSAGES

When calculating medications that are ordered in units, you may use either the proportional or the formula method.

The Proportional Method

EXAMPLE The physician ordered 4000 United States Pharmacopria (USP) units of heparin to be administered deep subcutaneously. On hand is heparin, 5000 USP units per milliliter.

Step 1. Use the following proportion to calculate the dosage.

$$\underset{\text{on hand}}{\text{Known unit}} : \underset{\text{form}}{\text{Known dosage}} = \underset{\text{ordered}}{\text{Dose}} : \underset{\text{to be given}}{\text{Unknown amount}}$$

$$5000\,\text{U} \ : \ 1\,\text{ml} \qquad = 4000\,\text{U} \ : \ x\,\text{ml}$$

$$5000x = 4000$$

$$x = \frac{4000}{5000} \quad = \frac{4}{5} \ \text{ml or } 0.8\,\text{ml}$$

You may use a tuberculin syringe to draw up 0.8 mL.

The Formula Method

EXAMPLE The physician ordered 450,000 units of Bicillin for deep IM injection. Available is Bicillin, 600,000 units per milliliter.

Step 1. Use the following formula to calculate the dosage.

$$\frac{\text{Dose ordered (desired)}}{\text{Dose on hand}} \times \text{Quantity (Q)} = \text{Amount to give}$$

$$\frac{450,000 \text{ U}}{600,000 \text{ U}} \times 1 \text{ ml} =$$

$$\frac{450,000}{600,000} \times 1 \text{ ml} = \frac{\overset{3}{45}}{\underset{4}{60}} \times 1 \text{ ml} = \frac{3}{4} \text{ ml or } 0.75 \text{ ml}$$

■ ■ PRACTICE PROBLEMS

2. a. The physician ordered 500 mg (800,000 units) of a medication. On hand you have 250 mg (400,000 units). How many tablets will you give?

   b. The physician ordered 500 units of heparin sodium subcutaneously. On hand you have 1,000 units/mL. How many milliliters will you give?

   c. The physician ordered a medication, 600,000 units for deep IM injection. The dose on hand is 1,200,000 units per 2 milliliters. How many milliliters will you administer to your patient?

■ ■ REVIEW PROBLEMS

1. Using the proportional or formula method, calculate the following adult dosages:

   a. The physician orders 125 mg of a medication. On hand you have 250 mg tablets. You will give _____ tablets to your patient.

   b. The physician orders 250 mg of a liquid medication. On hand you have 300 mg/5 mL. How many milliliters will you give? _____

   c. The physician orders 500 mg of a medication. On hand you have 1 gram tablets. The patient will receive _____ tabs.

   d. The physician orders 0.250 mg of Lanoxin. On hand you have 0.125 mg tablets. You will give your patient _____ tabs.

   e. The physician orders 62.5 mg of a medication. On hand you have 125 mg tablets. You will give your patient _____ tab.

   f. The physician orders 75 mg of Robaxin. On hand you have 100 mg/mL. How many milliliters will you give? _____

g. The physician orders 60 mg of Depo-Medrol. On hand you have 80 mg/mL. How many milliliters will you give? _____

h. The physician orders 10 mg of a medication. On hand you have 5 mg/mL. How many milliliters will you give? _____

i. The physician orders 1500 mcg of vitamin B_{12}. On hand you have 1000 mcg/mL. How many milliliters will you give? _____

j. The physician orders 500 mg of a medication. On hand you have a 2 mL ampule that contains 500 mg/mL. How many milliliters will you give? _____

■ ■ SELF-ASSESSMENT

This exercise is designed to assess your understanding of calculating adult dosages. Correctly calculate the following adult dosages. To verify your answers, you may check with your instructor or go to the student companion website.

1. The physician ordered Lanoxin tabs, 0.125 mg. Available are Lanoxin tabs, 0.25 mg. How many tablets will you give? _____

2. The physician ordered Coumadin tabs, 2.5 mg. Available are Coumadin tabs, 5 mg. How many tablets will you give? _____

3. The physician ordered acetaminophen tabs, 650 mg. Available are acetaminophen tabs, 325 mg. How many tablets will you give? _____

4. The physician ordered Carafate tabs, 500 mg. Available are Carafate, 1 gram tabs. How many tablets will you give? _____

5. The physician ordered Duricef tabs, 1500 mg. Available are Duricef tabs, 1 gram. How many tablets will you give? _____

6. The physician ordered Diuril tabs, 250 mg. Available are Diuril tabs, 0.25 g. How many tablets will you give? _____

7. The physician ordered amoxicillin caps, 500 mg. Available are amoxicillin caps, 250 mg. How many capsules will you give? _____

8. The physician ordered Lasix oral solution, 30 mg to be given as a single dose. Available is Lasix oral solution, 60 mL bottle that contains 10 mg/mL. How many milliliters will you give? _____

9. The physician ordered Demerol, 50 mg IM. On hand is Demerol, 100 mg per 2 mL. How many milliliters will you give? _____

10. The physician ordered Vistaril, 75 mg IM. On hand is Vistaril, 50 mg per mL. How many milliliters will you give? _____

11. The physician ordered Bicillin, 600,000 units for deep IM injection. On hand is Bicillin, 1,200,000 units per 2 mL. How many milliliters will you give? _____

12. The physician ordered Tigan, 200 mg IM. On hand is Tigan, 100 mg per mL. How many milliliters will you give? _____

13. The physician ordered 30 units of a medication. Available is 40 units per milliliter. How many milliliters will you give? _____

UNIT 6
Calculating Children's Dosages

OBJECTIVES

Upon completing this unit, you should be able to:

- Define the terms listed in the vocabulary.
- State the guidelines for administering medications to a pediatric patient.
- Calculate children's dosages according to kilogram of body weight.
- Work the practice problems and review problems correctly.
- Successfully complete the Self-Assessment.

VOCABULARY

child Any human between infancy and puberty.

infancy (in'fan-see). The stage of life from the time of birth through the completion of 1 year of age.

puberty (pyoo'ber-tee). The stage of life when sexual reproduction becomes possible.

INTRODUCTION

Each child is an individual, with differences in age, size, and weight. A child is any human between infancy and puberty. Infancy is the stage of life from the time of birth through the completion of one year. Puberty is the stage of life at which members of both sexes become functionally capable of reproduction. It is a period of rapid physical, mental, and emotional changes that occur from ages 13 to 15 in boys and ages 9 to 16 in girls. Because children do not develop in the same way during a given time span, medication dosage for pediatric patients is individualized.

One method used to calculate children's dosage is by kilogram of body weight. The body weight method is the method of choice, because most medications are ordered in this way, and it is easier to calculate.

GUIDELINES FOR ADMINISTERING PEDIATRIC MEDICATIONS

1. Follow the following seven rights of proper drug administration:
   - The right patient
   - The right drug
   - The right dose
   - The right route
   - The right time
   - The right technique
   - The right documentation

Correctly Document the Administration of a Medication: The physician ordered 500 mg of amoxicillin for Emily Justice, to be taken stat, and then 250 mg every 8 hours for seven days. On hand, you have 250 mg amoxicillin capsules. What will you administer to this patient?

| 11/28/20XX 9:00 a.m. | Administered two 250 mg capsules to Emily Justice. Patient took the oral medication with 8 ounces of water. Asked Emily to remain in waiting room for 30 minutes. Checked to be sure that she did not have any adverse reactions to medication. Patient free to go at 9:45 a.m. Jane Rice, RN, CMA-C-- |

7 Rights of Proper Drug Administration:

Rights Patient's Name:	Emily Justice
Right Drug:	Amoxicillin
Right Dose:	500 mg
Right Route:	Oral
Right Time:	9:00 a.m.
Right Technique:	Oral medication with 8 ounces of water. Checked to be sure patient did not have any adverse reactions to medication.
Right Docmentation:	See previous example.
Your Initials/Signature and Title:	Jane Rice, RN, CMA-C

2. Carefully assess each pediatric patient for the following:
   - Age
   - Weight
   - Physical state
   - Disease process
   - Mental and emotional state
   - Level of understanding
   - Allergies

3. Gain parental cooperation in the following ways:
   - Identify yourself, and call the parent and the child by name. Explain the procedure.
   - Whenever possible, allow the parent to assist you.
   - At times, it may be necessary to ask a parent to leave the room, as the parent's behavior may be upsetting to the child. When this is the case, explain to the parent and child that the procedure will only take a few minutes and you will ask another medical assistant to assist you.

4. Establish rapport with the child in the following ways:
   - Use a positive straightforward approach. Do not waste time. The longer it takes to accomplish a procedure, the more apprehensive the child will become.
   - Explain the procedure at the level of the child's understanding.
   - Whenever possible, allow the child to assist you.
   - Show approval for positive behavior by the child. Clap, laugh, and reward with a "treat" if possible.

5. Route of administration:

   The route of administration will depend on the child's age; weight; body size; physical, mental, and emotional state; disease process; level of understanding; specific properties of the medication; and the physician's order.

   - *Oral route.* Never force or give an oral medication to a crying child.

     Liquid medications may be administered by dropper or an appropriate device such as an oral syringe, calibrated medication cup, or spoon. See Figures 6-1A, B, & C.

     Solid medications are generally not ordered until the child is old enough to understand and cooperate by actually swallowing the medication. When a tablet is ordered, always check with the pharmacist to see if it can be crushed and then mixed with an appropriate food or liquid for ease of administration. It is best to give medicine to a baby before feedings. Give the medication directly into the side of the baby's mouth using a syringe or dropper from the medicine bottle. Do not mix any medicine in a baby's formula (bottle). The baby may not finish the bottle or may spit up the formula, resulting in the baby not receiving the correct amount of medication.

   - *Parenteral route.* Two people will be needed when administering an injection to a child—one to assist in maintaining a proper body position and the other to give the injection. Administer subcutaneous and/or intramuscular medications with extreme care.

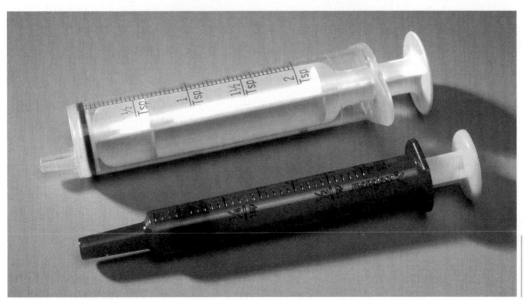

FIGURE 6-1A

Oral syringe
*Source: Delmar/
Cengage Learning*

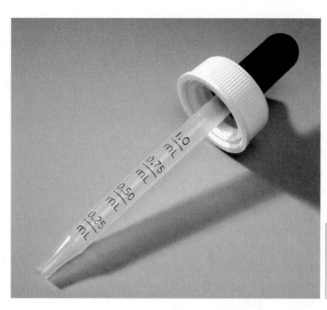

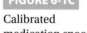

FIGURE 6-1B
Calibrated
medication dropper
*Source: Delmar/Cengage
Learning*

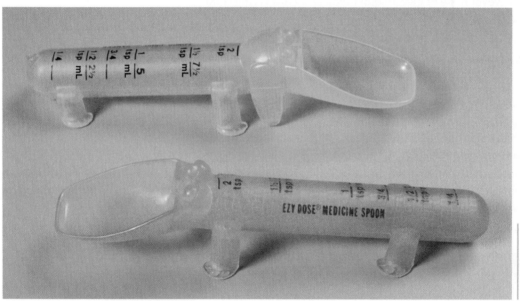

FIGURE 6-1C
Calibrated
medication spoons
*Source: Delmar/Cengage
Learning*

- *Rectal route.* Consider the significance the child places on this part of his/her body. A toddler who is in the process of toilet training may resist this form of drug administration, whereas older children may feel as though it is an invasion of privacy and may react with embarrassment and resentment.

6. New dosage forms of medications:

- Through the advancement in dosage technology, new dosage forms for the delivery and receipt of medications are now available. Examples of these forms include melting tablets, fixed-dose combinations, inhaled insulin, long-lasting injections, long-acting formulations, and delivery devices designed for easier use.

- A benefit of this new dosage form for children is in the administration of corticosteriods for asthma. The dosage can now be delivered as a fine mist, produced by a user-friendly jet nebulizer, which is inhaled through a face mask or mouthpiece. Another type of delivery device allows asthma patients to use their own breath to inhale premeasured doses of medication. Hand-breadth coordination or spacers are not required.

- Another benefit is that children with attention deficit hyperactivity disorder (ADHD) can now take 12-hour formulations of methylphenidate (Ritalin) before going to school. Thus, there is no need for storage of medication at school or for the children to have to see the school nurse for supervised administration, thereby identifying them as chidren with ADHD. Also, long-acting formulations can be helpful to adolescents because their day is usually longer than a young child's, due to after-school activities. In addition, children with ADHD do not have to keep up with the need to take a certain pill at a given time.

7. **Caution:** When calculating children's dosages, be extremely careful. It is advisable to have someone check your mathematics. Be sure to compare the normal dose range with the dosage you plan to administer. If there is any doubt, contact the physician or a pharmacist.

CALCULATING CHILDREN'S DOSAGES

The body weight method uses calculations based upon the child's weight in kilograms. Remember that 1 kilogram (kg) is equal to 2.2 pounds (lb). One pound is equal to 16 ounces (oz).

$1 \text{ kg} = 2.2 \text{ lb}$ and $1 \text{ lb} = 16 \text{ oz}$

Kilogram of Body Weight

As a medical assistant, you may be responsible for calculating the amount of dosage the physician orders according to kilogram of the child's body weight.

There are two methods of calculating dosage according to kilogram of body weight.

- **Method One**

Step 1. To convert pounds to kilograms, divide the number of pounds by 2.2 ($1 \text{ kg} = 2.2 \text{ lb}$).

Step 2. Multiply the dose ordered by kilogram of body weight.

Step 3. If the dose is ordered in divided doses, divide the number of times into the answer you obtained in Step 2.

EXAMPLE The physician orders ceftriaxone sodium (Rocephin), 50 mg/kg of body weight, in divided doses every 12 hours (not to exceed 4 g), for Alice Potts, who weighs 66 pounds. How many milligrams will Alice receive?

Step 1. Convert pounds to kilograms.

$$\frac{66 \text{ lb}}{2.2} = x \text{ kg}$$

$$\begin{array}{r} 30 \\ 2.2\overline{)66.0} \\ \underline{66} \\ 0 \\ \underline{0} \end{array}$$

$66 \text{ lb} = 30 \text{ kg}$

Step 2. Multiply the dose ordered by kilogram of body weight.

50 mg/kg
$50 \times 30 = 1500 \text{ mg} = 1.5 \text{ g}$

Step 3. Ordered in divided doses.

Divide 1500 by 2 to arrive at the divided dose = 750 mg.

Alice will receive 750 mg of Rocephin every 12 hours, as ordered by the physician.

- **Method Two: Using the proportional method to calculate kilogram of body weight.**

EXAMPLE The physician orders ceftriaxone sodium (Rocephin), 50 mg/kg of body weight, in divided doses every 12 hours (not to exceed 4 g), for Alice Potts, who weighs 66 pounds. How many milligrams will Alice receive?

Step 1. To convert 66 pounds to kilograms, set up the proportion as follows:

2.2 lb : 1 kg = 66 lb : x kg

Step 2. Now solve for x:

$$2.2 : 1 = 66 : x$$
$$2.2x = 66$$
$$x = 30$$

Step 3. Now calculate the prescribed dosage by placing 30 in the appropriate place:

50 mg/30 kg
50 × 30 = 1500 mg = 1.5 g

Step 4. To determine the amount of each dose, divide 1500 by 2 (every 12 hours).

1500 ÷ 2 = 750 mg

Alice will receive 750 mg of Rocephin every 12 hours, as ordered by the physician.

PRACTICE PROBLEMS

1. Calculate the following dosages according to kilogram of body weight:
   a. The physician orders cefadroxil (Duricef), 30 mg/kg of body weight, for John Knight, who weighs 44 pounds. The dose is to be divided and given every 12 hours. How many milligrams will you give? _____
   b. The physician orders codeine sulfate, 0.5 mg/kg of body weight for pain. The patient weighs 50 pounds. The medication may be given every 4 to 6 hours. How many milligrams will the patient receive? _____

REVIEW PROBLEMS

1. Calculate the following dosages according to kilogram of body weight:
   a. The physician orders Augmentin, 20 mg/kg/day for Sally Brown, who weighs 72 pounds. The dose is to be divided and given every 8 hours. What is the total dose? _____ What is the amount to be given every 8 hours? _____
   b. The physician orders a medication, 40 mg/kg for Michael Lee, who weighs 78 pounds. The dose is to be divided in four equal doses. What is the total dose? _____ What is the amount to be given in four equal doses? _____
   c. The physician orders a medication, 2.0 mg/kg every 8 hours for a child who weighs 86 pounds. What is the correct dosage? _____

■ ■ SELF-ASSESSMENT

This exercise is designed to assess your understanding of calculating children's dosages. Correctly calculate the following children's dosages. To verify your answers, you may check with your instructor or go to the student companion website.

1. The child weighs 66 pounds and the physician has ordered a medication to be given 30 mg/kg of body weight. What dosage will be given to the child? _____

2. The child weighs 44 pounds and the physician has ordered a medication to be given 30 mg/kg of body weight. What dosage will be given to the child? _____

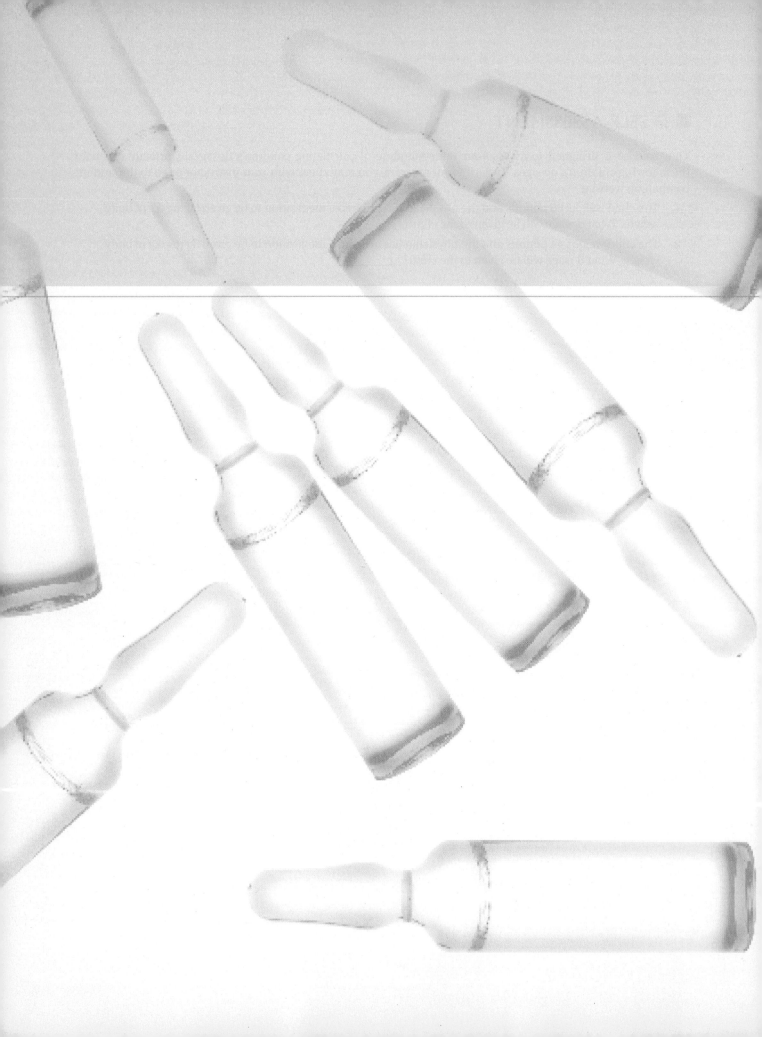

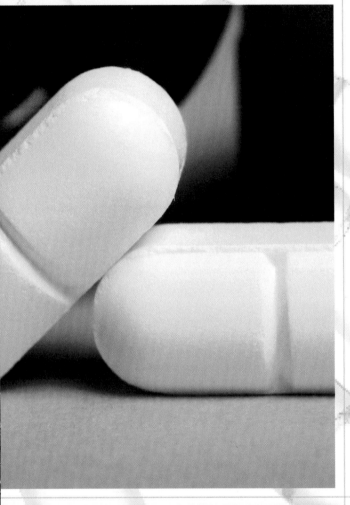

SECTION TWO

Introduction to Pharmacology

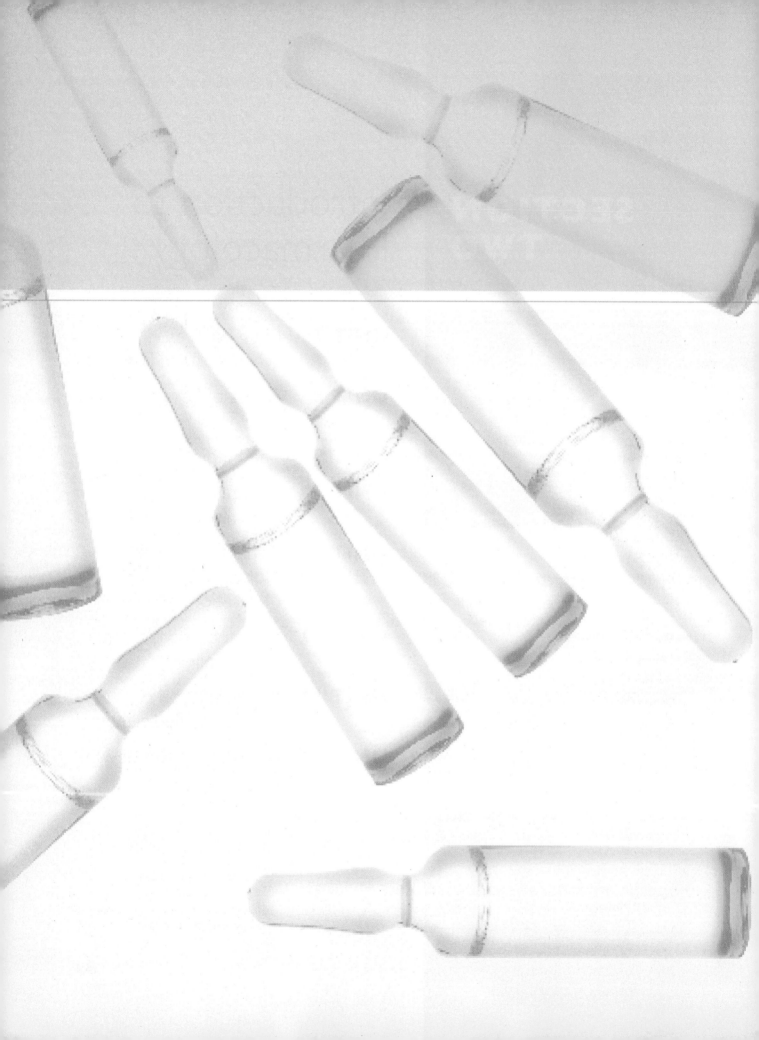

UNIT 7
Drug Sources, Schedules, and Dosages

OBJECTIVES

Upon completing this unit, you should be able to:

- Define the terms listed in the vocabulary.
- Define *pharmacology*.
- State the five medical uses for drugs.
- Give the three names assigned to a drug.
- List the five main sources for drugs, giving examples from each source.
- State the importance of the Federal Food, Drug, and Cosmetic Act.
- Explain the significance of the Controlled Substances Act (CSA).
- Define the five controlled substances schedules, and give examples of drugs listed in each.
- Explain storage and recordkeeping for controlled substances.
- Make use of the drug references/resources described in this unit.
- Define dosage.
- List the factors that affect drug dosage.
- Define the terms used in describing various types of dosages.
- Answer the review questions correctly.

VOCABULARY

abuse (a-byoose). The excessive or improper use of a substance, person, or animal.

addiction (a-dik'shun). The physical or psychological dependency on a substance.

administer (ad-min'is-ter). To give.

bioassay (bi"o-as'ā). The process of determining the strength and quality of a drug by testing it on an animal or on an isolated organ.

biologics (bi-ol'oj-iks). A term used more restrictively for a class of medications (either approved or in development) that are produced by means of biological processes involving recombinant DNA technology. Biologics include a wide range of medicinal products such as vaccines, blood and blood components, and recombinant therapeutic proteins.

biotechnology (bi'o-tek-nol-a-gee). The biological and engineering study of the relationship between human beings and machines.

controlled substance (kon-tro'led sub'stans). A drug that has the potential for addiction and abuse (for example, opium and cocaine and their derivatives, narcotics, stimulants, and depressants).

dispense (dis-pens'). To prepare and give out.

genetic engineering (jen-et'ik en"ja-neer'ing). The synthesis, alteration, or repair of genetic material through the application of engineering principles.

narcotic (nar-kot'ik). Producing sleep or stupor. A narcotic drug is one that depresses the central nervous system and, in moderate dosages, relieves pain, and produces sleep. Most narcotics are habit-forming.

pharmacopeia (far"ma-ko-pe'a). Authorized publication on drugs and their preparations. Generally refers to a book containing formulas and information that provides a standard for preparation and dispensation of drugs.

practitioner (prak-tish'un-er). One who has met the professional and legal requirements of a certain occupation or profession.

prescribe (pre-skribe). To order or recommend the use of a drug, diet, or other form of therapy.

INTRODUCTION

Pharmacology is the study of drugs; the science that is concerned with the history, origin, sources, physical and chemical properties, and uses of drugs and their effects on living organisms. Because of the complexity of the subject, pharmacology has evolved into the following subdivisions:

- *Pharmacodynamics.* The study of drugs and their actions on living organisms. It involves the biochemical and physiological effects of drugs upon living organisms, as well as their actions.
- *Pharmacognosy.* The science of natural drugs and their physical, botanical, and chemical properties.
- *Pharmacogenetics.* A new science of personalizing drug treatment according to genetic variation of the individual patient. Genetic variation can occur at many levels, including drug absorption, distribution, metabolism, receptor target, and elimination. When pharmaceutical companies embrace this new gene–environment interface, drugs will be created to a specific patient's needs.
- *Pharmacokinetics.* The study of the metabolism and action of drugs within the body. It involves the time required for absorption to take place, duration of action, distribution of the drug in the body, and the method of excretion.
- *Pharmacotherapeutics.* The study of drugs and their relationships to the treatment of disease. It involves determining which drug is most or least appropriate for a specific disease and the required dosage to achieve beneficial results.
- *Toxicology.* The study of poisons; the science concerned with toxic substances. It involves the study of the chemistry and pharmacological actions of substances and the establishment of antidotes, treatment, prevention, and methods for controlling exposure to harmful substances.

DRUGS

A *drug* can be defined simply as a medicinal substance that may alter or modify the functions of a living organism. In general, drugs have the following five medical uses:

- *Therapeutic use.* Certain drugs, such as antihistamines, may be used in the treatment of an allergy to relieve the symptoms or to sustain the patient until other measures are instituted.
- *Diagnostic use.* Certain drugs, such as Ethiodol, are used in conjunction with radiology to allow the physician to pinpoint the location of a disease process.
- *Curative use.* Certain drugs, such as antibiotics, kill or remove the causative agent of a disease.
- *Replacement use.* Certain drugs, such as hormones and vitamins, are used to replace substances normally found in the body.
- *Preventive or prophylactic use.* Certain drugs, such as immunizing agents, are used to ward off or lessen the severity of a disease.

Drug Names

Most drugs have the following three types of names: chemical, generic, and trade or brand name. The *chemical* name is usually the formula that denotes the composition of the drug. It is made up of letters and numbers that represent the drug's molecular structure. The *generic* name is the drug's *official* name, and is descriptive of its chemical structure. It is assigned to the drug by the U.S. Adopted Names (USAN) Council.

A generic drug can be manufactured by more than one pharmaceutical company. When that is the case, each company markets the drug under its own unique *trade* or *brand* name. A trade or brand name is registered by the U.S. Patent Office as well as approved by the U.S. Food and Drug Administration (FDA). The ® symbol that follows the drug's trade name denotes the fact that this name is the registered trademark used by the manufacturer. Some trade (brand) names are followed by the letters™, which also indicates that the name is registered and protected by laws that govern the use of trademarks.

EXAMPLE *Chemical* name: 4-hydroxyl-2-methyl-N-2-pyridinyl-2H-1,2,-benzothiazine-3-carboxamide 1,
1-dioxide (*Note:* the chemical name is *not* included on the medication label.)

Generic name: piroxicam

Trade or *brand* name: Feldene (first letter capitalized)

See Figure 7-1.

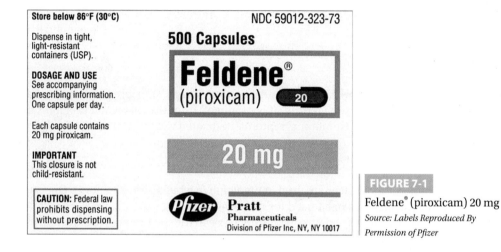

Store below 86°F (30°C)

NDC 59012-323-73

Dispense in tight,
light-resistant
containers (USP).

500 Capsules

DOSAGE AND USE
See accompanying
prescribing information.
One capsule per day.

Feldene®
(piroxicam)   20

Each capsule contains
20 mg piroxicam.

20 mg

IMPORTANT
This closure is not
child-resistant.

CAUTION: Federal law
prohibits dispensing
without prescription.

Pfizer **Pratt**
Pharmaceuticals
Division of Pfizer Inc, NY, NY 10017

FIGURE 7-1

Feldene® (piroxicam) 20 mg
*Source: Labels Reproduced By
Permission of Pfizer*

SOURCES OF DRUGS

Drugs prepared from roots, herbs, bark, and other forms of plant life are among the earliest known pharmaceuticals. Their origin can be traced back to primitive cultures where they were first used to evoke magical powers and to drive out evil spirits. In South America, the Carib Indians coated the tips of their arrows with a poisonous substance obtained from trees, thereby improving their chances of success in hunting. The pharmacologically active ingredients of this substance (curare) facilitate muscle relaxation and, like many of the compounds discovered by primitive groups, is still used by drug manufacturers as a component of modern-day medications.

Having discovered that certain plants were pharmacologically useful, early man began a search for other potential sources of drugs that continues to this day. In addition to plants, drugs are now derived from animals and minerals, and are produced in laboratories utilizing chemical and biochemical processes (see Figure 7–2).

Plants

The leaves, roots, stems, or fruit of certain plants may contain medicinal properties. The dried leaf of the purple foxglove plant is a source for *digitalis*, a cardiac glycoside used in the treatment of congestive heart failure.

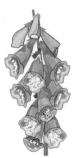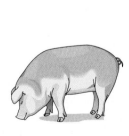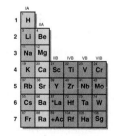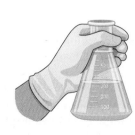

FIGURE 7-2

Drugs are obtained from a variety of sources:
(a) plant, (b) animal,
(c) mineral, and
(d) synthetic, as well as bioengineering,
(not shown).
*Source: Delmar/Cengage
Learning*

The kelp plant is a rich source of iodine, a nonmetallic element. *Iodine* not only is used as a disinfectant but is essential for the proper development and functioning of the thyroid gland. Another example of a drug derived from a plant source is Cenestin (synthetic conjugated estrogens), which is synthesized from soy and yam plants. This drug is prescribed for menopausal and postmenopausal women for estrogen replacement therapy.

Researchers have concluded that an extract from the saw palmetto plant (*Serenoa repens*) appears to be effective in easing the symptoms of benign prostatic hyperplasia (BPH). Benign prostatic hyperplasia is a common age-related swelling of the prostate gland that is thought to affect up to 40 percent of men age 70 and older. This condition is characterized by frequent urges to urinate, and, if untreated, can lead to bladder infections and kidney damage.

Animals

There are only a few drugs that are made from the fluids, tissues, organs, and/or glands of animals. Premarin (conjugated estrogens) is an example of such a drug. It is produced from the urine of a pregnant mare and has been prescribed for moderate to severe vasomotor symptoms associated with menopause.

Minerals

Some naturally occurring mineral substances are used in medicine in a highly purified form. One such mineral is *sulfur*, a nonmetallic element, which has been used for many years as a key ingredient in certain bacteriostatic drugs. Now prepared synthetically, sulfa drugs have widespread use in the treatment of urinary and intestinal tract infections.

Synthetic Drugs

By combining various chemicals, scientists can produce compounds that are identical to a natural drug, or they can create entirely new substances. These drugs are synthetic medications prepared in pharmaceutical laboratories.

The majority of drugs on the market are synthetically produced. Two advantages of synthetically prepared drugs are that they can be produced in great volume and, consequently, are usually less expensive than organically derived medications. For example, Chloromycetin may be produced naturally by organic means, or it may be created synthetically from ingredients that make up its chemical formula. Other drugs, such as sulfathiazole, cannot be produced by organic means and are available only as a result of synthetic processes.

Genetically Engineered Pharmaceuticals and Biologics

Genetic engineering is a biotechnology that has revolutionized agriculture, industry, health, and medicine. Scientists are capable of creating new strains of bacteria using a technique known as *gene splicing*. The range of applications of recombinant DNA technology in pharmaceuticals grows every day. Recombinant technology can harness bacteria to make certain drugs or hormones. This technique has been used to make human insulin (Humulin) using *Escherichia coli* (*E. coli*) (see Figure 7-3). Examples of other drugs that have been produced using biotechnology are Activase (alteplase, recombinant), a tissue plasminogen activator that may be used for patients with heart attacks, acute ischemic strokes, and/or acute massive pulmonary embolism; Nutropin (somatropin-rDNA origin), a human growth hormone; and Pulmozyme (dornase alfa, recombinant), for the management of cystic fibrosis.

Biologics include a wide range of medicinal products such as vaccines, blood and blood components, and recombinant therapeutic proteins. Biologics can be composed of sugars, proteins, or nucleic acids, or complex combinations of these substances, or may be living entities such as cells and tissues. Biologics may be isolated from a variety of natural sources, such as human, animal, or microorganism. They can be produced by biotechnology methods and other technologies. Gene-based and cellular biologics often are at the forefront of biomedical research. These may be used to treat a variety of medical conditions for which no other treatments are available. Biologics are usually given by injection or intravenous infusion in a physician's office (see Table 7-1).

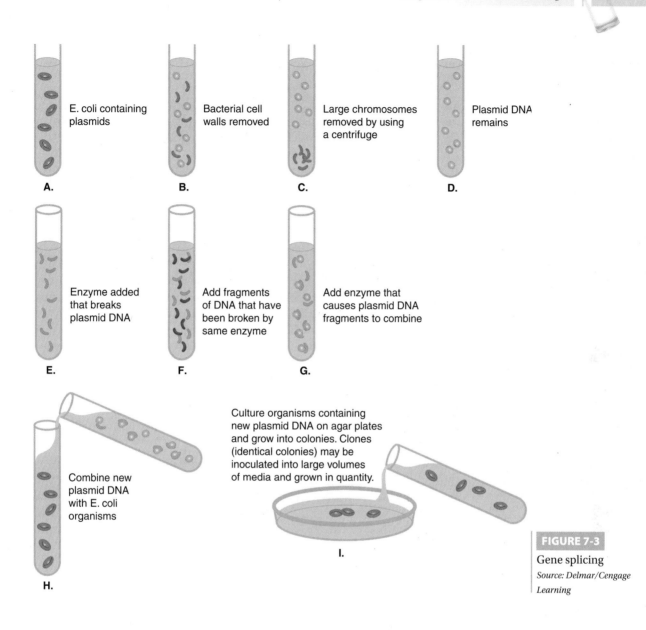

FIGURE 7-3

Gene splicing

Source: Delmar/Cengage Learning

TABLE 7-1 Examples of Biologics Made with Recombinant DNA Technology

GENERIC NAME	TRADE NAME	INDICATION
abatacept	Orenica	rheumatoid arthritis
adalimumab	Humira	rheumatoid arthritis, ankylosing spondylitis, psoriatic arthritis
alefacept	Amevive	chronic plaque psoriasis
erythropoietin	Epogen	anemia arising from cancer chemotherapy, chronic renal failure
etanercept	Enbrel	rheumatoid arthritis, ankylosing spondylitis, psoriatic arthritis, psoriasis
infliximab	Remicade	rheumatoid arthritis, ankylosing spondylitis, psoriatic arthritis, psoriasis, Crohn's disease
trastuzumab	Herceptin	breast cancer

DRUG LEGISLATION

Qualified medical **practitioners** who **prescribe**, **dispense**, or **administer** drugs must comply with federal and state laws governing the manufacture, sale, possession, administration, and dispensing and prescribing of drugs. All drugs available for legal use are controlled by the Federal Food, Drug, and Cosmetic Act. This law protects the public by ensuring the purity, strength, and composition of food, drugs, and cosmetics. It also prohibits the movement, in interstate commerce, of adulterated and misbranded food, drugs, devices, and cosmetics. Enforcement of the Federal Food, Drug, and Cosmetic Act is the responsibility of the Food and Drug Administration, which is a part of the Department of Health and Human Services (DHHS) of the U.S. government.

Controlled Substances Act (CSA)

The Controlled Substances Act controls the manufacture, importation, compounding, selling, dealing in, and giving away of drugs that have the potential for **addiction** and **abuse**. These drugs, known as **controlled substances**, include opium and cocaine and their derivatives, **narcotics**, stimulants, and depressants. The Drug Enforcement Administration (DEA) of the U.S. Justice Department enforces the act, which is also known as the Comprehensive Drug Abuse Prevention and Control Act. Under federal law, medical practitioners who prescribe, administer, or dispense controlled substances must register with the DEA, and physicians are required to renew their registration every three years (see Figure 7-4).

Form-224
APPLICATION FOR REGISTRATION
Under the Controlled Substances Act
APPROVED OMB NO 1117-0014
FORM DEA-224 (10-06)
Previous editions are obsolete

INSTRUCTIONS
Save time - apply on-line at ***www.deadiversion.usdoj.gov***
1. To apply by mail complete this application. Keep a copy for your records.
2. Print clearly, using black or blue ink, or use a typewriter.
3. Mail this form to the address provided in Section 7 or use enclosed envelope.
4. Include the correct payment amount. FEE IS NON-REFUNDABLE.
5. If you have any questions call 800-882-9539 prior to submitting your application.
IMPORTANT: DO NOT SEND THIS APPLICATION **AND** APPLY ON-LINE.

DEA OFFICIAL USE :
Do you have other DEA registration numbers? ☐ NO ☐ YES

MAIL-TO ADDRESS
Please print mailing address changes to the right of the address in this box.
FEE FOR THREE (3) YEARS IS $551
FEE IS NON-REFUNDABLE

SECTION 1 APPLICANT IDENTIFICATIION ☐ Individual Registration ☐ Business Registration
Name 1 (Last Name of individual -OR- Business or Facility Name)
Name 2 (First Name and Middle Name of individual - OR- Continuation of business name)
Street Address Line 1 (if applying for fee exemption, this must be address of the fee exempt institution)
Address Line 2
City State Zip Code
Business Phone Number Point of Contact
Business Fax Number Email Address

DEBT COLLECTION INFORMATION
Mandatory pursuant to Debt Collection Improvements Act
Social Security Number (*if registration is for individual*)
Provide SSN or TIN. See additional information note #3 on page 4.
Tax Identification Number (*if registration is for business*)

FOR Practitioner or MLP ONLY:
Professional Degree : *select from list only*
Professional School :
Year of Graduation :
National Provider Identification:
Date of Birth (*MM-DD-YYYY*): MM-DD-YYYY

SECTION 2 BUSINESS ACTIVITY
Check one business activity box only
☐ Central Fill Pharmacy
☐ Retail Pharmacy
☐ Nursing Home
☐ Automated Dispensing System
☐ Practitioner (DDS, DMD, DO, DPM, DVM, MD or PHD)
☐ Practitioner Military (DDS, DMD, DO, DPM, DVM,MD or PHD)
☐ Mid-level Practitioner (MLP) (DOM, HMD, MP, ND, NP, OD, PA, or RPH)
☐ Euthanasia Technician
☐ Ambulance Service
☐ Animal Shelter
☐ Hospital/Clinic
☐ Teaching Institution

FOR Automated Dispensing System (ADS) ONLY:
DEA Registration # of Retail Pharmacy for this ADS
An ADS is automatically fee-exempt. Skip Section 6 and Section 7 on page 2. You must attach a notorized affidavit.

SECTION 3 DRUG SCHEDULES
Check all that apply
☐ Schedule II Narcotic
☐ Schedule II Non-Narcotic
☐ Schedule III Narcotic
☐ Schedule III Non-Narcotic
☐ Schedule IV
☐ Schedule V
☐ Check this box if you require official order forms - for purchase or transfer of schedule 2 narcotic and/or schedule 2 non-narcotic controlled substances.
NEW - Page 1

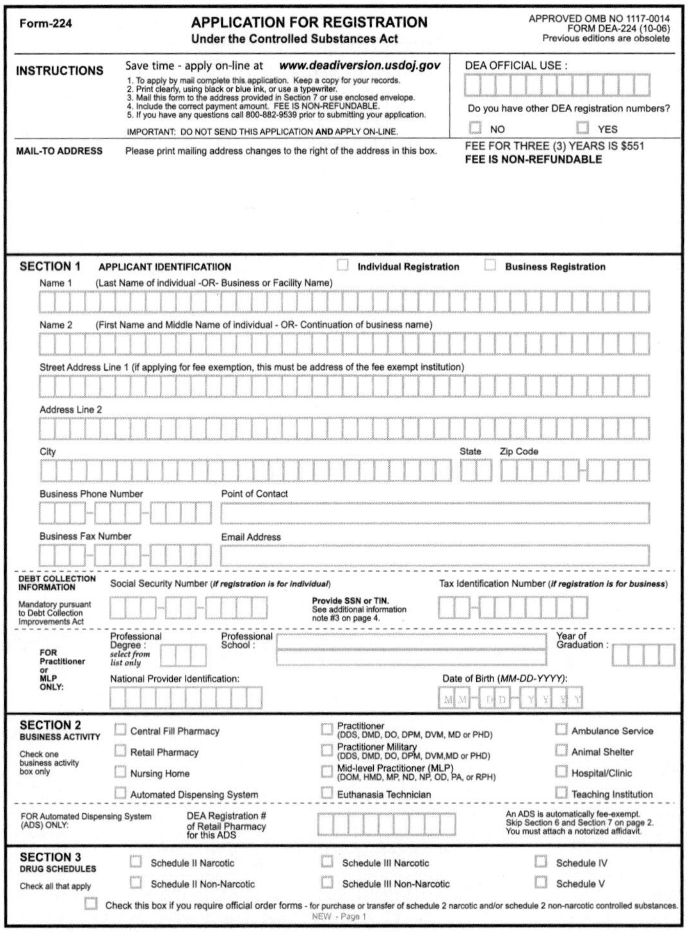

FIGURE 7-4

DEA Form 224 is the form that physicians use to register for a DEA number to prescribe controlled substances. *Source: Delmar/Cengage Learning*

Drug Schedules

Controlled substances are classified according to five drug schedules. Table 7-2 lists the five drug schedules, with a description of each, and examples of the controlled substances in the classification. See Figure 7-5 for an example of how controlled substances are labeled. Note the circled ℂ and CIII.

Controlled substance analogues are a class of substances created by the Anti-Drug Abuse Act of 1986. A *controlled substance analogue* is a substance with a chemical structure substantially similar to the chemical structure of a controlled substance in Schedule I or II.

Registration

Any person who handles or intends to handle controlled substances must obtain a registration issued by the DEA. A unique number is assigned to the importer, exporter, manufacturer, distributor, hospital, pharmacy, practitioner, and researcher. Exceptions include physicians who are interns, residents, from a foreign country or

TABLE 7-2 Drug Schedules with Description and Examples of Controlled Substances

SCHEDULE	DESCRIPTION WITH EXAMPLES
Schedule I (ℂ)	Drugs that have a high potential for abuse and are not accepted for medical use within the United States. Examples: hashish, hashish oil, heroin, LSD, marijuana, mescaline, nicocodeine, peyote, psilocybin, psilocyn.
Schedule II (ℂ)	Drugs that have a high potential for abuse, but do have an accepted medical use within the United States. Examples: Amytal, cocaine, codeine, Demerol, Dexedrine, Dilaudid, morphine, opium, Numorphan, Nembutal, Percocet, Preludin, Ritalin, Seconal, Sublimaze.
Schedule III (ℂ)	Drugs that have a low-to-moderate potential for physical dependency, yet they have a high potential for psychological dependency. They do have an accepted medical use within the United States. Examples: anabolic steroids, barbiturates, Doriden, Marinol, Nalline, Noludar, paregoric, Tylenol with codeine.
Schedule IV (ℂ)	Drugs that have a low potential for abuse relative to Schedule III drugs. They do have an accepted medical use within the United States. Examples: Ativan, barbital, chloral hydrate, Clonopin, Equanil, Librium, Placidyl, Serax, Valium, Xanax.
Schedule V (ℂ)	Drugs that have the lowest abuse potential of controlled substances. They do have an accepted medical use within the United States. Examples: Actifed with codeine, Donnagel, Lomotil, Robitussin A-C syrup.

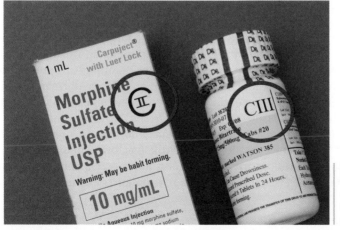

FIGURE 7-5

An example of how controlled substances are labeled.

Source: Delmar/Cengage Learning

on the staff of a Veterans Administration facility, and who prescribe and dispense controlled substances using a special code under the registration of a hospital or other health care institution.

Record Keeping

Controlled substances may be dispensed by a practitioner by direct administration, by prescription, or by dispensing from office supplies. Records of Schedule II substances must be maintained separately from all other records. Schedule III, IV, and V records must be maintained separately or otherwise be readily retrievable from the ordinary professional and business records. This also includes computer-generated records. This data system is maintained on a daily basis and kept for a minimum of two years (three years in some states). The Controlled Substances Act does not require practitioners to maintain copies of prescriptions, but certain states require the use of multiple-copy prescriptions for Schedule II and other specified controlled substances.

Security

Controlled substances must be kept separate from other drugs. They must be placed in a double-locked compartment, such as a securely locked box, or placed in a locked safe or a substantially constructed cabinet. The number of employees with access to controlled substances must be kept to a minimum. The person responsible for administering controlled substances must keep the narcotic keys protected from possible misuse.

DRUG REFERENCES RESOURCES

The *United States Pharmacopeia—National Formulary* (USP-NF) is recognized by the U.S. government as the official list of standardized drugs. Published yearly by the United States Pharmacopeial Convention, this reference book includes only those drugs that have been tested and certified as having met established standards of quality, purity, and potency. Such testing may involve *assay*, whereby the ingredients of the drug are identified and measured, and **bioassay**, wherein the dosage necessary to produce a therapeutic effect is established utilizing animal studies. Each revision of the *United States Pharmacopeia—National Formulary* (USP-NF) includes new drugs and drops those older products that have been replaced by safer or more effective drugs.

Upon release by the FDA, the drug may be listed in *New Drugs* until it has been proved to be of sufficient value to be included in the USP-NF. The Federal Food, Drug, and Cosmetic Act specifies that a drug is official when it is listed in the USP-NF.

New Drugs, published annually by the Council on Pharmacy of the American Medical Association (AMA), lists all drugs that have reached a certain frequency of use. Listing does not imply endorsement of any drug by the AMA. This publication provides health professionals with an up-to-date listing of drugs new to the market.

The *Physicians' Desk Reference* (PDR) is a useful drug information book for physicians and health professionals. Published annually by Healthcare Divison of Thomson Reuters in cooperation with pharmaceutical companies, it is an excellent drug reference book. Supplements to the PDR are provided to purchasers of the book as they become available throughout the year, thereby keeping this reference current.

The PDR *Nurse's Drug Handbook* is an authoritative source of information on prescription medications. Published annually by Cengage Delmar Learning, it is organized for quick, easy access by generic name. Dosage forms and routes are delineated and correlated, when appropriate, with the target disease state. Boldface italics highlight life-threatening side effects. For fast emergency reference, symptoms and treatment of overdose are summarized in each drug's Overdose Management section. Nursing considerations are presented in nursing process format, with assessment, intervention, teaching, and evaluation guidelines all clearly labeled. Specific criteria for evaluating the outcomes of drug therapy are easily found in the Outcomes/Evaluate section. Instant Internet updates are available at the handbook's website at www.cengage.com.

Another source of information about a particular drug is the *product information insert* that most manufacturers provide with their products. This is a brief description of the drug, its clinical pharmacology, indications and usage, contraindications, warnings, precautions, drug interactions, adverse reactions, overdosage, dosage, and administration. The package insert can be a valuable source of information about new drugs that might not be listed elsewhere.

The Internet can be used as an effective drug resource for health care professionals. Professionals can use many websites, but the official site is the Drugs section of the U.S. Food and Drug Administration, Department of Health and Human Services, Center for Drug Evaluation and Research (CDER) at Drugs@FDA. This site includes a catalog of FDA-approved drug products, both prescription and over the counter. On this site, you can search by drug name, active ingredient, application number, or use the alphabetical listing (A–Z) indicated on the home page and browse by drug name. In addition to drug information, you will find FAQ, Instructions, a Glossary, Drugs@FDA demo, and What's New in Drugs@FDA. Details about drugs are organized by FDA Application Number and can contain drug product labels that include:

- description of the drug
- clinical pharmacology
- indications
- contraindications
- warnings
- precautions
- adverse events (side effects)
- drug abuse and dependence
- dosage and administration
- use in pregnancy: use in nursing mothers
- use in children and older patients
- how the drug is supplied
- safety information for patients

At Drugs@FDA you can find daily updates regarding current marketing status, such as whether the drug has been discontinued. A drug may be listed as discontinued when it has been taken off the market or it may no longer be manufactured by a given pharmaceutical company under its brand name. The generic equivalent may still be available, as it may be manufactured by another pharmaceutical company.

EXAMPLE The anti-inflammatory drug Dolobid, by Merck & Co. Inc., has been discontinued, but diflunisal, the generic equivalent is available and produced by Teva Pharmaceuticals USA.

Safety Precautions:

*When researching the Web for drug information, it is important for you to use an official Internet site, such as DRUG@FDA. Be careful of the many unreliable medical and drug sites available on the Web. When it comes to obtaining accurate medical or drug information, **do not** rely on a "blog" or someone's personal opinion.*

DRUG DOSAGE

The *dosage* is the amount of medicine that is prescribed for administration. It is determined by a physician or a qualified practitioner who considers the following factors in the decision:

- Weight, sex, and age of the patient

  Age. The usual adult dose is generally suitable for the 20 to 60 age group. Infants, young children, adolescents, and the aged require individualized dosage.

Pediatric patients are usually divided into age groups:

Newborn—0 to 4 weeks

Infant—5 to 52 weeks

Child—1 to 16 years

Adolescent—12 to 16 years

Pediatric patients require a smaller amount of a medication because of differences in gastrointestinal function, body composition, metabolism, and reduced renal function. The dosage is often determined by the size of the child rather than by age (see Unit 6).

Geriatric patients are not necessarily divided into a specific age group, because of the wide variance in the aging process. A person who is 60 years old or older may or may not be considered a geriatric patient. Therefore, the physician will consider all factors, including the mental and physical state of the individual, to determine an appropriate dosage regimen. The geriatric patient requires special considerations because of the following factors:

1. Decreased gastrointestinal function may cause poor absorption. Geriatric patients often suffer from constipation.

2. Impaired or reduced metabolism

3. Changes in body composition; limitations, deformities

4. Alterations in circulation, liver function, and kidney function

5. Changes in body functioning; systems, eyes, ears, and speech

6. Sensitivity to drugs

7. Number of medications the patient is taking; drug interactions

8. Psychosocial changes:

Alertness	*Forgetfulness*
Confusion	*Misunderstanding of directions*
Attitude	*Memory loss*

9. Disease process; multiple conditions

10. Self-medication; over-the-counter (OTC) drugs

11. Cost

12. Living conditions; alone, with mate, in nursing home or other care facility

13. Poor water intake

- Pregnancy and lactation
- The physical and emotional condition of the patient
- The disease process
- The presence of another disease process
- The causative microorganism and the severity of the infection
- The patient's past medical history, allergies, and idiosyncrasies
- The safest method, route, time, and amount to effect the desired maximum result

Terms used to describe dosages:

- An *initial* dose is the first dose.
- An *average dose* is the amount of medication proven most effective with minimum toxic effect.
- A *loading dose* is an initial larger dose of a drug that may be given at the beginning of a course of treatment to bring the level of the drug to a therapeutic level in the body more rapidly. A loading dose is most useful for drugs that are eliminated from the body relatively slowly. Such drugs need only a low maintenance dose to keep the amount of the drug in the body at the appropriate level.

- A *maintenance dose* is the amount that will keep concentrations of the drug at a therapeutic level in the patient's bloodstream.
- A *minimum dose* is the smallest dose that will be effective.
- A *maximum dose* is the largest amount of a medication that can be given safely to a patient.
- A *therapeutic dose* is the amount needed to produce the desired effect.
- A *divided dose* is a fractional portion administered at short intervals.
- A *unit dose* is a premeasured amount of the medication, individually packaged on a per-dose basis.
- A *cumulative dose* is the summation of a drug present in the body after repeated medication.
- A *lethal dose* is the amount of medication that could kill a patient.
- A *toxic dose* is the amount of a drug that causes signs and symptoms of drug toxicity.

◼ ◼ REVIEW QUESTIONS

Directions. Select the best answer to each of the following multiple choice questions, circling the letter of your choice:

1. _____ means to give.
   a. Dispense   b. Administer   c. Prescribe   d. Addictive

2. _____ is the study of drugs; the science that is concerned with the history, origin, sources, physical and chemical properties, and uses of drugs and their effects upon living organisms.
   a. Pharmacognosy   c. Pharmacology
   b. Pharmacokinetics   d. Pharmacodynamics

3. Certain drugs that are used to ward off or lessen the severity of a disease are called _____.
   a. preventive or prophylactic agents   c. diagnostic agents
   b. therapeutic agents   d. replacement agents

4. The _____ name of a drug is its official name.
   a. chemical   b. generic   c. trade or brand   d. medical

5. Humulin is a type of insulin that is obtained _____.
   a. from plants
   b. from animals
   c. through the process of genetic engineering
   d. from minerals

6. The Federal Food, Drug, and Cosmetic Act _____.
   a. protects the public
   b. prohibits the movement, in interstate commerce, of adulterated and misbranded food, drugs, devices, and cosmetics
   c. both a and b
   d. none of these

7. _____ includes drugs that have an accepted medical use with certain restrictions.
   a. Schedule I   c. Schedule III   e. Schedule V
   b. Schedule II   d. Schedule IV

8. Federal law requires that all controlled substances be _____.
   a. kept with other drugs
   b. stored in a substantially constructed metal box or compartment that is equipped with a double lock
   c. kept separate from other drugs
   d. both b and c

9. The Federal Food, Drug, and Cosmetic Act specifies that a drug is official when it is listed in the _____.

   a. *National Formulary*

   b. *Physicians' Desk Reference*

   c. *United States Pharmacopeia—National Formulary*

   d. all of these

10. The _____ is published annually by Delmar Cengage Learning.

    a. *National Formulary*   c. *United States Pharmacopeia*

    b. *PDR Nurse's Drug Handbook*   d. all of the above

11. Drugs included on the FDA website are organized by the:

    a. application date

    b. application number

    c. reapplication date

    d. reapplication number

12. The amount of medicine that is prescribed for administration is known as the _____.

    a. schedule   b. dosage   c. medication   d. route

13. Factors that affect drug dosage are _____.

    a. weight, sex, and age   c. disease process

    b. pregnancy and lactation   d. all of the above

14. Pediatric patients require a _____ amount of a medication than adults.

    a. smaller   c. greater

    b. larger   d. none of the above

15. The geriatric patient requires special considerations because of _____.

    a. decreased gastrointestinal function

    b. changes in body composition

    c. changes in body function

    d. all of the above

16. _____ is the summation of a drug present in the body after repeated medication.

    a. Maximum dose   c. Cumulative dose

    b. Maintenance dose   d. Average dose

Matching. Place the correct letter from Column II on the appropriate line of Column I:

Column I

17. _____ abuse
18. _____ toxicology
19. _____ pharmacodynamics
20. _____ pharmacokinetics
21. _____ addictive
22. _____ administer
23. _____ Herceptin
24. _____ narcotic
25. _____ prescribe

Column II

A. to give

B. pertaining to habit-forming

C. a biologic indicated for breast cancer

D. to order or recommend the use of a drug, diet, or other form of therapy

E. producing sleep or stupor

F. the excessive or improper use of a substance, person, or animal

G. the study of drugs and their actions on living organisms

H. the study of the metabolism and actions of drugs within the body

I. the study of poisons

J. the study of drugs and their relationships to the treatment of disease

UNIT 8
Forms of Drugs and How They Act

OBJECTIVES

Upon completing this unit, you should be able to:

- Define the terms listed in the vocabulary.
- List the forms in which drugs are prepared, and give examples of these preparations.
- List the routes used for drug administration.
- Classify drugs according to preparation and therapeutic action.
- Define selected classifications of drugs and give examples of each.
- List the three general ways that drugs may be grouped.
- Define the actions of drugs according to the descriptive terms listed in this unit.
- Describe the factors that affect drug action.
- Describe the undesirable actions of drugs.
- Answer the review questions correctly.

VOCABULARY

form (form). The shape, structure, and size of anything that distinguishes it from another object.

homogeneous (ho"mo-je'ne-us). Similar or same in structure, composition, or nature.

solvent (sol'vent). That in which a substance is dissolved.

suspended (sus-pend'ed). Large particles of a drug are dispersed or scattered in a liquid.

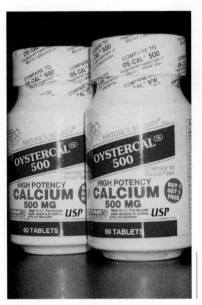

FIGURE 8-1

Oystercal™ 500. High Potency Calcuim 500 mg, usp, 60 tablets

Source: Delmar/Cengage Learning

INTRODUCTION

Drugs are compounded in three basic types of preparations: liquids, solids, and semisolids. The ease with which a drug's ingredients can be dissolved largely determines the variety of **forms** manufactured. Some drug agents are soluble in water, others in alcohol, and others in a mixture of several **solvents**.

The method for administering a drug depends upon its form, its properties, and the effects desired (see Figure 8-1). When given orally, a drug may be in the form of a liquid, powder, tablet, capsule, or caplet. If it is to be injected, it must be in the form of a liquid. For topical use, the drug may be in the form of a liquid, a powder, or a semisolid. Oral and injectable medications are examples of preparations designed for *internal use*.

Liquid Preparations

Liquid preparations are those containing a drug that has been dissolved or **suspended**. Depending upon the solvent used, the drug may be further classified as an aqueous (water) or alcohol preparation. When prescribed for internal use, liquid preparations other than emulsions are rapidly absorbed through the stomach or intestinal walls. The following are types of liquid preparations:

- *Emulsions*. Emulsions consist of fine droplets of an oil in water or water in oil. They separate into layers after standing for long periods of time and must be shaken vigorously before they are ready for use. An example of an emulsion is castor oil.

- *Solutions*. One or more drugs can be dissolved in an appropriate solvent to make a solution. The solution will appear to be clear and **homogeneous**. An example of a solution is normal saline.

- *Mixtures and suspensions*. Drugs that have been mixed with a liquid, but not dissolved, are called mixtures or suspensions. These preparations must be shaken before being administered to the patient. Pepto-Bismol Liquid is an example.

- *Syrups*. Drugs dissolved in a solution of sugar and water and then flavored are called syrups. An example is Benylin DM cough syrup.

- *Elixirs*. Drugs dissolved in a solution of alcohol and water that has been sweetened and flavored are elixirs. When prepared in this manner, the bitter or salty taste of the drug is disguised. For this reason, elixirs are frequently used for children's medications. An example of an elixir is Donnatal (phenobarbital, hyoscyamine sulfate, atropine sulfate, and scopolamine hydrobromide). Donnatal is also available in tablets, Extentabs, and capsules.

- *Tinctures.* Tinctures are drugs dissolved in alcohol or alcohol and water. For the most part, they are made to represent 10 percent of the drug agent. An example is tincture of digitalis. Another example, tincture of iodine, is an exception to the 10 percent rule. It may be found as a 7 percent or as a 2 percent tincture.

- *Spirits.* Alcoholic solutions of volatile (easily vaporized) drugs are called spirits. A spirit is also called an essence. Examples are spirits of peppermint and aromatic spirits of ammonia.

- *Fluidextracts.* Drugs that have been processed to a concentrated strength using alcohol as the solvent are called fluidextracts. Examples include fluidextract of ergot, fluidextract of ipecac, and cascara sagrada fluidextract.

- *Lotions.* Aqueous preparations of suspended ingredients used externally (without massage) to treat skin conditions are lotions. They may be a clear solution, suspension, or emulsion. Examples are calamine lotion and Caladryl.

- *Liniments.* Liniments are drugs that are used externally, with massage, to produce a feeling of heat to the area. An example is methyl salicylate.

- *Sprays.* As the name implies, sprays are drugs prepared to such a consistency that they may be administered by an atomizer. They are used primarily to treat nose and throat conditions. Some drugs administered by this method function as astringents and produce a shrinking or contracting effect. Others function as antiseptics and inhibit the growth of bacteria. Oil is usually used as a solvent. An example of a spray is Neo-Synephrine.

- *Aerosols.* These preparations may contain medications, ointments, creams, lotions, powders, or liquids. They utilize a propellant, such as butane, and are packaged in pressurized units. An example is Azmacort inhaler in a metered-dose aerosol unit. Azmacort is an anti-inflammatory steroid.

Solid and Semisolid Preparations

Tablets, capsules, caplets, troches or lozenges, suppositories, and ointments are examples of solid and semisolid preparations. These products offer great flexibility as a means of dispensing different dosages of drugs (see Figure 8-2). The following describes these products in detail:

- *Capsules* are small, two-part containers (hard or soft shell), which are usually made of a gelatin substance that is designed to dissolve in the stomach or gastrointestinal tract. Some capsules contain drug-impregnated beads (sustained-action) that are designed to release the medication at different rates.

- *Gelcaps* are oil-based medications that are enclosed in soft gelatin capsules.

- *Caplets* have the size and shape of a capsule, but the consistency of a tablet. They are coated, solid preparations for oral administration.

- *Tablets* are medication, in the form of a powder, that has been compressed into a small, disklike shape. Tablets come in various sizes, shapes, colors, and compositions. The following are some of the descriptive names for certain tablets:

    Enteric-coated tablets are designed to pass through the stomach without dissolving. Their special coating will dissolve in the small intestine.

    Buccal tablets are formulated to be dissolved and absorbed when placed between the cheek and gum. Advise the patient not to chew the tablet.

    Sublingual tablets are designed to be placed under the tongue where they dissolve and are absorbed. Advise the patient not to chew the tablet.

    Layered tablets may contain two or more layers of ingredients, or the same ingredient that has been treated to provide a different absorption rate.

    Scored tablets are those whose surface has been bisected by a groove to make it easy for the user to break them into halves or quarters to vary the dosage (see Figure 8-3).

- *Chewable* tablets are designed to be chewed. They contain a base of flavored and/or colored mannitol (a sugar alcohol). They are a preferred dosage form for antacids, some vitamins, and for children. A new

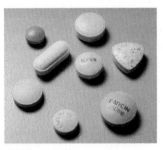
Tablets

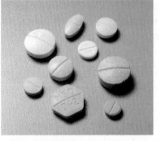
Scored Tablets

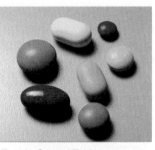
Enteric-Coated Tablets

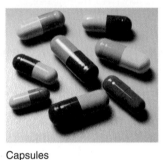
Capsules

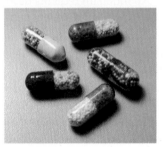
Controlled-Release Capsules

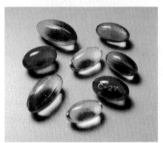
Gelatin Capsules

FIGURE 8-2

Types of tablets and capsules *Source: Delmar/Cengage Learning*

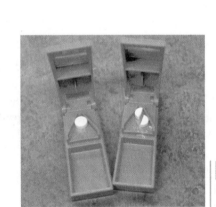

FIGURE 8-3

Scored tablets may be broken, if necessary.
Source: Delmar/Cengage Learning

form of chewable tablets is called *quick dissolve.* This unique form dissolves quickly in the mouth. An example of this form is Maalox Quick Dissolve, which is used to relieve heartburn and acid indigestion fast.

- *Effervescent* tablets are made with granular effervescent salts and other materials that release gas. When placed in water, they dispense active ingredients into the solution. An example of this form is Alka-Seltzer effervescent tablets.

- *Vaginal* tablets are designed to be placed into the vagina via an applicator. They dissolve in the vagina and are absorbed into the vaginal mucosa. An example of this form is Mycostatin antifungal vaginal tablets.

- *Troches or lozenges* are hard, circular, or oblong discs that consist of a medication in a candy-like base. These medications are designed to dissolve in the mouth and are commonly used to relieve the discomfort of a sore throat. Advise the patient not to chew the troche or lozenge but to let it dissolve in the mouth. The effectiveness of this medication is destroyed by drinking liquids too soon after use.

Other routes of administration are direct application to the skin (lotions, creams, liniments, ointments, and transdermal systems); sublingual (tablets, liquid: drops); buccal (tablets); rectal (suppositories, ointments); vaginal (suppositories, creams, tablets); inhalation (sprays, aerosols); and instillation (liquid: drops).

CLASSIFICATION OF DRUGS/THERAPEUTIC ACTION

Drugs are classified in many ways. Two of these ways are by preparation and by therapeutic action. The therapeutic action of the drug involves the process of treating, relieving, or obtaining results through the action of the medication upon the body. Table 8-1 includes selected classifications, a pronunciation guide, actions, and examples.

TABLE 8-1   Selected Drug Classifications

CLASSIFICATION	ACTION	EXAMPLES
Analgesic (an′al-je′sik)	An agent that relieves pain without causing loss of consciousness	acetaminophen (Tylenol), aspirin, ibuprofen (Advil, Motrin)
Anesthetic (an″es-thet′ik)	An agent that produces a lack of feeling; may be local or general depending upon the type and how administered	lidocaine HCl (Xylocaine), procaine HCl (Novocain)
Antacid (ant-as′id)	An agent that neutralizes acid	Gelusil, Mylanta, Aludrox, milk of magnesia
Antianxiety (an″ti-ang-zi′e-te)	An agent that relieves anxiety and muscle tension	benzodiazepines: chlordiazepoxide HCl (Librium) and diazepam (Valium)
Antiarrhythmic (an″te-a-rith′mik)	An agent that controls cardiac arrhythmias	lidocaine HCl (Xylocaine), propranolol HCl (Inderal)
Antibiotic (an″ti-bi-ot′ik)	An agent that is destructive to or inhibits growth of microorganisms	cephalosporins (Rocephin), penicillins (Zosyx, Augmentin)
Anticholinergic (an″ti-ko″lin-er′jik)	An agent that blocks parasympathetic nerve impulses	atropine, scopolamine
Anticoagulant (an″ti-ko-ag′u-lant)	An agent that prevents or delays blood clotting	heparin sodium, warfarin sodium (Coumadin)
Anticonvulsant (an″ti-kon-vul′sant)	An agent that prevents or relieves convulsions	carbamazepine (Tegretol), ethosuximide (Zarontin), phenytoin (Dilantin)
Antidepressant (an″ti-dep-res′ant)	An agent that prevents or relieves the symptoms of depression	imipramine HCl (Tofranil), monoamine oxidase inhibitors (MAOI): isocarboxazid (Marplan), phenelzine sulfate (Nardil)
Antidiarrheal (an″ti-di-a-re′al)	An agent that prevents or relieves diarrhea	Kaopectate, Lomotil, Pepto-Bismol
Antidote (an-ti′dot)	An agent that counteracts poisons and their effects	naloxone
Antiemetic (an″ti-e-met′ik)	An agent that prevents or relieves nausea and vomiting	Dramamine, Marinol, Phenergan, Reglan, Tigan
Antifungal (an″ti-fung′gal)	An agent that destroys or inhibits the growth of fungi	Diflucan, Lamisil, Lotrimin-AF, Monistat-3, Nizoral, Terazol

(continues)

TABLE 8-1 *(continued)*

CLASSIFICATION	ACTION	EXAMPLES
Antihistamine (an″ti-his′ta-min)	An agent that acts to prevent the action of histamine	Allegra, Benadryl, Dimetane
Antihyperlipidemic (an″ti-hi″per-li-pe′mik)	An agent that is used to lower abnormally high blood levels of fatty substances (lipids)	Lipitor, Lopid, Mevacor, Zocor
Antihypertensive (an″ti-hi″per-ten′siv)	An agent that prevents or controls high blood pressure	clonidine HCl (Catapres), methyldopa (Aldomet), metoprolol tartrate (Lopressor)
Anti-inflammatory (an′ti-in-flam′a-to-re)	An agent that prevents inflammation	aspirin, ibuprofen (Advil, Motrin), naproxen (Naprosyn)
Antimanic (an″ti-man′ik)	An agent used for the treatment of the manic episode of manic-depressive disorder	lithium
Antineoplastic (an″ti-ne″o-plas′tik)	An agent that prevents the replication of neoplastic cells	busulfan (Myleran), cisplatin (Platinol)
Anti-Parkinsonian (an″ti-par″kin-son′e-an)	An agent used for palliative relief of major symptoms of Parkinson's disease	L-Dopa, Requip, Symmetrel
Antipyretic (an″ti-pi-ret′ik)	An agent that reduces fever	acetaminophen (Tylenol), aspirin
Antituberculosis (an″ti-tu-ber″ku-lo′sis)	An agent used in the treatment of tuberculosis	Myambutal, Mycobutin, Priftin, PZA, Rifadin, Streptomycin
Antitumor necrosis factor (an″ti-tu′mor ne-kro′sis fak-or)	An agent that seems to slow, if not halt altogether, the destruction of the joints by disrupting the activity of tumor necrosis factor (TNF)	Enbrel
Antitussive (an″ti-tus′iv)	An agent that prevents or relieves cough	benzonatate (Tessalon), codeine
Antiulcer (an″ti-ul′ser)	An agent used in the treatment of active duodenal ulcer and for pathological hypersecretory conditions	Axid, Pepcid, Tagamet, Zantac
Antiviral (an″ti-vir′al)	An agent that combats a specific viral disease	Denavir, Famivir, Relenza, Retrovir, Tamiflu, Zovirax
Bronchodilator (brong″ko-dil-a′tor)	An agent that dilates the bronchi	isoproterenol HCl (Isuprel)
Cardiac glycoside (kar′de-ak gli″ko-si′de)	An agent that exerts a positive inotropic effect on the heart	Digitalis preparation Lanoxin
Contraceptive (kon″tra-sep′tiv)	Any device, method, or agent that prevents conception	Enovid-E-21, Ortho-Novum 10/11-21; 10/11-28, Triphasil-28
COX-2 inhibitor (kok-2 in-hib″i-tor)	An agent that inhibits cyclooxygenase (COX-2)—an enzyme found in joints and other areas affected by inflammation	Celebrex, Mobic
Decongestant (de″con-gest′ant)	An agent that reduces nasal congestion and/or swelling	oxymetazoline (Afrin), phenylephrine HCl (Neo-Synephrine), pseudoephedrine HCl (Sudafed)

(continues)

TABLE 8-1 (*continued*)

CLASSIFICATION	ACTION	EXAMPLES
Disease-modifying antirheumatic drugs (DMARDs) (di-zez-mod"i-fiving an"ti-roo-mat'ik drugs)	An agent that may influence the course of the disease progression of rheumatoid arthritis	Arava, Cuprimine, Cytoxan, Rheumatrex, Ridaura
Diuretic (di"u-ret'ik)	An agent that increases the excretion of urine	chlorothiazide (Diuril), furosemide (Lasix), mannitol (Osmitrol)
Emetic (e-met'ik)	An agent used to induce vomiting	Apomorphine HCl, ipecac syrup
Expectorant (ek-spek'to-rant)	An agent that facilitates removal of secretion from broncho-pulmonary mucous membrane	guaifenesin (Robitussin)
Gastric acid—pump inhibitor (gas'trik as'id-pump in-hib"i-tor)	An agent that suppresses gastric acid secretion by specific inhibition of the H1/K1 ATPase enzyme system; used for gastroesophageal reflux disease (GERD)	Aciphex, Prevacid, Prilosec, Protonix
Hemostatic (he"mo-stat'ik)	An agent that controls or stops bleeding	Amicar, vitamin K
Hypnotic (hip-not'ik)	An agent that produces sleep or hypnosis	chloral hydrate, secobarbital (Seconal)
Hypoglycemic (hi"po-gli-se'mik)	An agent that lowers blood glucose level	chlorpropamide (Diabinese), insulin
Immunologic (im"u-no-log'ik)	An agent administered to induce immunity and thereby prevent infectious diseases	Diphtheria, tetanus and pertussis (DTaP), mumps, rubeola, rubella (MMR), Engerix-B, Havrix, Infanrix, Varivax
Laxative (lak'sa-tiv)	An agent that loosens and promotes normal bowel elimination	Metamucil powder
Leukotriene receptor antagonist (Blockers) (loo'ko-tri-en ri-sep'tor an-tag¢ o-nist)	An agent that is used for the treatment and management of asthma	Accolate, Singulair
Mucolytic (mu"ko-lit'ik)	An agent that breaks chemical bonds in mucus, thereby lowering the viscosity	acetylcysteine
Muscle relaxant (mus'el re-lak'sant)	An agent that produces relaxation of skeletal muscle	Norflex, Paraflex, Robaxin, Skelaxin, Valium
Neuroleptic (nu"ro-lep'tik)	An agent that modifies psychotic behavior	Clozaril, Haldol, Risperdal, Stelazine, Zyprexa
Sedative (sed'a-tiv)	An agent that produces a calming effect without causing sleep	amobarbital (Amytal), butabarbital sodium (Buticaps), phenobarbital
Selective serotonin reuptake inhibitors (SSRIs) (si-lek'tiv ser"o-ton'in re-up-tak in-hib"i'tor)	An agent that selectively inhibits serotonin reuptake and results in a potentiation of serotonergic neurotransmissions	Luvox, Paxil, Prozac, Zoloft

(*continues*)

TABLE 8-1 (continued)		
CLASSIFICATION	ACTION	EXAMPLES
Serotonin nonselective reuptake inhibitor (SNRI) (ser″o-ton′in non-si-lek′tiv re-up-tak in-hib″i′tor)	An agent that inhibits the reuptake of both serotonin and norepinephrine.	Effexor
Thrombolytic (throm-bo-lit′ik)	An agent that dissolves an existing thrombus when administered soon after its occurrence.	Activase, Kabikinase, Streptase
Vasodilator (vas″o-di-la′tor)	An agent that produces relaxation of blood vessels; lowers blood pressure.	isorbide dinitrate (Isordil), nitroglycerin
Vasopressor (vas″o-pres′or)	An agent that produces contraction of muscles of capillaries and arteries; elevates blood pressure.	norepinephrine (Levophed)

PRINCIPAL ACTIONS OF DRUGS

Drugs may be used as a cure for disease. They may also be used to restore a disturbed or diseased physical state to one that is normal or improved. In the latter case, drugs assist the body to overcome its own difficulties by causing a change in cell activity without altering basic cell functions. In general, drugs may be grouped as follows:

- Those that act directly upon one or more tissues of the body.
- Those that act upon microorganisms invading the body (chemotherapy and antibiotics).
- Those that replace body chemicals and secretions (hormones).

Certain drugs are prescribed because of the selective actions that result when they are administered. The following descriptive terms have been applied to drugs because of the action that takes place:

- *Selective action* is a term applied to drugs that act upon certain tissues or on specific organs of the body. They are principally the stimulants and depressants.

    Stimulants are drugs that increase cell activity. An example is caffeine, which acts to stimulate the cerebrum.

    Depressants are drugs that decrease cell activity. An example is morphine, which acts to depress the respiratory center in the brain.

- *Agonist* action is the term applied to a drug that has affinity for the cellular receptors (specific sites in certain cells) of another drug or natural substance and initiates/produces a drug response.

- *Antagonist* action is the term applied to a drug that binds to a cellular receptor for a hormone, neurotransmitter, or another drug, blocking the action of that substance without producing any drug effect itself.

● *Note*

A receptor is a receiver, a cell component that combines with a hormone, neurotransmitter, or drug to alter the function of the cell. ●

- *Local action* is the term applied to an external drug designed to act on the area to which it is administered. An example is methyl salicylate, a medication that is often applied to sore muscles or painful joints by rubbing it into the affected area.

- *Remote action* is the term applied to a drug affecting a part of the body that is distant from the site of administration. An example is the action of an apomorphine injection into the arm to stimulate the vomiting center in the brain.

- *Specific action* is the term applied to a drug that has a particular effect on a certain pathogenic organism. An example is the action of primaquine on the malarial parasite.

- *Synergistic action* is the term that is used when one drug potentiates or increases the action of another. An example is the action of Demerol and Phenergan given as a preoperative. Phenergan increases the effect of Demerol.

- *Systemic action* is the term applied to a drug that, when in the bloodstream as a result of injection or absorption, is carried throughout the body.

FACTORS THAT AFFECT DRUG ACTION

The principal factors that affect drug action are absorption, distribution, biotransformation, and elimination. These factors depend upon the individual patient, the form and chemical composition of the drug, and the method of administration.

- *Absorption* is the process whereby the drug passes into body fluids and tissues. The rate of absorption depends upon the route of administration, the drug, differences in gastrointestinal function (pediatrics and geriatrics), and individual differences.

- *Distribution* is the process whereby the drug is transported from the blood to the intended site of action, site of biotransformation, site of storage, and site of elimination. The rate and extent of distribution depend upon the physical and chemical properties of the drug, the ability of the drug to bind to plasma proteins, and individual differences (such as cardiovascular function).

- *Biotransformation* is the chemical alteration that a substance (drug) undergoes in the body. Through this process, enzymes may be activated to break down the drug and prepare it for elimination. Most biotransformation occurs in the liver.

- *Elimination* is the process whereby a substance is excreted from the body. Many drugs are eliminated via the kidneys, whereas others may be eliminated via the gastrointestinal tract, respiratory tract, the skin, mucous membranes, and mammary glands (breast-feeding).

UNDESIRABLE ACTIONS OF DRUGS

Most drugs have the potential for causing an action other than their intended action. For example, certain antibiotics that are administered orally may disrupt the normal bacterial flora of the gastrointestinal tract and cause gastric discomfort. This type of reaction is known as a *side effect*. A side effect is an undesirable action of the drug and may limit the usefulness of the drug.

An *adverse reaction* is an unfavorable or harmful unintended action of a drug. Using a drug reference source, look up Demerol and note the adverse reactions. Light-headedness, dizziness, sedation, nausea, and sweating are the most frequent adverse reactions to Demerol. To report an adverse reaction to a drug, you may call 1-800-FDA-1088.

A drug *interaction* may occur when one drug potentiates or diminishes the action of another drug. These actions may be desirable or undesirable. Drugs may also interact with various foods, alcohol, tobacco, and other substances. It is recommended that a pharmacist be consulted any time there is the possibility of a drug interaction.

REVIEW QUESTIONS

Directions. Select the best answer to each of the following multiple-choice questions, circling the letter of your choice:

1. The term solvent means _____.
   a. similar or same in structure
   b. strength of a substance
   c. that in which a substance is dissolved
   d. the substance that is dissolved to form a solution

2. The method for administering a drug is dependent upon _____.
   a. its form   c. the effects desired
   b. its properties   d. all of the above

3. Drugs are compounded in three basic types of preparations. These types are _____.
   a. hypodermic, oral, and sublingual
   b. oral, parenteral, and topical
   c. liquids, solids, and semisolids
   d. intradermal, intramuscular, and intravenous

4. _____ are drugs dissolved in a solution of sugar and water and then flavored.
   a. Elixirs   b. Syrups   c. Tinctures   d. Fluidextracts

5. Pepto-Bismol liquid is an example of a(an) _____.
   a. emulsion   b. solution   c. suspension   d. elixir

6. Tablets that are designed to dissolve in the intestines and not in the stomach are known as _____.
   a. buccal   c. sublingual
   b. layered   d. enteric-coated

7. _____ tablets are designed to be placed under the tongue where they dissolve and are absorbed.
   a. Scored   c. Sublingual
   b. Layered   d. Enteric-coated

8. The following are all true statements about suppositories except that they are _____.
   a. semisolid preparations
   b. usually lubricated with a water-soluble jelly before insertion
   c. will not melt when subjected to body heat
   d. classified as drugs for external use

9. _____ is a small adhesive patch or disk that may be attached to the body near the treatment site.
   a. Ocular therapeutic system   c. Transdermal system
   b. Implanted device   d. all of these

10. _____ is an agent that relieves pain without causing loss of consciousness.
    a. Anesthetic   b. Hypnotic   c. Sedative   d. Analgesic

11. Xylocaine and Novocain are examples of _____.
    a. analgesics   b. anesthetics   c. hypnotics   d. sedatives

12. An agent that blocks parasympathetic nerve impulses is known as an _____.
    a. anticonvulsant b. anticholinergic c. antidepressant   d. antidiarrheal

13. Coumadin is an example of an _____.
    a. antiarrhythmics b. anticholinergics c. anticoagulants   d. anticonvulsants

14. Allegra and Benadryl are examples of _____.

    a. antihistamine   b. antiemetic   c. antihypertensive   d. antitussive

15. An agent that prevents the replication of neoplastic cells is known as an _____ agent.

    a. antipyretic   c. antineoplastic

    b. anti-inflammatory   d. antimanic

16. Aspirin and acetaminophen are examples of _____.

    a. analgesics and antipyretics   c. antihistamines and antiemetics

    b. antitussives and decongestants   d. antidotes and antibiotics

17. The most frequently utilized routes of administering medications to a patient are _____.

    a. sublingual and buccal   c. rectal and vaginal

    b. oral and parenteral   d. inhalation and instillation

18. Medications applied directly to the skin may be in the form of _____.

    a. lotions, creams   c. transdermal systems

    b. liniments, ointments   d. all of the above

19. An agent that lowers blood glucose level is known as a _____ agent.

    a. hyperglycemic   b. hypnotic   c. hypoglycemic   d. hypertensive

20. Diuril and Lasix are examples of _____.

    a. muscle relaxants   c. antidiuretics

    b. diuretics   d. antiemetics

21. An agent that modifies psychotic behavior is known as a _____.

    a. sedative   b. hypnotic   c. muscle relaxant   d. neuroleptic

22. _____ action occurs when the drug is absorbed into the bloodstream.

    a. Local   b. Remote   c. Systemic   d. Antagonist

23. A _____ is a receiver, a cell component that combines with a hormone, neurotransmitter, or drug to alter the function of the cell.

    a. receptor   c. depressant

    b. stimulant   d. none of the above

24. _____ is the process whereby the drug passes into body fluids and tissues.

    a. Absorption   b. Distribution   c. Biotransformation   d. Elimination

25. A(An) _____ is an unfavorable or harmful unintended action of a drug.

    a. interaction   c. adverse reaction

    b. side effect   d. specific action

Matching. Place the correct letter from Column II on the appropriate line of Column I:

Column I	*Column II*
26. _____ form	A. that in which a substance is dissolved
27. _____ homogeneous	B. drugs that decrease cell activity
28. _____ stimulants	C. similar or same in structure, composition, or nature
29. _____ depressants	D. the shape, structure, and size of anything that distinguishes it from another
30. _____ solvent	E. drugs that increase cell activity
	F. the color and consistency of a substance

OBJECTIVES

Upon completing this unit, you should be able to:

- Define the terms listed in the vocabulary.
- Describe the various types of medication orders.
- State who may administer medications.
- Describe the nine parts of a prescription.
- State the two main classes of medicines according to federal law.
- Describe and give the benefits of e-prescribing.
- Describe what happens to a prescription after a pharmacist fills it.
- List eight steps for safeguarding the prescription.
- List your responsibilities with regard to a patient's request for a prescription refill.
- List five ways in which qualified people may protect themselves when taking a verbal order.
- List seven guidelines for understanding the medication order.
- Understand medication labels (prescription and nonprescription).
- Read and write the common medical abbreviations given in this unit.
- Answer the review questions correctly.

VOCABULARY

agent (a'jant). One who acts for another. A representative who performs authorized acts in the name of another while under the directions and control of the principal party.

compounding (kom-pound'ing). The process of combining and mixing.

e-prescribing or **electronic prescribing**. The use of online, computerized software to create and sign prescriptions.

pharmacist (far'ma-sist). One who is licensed to prepare and dispense drugs.

INTRODUCTION

It is the physician's responsibility to diagnose the cause of an illness and to prescribe a medication. Today, medications play an important role in the treatment of diseases. Because thousands of drugs are on the market and various drugs can be prescribed for each disease process, physicians determine which drugs they wish to prescribe. The drug prescribed is generally referred to as a *medication order*. Once prescribed, any legally approved health professional has the responsibility to carry out the physician's medication order. Thus, it is essential that those whose duties include giving medications be knowledgeable about all aspects of drug administration. In this unit, emphasis is given to the medication order.

THE MEDICATION ORDER

The medication order is given for a specific patient. A physician or duly authorized prescriber generally writes a medication order. In a hospital setting or other health care facility that is equipped with computers, the medication ordering process of computerized physician order entry (CPOE) ensures complete, unambiguous, and legible orders. Also, the computer can assist the physician at the time of ordering by suggesting appropriate doses and frequencies, displaying relevant laboratory data, and screening orders for allergies and drug–drug and drug–laboratory interactions. No matter the method of ordering, a proper medication order includes the following information:

- The name of the patient. Full name is preferable.
- The name of the medication. Generic name is preferred. Brand name may be added for clarity. (The use of brand name alone is acceptable when a combination product containing two or more drugs within one formulation [Bactrim DS] is prescribed and for extended or sustained release formulations such as Cardizem CD 120 mg.)
- The dose and route of the medication.
- Frequency of the medication administration.
- The date and time the medication order was written.
- Specific directions for administration.
- Signature of the duly authorized prescriber.

Legibility and Completeness of the Medication Order

Medication orders that are illegible, unclear, or incompletely written will not be carried out until rewritten or clarified in writing. The individual who wrote the original order will be contacted. If that person is unavailable, the covering provider will be contacted.

There are acceptable and unacceptable abbreviations used in the writing of a medication order. The following are the abbreviations that have been listed in these categories:

Acceptable	*Unacceptable*
Write out microgram or abbreviate mcg	Abbreviate μg for microgram
Write out units	Abbreviate u or U for unit
Write out days or doses for duration	Abbreviate d or D for days or doses
Use a leading 0 before a decimal point (0.2 mg)	Use trailing 0 after a decimal point (2.0 mg)

The Prescription

The prescription is a written legal document that gives directions for compounding, dispensing, and administering a medication to a patient. There are eight parts to a prescription; see Figure 9-1. The purpose of a prescription

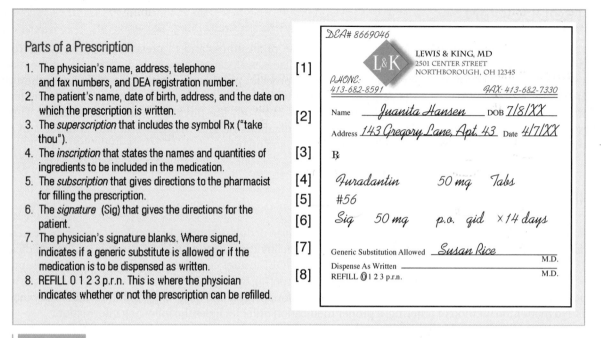

Parts of a Prescription

1. The physician's name, address, telephone and fax numbers, and DEA registration number.
2. The patient's name, date of birth, address, and the date on which the prescription is written.
3. The *superscription* that includes the symbol Rx ("take thou").
4. The *inscription* that states the names and quantities of ingredients to be included in the medication.
5. The *subscription* that gives directions to the pharmacist for filling the prescription.
6. The *signature* (Sig) that gives the directions for the patient.
7. The physician's signature blanks. Where signed, indicates if a generic substitute is allowed or if the medication is to be dispensed as written.
8. REFILL 0 1 2 3 p.r.n. This is where the physician indicates whether or not the prescription can be refilled.

[1]

[2]

[3]

[4]

[5]

[6]

[7]

[8]

> DEA# 8669046
>
> **L&K** LEWIS & KING, MD
> 2501 CENTER STREET
> NORTHBOROUGH, OH 12345
>
> PHONE:
> 413-682-8591   FAX: 413-682-7330
>
> Name *Juanita Hansen* DOB 7/8/XX
>
> Address *143 Gregory Lane, Apt. 43* Date 4/7/XX
>
> Rx
>
> *Furadantin   50 mg   Tabs*
>
> *#56*
>
> *Sig   50 mg   p.o.   qid   × 14 days*
>
> Generic Substitution Allowed *Susan Rice*
> _____ M.D.
> Dispense As Written _____
> REFILL ⓪ 1 2 3 p.r.n. M.D.

FIGURE 9-1

Prescriptions are written legal documents that give directions for compounding, dispensing, and administering a medication. Prescriptions have eight distinct elements. *Source: Delmar/Cengage Learning*

is to control the sale and use of drugs that can be safely and effectively used only under the supervision of a licensed physician. Federal law divides medicines into two main classes: prescription medicines (dangerous, powerful, or habit-forming) and over-the-counter (OTC) medicines. The prescription is written by the physician and signed with an ink pen or is e-prescribed. The **pharmacist** fills the prescription according to the physician's order. Once the prescription has been filled, the assigned prescription number and all other information may be entered into a computer. The hard copy of the prescription is filed and kept for a minimum of seven years. Schedule II–controlled substance prescriptions are kept separate from other prescriptions and are stamped with a red C. Schedule III through V prescriptions are stamped with a red C and filed.

E-Prescribing or Electronic Prescribing

E-prescribing or **electronic prescribing** is the use of online, computerized software to create and sign prescriptions. Electronic prescribing, as defined by the National Council for Prescription Drug Programs (NCPDP), a standards development organization, has the following two parts:

Part 1: Two-way [electronic] communication between physicians and pharmacies involving new prescriptions, refill authorizations, change requests, cancel prescriptions, and prescription fill messages to track patient compliance. Electronic prescribing is not faxing or printing paper prescriptions.

Part 2: Potential for information sharing with other health care partners including eligibility/formulary information and medication history.

There are numerous e-prescribing software programs that physicians can implement to change from handwriting prescriptions to electronic prescribing. An estimated 75 percent of U.S. doctors will be writing electronic prescriptions by the year 2014. The economic stimulus bill President Barack Obama signed in 2009 included about $19 billion to promote the use of health care information technology, including e-prescribing.

E-prescribing is intended to bring safety and efficiency benefits to the prescribing process for patients and physicians. Patients will benefit because of the safety features of e-prescribing. These include the elimination of medication errors due to poor handwriting and the automated drug safety checks provided by e-prescribing software.

E-prescribing allows physicians to access information about medications the patient may be taking, any potential interactions or allergies, and whether the drug is in the patient's health care formulary (see Figure 9-2). Physicians would then electronically send prescriptions to the patient's pharmacy. The e-prescription can be received by participating pharmacies as an e-mail or as a fax. Either way, the pharmacist receives the information in a legible format, minimizing the risk for errors. The electronic script can be checked automatically for potential errors, such as an inconsistency in the prescribed dosage or duplicate therapies. If the program can access the patient's insurance formulary, the billing process can also be streamlined.

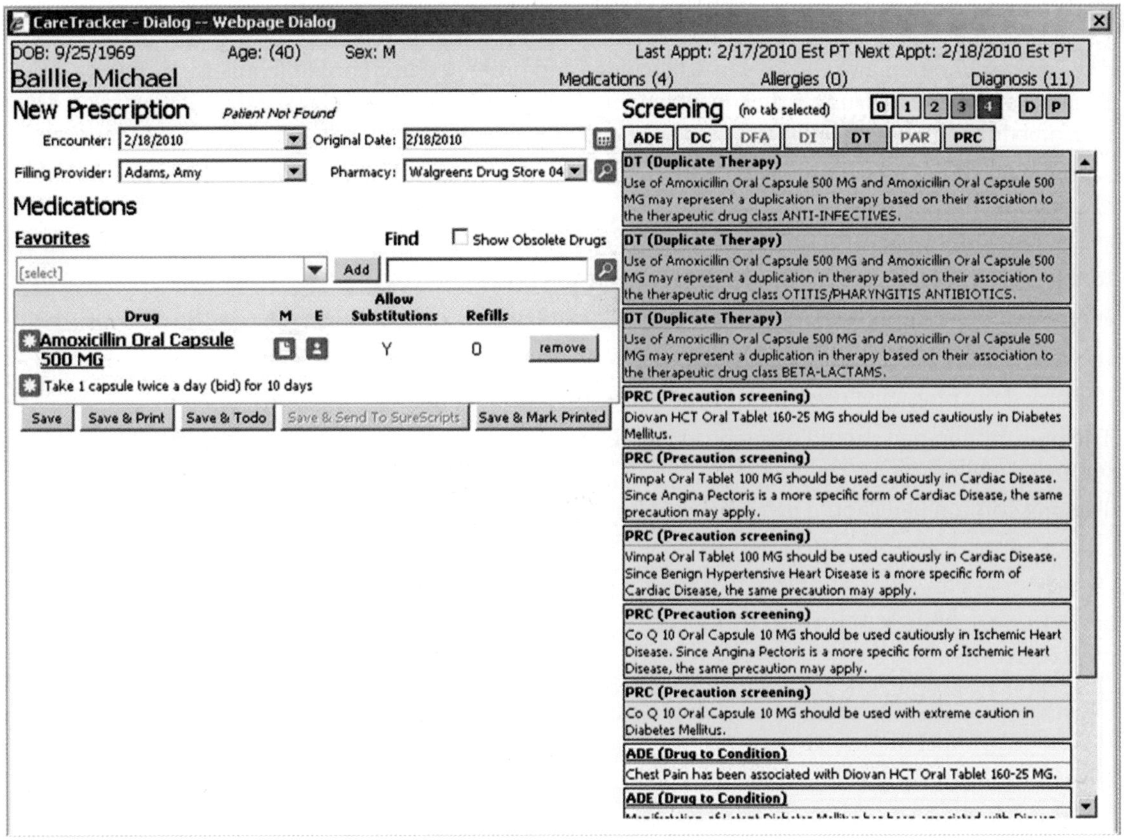

FIGURE 9-2

E-prescribing allows the physician to access information about medications the patient may be taking, any potential drug interactions or allergies. *Courtesy of Ingenix®CareTracker*

Prescription Refill

Prescription refill policies may vary from one office to another. It is always best to become familiar with the policy your physician establishes. The following are general guidelines regarding a patient's request for a prescription refill:

- Write down the patient's full name, telephone number, the medication requested, and the name of the pharmacy the patient uses.

- Inform the patient that you will have to ask the physician about the request for a refill. Give an approximate time the patient can expect an answer.

- Pull the patient's chart.
  1. Check the record for the date of the last prescription filled.
  2. Check the record for the date of the last visit.
  3. Check the record to see when the patient was to return to the office.
- Place the written request along with the chart in the appropriate location for the physician to approve or deny the request. *Prescriptions may not legally be refilled without the physician's authorization.*
- Notify the patient of the physician's decision.

 ## Safeguarding the Prescription

1. The prescription pad must be kept in a safe place and protected from possible misuse by any person. Because of the rise in drug abuse and stolen and forged prescriptions, it is essential that extra care be given to protecting the prescription pad.

2. A physician should never sign a prescription until ready to actually give the prescription to the patient.

3. The actual amount of prescribed medication should be written out as well as expressed in numerical form. In this way, a person cannot change the number that is prescribed.

4. Preprinted prescriptions should be stored in a locked drawer or compartment.

5. It is best to have prescription blanks numbered and printed in a colored ink that is nonreproducible.

6. It is best if the physician uses only one prescription pad at a time.

7. The prescription pad should never be left in an examining room where a person has easy access to removing a blank.

8. The prescription pad should never be used for anything other than its legal purpose.

Other Types of Medication Orders

- *Verbal order* (VO). One expressed by speech and not written out. In the physician's office, a physician often employs this method of giving a medication order. Licensed or certified health care providers should protect themselves by:
  1. Writing down the order exactly as heard.
  2. Repeating the order back to the physician.
  3. Making sure that they understand the order and are knowledgeable about the medication to be administered.
  4. Following the "seven rights" of proper drug administration. (See Unit 10.)
  5. Carefully documenting all appropriate information about the administration.
- *Telephone order* (TO). A type of verbal order that is transmitted via a telecommunications system. In some states, only physicians are allowed to give medication orders to a pharmacist via the telephone. In other states, a qualified **agent** may call in a physician's order to a pharmacist. It is essential that you know your legal role in receiving and transmitting medication orders. You may wish to gather this information from the Secretary of State, or the Medical Association where you are or will be employed.

- *PRN order.* With this type of order, medication is given "as necessary" or "when needed," within the specific time frame.
- *Routine order.* A prescribed, detailed course of action that is to be followed regularly. This type of order is not permissible for narcotic drugs or barbiturates.
- *Single order.* An order that is given one time only.
- *Stat order.* An order for *immediate* administration of a medication.
- *Facsimile or electronic orders.* An order transmitted by a facsimile machine (fax) or electronically by an authorized prescriber or the prescriber's authorized agent. If the electronic prescription is transmitted by an authorized agent, the transmission must include the full name and title of the agent. The pharmacist must ensure that the facsimile machine used to receive facsimile prescriptions, or the computer device used to receive electronically transmitted prescriptions, is located within the pharmacy prescription area. The pharmacist receiving the transmission must be sure that the order contains the identification number of the facsimile machine used to transmit the prescription and the date and time of the transmission. If a pharmacist is receiving an electronic prescription, the permit holder must ensure that the electronic system utilized in the pharmacy has adequate security and system safeguards designed to prevent and detect unauthorized access, modification, or manipulation of the prescription. Pharmacists are required to seek verbal verification of facsimile or electronic prescriptions from prescribers whenever the pharmacist has a question regarding the authenticity, accuracy, or appropriateness of the prescription.

Today, the electronic medical record (EMR) or electronic health record (EHR) is being utilized more by physicians and health care providers than in previous years. Sections contained within the medical record will vary according to the physician's preference, type of practice, cost, and regulatory requirements. Many of the EMR software programs have a prescription component that can be accessed by clicking on a prescription tab. The program can store thousands of drug names with their usual dosages (see Figure 9–3A). With just a few clicks, an entire prescription can be created (see Figure 9–3B).

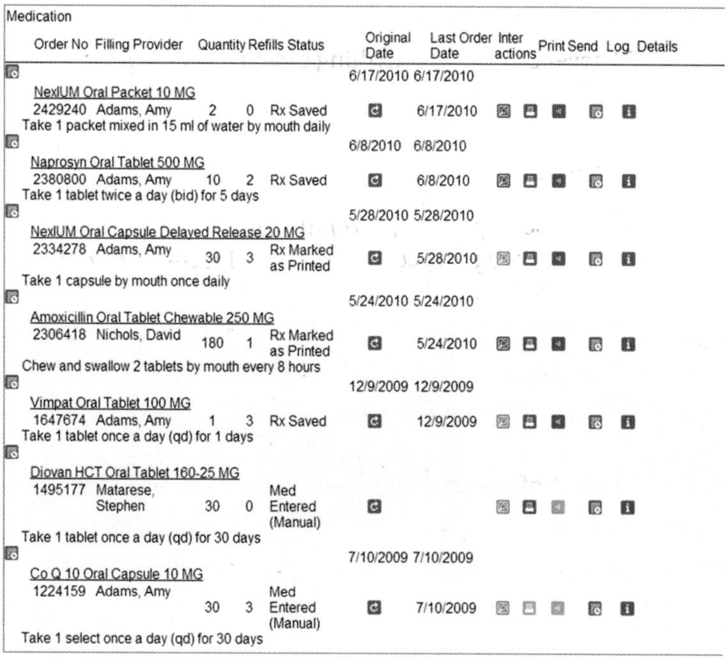

Medication						Original Date	Last Order Date	Inter actions	Print	Send	Log	Details
Order No	Filling Provider	Quantity	Refills	Status								
						6/17/2010	6/17/2010					
NexIUM Oral Packet 10 MG												
2429240	Adams, Amy	2	0	Rx Saved			6/17/2010					
Take 1 packet mixed in 15 ml of water by mouth daily												
						6/8/2010	6/8/2010					
Naprosyn Oral Tablet 500 MG												
2380800	Adams, Amy	10	2	Rx Saved			6/8/2010					
Take 1 tablet twice a day (bid) for 5 days												
						5/28/2010	5/28/2010					
NexIUM Oral Capsule Delayed Release 20 MG												
2334278	Adams, Amy	30	3	Rx Marked as Printed			5/28/2010					
Take 1 capsule by mouth once daily												
						5/24/2010	5/24/2010					
Amoxicillin Oral Tablet Chewable 250 MG												
2306418	Nichols, David	180	1	Rx Marked as Printed			5/24/2010					
Chew and swallow 2 tablets by mouth every 8 hours												
						12/9/2009	12/9/2009					
Vimpat Oral Tablet 100 MG												
1647674	Adams, Amy	1	3	Rx Saved			12/9/2009					
Take 1 tablet once a day (qd) for 1 days												
Diovan HCT Oral Tablet 160-25 MG												
1495177	Matarese, Stephen	30	0	Med Entered (Manual)								
Take 1 tablet once a day (qd) for 30 days												
						7/10/2009	7/10/2009					
Co Q 10 Oral Capsule 10 MG												
1224159	Adams, Amy	30	3	Med Entered (Manual)			7/10/2009					
Take 1 select once a day (qd) for 30 days												

FIGURE 9-3A

EMR software programs can store thousands of drug names with their usual dosages. *Courtesy of Ingenix ®CareTracker*

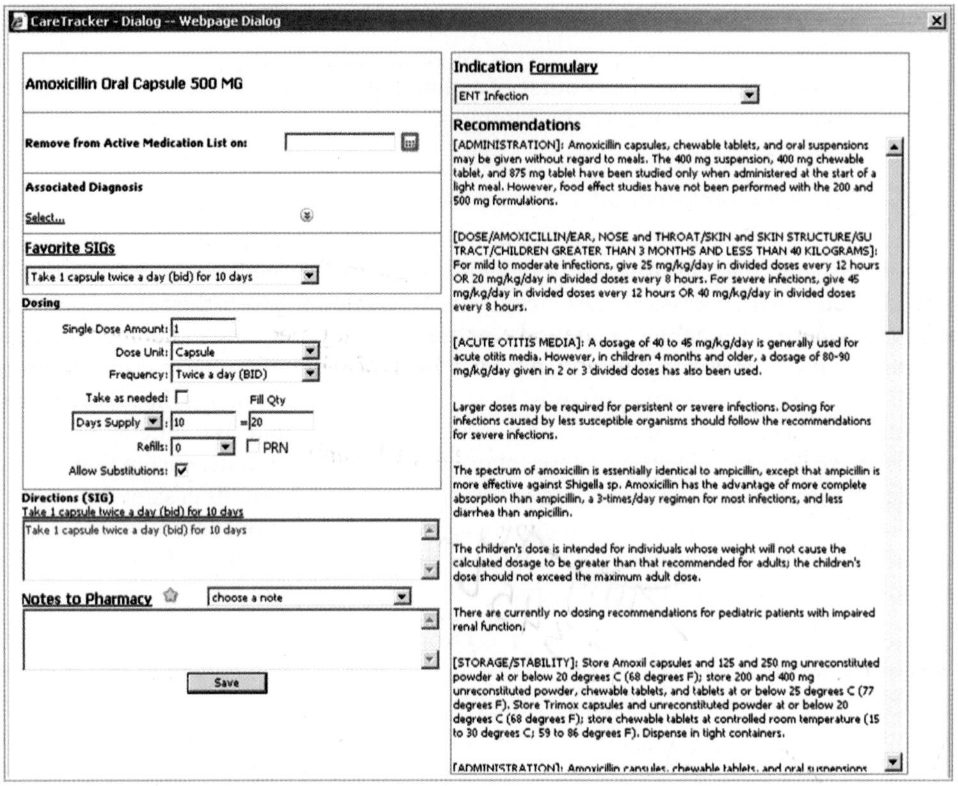

FIGURE 9-3B

An example of an electronic prescription screen. With just a few clicks, an entire prescription can be created. *Courtesy of Ingenix®CareTracker*

Guidelines for Understanding the Medication Order

1. Become knowledgeable about the medications that your physician prescribes.
   - Make a list of the drugs.
   - Make a drug card for each drug. Learn the following information:

Name of Drug:	Trade/Brand ______
	Generic ______
Actions:	
Indications/Uses:	
Adverse Reactions:	
Dosage & Administration:	

   - File each drug card (in alphabetical order or according to classification) in a small metal box.
2. Write down each verbal order exactly as heard.
3. Repeat the order back to the physician.
4. Make sure you understand the medication order before administering any drug.
5. If there are any questions, ask before giving.

6. If you are ever in doubt, seek the assistance of your physician.

7. Be knowledgeable about new drugs on the market, especially any new drugs that your physician may order for specific disease processes.

THE MEDICATION LABEL

The medication label can be a source of valuable information for the medical assistant and the patient. Regardless of whether one is administering a prescription drug or taking a nonprescription product, an understanding of the information provided on the label is essential to the safe and effective use of any medicine. In addition to the name and address of the manufacturer, the following are the most important items of information that may be on a medication label:

- The trade or brand name for the medication.
- The generic name (or listing of active and inactive ingredients).

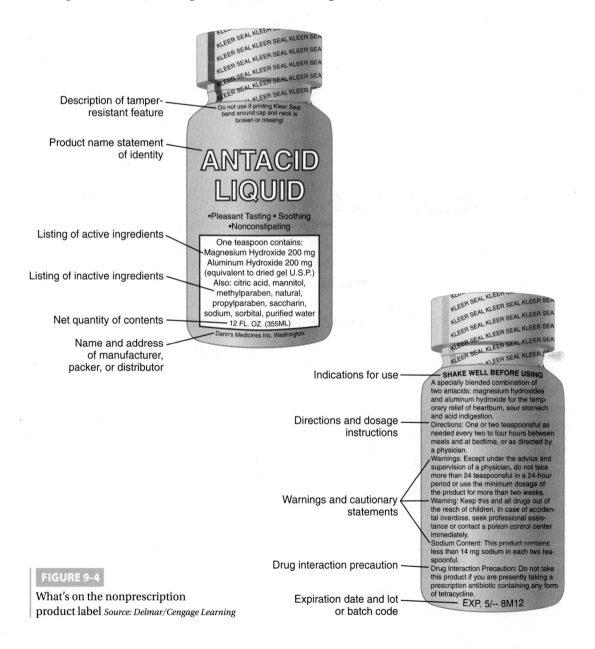

FIGURE 9-4

What's on the nonprescription product label *Source: Delmar/Cengage Learning*

- The National Drug Code (NDC) numbers that can be used to identify the manufacturer, the product, and the size of the container.
- The dosage strength in a given amount of the medication.
- The usual dosage and frequency of administration.
- The route of administration.
- Precautions and warnings.
- The expiration date for the medication and the lot or batch code.

The prescription label may also have directions for storage and the directions for mixing or reconstituting a powdered form of the drug. Prescription medications that are listed in the Federal Controlled Substances Act are so identified on the label by the symbols Ⅽ, Ⅽ, Ⅽ, Ⅽ, and Ⅽ.

Nonprescription medications, also known as over-the-counter products, are intended for use without medical supervision. As such, the labeling of these products is very important to their safe and proper use by the consumer. Figure 9-4 illustrates the required or recommended label information contained on a typical nonprescription product.

Understanding the Medication Label

Refer to Figure 9-5 (sample of a medication label: Feldene®), and note the following information as it relates to this label.

1. The trade or brand name for the medication: **Feldene**.
2. The generic name: **piroxicam**.
3. The National Drug Code numbers that can be used to identify the manufacturer, the product, and the size of the container: **59012-323-73**.
4. The dosage strength in a given amount of the medication: **20 mg**.
5. The usual dosage and frequency of administration: **See accompanying prescribing information. One capsule per day**.
6. The form in which the drug is supplied: **capsules**.
7. **Important**: This closure is not child-resistant.
8. The manufacturer's name: **Pfizer**.
9. The total number and/or volume of the drug contained: **500 capsules**.

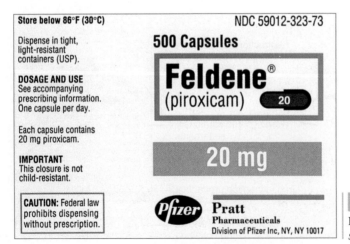

FIGURE 9-5

Feldene® (piroxicam) 20 mg

Source: Label reproduced by permission of Pfizer

Warning Labels for Prescription Medication Containers

Warning labels are placed on prescription medication containers and patients should be advised to read and adhere to the precautions or instructions (see Figure 9-6).

Precautions or instructions are stated in phrases or sentences similar to the following:

- Finish all this medication unless otherwise directed by physician.
- Refrigerate—shake well. Discard after _____.
- For the eye.
- Obtain medical advice before taking nonprescription drugs, as some may affect the action of this medication.
- Take medication on an empty stomach, 1 hour before or 2 to 3 hours after a meal, unless otherwise directed by your doctor.
- Do not take dairy products, antacids, or iron preparations within 1 hour of this medication.
- For the ear.
- Some nonprescription drugs may aggravate your condition. Read all labels carefully. If a warning appears, check with your doctor.
- May cause drowsiness. Alcohol may intensify this effect. Use care when operating a car or dangerous machinery.
- May cause drowsiness or dizziness.

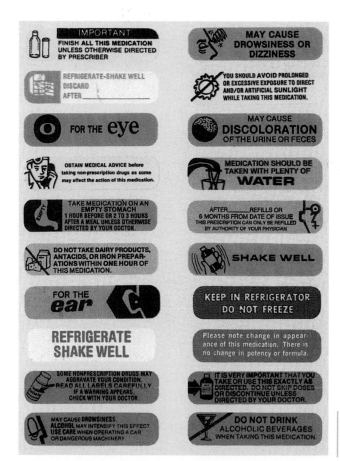

FIGURE 9-6

Examples of instruction and warning labels for prescription medications *Source: Delmar/Cengage Learning*

TABLE 9-1 Abbreviations and Their Meanings

ABBREVIATION	MEANING	ABBREVIATION	MEANING
aa	of each	noct	at night
a.c.	before meals	NPO	nothing by mouth
ad lib	as desired	NS	normal saline
AM, am	morning	os	mouth
amp	ampule	oz	ounce
amt	amount	O_2	oxygen
aq	aqueous	p	after
b.i.d.	twice a day	p.c.	after meals
c̄	with	PM, pm	afternoon or evening
cap	capsule	po, PO	by mouth
DAW	dispense as written	prn, PRN	whenever necessary
disp	dispense	pt	pint
dL	deciliter	q	every
DW	distilled water	qh	every hour
elix	elixir	q2h	every 2 hours
et	and	q3h	every 3 hours
ext	extract	q.i.d.	four times a day
fl, fld	fluid	qs	quantity sufficient
g	gram	qt	quart
h, hr	hour	R	right, rectal
H_2O	water	Rx	take, thou
ID	intradermal	s̄	without
IM	intramuscular	Sig	label
IV	intravenous	SL	sublingual
kg	kilogram	sol	solution
L	liter	SOS	once if necessary
lb	pound	sp	spirits
mcg, ▪	microgram	stat, STAT	immediately
mEq	milliequivalent	supp	suppository
mL	milliliter	syr	syrup
MOM	milk of magnesia	tab	tablet
MS	morphine sulfate	T, tbsp	tablespoon
n	normal	t, tsp	teaspoon
NaCl	sodium chloride	t.i.d.	three times a day
NKA	no known allergies	tinc	tincture
NKDA	no known drug allergies	ung	ointment

- You should avoid prolonged or excessive exposure to direct and/or artificial sunlight while taking this medication.
- May cause discoloration of the urine or feces.
- Medications should be taken with plenty of water.
- Please note change in appearance of this medication. There is no change in potency or formula.
- It is very important that you take or use this exactly as directed. Do not skip doses or discontinue unless directed by your doctor.
- Do not drink alcoholic beverages when taking this medication.

ABBREVIATIONS

Abbreviations are the shorthand of the medical field. They are a clear and concise means for writing orders. This medical shorthand is an international language used by professional and nonprofessional people who are concerned with patient care. All of the abbreviations listed in Table 9-1 should be learned to properly fulfill your role in the administration of medications.

It is important for you to understand that there are many abbreviations, symbols, and dose designations that have been reported to the Institute for Safe Medication Practises (ISMP) because they are frequently misinterpreted and involved in harmful medication errors. They should never be used when communicating medical information. This includes internal communications, telephone/verbal prescriptions, computer-generated labels, and labels for drug computer order entry screens. Also, The Joint Commission has established a National Patient Safety Goal that specifies that certain abbreviations must appear on an accredited organization's do-not-use list (see Figure 9-7).

Institute for Safe Medication Practices

ISMP's List of *Error-Prone Abbreviations, Symbols,* and *Dose Designations*

The abbreviations, symbols, and dose designations found in this table have been reported to the Institute for Safe Medication Practices (ISMP) through the ISMP Medication Errors Reporting Program (MERP) as being frequently misinterpreted and involved in harmful medication errors. They should NEVER be used when communicating medical information. This includes internal communications, telephone/verbal prescriptions, computer-generated labels, labels for drug storage bins, medication administration records, as well as pharmacy and prescriber computer order entry screens.

The Joint Commission (TJC) has established a National Patient Safety Goal that specifies that certain abbreviations must appear on an accredited organization's do-not-use list; we have highlighted these items with a double asterisk (**). However, we hope that you will consider others beyond the minimum TJC requirements. By using and promoting safe practices and by educating one another about hazards, we can better protect our patients.

Abbreviations	Intended Meaning	Misinterpretation	Correction
μg	Microgram	Mistaken as "mg"	Use "mcg"
AD, AS, AU	Right ear, left ear, each ear	Mistaken as OD, OS, OU (right eye, left eye, each eye)	Use "right ear," "left ear," or "each ear"
OD, OS, OU	Right eye, left eye, each eye	Mistaken as AD, AS, AU (right ear, left ear, each ear)	Use "right eye," "left eye," or "each eye"
BT	Bedtime	Mistaken as "BID" (twice daily)	Use "bedtime"
cc	Cubic centimeters	Mistaken as "u" (units)	Use "mL"
D/C	Discharge or discontinue	Premature discontinuation of medications if D/C (intended to mean "discharge") has been misinterpreted as "discontinued" when followed by a list of discharge medications	Use "discharge" and "discontinue"
IJ	Injection	Mistaken as "IV" or "intrajugular"	Use "injection"
IN	Intranasal	Mistaken as "IM" or "IV"	Use "intranasal" or "NAS"
HS	Half-strength	Mistaken as bedtime	Use "half-strength" or "bedtime"
hs	At bedtime, hours of sleep	Mistaken as half-strength	
IU**	International unit	Mistaken as IV (intravenous) or 10 (ten)	Use "units"
o.d. or OD	Once daily	Mistaken as "right eye" (OD-oculus dexter), leading to oral liquid medications administered in the eye	Use "daily"
OJ	Orange juice	Mistaken as OD or OS (right or left eye); drugs meant to be diluted in orange juice may be given in the eye	Use "orange juice"
Per os	By mouth, orally	The "os" can be mistaken as "left eye" (OS-oculus sinister)	Use "PO," "by mouth," or "orally"
q.d. or QD**	Every day	Mistaken as q.i.d., especially if the period after the "q" or the tail of the "q" is misunderstood as an "i"	Use "daily"
qhs	Nightly at bedtime	Mistaken as "qhr" or every hour	Use "nightly"
qn	Nightly or at bedtime	Mistaken as "qh" (every hour)	Use "nightly" or "at bedtime"
q.o.d. or QOD**	Every other day	Mistaken as "q.d." (daily) or "q.i.d." (four times daily) if the "o" is poorly written	Use "every other day"
q1d	Daily	Mistaken as q.i.d. (four times daily)	Use "daily"
q6PM, etc.	Every evening at 6 PM	Mistaken as every 6 hours	Use "6 PM nightly" or "6 PM daily"
SC, SQ, sub q	Subcutaneous	SC mistaken as SL (sublingual); SQ mistaken as "5 every;" the "q" in "sub q" has been mistaken as "every" (e.g., a heparin dose ordered "sub q 2 hours before surgery" misunderstood as every 2 hours before surgery)	Use "subcut" or "subcutaneously"
ss	Sliding scale (insulin) or ½ (apothecary)	Mistaken as "55"	Spell out "sliding scale;" use "one-half" or "½"
SSRI	Sliding scale regular insulin	Mistaken as selective serotonin reuptake inhibitor	Spell out "sliding scale (insulin)"
SSI	Sliding scale insulin	Mistaken as Strong Solution of Iodine (Lugol's)	
i/d	One daily	Mistaken as "tid"	Use "1 daily"
TIW or tiw	3 times a week	Mistaken as "3 times a day" or "twice in a week"	Use "3 times weekly"
U or u**	Unit	Mistaken as the number 0 or 4, causing a tenfold overdose or greater (e.g., 4U seen as "40" or 4u seen as "44"); mistaken as "cc" so dose given in volume instead of units (e.g., 4u seen as 4cc)	Use "unit"

Dose Designations and Other Information	Intended Meaning	Misinterpretation	Correction
Trailing zero after decimal point (e.g., 1.0 mg)**	1 mg	Mistaken as 10 mg if the decimal point is not seen	Do not use trailing zeros for doses expressed in whole numbers"
"Naked" decimal point (e.g., .5 mg)**	0.5 mg	Mistaken as 5 mg if the decimal point is not seen	Use zero before a decimal point when the dose is less than a whole unit

FIGURE 9-7

ISMP's list of error-prone abbreviations, symbols, and dose designations *Source: ISP 2008*

Institute for Safe Medication Practices

ISMP's List of *Error-Prone Abbreviations, Symbols,* and *Dose Designations* (continued)

Dose Designations and Other Information	Intended Meaning	Misinterpretation	Correction
Drug name and dose run together (especially problematic for drug names that end in "l" such as Inderal40 mg; Tegretol300 mg)	Inderal 40 mg Tegretol 300 mg	Mistaken as Inderal 140 mg Mistaken as Tegretol 1300 mg	Place adequate space between the drug name, dose, and unit of measure
Numerical dose and unit of measure run together (e.g., 10mg, 100mL)	10 mg 100 mL	The "m" is sometimes mistaken as a zero or two zeros, risking a 10- to 100-fold overdose	Place adequate space between the dose and unit of measure
Abbreviations such as mg. or mL. with a period following the abbreviation	mg mL	The period is unnecessary and could be mistaken as the number 1 if written poorly	Use mg, mL, etc. without a terminal period
Large doses without properly placed commas (e.g., 100000 units; 1000000 units)	100,000 units 1,000,000 units	100000 has been mistaken as 10,000 or 1,000,000; 1000000 has been mistaken as 100,000	Use commas for dosing units at or above 1,000, or use words such as 100 "thousand" or 1 "million" to improve readability
Drug Name Abbreviations	**Intended Meaning**	**Misinterpretation**	**Correction**
ARA A	vidarabine	Mistaken as cytarabine (ARA C)	Use complete drug name
AZT	zidovudine (Retrovir)	Mistaken as azathioprine or aztreonam	Use complete drug name
CPZ	Compazine (prochlorperazine)	Mistaken as chlorpromazine	Use complete drug name
DPT	Demerol-Phenergan-Thorazine	Mistaken as diphtheria-pertussis-tetanus (vaccine)	Use complete drug name
DTO	Diluted tincture of opium, or deodorized tincture of opium (Paregoric)	Mistaken as tincture of opium	Use complete drug name
HCl	hydrochloric acid or hydrochloride	Mistaken as potassium chloride (The "H" is misinterpreted as "K")	Use complete drug name unless expressed as a salt of a drug
HCT	hydrocortisone	Mistaken as hydrochlorothiazide	Use complete drug name
HCTZ	hydrochlorothiazide	Mistaken as hydrocortisone (seen as HCT250 mg)	Use complete drug name
MgSO4**	magnesium sulfate	Mistaken as morphine sulfate	Use complete drug name
MS, MSO4**	morphine sulfate	Mistaken as magnesium sulfate	Use complete drug name
MTX	methotrexate	Mistaken as mitoxantrone	Use complete drug name
PCA	procainamide	Mistaken as patient controlled analgesia	Use complete drug name
PTU	propylthiouracil	Mistaken as mercaptopurine	Use complete drug name
T3	Tylenol with codeine No. 3	Mistaken as liothyronine	Use complete drug name
TAC	triamcinolone	Mistaken as tetracaine, Adrenalin, cocaine	Use complete drug name
TNK	TNKase	Mistaken as "TPA"	Use complete drug name
ZnSO4	zinc sulfate	Mistaken as morphine sulfate	Use complete drug name
Stemmed Drug Names	**Intended Meaning**	**Misinterpretation**	**Correction**
"Nitro" drip	nitroglycerin infusion	Mistaken as sodium nitroprusside infusion	Use complete drug name
"Norflox"	norfloxacin	Mistaken as Norflex	Use complete drug name
"IV Vanc"	intravenous vancomycin	Mistaken as Invanz	Use complete drug name
Symbols	**Intended Meaning**	**Misinterpretation**	**Correction**
ℨ	Dram	Symbol for dram mistaken as "3"	Use the metric system
ℳ	Minim	Symbol for minim mistaken as "mL"	
x3d	For three days	Mistaken as "3 doses"	Use "for three days"
> and <	Greater than and less than	Mistaken as opposite of intended; mistakenly use incorrect symbol; "< 10" mistaken as "40"	Use "greater than" or "less than"
/ (slash mark)	Separates two doses or indicates "per"	Mistaken as the number 1 (e.g., "25 units/10 units" misread as "25 units and 110" units)	Use "per" rather than a slash mark to separate doses
@	At	Mistaken as "2"	Use "at"
&	And	Mistaken as "2"	Use "and"
+	Plus or and	Mistaken as "4"	Use "and"
°	Hour	Mistaken as a zero (e.g., q2° seen as q 20)	Use "hr," "h," or "hour"

**These abbreviations are included on TJC's "minimum list" of dangerous abbreviations, acronyms, and symbols that must be included on an organization's "Do Not Use" list, effective January 1, 2004. Visit www.jointcommission.org for more information about this TJC requirement.

Institute for Safe Medication Practices
www.ismp.org

FIGURE 9-7

(continued)

■ ■ REVIEW QUESTIONS

Directions. Select the best answer to each of the following multiple-choice questions, circling the letter of your choice:

1. The medication order is given by the physician for a specific patient and it includes _____.
   a. the drug to be given
   b. the dosage and form of the drug
   c. the time and route
   d. all of the above

2. The prescription is a written legal document that gives directions for _____.
   a. compounding, dispensing, and administering a medication
   b. compounding, dispensing, and selling a medication
   c. distributing, dispensing, and selling a medication
   d. none of the above

3. The hard copy of the prescription is filed and kept for _____.
   a. five years
   b. six years
   c. seven years
   d. two years

4. Schedule II–controlled substances prescriptions are _____.
   a. stamped with a C and filed with other prescriptions
   b. kept separate from other prescriptions
   c. stamped with a red C
   d. b and c

5. To safeguard the prescription pad, one should _____.
   a. use it as a scratch pad
   b. leave it in the examining room
   c. keep it in a safe place
   d. keep it in an unsafe place

6. The _____ states the names and quantities of ingredients to be included in the medication.
   a. superscription
   b. inscription
   c. subscription
   d. signature

7. The _____ gives directions to the pharmacist for filling the prescription.
   a. superscription
   b. inscription
   c. subscription
   d. signature

8. Stat order is one that is _____.
   a. a type of protocol
   b. given "as necessary"
   c. given immediately
   d. given one time only

9. All of the following are ways that one may become knowledgeable about the medications that one's physician orders except _____.
   a. make a list of drugs
   b. make a drug card for each drug
   c. learn the appropriate information about each drug
   d. don't keep up with new drugs

10. The abbreviation b.i.d. means _____.
    a. three times a day
    b. twice a day
    c. four times a day
    d. daily

11. The abbreviation oz means _____.
    a. ounce
    b. pound
    c. mouth
    d. none of the above

12. The abbreviation for after meals is _____.

    a. a.c.   b. p.c.   c. c̄   d. am

13. The abbreviation Sig means _____.

    a. one-half   c. label

    b. take thou   d. signature

14. An understanding of the information provided on a label is essential for _____.

    a. safe and uneffective use of any medicine

    b. safe and effective use of any medicine

    c. safe and ineffective use of any medicine

    d. none of these

15. The National Drug Code numbers on a label identify _____.

    a. the manufacturer   c. the size of the container

    b. the product   d. all of these

16. Prescription medications that are listed in the Federal Controlled Substances Act are identified by the symbols and/or abbreviations _____.

    a. FCSA   c. ℂ, ℂ, ℂ, ℂ, and ℂ

    b. NDS   d. all of these

17. The electronic medical record (EMR) can vary according to which of the following?

    a. physician's preference

    b. type of practice

    c. cost

    d. all of these

Matching. Place the correct letter from Column II on the appropriate line of Column I:

Column I	*Column II*
18. _____ agent	A. a written legal document that gives directions for compounding, dispensing, and administering a medication to a patient
19. _____ compounding	B. states the names and quantities of ingredients to be included in the medication
20. _____ pharmacist	C. includes the symbol R$_x$ ("take thou")
21. _____ prescription	D. gives the directions for the patient
22. _____ inscription	E. the use of online, computerized software to create and sign prescriptions
23. _____ subscription	F. one who acts for another
24. _____ signature	G. one who is licensed to prepare and dispense drugs
25. _____ e-prescribing	H. the process of combining and mixing
	I. gives directions to the pharmacist for filling the prescription

UNIT 10
Medication Administration Essentials

OBJECTIVES

Upon completing this unit, you should be able to:

- Define the terms listed in the vocabulary.
- Describe the legal implications for a person who prepares and administers medications.
- State the "seven rights" of proper drug administration.
- List the essential medication guidelines.
- Describe the universal precautions.
- Describe the standard precautions.
- List the guides that should be followed and precautions to be taken for the safe storage of medications in the physician's office.
- List the emergency medications, supplies, and equipment that must be readily available.
- List the data that should be recorded about drug administration.
- Give the ethical considerations for working around drugs.
- List the five actions that may constitute a medication error.
- List the five steps to take in case a medication error occurs.
- Answer the review questions correctly.

VOCABULARY

allergy (al-er-gee). An individual hypersensitivity to a substance; usually an antibody-antigen reaction.

ethical (eth′i-k″l). Pertaining to a system of moral principles or standards that govern conduct.

illegal (i-lee′gal). Pertaining to things unlawful; not legal.

meniscus (men-is-kus). A term used to describe the convex or concave upper surface of a column of liquid in a container; crescent-shaped.

opaque (o-pake′). Dark; not transparent.

precipitate (pre-sip′i-tait). A substance, in the form of fine particles, that separates from a solution if allowed to stand for a period of time.

unethical (un-eth′ik″l). Pertaining to any action that goes against a system of moral principles or standards that govern conduct.

LEGAL IMPLICATIONS

Members of the health care profession who prepare and administer medications have an **ethical** and legal responsibility for their own actions. Under the law, these individuals are required to be licensed, registered, or otherwise authorized by a physician.

Each state has enacted laws governing the practice of medicine, nursing, and pharmacy. These laws vary from state to state; therefore, it is essential that one become familiar with the laws of the state in which one is employed before giving any medication. In some states, the only health professional authorized to give injections, other than a physician, is the registered nurse. On the other hand, legislation in some states gives physicians broad authority to delegate responsibility for giving medications. An example taken from such legislation is worded as follows:

> . . . the right to delegate certain duties to any qualified and properly trained person or persons acting under the physician's supervision any medical act which a reasonable and prudent physician would find is within the scope of sound medical judgment to delegate if, in the opinion of the delegating physician, the act can be properly and safely performed by the person to whom the medical act is delegated . . .

This person acts as the *agent* of the physician. As an agent of the physician, one is responsible and accountable for the acts performed and may be subject to penalty in case of default.

Regardless of the differences in state authorization laws, the courts will not permit the careless actions of health care workers to go unpunished, especially when such actions result in harm to or the death of the patient. Under the law, those administering medications are expected to be familiar with the drugs administered and the effects they might have on a patient. In that, thousands of drugs are on the market, and the task of keeping up with current information on each medication is overwhelming. Therefore, it is necessary to be aware of new drugs that your physician may prescribe and to keep up-to-date reference books available so that you can look up any drug with which you are not familiar.

The "Seven Rights" of Proper Drug Administration

The "seven rights" of proper drug administration should be employed each time you prepare and administer a medication to a patient. These rights have been developed as a checklist of activities to ensure the safe delivery of a medication to a patient.

- *Right Patient: Know your patient.* Before administering any medication, always be sure that you have the right patient. A good safety practice is to correctly identify the patient on each occasion when you administer a medication. In a physician's office, call the patient by name or ask the patient to state his or her name.

- *Right drug: Know the drugs that you administer.* To be sure that the correct drug has been selected, compare the medication order with the label on the medication. A frequent check of the medication label is a good way to avoid a medication error. One should make a practice of reading the label on each of the following three occasions:

  1. When the medication is taken from the storage area.

  2. Just before removing it from its container.

  3. Upon returning the medication container to storage or prior to discarding the empty container.

- *Right dose: Know mathematics and dosage calculations.* It is essential that the patient receive the right dose. If the dose ordered and the dose on hand are *not the same*, carefully determine the correct dose through mathematical calculation. When calculating dosage, it is advisable to have another qualified person verify the accuracy of your calculations *before the medication is administered*.

- *Right route: Know the routes used for drug administration.* Check the medication order to be sure that you have the right route of administration.

- *Right time: Know the time the medicine is to be given.* Check the medication order to ensure that a drug is administered according to the time interval prescribed. For a drug to be maintained at the proper blood level, care must be taken to administer it at the right time.

- *Right technique: It is important that you know the proper technique for each drug that you are to administer.* This includes following the cornerstone "five rights" of proper drug administration (patient, drug, dose, route, time) and any specific directions to follow. You must consider all safety measures, such as maintaining sterile technique during injection administration, any specific techique of preparation of the medicine, such as not shaking an insulin bottle, and specific directions as indicated on the medication, such as taking the first thing in the morning, and not taking with any other medication, food, or liquid except 8 ounces of water. The patient is to sit up straight for 30 minutes.

- *Right documentation: A patient's chart is a legal document.* It is essential that the following data about drug administration be entered correctly: the patient's name; the date and time of administration; the name of the medication and the amount (dosage) administered; the *route* by which the medication was administered; the injection site used; any adverse reactions experienced by the patient; any complication in administering the drug (e.g., patient refusing to take the medication, difficulty in swallowing, and so forth). If the medication was *not given*, state why, and dispose of the medication according to agency policy.

ESSENTIAL MEDICATION GUIDELINES

Regardless of a medication's form or the route by which it is administered, certain basic guidelines must be followed. These guidelines are the following:

- Practice medical asepsis. Wash your hands before and after administering a medication (see Figure 10-1).
- Work in a well-lighted area that is free from distractions.
- Follow the "seven rights" of proper drug administration.
- Always check for any allergy before administering any medication.
- Give only drugs that are ordered by a licensed physician or practitioner authorized to prescribe medications.

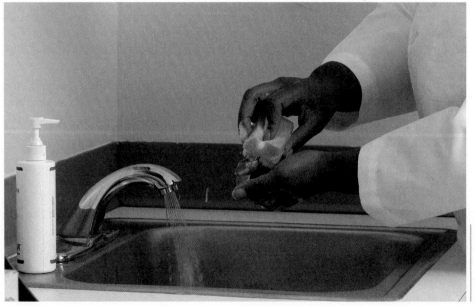

FIGURE 10-1

A medical assistant performs the medical asepsis hand wash.

Source: Delmar/Cengage Learning

- *Never* give a medication if there is any question about the order.
- Be completely familiar with the drug that you are administering before giving it to your patient.
- Always check the expiration date on the medication label.
- Never give a drug if its normal appearance has been altered in any way (color, structure, consistency, or odor).
- Give only those medications that you have actually prepared for administration.
- Do not allow someone else to give a medication that you have prepared.
- Once you have prepared a medication for administration, do not leave it unattended.
- Be careful in transporting the medication to the patient.
- When administering oral medications, stay with the patient until you are certain that the medication has been taken.
- Shake (to mix) all liquid medications that contain a **precipitate** before pouring.
- When pouring a liquid medication, hold the measuring device at eye level with the label toward the palm (in case of an accidental spill, this protects the label from becoming soiled) and read the correct amount at the lowest level of the **meniscus** (see Figure 10-2).
- Do not contaminate the cap of a bottle while pouring a medication. Place the cap with the rim pointed upward to prevent contamination of the portion that comes into contact with the medication.
- Keep all drugs not being administered in a safe storage place.
- Carefully follow the procedural steps for the type of medication that you are giving or the type of procedure you are performing.

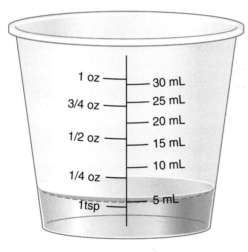

FIGURE 10-2

Always measure the volume of a liquid medication at the *lowest point* of the meniscus. This medicine cup contains 5 mL of liquid. *Source: Delmar/Cengage Learning*

Universal Precautions

Universal precautions are simple infection-control measures that reduce the risk of transmission of bloodborne pathogens through exposure to blood or body fluids among patients and health care workers. Under the universal precautions principle, blood and body fluids from all people should be considered as infected with HIV, regardless of the known or supposed status of the person. Improving the safety of injections is an important component of universal precautions.

Any percutaneous or permucosal exposure to blood or body fluids represent a potential source of HIV infection. These include skin-piercing procedures with contaminated objects and exposures of broken skin, open wounds, cuts, and mucosal membranes (mouth or eyes) to the blood or body fluid of an infected person.

"Universal precautions," as defined by the Centers for Disease Control and Prevention (CDC), are a set of precautions designed to prevent transmission of the human immunodeficiency virus(HIV), hepatitis B virus (HBV), and other bloodborne pathogens when providing first aid and health care. Under universal precautions, blood and certain body fluids of all patients are considered potentially infectious for HIV, HBV and other blood-borne pathogens.

The following are some of the universal precautions recommended by the CDC.

1. All health care workers should routinely use appropriate barrier precautions to prevent skin and mucous-membrane exposure when contact with blood or other body fluids of any patient is anticipated. Gloves should be worn for touching blood and body fluids, mucous membranes, or nonintact skin of all patients; for handling items or surfaces soiled with blood or body fluids; and for performing venipuncture and other vascular access procedures. Gloves should be changed after contact with each patient. Masks and protective eyewear or face shields should be worn during procedures that are likely to generate droplets of blood or other body fluids to prevent exposure of mucous membranes of the mouth, nose, and eyes. Gowns or aprons should be worn during procedures that are likely to generate splashes of blood or other body fluids.

2. Hands and other skin surfaces should be washed immediately and thoroughly with soap and water if contaminated with blood or other body fluids. Hands should be washed immediately after gloves are removed.

3. All health care workers should take precautions to prevent injuries caused by needles, scalpels, and other sharp instruments or devices during procedures; when cleaning used instruments; during disposal of used needles; and when handling sharp instruments after procedures. To prevent needlestick injuries, needles should not be recapped, purposely bent or broken by hand, removed from disposable syringes, or otherwise manipulated by hand. After they are used, disposable syringes and needles, scalpel blades, and other sharp items should be placed in puncture-resistant containers for disposal; the puncture-resistant containers should be located as close as practical to the use area. Large-bore reusable needles should be placed in a puncture-resistant container for transport to the reprocessing area. Use of new, single-use disposable injection equipment for all injections is highly recommended. Sterilizable injection equipment should only be considered if single-use equipment is not available and if sterility can be documented with time, pressure (steam), and temperature indicators. Sterilization indicators placed within a pack will register that the proper pressure and temperature were present for the required time to allow steam to penetrate to the inner parts of the pack.

4. Mouth-to-mouth resuscitation mouthpieces, resuscitation bags, or other ventilation devices should be available for use in areas in which the need for resuscitation is predictable.

5. Health care workers who have exudative lesions or weeping dermatitis should refrain from all direct patient care and from handling patient-care equipment until the condition improves.

6. Pregnant health care workers are not known to be at greater risk of contracting HIV infection than health care workers who are not pregnant; however, if a health care worker develops HIV infection during pregnancy, the infant is at risk of infection through perinatal transmission. Because of this risk, pregnant health care workers should be especially familiar with and strictly adhere to precautions to minimize the risk of HIV transmission.

Standard Precautions

The CDC recommends a set of infection control guidelines to help protect health care providers, patients, and their visitors from infectious diseases. For all patients, all health care professionals should utilize standard precautions for infection control.

Standard precautions combine many of the basic principles of universal precautions with techniques known as body substance isolation (BSI), a system that maintains that personal protective equipment should be worn during contact with all body fluids whether or not blood is visible. Advantages of the standard precautions are that they include all of the major recommendations of universal precautions and body substance isolation, while incorporating information intended to protect all patients, all health care providers, and all visitors.

According to the CDC, standard precautions are "designed to reduce the risk of transmission of microorganisms, from both recognized and unrecognized sources of infection in hospitals." Standard precautions apply to:

1. blood.
2. all body fluids, secretions, and excretions regardless of whether or not they contain visible blood.
3. nonintact skin.
4. mucous membranes.

To be effective, standard precautions must be practiced conscientiously at all times. Although standard precautions were intended primarily for use in acute care facilities such as hospitals, they should be used by all health care professionals, including those in ambulatory care settings. Figure 10-3 provides a comprehensive review of the standard precautions.

Safe Storage of Medications

All medications not being administered should be kept in a safe storage place. This place may vary from office to office, but certain guides and precautions should be followed.

- Ideally, there should be one room designated as the medication room. This room should be:
  1. well-lighted, away from the flow of patient traffic.
  2. contain a sink and a refrigerator.
  3. have enough cabinet space so that internal drugs, external drugs, and poisonous substances can be kept separate. There should be a drawer or metal box for controlled substances. This drawer or metal box has to be equipped with a double lock.
- There are several ways that drugs may be categorized for safe storage:
  1. Drugs for internal use, external use, and eye use, and poisonous substances must be stored separately.
  2. Drugs may be stored according to:

     Preparation: solid, semisolid, and liquid

     Route: oral, parenteral, application to skin, sublingual, buccal, rectal, vaginal, inhalation, and instillation

     Therapeutic action: classifications (analgesics, antiemetic, etc.)

     Alphabetical order: generic name; trade or brand name

     Principal actions: stimulants, depressants, etc.

     Actions of drugs: according to body systems (cardiovascular, etc.)
- Certain medications must be stored in dark (**opaque**) containers.
- Certain medications must be refrigerated.
- Certain medications must be stored in glass containers.
- All controlled substances must be stored in a substantially constructed metal box or compartment that is equipped with a double lock. The narcotic key must be kept safe from possible misuse.
- All poisonous substances (cleaning materials, etc.) should be labeled in *red.*
- Pharmaceutical drug samples should be properly stored according to the policy of your office. In most offices, these are kept separate from the other medications. Controlled substances samples must be locked up and dispensed only by the physician.
- All medications, supplies, and equipment must be checked on a regular basis to guarantee their freshness.

STANDARD PRECAUTIONS

Assume that every person is potentially infected or colonized with an organism that could be transmitted in the health care setting.

Hand Hygiene

Avoid unnecessary touching of surfaces in close proximity to the patient.

When hands are visibly dirty, contaminated with proteinaceous material, or visibly soiled with blood or body fluids, wash hands with soap and water.

If hands are not visibly soiled, or after removing visible material with soap and water, decontaminate hands with an alcohol-based hand rub. Alternatively, hands may be washed with an antimicrobial soap and water.

Perform hand hygiene:
    Before having direct contact with patients.
    After contact with blood, body fluids or excretions, mucous membranes, nonintact skin, or wound dressings.
    After contact with a patient's intact skin (e.g., when taking a pulse or blood pressure or lifting a patient).
    If hands will be moving from a contaminated body site to a clean body site during patient care.
    After contact with inanimate objects (including medical equipment) in the immediate vicinity of the patient.
    After removing gloves.

Personal Protective Equipment (PPE)

Wear PPE when the nature of the anticipated patient interaction indicates that contact with blood or body fluids may occur.

Before leaving the patient's room or cubicle, remove and discard PPE.

Gloves

Wear gloves when contact with blood or other potentially infectious materials, mucous membranes, nonintact skin, or potentially contaminated intact skin (e.g., of a patient incontinent of stool or urine) could occur.

Remove gloves after contact with a patient and/or the surrounding environment using proper technique to prevent hand contamination. Do not wear the same pair of gloves for the care of more than one patient.

Change gloves during patient care if the hands will move from a contaminated body site (e.g., perineal area) to a clean body site (e.g., face).

Gowns

Wear a gown to protect skin and prevent soiling or contamination of clothing during procedures and patient care activities when contact with blood, body fluids, secretions, or excretions is anticipated.

Wear a gown for direct patient contact if the patient has uncontained secretions or excretions.

Remove gown and perform hand hygiene before leaving the patient's environment.

Mouth, nose, eye protection

Use PPE to protect the mucous membranes of the eyes, nose, and mouth during procedures and patient care activities that are likely to generate splashes or sprays of blood, body fluids, secretions, and excretions.

During aerosol-generating procedures, wear one of the following: a face shield that fully covers the front and sides of the face, a mask with attached shield, or a mask and goggles.

Respiratory Hygiene/Cough Etiquette

Educate health care personnel to contain respiratory secretions to prevent droplet and fomite transmission of respiratory pathogens, especially during seasonal outbreaks of viral respiratory tract infections.

Offer masks to coughing patients and other symptomatic people (e.g., people who accompany ill patients) upon entry into the facility.

Patient Care Equipment and Instruments/Devices

Wear PPE (e.g., gloves, gown), according to the level of anticipated contamination, when handling patient care equipment and instruments/devices that are visibly soiled or may have been in contact with blood or body fluids.

Care of the Environment

Include multiuse electronic equipment in policies and procedures for preventing contamination and for cleaning and disinfection, especially those items that are used by patients, those used during delivery of patient care, and mobile devices that are moved in and out of patient rooms frequently (e.g., daily).

Textiles and Laundry

Handle used textiles and fabrics with minimum agitation to avoid contamination of air, surfaces and people.

FIGURE 10-3

Standard precautions for Infection Control issued by the Centers for Disease Control and Prevention.

Reprinted with permission from Brevis Corporation (www.brevis.com)

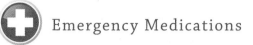 Emergency Medications

The following emergency supplies and medications must be readily available when administering any medication to a patient. These materials should be stored separately from other drugs either on a tray or crash cart, or in a box or cabinet. These supplies and medications are to be checked on a regular basis. Replace any used items and discard any outdated drugs or supplies.

epinephrine (ep-i-nef-rin)

A vasoconstrictor. Relieves anaphylactic shock.

aminophylline (am-in-off'ilin)

A bronchodilator. Relaxes smooth muscle of the respiratory tract.

Benadryl (ben'a-dril)—diphenhydramine

An antihistamine that relieves allergic symptoms.

Phenergan (fen'ar-gan)—promethazine

An antiemetic. Relieves symptoms of nausea and vomiting.

dextrose (deks'trose) **50%**

Used for hypoglycemia to counteract hyperinsulinism.

digoxin (di-jox'in)

Cardiac drug. Used for congestive heart failure, arrhythmias. Slows and strengthens heartbeat.

Dilantin (di-lan'tin)—phenytoin

Anticonvulsant. Used in grand mal and partial seizure epilepsy and cardiac arrhythmias induced by digitalis.

glucagon (gloo-ka'gon)

Hyperglycemic agent. Used for hypoglycemia.

hydrocortisone (hi''dro-cort'i-zon)

An anti-inflammatory. Used to suppress swelling and shock.

Lasix (las'ik)—furosemide

Promotes excretion of urine.

lidocaine (lie-doh'cane)

Antiarrhythmic. Used for ventricular arrhythmias.

morphine sulfate (mor'fen sul'fat)

Narcotic analgesic. Used for severe pain.

Naloxone hydrochloride (na'lak-son hy-dro'klar-id)

Antidote. Used in narcotic overdose.

nitroglycerin (ni''tro-glis'er-in)

Vasodilator. Dilates coronary arteries. Used in treatment of angina pectoris.

sodium bicarbonate (so'de-um bi-kar'bo-nat)

Alkalinizing agent. Used for metabolic acidosis caused by diseases, drugs, or chemicals.

Valium (val'e-um)—diazepam

Antianxiety, muscle relaxant. Used to calm very anxious patients and to relax muscles. Also used for status epilepticus.

Supplies and Equipment

Intravenous materials such as IV fluids, tourniquet, syringes and needles, alcohol swabs, sterile dry cotton balls

Blood pressure monitoring equipment: stethoscope and sphygmomanometer

Adult, child, infant disposable mask resuscitators

Automated external defibrillator (AED)

CPR equipment (such as face shields, compact barrier, mouth shields, Ambu-Bag)

Elastic and gauze bandages

Gloves

Goggles/face shields

Laryngoscope, endotracheal tubes

Nebulizers

Ophthalmoscope

Oral airways

Otoscope

Oxygen

Oxygen mask or cannula

Penlight

Suction equipment

DOCUMENTATION OF DRUG ADMINISTRATION

The recording process is the vital link between the physician, the patient, and the medical assistant. It is an account of essential data that are collected and preserved. The patient's chart is a legal document; therefore, all data should be carefully recorded. The data should be accurate and clearly stated. It is important that the following data about drug administration be entered in the patient's chart.

- The patient's name
- The date and time of administration
- The name of the medication and the amount (dosage) administered
- The route by which the medication was administered and the injection site used
- The right technique used. It is important that you know the proper technique for administering the various forms of medications presented in Units 11 through 14, the proper route to use, any specific directions to follow, and all safety measures as presented in Section 2 of this text.
- Any adverse reactions experienced by the patient
- Any complications in administering the drug (patient refusing to take the medication, difficulty in swallowing, and so forth)
- If the medication was *not given*, state why, and dispose of the medication according to agency policy
- Patient data, such as blood pressure, pulse, and respiration.

Example of Documenting Drug Administration Data

Ramona Sawyer   age 33
6/22/xx   9:30 am
Benadryl 25 mg PO
For contact dermatitis, right palm
T 98.6 F
P 74
R 16
B/P 118/76

                              J. Rice, RN, CMA

- The effectiveness of the drug (for example, a patient with Parkinson's disease shows improvement after three weeks of treatment with Levodopa)
- Your name or initials and title

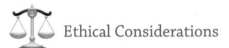

Ethical Considerations

Anyone who has access to medications may be tempted to use them for personal benefit. To do so is not only unethical, it is illegal. The conversion to personal use of medications intended for another is both unethical and may cause harm to the patient. It is also unethical and illegal to take any medication, even aspirin, that belongs to your employer without proper authorization.

MEDICATION ERROR

Medication errors should not happen when personnel follow the "seven rights" of proper drug administration and the essential medication guidelines; however, honest mistakes will be made periodically. A medication error occurs when any of the following actions are taken.

- A drug is given to the wrong *patient*.
- The wrong *drug* is given.
- The wrong *dose* is administered.
- The drug is given via the wrong *route*.
- The drug is given at the wrong *time*.
- The wrong *technique* was used.
- The wrong *data* was documented.

When a medication error occurs, this is the procedure to follow:

1. Recognize that an error has been made.
2. Stay calm. Assess the patient's condition and/or reactions to the medication.
3. Report the error immediately to the appropriate physician. Give the details of the mistake and the patient's reactions.
4. Follow the physician's order for correcting the error.

5. Document the error in the patient's record and complete an institution's incident form.
   - Describe the type of error.
   - Describe the patient's reactions.
   - Describe the steps taken to correct the error.
   - State the date, time, and your name.

Reactions to Medications

Reactions to medications can be favorable or unfavorable. Usually, the drug used will produce its intended response; however, potentially dangerous reactions can occur. When administering medications, one should make a written report describing the patient's responses to the drug. Written documentation is particularly important in those cases that involve an adverse reaction to a medication. Documentation of drug reactions should include the patient's name, prescriber's name, date, time, medication used, the nature of the reaction, and the name of the person who administered the medication.

You may voluntarily report an adverse event and problem to the FDA through their MedWatch program. The purpose of the MedWatch program is to enhance the effectiveness of post-marketing surveillance of medical products as they are used in clinical practice and to rapidly identify significant health hazards associated with these products. The program has four goals:

1. To increase awareness of drug and device-induced disease.
2. To clarify what should (and should not) be reported to the agency.
3. To make it easier to report by operating a single system for health professionals to report adverse events and product problems to the agency.
4. To provide regular feedback to the health care community about safety issues involving medical products.

Adverse events and product problems that occur with vaccines should not be reported to the MedWatch program or on the MedWatch form but should be sent to the joint FDA/CDC Vaccine Adverse Event Reporting System (VAERS). To report such an event, one may call 1-800-822-7967 for a copy of the VAERS form.

The FDA MedWatch program offers advice about voluntary reporting and you may obtain additional information by visiting www.fda.gov/medwatch or calling 1-800-FDA-1088.

■ ■ REVIEW QUESTIONS

Directions. Select the best answer to each of the following multiple-choice questions, circling the letter of your choice:

1. _____ is an individual hypersensitivity to a substance.

   a. Antibody   b. Antigen   c. Allergy   d. none of the above

2. Individuals who prepare and administer medications are expected to be _____.

   a. licensed   c. authorized by a physician to do so

   b. registered or certified   d. all of the above

3. Acting as an agent of the physician, one must be _____.

   a. qualified   b. responsible   c. accountable   d. all of the above

4. When reading a medication label, you should _____.

   a. always check for the expiration date of the medicine

   b. compare the medication order with the label

   c. read the label four times

   d. a and b

5. When administering a medication in a physician's office, the best method of identifying the patient is _____.

    a. checking the patient's identification bracelet

    b. calling the patient by name

    c. asking the patient to state his or her name

    d. b and c

6. Whish is most essential for a medication to be maintained at the proper blood level, for it to be given _____.

    a. by the right route   c. in the right dose

    b. at the right time   d. in the right drug

7. When reading the correct amount of a liquid medication that has been poured in a measuring device, _____.

    a. read at the top of the meniscus   c. read at the lowest level of the meniscus

    b. read at the level of the meniscus   d. all of these

8. _____ is a substance, in the form of fine particles, that separates from a solution if allowed to stand for a period of time.

    a. Meniscus   b. Precipitate   c. Solvent   d. Solute

9. Essential medication guidelines include all of the following except _____.

    a. working in a dim-lighted area   c. following the six rights

    b. always checking for allergies   d. being completely familiar with each drug

10. All of the following are true statements about safe drug storage except that _____.

    a. certain medications must be refrigerated

    b. controlled substances must be stored along with other drugs

    c. emergency supplies and medications must be readily available

    d. all poisonous substances should be labeled in red

11. All of the following are true statements about the recording process except that _____.

    a. it provides a vital link between the physician, patient, and medical assistant

    b. all data should be accurate and clearly stated

    c. all data should be written in ink or typed

    d. the patient's chart is not a legal document

12. It is _____ to take any medication that belongs to your employer.

    a. ethical   b. unethical   c. illegal   d. b and c

13. A medication error occurs when _____.

    a. the right dose is administered   c. the right route is used

    b. the right drug is given   d. the drug is given to the wrong patient

14. When a medication error occurs, do all of the following except _____.

    a. stay calm, assess the patient's condition

    b. tell the patient that you have made an error

    c. report the error to the physician

    d. document the error in the patient's record

Matching. Place the correct letter from Column II on the appropriate line of Column I:

Column I			*Column II*

15. _____ meniscus

16. _____ precipitate

17. _____ allergy

18. _____ "seven rights"

19. _____ recording process

20. _____ opaque

21. _____ illegal

22. _____ ethical

23. _____ unethical

24. _____ patient's chart

25. _____ emergency medications

A. a checklist of activities to ensure the safe delivery of a medication to a patient

B. the vital link between the physician, the patient, and the medical assistant

C. pertaining to a system of moral principles or standards that govern conduct

D. pertaining to things unlawful; not legal

E. dark; not transparent

F. the convex or concave upper surface of a column of liquid in a container

G. a substance in the form of fine particles

H. an individual hypersensitivity to a substance

I. a legal document

J. epinephrine, Benadryl, and hydrocortisone

K. pertaining to any action that goes against a system of moral principles or standards that govern conduct

L. a checklist of activities to ensure the unsafe delivery of a medication to a patient

UNIT 11
Administration of Nonparenteral Medications

OBJECTIVES

Upon completing this unit, you should be able to:

- Define the terms listed in the vocabulary.
- List several advantages and disadvantages of the oral route of drug administration.
- Describe the measuring devices most commonly used when administering oral medications.
- Administer oral medications.
- State the guidelines that should be followed whenever it is necessary to crush a solid medication.
- Perform an eye instillation.
- Perform an ear instillation.
- Describe the administration of nasal medications.
- Describe a transdermal system.
- Describe inhalation and give three uses of inhalation therapy.
- State the implications for patient care when an inhaler is prescribed.
- List the signs and symptoms of hypoxemia.
- List the symptoms of oxygen toxicity.
- Describe the methods used for oxygen delivery.
- Describe oxygen safety precautions.
- Describe the administration of drugs by local application.
- Answer the review questions correctly.

VOCABULARY

angina pectoris (an-ji'na pek'to-ris). A severe pain about the heart. The pain may radiate to the left shoulder, down the left arm, and up to the jaw or through to the back.

cannula (kan'u-la). Tubing used to deliver oxygen at levels from 1 to 6 L/min.

canthus (kan'thus). The angle at either end of the slit between the eyelids; the corner of the eye.

enema (en'e-ma). The means of delivering a solution or medication into the rectum and colon.

hypoxemia (hi-poks-ee'-mee-a). A deficient amount of oxygen in the blood.

inhalation (in"ha-la'shun). The act of drawing breath, vapor, or gas into the lungs.

inhaler (in"hal'er). A small handheld apparatus, usually an aerosol unit, that contains a microcrystalline suspension of medication.

insertion (in-sur'shun). The placement or implanting of something into something else.

instillation (in"stil-ay'-shun). The process of slowly pouring or dropping a liquid onto or into a body cavity or its surface.

inunction (in-ungk'shun). The application of a drug by rubbing it onto the skin.

irrigation (ir"a-ga'shun). The cleansing of a canal by flushing with water or other fluids.

nitroglycerin (ni"tro-glis'er-in). A glyceryl trinitrate that is a vasodilator. It is used in the treatment of *angina pectoris*.

ointment (oynt'ment). A semisolid preparation consisting of a drug combined with a base of petroleum jelly or lanolin.

oxygen (ok'si-jen). A colorless, odorless, tasteless gas that is essential for life.

(continues)

123

> **suppository** (su-poz'i-to-re). A semisolid substance for introduction of medication into the rectum, vagina, or urethra, where it dissolves.
>
> **transdermal system** (trans-der-mal sis'tem). A small adhesive patch or disk, which contains a drug, that may be applied to the body near the treatment site.

INTRODUCTION

Nonparenteral medications are those that are administered by any route other than by injection. In this chapter, nonparenteral methods of medication described are oral, ophthalmic, otic, nasal, rectal, special delivery, by inhalation, by local application, and administration of oxygen.

ORAL MEDICATIONS

The method by which a medicine is to be administered is determined by the condition of the patient, the disease or illness, the rate of absorption desired, and the form of the drug available. The most common method of administering a medication is by mouth. Sometimes referred to as the *administration of oral medications*, the use of the oral route of giving a drug offers the safest, most convenient, and most economical method available.

Drugs administered by mouth may be in a solid or a liquid form. Some of the solid forms are tablets, capsules, and caplets. These drugs are usually swallowed with a drink of water.

Not all drugs administered by mouth are swallowed. Although they are oral medications, those drug forms that are not swallowed are referred to as *sublingual* or *buccal medicines*. These terms refer to the route by which the drug is absorbed into the body. Sublingual medications, such as nitroglycerin tablets, are placed under the tongue. Buccal tablets are placed between the cheek and gum and allowed to dissolve. Another solid medication that is allowed to dissolve in the mouth is the *lozenge*, which is used for coughs and sore throats.

Liquid preparations include solutions, suspensions, elixirs, and syrups. These forms of medication are absorbed more rapidly than solid forms. Liquid medications are often artificially colored and flavored to disguise their true appearance and taste. A drug that has an agreeable taste and appearance often has a favorable psychological effect upon the patient.

Weight and volume are both used in measuring the amount of medication to be administered. The volume of a liquid medication may be measured in milliliters, cubic centimeters, drams, ounces, and by such household measures as teaspoons. Both solid and liquid forms of drugs can be measured in terms of weight. Dosages may be in micrograms, milligrams, grams, grains, milliequivalents, or units.

The amount of medication in the average dose for adults and children is based upon the age and weight of the individual. The average adult patient is between 20 and 60 years of age and weighs 150 pounds.

Oral medications are easily and economically administered with a high degree of safety. There are, however, several disadvantages associated with the oral route. For instance, the drug may

- Have an objectionable odor.
- Have an objectionable taste.
- Cause discoloration of the teeth, mouth, and tongue.
- Irritate the gastric mucosa.
- Be altered by digestive enzymes.
- Be poorly absorbed from the digestive system, due to illness or nature of the medication.
- Come in a form (tablet, capsule, or caplet) that is too large for the patient to swallow.
- Be difficult or impossible to take because of nausea and/or vomiting.
- Be refused by the patient.
- Have less predictable effects upon the body when given orally than when given by the parenteral route (by injection).

EQUIPMENT AND SUPPLIES

The equipment and supplies used in the administration of oral medications may include the following items:

- Medication order
- Medication record system
- Medication cart
- Medication cabinet
- Medication tray
- Medicine cup (plastic, glass, or paper)
- Medicine dropper
- Water cup (plastic, paper)
- Drinking straws
- Syringes
- Tablet crusher
- Other: refrigerator, sink, soap, paper towels, and a pen

Three measuring devices commonly used in the administration of oral medications are the medicine cup, the water cup, and the medicine dropper. The medicine cup (see Figure 11-1) comes in various sizes and shapes, depending upon its manufacturer and its intended use. In the illustration provided, note that the cup is calibrated in fluid ounces (oz), fluid drams (dr), milliliters (mL), teaspoons (tsp), and tablespoons (tbs).

The water cup is a small plastic or paper cup that is disposable and holds 3 ounces of liquid. The medicine dropper may be calibrated in milliliters or drops. Medicine droppers are often provided as a part of the container with many medications (see Figure 11-2). Uncalibrated droppers may be provided when the medicine

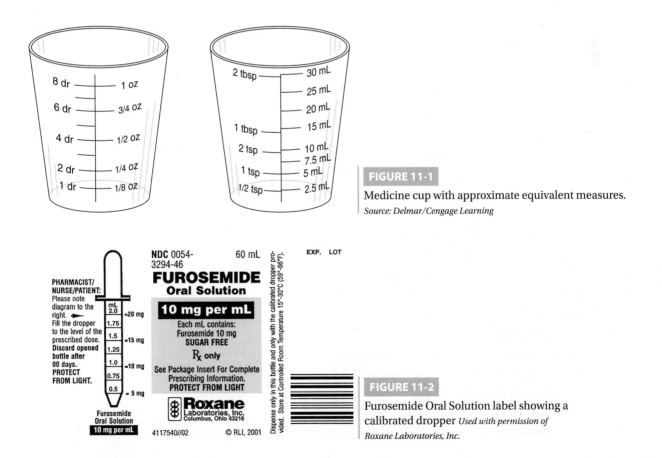

FIGURE 11-1

Medicine cup with approximate equivalent measures.

Source: Delmar/Cengage Learning

FIGURE 11-2

Furosemide Oral Solution label showing a calibrated dropper *Used with permission of Roxane Laboratories, Inc.*

is administered only in drops. The size of the drop varies with the size of the dropper opening, the angle at which it is held, the force exerted on the rubber bulb, and the viscosity of the medication.

It is important that you select the appropriate container for a medication and measure the prescribed dosage accurately. The selection of the container depends upon the physical structure of the medication (solid or liquid), the amount of medication prescribed, the size of the container, and the calibrations on the container.

ADMINISTRATION OF ORAL MEDICATIONS

Earlier chapters of this section provided information on drug sources, standards, dosages, the forms of drugs, and drug actions. Also covered were responsibilities in the administration of medications, and the types of medicine orders. With this background, it is now time to apply this knowledge to the preparation and administration of oral medications.

Before beginning, however, note that because oral medications may be in solid or liquid form, different procedures are employed, depending upon which form is used. In addition, medications may be supplied in unit-dose or multiple-dose containers. Thus, different procedural steps are necessary when there is a difference in the way medications are supplied.

Using A Multiple-Dose Solid Medication

- Remove the cap from the container in which the medicine is supplied. (Touch only the outside of the cap to avoid contamination.)
- Dispense the prescribed amount of solid medicine into the container's cap. (Do not touch the medication.)
- Transfer the medication from the cap to the disposable paper cup.
- Recap the medication container.
- Dispense only one medication at a time.

Using a Multiple-Dose Liquid Medication

- Shake the preparation if it is a precipitate (or if the instructions call for it to be shaken).
- Remove the cap from the medication bottle.
- Place the cap, open side up, on a flat surface. (This prevents contamination of the part of the cap that is in contact with the medicine bottle.)
- With the label covered by the palm of your hand (to safeguard the label from becoming stained), pour the liquid medicine into an appropriate measuring device.
- When pouring, always hold the measuring device at eye level (see Figure 11-3).
- When pouring, do not allow the bottle to come into contact with the measuring device.

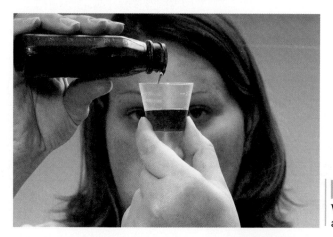

FIGURE 11-3

When pouring, always hold the measuring device at eye level. *Source: Delmar/Cengage Learning*

- Measure the medicine at the lowest level of the meniscus.
- After pouring, cleanse the bottle, if necessary. (If the label becomes soiled, a pharmacist must relabel the medication.)
- Recap the medication bottle.

Using a Unit-Dose Solid or Liquid Medication

- It is best to open a unit-dose medication when you are at the patient's side. (If the patient refuses the medication, an unopened unit-dose medication does not have to be discarded.) However, when you have to give $\frac{1}{2}$ tablet, you generally bisect the tablet before entering the patient's room and the $\frac{1}{2}$ tablet not given is properly discarded.
- Open the package according to the directions on its label.
- Without touching the medication, place it into the patient's hand (or pour it into an appropriate container).

Safety Precautions:

Following the administration of an oral medication, the medical assistant should observe the patient for any adverse reactions, check the medication label for the third time, and document the procedure. The final steps in the procedure involve the disposal and aftercare of the equipment and supplies. The medical assistant should:

- *Properly discard disposable materials.*
- *Return any unused supplies to the designated area.*
- *Clean and return reusable materials to the designated area.*
- *Perform the medical asepsis hand wash.*

Practice Session

Study the procedural steps for administration of oral medications. Then, with the permission of your instructor, practice the procedure. Where possible, have another student act as your patient. See Procedure 11-1, Administration of Oral Medications.

PROCEDURE 11-1
Administration of Oral Medications

Standard Precautions:

Purpose:
Correctly administer an oral medication after receiving a physician's order and oral medication, and assembling the necessary equipment and supplies.

Equipment/Supplies:
Proper medication
Medicine card
Water, milk, or juice for patient

Procedure Steps:
1. Verify the physician's order.
2. Follow the "seven rights" (Figure 11-4A).

(continues)

PROCEDURE 11-1 *continued*
Administration of Oral Medications

Procedure Steps (continued):

3. Perform medical asepsis hand wash.
4. Work in a well-lighted, quiet, clean area.
5. Assemble equipment and supplies.
6. Obtain the correct medication.
7. Compare the medication label with the order (first time).
8. Check the expiration date.
9. Calculate dosage if necessary.
10. Compare the medicine label with the order (second time).
11. Correctly prepare (a, b, or c) (Figure 11-4B).
    a. *Multiple-dose solid medication*
    b. *Unit-dose medication*
    c. *Liquid medication*
12. Compare the medication label with the order (third time).
13. Properly transport the medicine.
14. Identify the patient. Explain the procedure.
15. Assess patient. Take vital signs if indicated.
16. Assist patient to a comfortable position.
17. Provide water, milk, or juice (unless contraindicated).
18. Administer the medication. Be certain that the patient takes the medicine (Figure 11-4C).
19. Provide for the patient's safety: Observe the patient for any adverse reactions.
20. Document the procedure.
21. Care for equipment and supplies according to OSHA guidelines.
22. Wash hands.

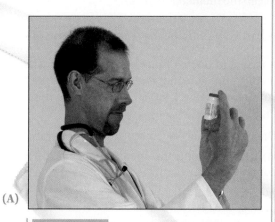

(A)

FIGURE 11-4

(A) Medical assistant checks for right drug, right dose, right route, and expiration date before pouring medication.

Source: Delmar/Cengage Learning

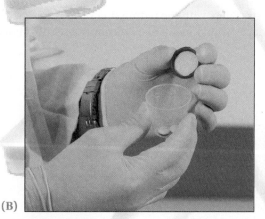

(B)

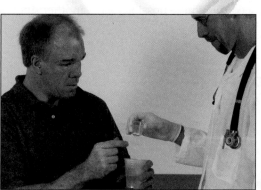

(C)

FIGURE 11-4

continued (B) The medical assistant pours tablets from the cover of the medicine container into a medicine cup prior to administering medicine to the patient. The medication is poured into the cover to avoid contamination of medicine. (C) The medical assistant administers the medication, being certain that the patient takes the medicine. *Source: Delmar/Cengage Learning*

Preparing and Administering a Crushed Medicine

There may be a time when your patient is not able to swallow a tablet and the medicine does not come in any other form. When this occurs, you may have to crush the solid medicine and mix it with either food or a liquid. To do this, you need to know which medicines can be crushed and which cannot. Certain medications, such as time released tablets, are designed to dissolve at a specified rate and should not be crushed. Some medicines should be taken with food and others on an empty stomach. Some should be followed by a full glass of water. Before you crush any medicine, ask the prescribing provider if you can crush the medicine and mix it with another substance. Whenever it is necessary to crash a solid medication, the following guidelines should be followed:

1. If you have any questions as to whether a medication should be crushed, ask the pharmacist or the prescribing physician before attempting to crush the medicine.

2. As a general rule, most compressed tablets may be crushed.

3. Buccal or sublingual tablets, sustained-release tablets, and enteric-coated tablets should not be crushed. To do so would alter the effect of these medications.

4. When possible, avoid crushing Ecotrin, E-Mycin, and Dulcolax, because these drugs may cause gastric irritation when crushed.

5. As a rule, hard capsules should not be crushed. Some capsules can be pulled apart to allow the dry powder to be removed.

6. Unit-dose medications should be crushed in the wrapper prior to opening.

The method used to crush a tablet depends upon the equipment available. A specially designed tablet crusher or a mortar and pestle are the best devices for crushing tablets. When these are not available, one may use two spoons to crush the medicine. Great care must be taken to ensure that none of the medication is lost in the crushing process (see Figures 11-5, 11-6, and 11-7).

If the patient's diet permits, one may use small amounts of food (applesauce, strained fruit, pudding, ice cream) as a vehicle for administering a crushed medicine. The patient should be informed that the prescribed medication is in the food or liquid. The entire amount of food or liquid used as a vehicle must be consumed; this is why small amounts should be used as some patients may not be able to tolerate regular portions.

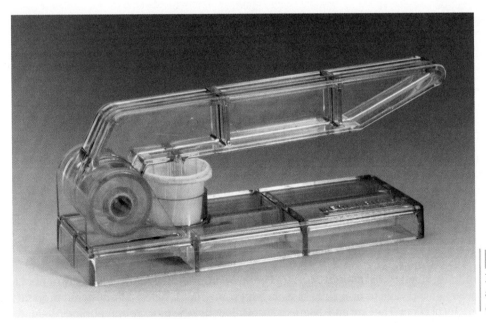

FIGURE 11-5

Deluxe Medi-Crush Pill and Tablet Crusher.

Courtesy of EDI-DOSE/EPS, Inc.

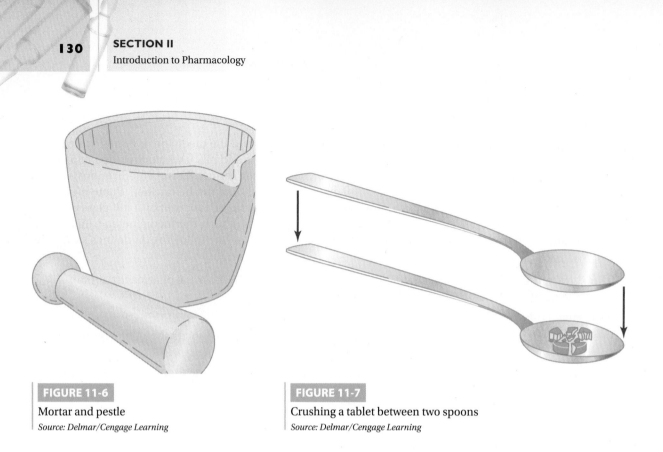

FIGURE 11-6
Mortar and pestle
Source: Delmar/Cengage Learning

FIGURE 11-7
Crushing a tablet between two spoons
Source: Delmar/Cengage Learning

Using a Syringe to Administer a Liquid Oral Medicine

When a patient is unable to take a liquid medicine from a cup or other container, one may use a syringe to administer the medication. Should it become necessary to use this method, be sure that you follow the correct procedure for administering a medication. After identifying the patient and explaining the procedure, it is best to squirt the medicine into the side of the patient's mouth, to prevent choking or having the patient spit the medicine back out. Care should be taken that the patient does not aspirate the medicine.

Safety Precautions:

When prepared by the pharmacist, oral preparations in syringes should be brightly labeled as a safety precaution against accidental intramuscular injection.

Devices Used for Administering Oral Medications to a Child

There are various devices that may be used to administer an oral medication to a child (see Figure 11-8). It is essential that you measure the exact prescribed dosage of medication that is to be administered. The calibrated devices are in teaspoons and milliliters. There are 5 milliliters to a teaspoon.

ADMINISTRATION OF OPHTHALMIC MEDICATIONS

Ophthalmic medications are administered by *instillation* (slowly pouring or dropping a liquid into a cavity or onto a surface) or by *application* (the act of applying; to bring into contact with something). When administered properly, ophthalmic medications have a local effect. The rate and extent of absorption into the mucous membranes depends upon the vascularity and the thickness of the membrane. See Procedure 11-2, Performing Eye Instillation.

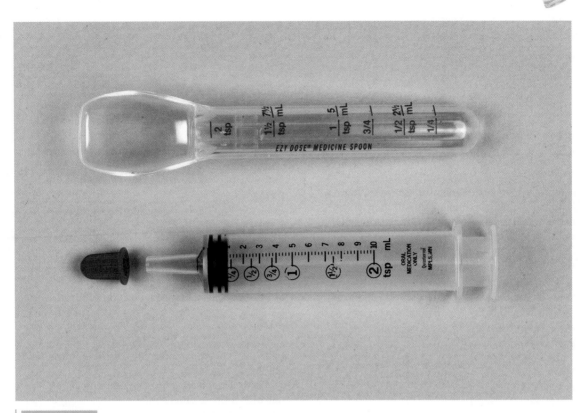

Devices for administering oral medications to children *Source: Delmar/Cengage Learning*

Safety Precautions:

Ophthalmic medications can cause systemic symptoms if the medicine is allowed to flow into the lacrimal sac, where the medicine is absorbed into the general circulation.

To apply eye ointment:

- Place the hand in which you are holding the ointment against the patient's forehead (directly over the eye to be medicated).
- Gently squeeze the prescribed medication along the conjunctival border.

● *Note*

Start at the inner canthus and spread the medication outward toward the outer canthus. ●

- Ask the patient to close the eyes and to gently roll the eyes around to distribute the ointment.
- Remove any excess ointment with a sterile gauze pad.

● *Note*

Instruct the patient not to rub the eyes, and to remain in the supine position for approximately 5 minutes. ●

PROCEDURE 11-2
Performing Eye Instillation

Standard Precautions:

Purpose:

To treat eye infections, soothe irritation, anesthetize, and dilate pupils. Ophthalmic medication is supplied in liquid or ointment form. Use separate medication for each eye, if both are affected.

Equipment/Supplies:

Sterile eye dropper
Sterile ophthalmic medication as ordered by the physician, either drops or ointment
Sterile cotton balls
Sterile gloves

Procedure Steps:

1. Wash hands.
2. Assemble supplies.
3. Check medication carefully as ordered by the physician, including expiration date. Read label three times.
4. Identify patient.
5. Explain procedure to the patient and inform the patient that instillation may temporarily blur vision.
6. Position the patient in a sitting or lying position.
7. Instruct the patient to stare at a fixed spot during instillation of the drops. Put on gloves.
8. Prepare medication using either drops or ointment.
9. Have the patient look up to the ceiling and expose the lower conjunctival sac of the affected eye by using fingers to pull down on the tissue (Figure 11-9).
10. Place the number of drops ordered in the center of the lower conjunctival sac or a thin line of ointment in the lower surface of the eyelid being careful not to touch the eyelid, eyeball, or eyelashes with the tip of the medication applicator. Carefully replace dropper in the bottle to avoid contamination.
11. Have the patient close the eye and roll the eyeball. RATIONALE: Movement distributes the medication evenly.
12. Blot excess medication from eyelids with cotton ball from inner to outer canthus.
13. Dispose of supplies.
14. Remove gloves.
15. Wash hands.
16. Document procedure.

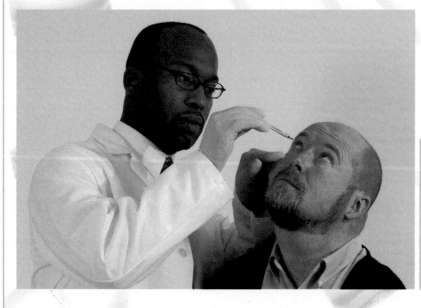

FIGURE 11-9

When medication is being instilled into a patient's eye, the patient should look up to the ceiling while the medical assistant pulls down on the lower eyelid.

Source: Delmar/Cengage Learning

ADMINISTRATION OF OTIC MEDICATIONS

Otic medications are usually administered by instillation. They may be used to treat infection and inflammation, to soften cerumen, to produce a local anesthetic effect, or to immobilize a trapped insect. Ear drops are usually contraindicated if the patient has a perforated eardrum, is hypersensitive to any ingredient in its formula, or has certain conditions such as herpes, other viral infections, or systemic fungal infections (see Procedure 11-3, Performing Ear Instillation).

PROCEDURE 11-3
Performing Ear Instillation

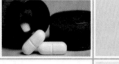

Standard Precautions:

Purpose:

To soften impacted cerumen, fight infection with antibiotics, or relieve pain.

Equipment/Supplies:

Otic medication as prescribed by the physician
Sterile ear dropper
Cotton balls
Gloves

Procedure Steps:

1. Wash hands and assemble supplies.
2. Identify patient.
3. Explain procedure to the patient.
4. Position patient to either lie on unaffected side or sitting position with head tilted toward unaffected ear. RATIONALE: Facilitates flow of medication.
5. Check otic medication three times against the physician's order and check expiration date of the medication. RATIONALE: Only otic medication can be used in the ear. Checking the medication three times minimizes medication error.
6. Draw up the prescribed amount of medication. Put on gloves.
7. Gently pull the top of the ear upward and back (adult) or pull earlobe downward and backward (child) (Figure 11-10).
8. Instill prescribed dose of medication (number of drops) into the affected ear by squeezing rubber bulb on dropper.

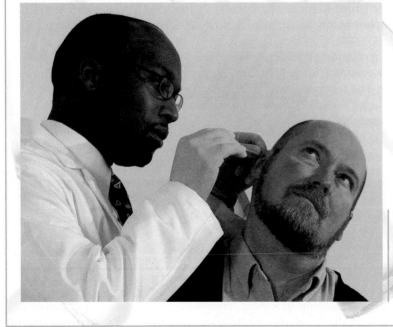

FIGURE 11-10

When drops are being instilled into a patient's ear, the patient should tilt the head so the affected ear is uppermost.

Source: Delmar/Cengage Learning

PROCEDURE 11-3 *continued*
Performing Ear Instillation

9. Have the patient maintain the position for about 5 minutes to retain medication.

10. When instructed by the physician, insert moistened cotton ball into external ear canal for 15 minutes. RATIONALE: Moistened cotton ball will not absorb medication and will help retain medication in ear.

11. Dispose of supplies.

12. Remove gloves.

13. Wash hands.

14. Document procedure.

ADMINISTRATION OF NASAL MEDICATIONS

Nasal medications are usually administered by instillation, spray, or nasal inhaler. They may be used to treat the symptoms of seasonal or perennial rhinitis, and to relieve nasal congestion due to colds and sinusitis. Nose drops, sprays, and inhalers are usually contraindicated in patients who are hypersensitive to any ingredient in their formula. These medications should be used as directed, and one must not exceed the recommended dosage. Continued long-term use of nasal sprays may lead to rebound congestion (swelling and congestion of the nasal mucosa).

Nasal medications are usually best administered by the patient. The patient should be instructed to clear the nasal passageway before instilling nose drops, or using a spray or inhaler. Caution patients not to use any over-the-counter drugs without advice from their physician.

ADMINISTRATION OF RECTAL MEDICATIONS

Rectal medications are usually administered by instillation or insertion. The medication may be in the form of a suppository, ointment, or enema. A **suppository** (a semisolid substance for introducing medication into the rectum, vagina, or urethra, where it dissolves) may be used as a contact laxative acting directly on the colonic mucosa to produce normal peristalsis throughout the large intestine; as a narcotic analgesic; as a local anesthetic inhibiting pain, burning, and itching; as an anti-inflammatory agent; as an antipyretic agent; as an antiemetic to relieve nausea and vomiting; and as a sedative.

An **enema** is the means of delivering a solution or medication into the rectum and colon. An enema may also be used to cleanse the lower bowel in preparation for radiography, sigmoidoscopy, proctoscopy, endoscopy, surgery, and many other special procedures. The ready-to-use Fleet enema may be utilized in a hospital, nursing home, extended care facility, home, or physician's office. It is not to be administered to children under 2 years of age or to patients with undiagnosed abdominal pain.

Safety Precautions:

By introducing an enema or suppository into the rectum, a vagal response may occur, which slows the heart rate, or could even cause it to stop.

An **ointment** is a semisolid preparation consisting of a drug combined with a base of petroleum jelly or lanolin. These forms are not water-soluble; however, some ointments are composed of ingredients that are water-soluble. Ointments are generally applied externally to the skin, but certain ointments are prepared for rectal administration. An example is Preparation H hemorrhoidal ointment that is used to help shrink swelling of hemorrhoidal tissues caused by inflammation and to give prompt, temporary relief in many cases from pain and itching. Before applying, remove the protective cover from the applicator. The applicator must be lubricated before each application and the applicator must be cleansed after each use.

SPECIAL DELIVERY MEDICATIONS

Today, because of technological advances, there are new ways by which a drug can be prepared and delivered to a patient. Some of these preparations are known as *special delivery systems* that provide the drug to a targeted area. Others are modified preparations of the conventional form of the drug.

A **transdermal system** is a small adhesive patch or disk that may be applied to the body near the treatment site. A transdermal system generally consists of four layers:

1. An impermeable back that keeps the drug from leaking out of the system
2. A reservoir containing the drug
3. A membrane with tiny holes in it that controls the rate of drug release
4. An adhesive layer or gel that keeps the device in place

The physician will evaluate each patient very carefully before prescribing any type of medication. There are warnings, precautions, adverse reactions, and other valuable information supplied by the manufacturer. It is essential that the prescribing physician and staff be totally familiar with all aspects of a drug before it is prescribed for a patient.

As a medical assistant, you may be responsible for instructing the patient in how to use and apply a transdermal system. It is important to read to the patient the instructions that accompany the medication. Each manufacturer of transdermal systems provides this information.

> ### ✚ Safety Precautions:
>
> *It is most important to teach the patient to remove the patch that is in place before applying a new one. It is best to rotate the site of application for each new patch.*

Transdermal systems may be used to administer **nitroglycerin**. Nitroglycerin is a smooth-muscle relaxant with vascular effects manifested predominantly by venous dilatation and pooling. The major beneficial effect of nitroglycerin in **angina pectoris** is a reduction in myocardial oxygen consumption, secondary to vascular smooth-muscle relaxation with resultant reduction in cardiac preload and afterload.

ADMINISTERING DRUGS BY INHALATION

The inhalation technique is used for the purpose of providing cold or warm air, usually in the form of medicated steam or aerosol therapy, for the patient to breathe at intervals prescribed by the physician. Drugs administered by this method produce either a local or systemic effect and are given by inhalation for the following reasons:

- To provide local treatment for infections of the respiratory tract when these areas can be treated only by vapor. For example, steam (moist) inhalations are used to relieve inflammation due to colds. The steam may or may not contain a drug.

- To provide systemic treatment for serious respiratory infections. For example, when oxygen is forced under pressure through a nebulizer containing penicillin or another antibiotic, fine particles of the drug are carried into the respiratory tract. The medium is the cold air.

- To supply a medication that can be absorbed into the bloodstream through the lungs, thereby producing a rapid systemic effect. An example is the use of aromatic spirits of ammonia. It is used to elicit stimulation of respiration and as "smelling salts" to stimulate people who have fainted.

Inhalation Methods

The act of drawing breath, vapor, or gas into the lungs is known as inhalation. Inhalation therapy may involve the administration of medicines, water vapor, and such gases as oxygen, carbon dioxide, and helium.

An inhaler may be used to deliver medications to the lungs. Medications that utilize an inhaler include bronchodilators, mucolytic agents, and steroids. Inhalers are useful in the delivery of treatment for chronic obstructive pulmonary disease (COPD) and reversible obstructive airway disease. An inhaler is a small handheld apparatus, usually an aerosol unit, that contains a microcrystalline suspension of medication (see Figure 11-11). When activated, it produces a fine mist or spray containing the medication. This suspension is then drawn into the respiratory tract, settling deep into the lungs and alveoli.

A metered-dose inhaler (MDI) is a device that delivers a specific amount of medication to the lungs, in the form of a short burst of aerosolized medicine that the patient inhales. It is most commonly used delivery system for treating asthma, chronic obstructive pulmonary disease (COPD), and other respiratory conditions. A metered-dose inhaler contains enough medication for a given number of puffs. This number is printed on the canister and it is important for the patient to keep a record of the number of times the inhaler is used. Even though the inhaler may continue to work beyond that number of uses, it should be discarded and not used again.

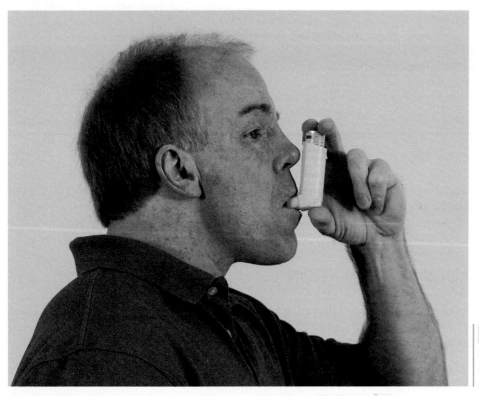

FIGURE 11-11

Self-administration with a metered-dose inhaler

Source: Delmar/Cengage Learning

Clinical Considerations for the Use of an Inhaler

- Patients should be instructed to follow the physician's order. The prescribed medicine and the type of inhaler to be used will determine the method of administration. The types of inhalers available for use are:
  — Handheld. This type includes nasal and oral inhalers.
  — Nebulizers. This type is for or large-volume (heated or cool) delivery, ultrasonic, and side-stream diffusion.
  — Intermittent positive-pressure breathing (IPPB) machines.
- Patients should be advised to avoid overuse of the inhaler. Tolerance, rebound bronchospasm, and adverse cardiac effects can occur from overuse.
- Patients should be cautioned against the continued use of a metered-dose canister after the stated number of uses.
- Patients should be instructed to notify their physician should the prescribed dose of medication fail to produce the desired effect.
- The patient should be instructed to perform good oral hygiene, including rinsing the mouth, after each inhalation treatment (to prevent the possible growth of fungi).
- Inhalation therapy may be contraindicated in patients with delicate fluid balance, cardiac arrhythmias, status asthmaticus, and hypersensitivity to the medication.

ADMINISTRATION OF OXYGEN

Oxygen is a colorless, odorless, tasteless gas that is essential for life. When the body does not have an adequate supply of oxygen, a state of hypoxemia develops, and irreversible damage to vital organs is possible. When a lack of oxygen threatens a person's survival, supplemental oxygen must be prescribed and administered immediately, and arterial blood gas analysis must be made after oxygen administration has been started. If there is no emergency or life-threatening situation, the arterial blood gas analysis must be made before the physician prescribes the dosage and method of administration. The normal adult range for oxygen in the arterial blood is 80 to 100 mm Hg (millimeters of mercury).

Signs and Symptoms of Hypoxemia

- Anxiety
- Cyanosis
- Pale, cold extremities
- Dyspnea
- Tachycardia
- Increased blood pressure
- Restlessness
- Confusion

Conditions or Diseases That May Require Oxygen Administration

- Apnea
- Carbon monoxide poisoning
- Drowning
- Congestive heart failure

- Chronic obstructive pulmonary disease
- Myocardial infarction
- Surgery
- Pulmonary edema
- Pneumonia
- Shock

Dosage

When oxygen is to be administered, dosage is based on individual needs. Because oxygen is a drug, the physician will prescribe the flow rate, concentration, method of delivery, and length of time for administration. Oxygen is ordered as liters per minute (LPM) and as percentage of oxygen concentration (%).

As a medical assistant, it is your responsibility to follow the physician's order, and to adhere to the guidelines for proper drug administration. Always assess the patient as an individual, explain the procedure, and carefully observe the patient for signs of improvement or symptoms of oxygen toxicity.

Oxygen toxicity may develop when 100 percent oxygen is breathed for a prolonged period. As with any other drug, toxicity depends upon dose, time, and the patient's response. The higher the dose, the shorter the time required to develop toxicity. Symptoms of oxygen toxicity are substernal pain, nausea, vomiting, malaise, fatigue, numbness, and a tingling of the extremities.

High concentrations of inhaled oxygen cause alveolar collapse, intra-alveolar hemorrhage, hyaline membrane formation, disturbance of the central nervous system, and retrolental fibroplasia in newborns.

> ## Safety Precautions:
>
> *Apnea can result when giving oxygen at a flow rate greater than 2 liters per minute to patients with COPD, especially those with emphysema. The patient who has emphysema has difficulty ridding the body of CO_2.*

METHODS OF OXYGEN DELIVERY

Many methods are available today for the delivery of oxygen. The more commonly prescribed methods include the use of nasal cannulas and masks (see Figures 11-12 and 11-13). Other methods of delivery involve the use of nasal catheters, isolettes, hoods, tents, and portable oxygen tanks (see Figure 11-14).

Nasal Cannula

When a low concentration of oxygen is desired, the nasal **cannula** is the simplest and most convenient method for the administration of oxygen (see Figure 11-15). Made of plastic, the nasal cannula consists of two hollow prongs through which the oxygen passes, and a strap or other device to secure it to the patient's head. The nasal prongs are placed into the patient's nostrils. Avoid a direct flow of O_2 against the patient's nasal mucosa, as this causes tissue dehydration. Flow rates greater than 3 to 4 liters per minute require humidification.

Masks

The common types of masks used for inhalation therapy are plastic disposable, partial rebreather, nonrebreather, and Venturi. These devices are employed when the patient requires high humidity and a precise amount of oxygen. To be effective, the mask must be fitted snugly to the patient (see Figure 11-16).

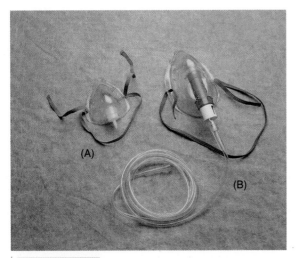

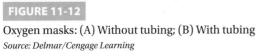

FIGURE 11-12

Oxygen masks: (A) Without tubing; (B) With tubing

Source: Delmar/Cengage Learning

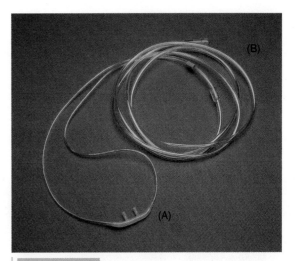

FIGURE 11-13

(A) Oxygen cannula with (B) tubing

Source: Delmar/Cengage Learning

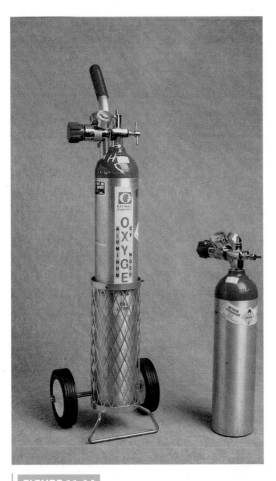

FIGURE 11-14

Oxygen tanks. Note gauge at top of tanks.

Source: Delmar/Cengage Learning

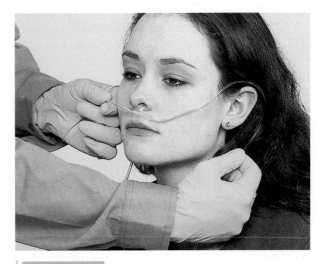

FIGURE 11-15

A medical assistant adjusts the nasal cannula around the patient's ears for oxygen administration.

Source: Delmar/Cengage Learning

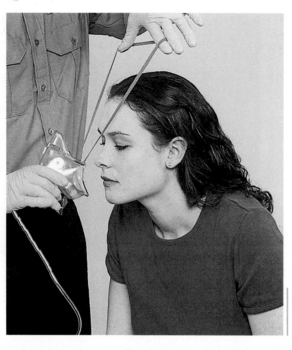

FIGURE 11-16
A medical assistant adjusts the oxygen mask around a patient's head. *Source: Delmar/Cengage Learning*

Safety Precautions:

Oxygen must be humidified before delivery to the patient in order to prevent drying of the respiratory mucosa.

Oxygen Safety Precautions

- Oxygen supports combustion. Thus, there is the danger of a fire being started when oxygen is in use. Extreme caution should be exercised, because ignition can be caused by friction, static electricity, or a lighted cigar or cigarette. When oxygen is being administered, an **OXYGEN IN USE—NO SMOKING** sign should be clearly displayed at the door of the room, and above the patient's bed.

- Electrical appliances, such as heating pads, blankets, razors, or other electrical devices should not be used while oxygen is being administered.

- One should use suction machines, X-ray and EKG equipment, and monitors with caution while administering oxygen.

- Check the patient's room for safety before initiating oxygen therapy. When possible, replace electrical devices with nonelectric units.

- Explain safety measures to the patient, to his or her roommate, and to visitors.

ADMINISTERING DRUGS BY LOCAL APPLICATION

Ointments, lotions, liniments, wet medicated dressings, poultices, and plasters are all applied directly to the skin. Drugs commonly used for local application to the mucous membranes of body cavities are administered by irrigation, instillation, and insertion into body openings.

Application to the Skin

Ointments are applied directly to the skin, or they may be applied as a dressing by spreading the medication on a piece of gauze. When the drug is applied by rubbing it onto the skin, the method is called inunction. Ointments may be used to relieve irritations and to treat various skin diseases. Zinc oxide is an example of an ointment used for local application.

Lotions are drugs that are swabbed onto the skin for antiseptic or astringent effects. Itching, dryness, and irritations caused by inflammation and diseases of the skin are relieved. Calamine lotion is an example of such a drug.

Liniments are drugs that usually have a counterirritant effect. They are applied by vigorously rubbing them onto the skin of the affected area to relieve soreness in muscles and joints. The psychological effect of massage is an important factor in the application of liniments. Camphor liniment and chloroform liniment are examples.

- Avoid excessive rubbing of counterirritant drugs into skin, as blistering may result.

- When applying ointments and lotions to infected areas, use extreme care not to aggravate the infection. Apply medication as directed. Use disposable gloves to avoid danger of infection to oneself, or if the drug may produce allergic reactions.

Medicated or wet dressings may be used for local treatment of skin disorders; they are gauze sponges, saturated with a drug in solution. The drug may act as an antiseptic or an astringent. Neomycin is an example of a drug that can be prepared as a solution and used as an antiseptic for local application.

> **Safety Precautions:**
>
> When medicated wet dressings are applied, the dressings must be changed frequently to produce the maximum desired effect.

Application to Body Cavities

Medications are applied to various body cavities to treat inflammation and infection in three ways: (1) irrigation, a flushing of the mucous lining with a solution for the purpose of removing secretions and soothing the tissues; (2) instillation, the introduction of a drug, usually in liquid form, into a body cavity (eye, ear, nose) for temporary retention; and (3) insertion, the placement of a suppository into the rectum or vaginal cavity, or a tablet into the mouth, vagina, or rectum.

Open cavities often treated by irrigation include the nose, mouth, ear, throat, vagina, and rectum. Normal saline and water is a commonly used solution for irrigations of the ear, nose, and throat. Other irrigations (douches) and installations require special strengths of solutions and medications.

The temperature of all irrigations and douches must be moderate, about 39°C to 40°C (102.2°F to 104°F), to avoid burning the patient.

Drugs may be inserted rectally or vaginally if a patient is likely to become nauseated by oral intake, or if the patient is extremely ill or unconscious. Drugs are also given by this method when the physician desires to promote a sustained local action.

■ ■ REVIEW QUESTIONS

Directions. Select the best answer to each of the following multiple-choice questions, circling the letter of your choice:

1. A disadvantage of the oral route of drug administration is that _____.
   a. the drug may irritate the gastric mucosa
   b. the drug does not alter the digestive enzymes
   c. the drug is easily and economically administered
   d. the patient usually takes the medication

2. Which of the following basic procedures must be observed before administering an oral medication?
   a. verify the accuracy of the physician's order
   b. work in a well-lighted, quiet, clean area
   c. perform the medical asepsis hand wash
   d. all of these

3. When pouring a liquid oral medication, it is important to _____.
   a. palm the label of the medication
   b. hold the measuring device at eye level
   c. allow the bottle to come into contact with the measuring device
   d. a and b

4. Following the administration of an oral medication, the medical assistant should _____.
   a. observe the patient for any adverse reactions
   b. check the medication label for the third time
   c. document the procedure
   d. all of these

5. When administering an ophthalmic medication, the medical assistant should _____.
   a. assist the patient into a side-lying position
   b. instruct the patient to tilt the head forward
   c. ask the patient to look up at the ceiling
   d. all of these

6. When instilling ear drops, the medical assistant should _____.
   a. check the medication three times against the physician's order
   b. check the expiration date
   c. draw up the correct amount of medicine into the dropper
   d. all of these

7. In a physician's office, the Fleet enema may be utilized to cleanse the lower bowel in preparation for _____.
   a. radiography   b. sigmoidoscopy   c. proctoscopy   d. all of these

8. To instill a Fleet enema, the medical assistant should _____.
   a. provide for privacy
   b. assist the patient into the supine position
   c. appropriately drape the patient
   d. a and c

9. A transdermal system is _____.
   a. a small patch or disk
   b. applied to the body near the treatment site
   c. used for the treatment of angina pectoris
   d. all of these

10. Before instructing a patient on how to apply or use a transdermal system, you should _____.
    a. be totally familiar with all aspects of the drug
    b. read the patient instructions that accompany the medication
    c. assume that all transdermal systems are the same
    d. a and b

11. _____ is the act of drawing breath, vapor, or gas into the lungs.

    a. Instillation   b. Irrigation   c. Inhalation   d. Inunction

12. A(an) _____ is a small, handheld apparatus, usually an aerosol unit, that contains a microcrystalline suspension of medication.

    a. disk   b. inhaler   c. patch   d. lens

13. When oxygen is to be administered, the physician will prescribe _____.

    a. the flow rate   c. method of delivery and length of time

    b. concentration   d. all of these

14. Symptoms of oxygen toxicity are _____.

    a. substernal pain, nausea, vomiting, malaise, fatigue, numbness, and tachycardia

    b. substernal pain, nausea, vomiting, malaise, and bradycardia

    c. sternal pain, nausea, vomiting, dizziness, and fatigue

    d. substernal pain, nausea, vomiting, malaise, fatigue, numbness, and tingling of the extremities

15. Oxygen must be humidified before delivery to the patient to _____.

    a. prevent combustion

    b. prevent drying of the respiratory mucosa

    c. prevent causing an infection

    d. none of these

16. In the physician's office, oxygen is generally stored in _____.

    a. units   b. cannisters   c. tanks   d. pipes

Matching. Place the correct letter from Column II on the appropriate line of Column I:

Column I	*Column II*
17. _____ angina pectoris	A. a medication that is used in the treatment of angina pectoris
18. _____ canthus	B. a deficient amount of oxygen in the blood
19. _____ hypoxemia	C. a severe pain about the heart
20. _____ instillation	D. the angle at either end of the slit between the eyelids
21. _____ nitroglycerin	E. the process of slowly pouring or dropping a liquid onto or into a body cavity or its surface
22. _____ 30 mL	F. $\frac{1}{2}$ fluid ounce
23. _____ 15 mL	G. 1 fluid ounce
24. _____ 5 mL	H. 1 tablespoon
25. _____ 4 fluid drams	I. 1 teaspoon
	J. $\frac{3}{4}$ fluid ounce

UNIT 12
Parenteral Equipment and Supplies

OBJECTIVES

Upon completing this unit, you should be able to:

- Define the terms listed in the vocabulary.
- Describe the syringes that are most frequently used for administering parenteral medications.
- Describe the component parts of a syringe.
- Name the parts of a syringe that must be kept sterile during the preparation and administration of a parenteral medication.
- Classify syringes as disposable, as nondisposable, or as a combination of these two types.
- Give the advantages of using a disposable syringe.
- Explain how to prevent needlestick injuries in health care settings.
- Describe the Needlestick Safety and Prevention Act.
- Describe various safety design devices.
- Give the National Institute for Occupational Safety and Health's (NIOSH) recommendations for health care workers on how to protect themselves and their coworkers.
- Correctly read the calibrated scales of a 3-mL, 5-mL, tuberculin, and U-100 insulin syringe.
- Describe the component parts of a needle.
- Select an appropriate-sized needle and syringe for the following types of injections: intramuscular, subcutaneous, and intradermal.
- Name the diseases commonly transmitted by a contaminated syringe needle.
- Dispose of used needles and syringes safely.
- Demonstrate the procedure for handling a sterile syringe-needle unit, loading and unloading a Tubex injector, removing medication from a vial, removing medication from an ampule, mixing two medications in one syringe, and reconstituting a powder medication for administration.
- Answer the review questions correctly.

VOCABULARY

ampule (am'pool). A small, sterile, prefilled glass container that holds a hypodermic solution. It usually contains a unit dose of medication.

cartridge (kar'trij). A cylindrical case made of glass, plastic, or other material that is prefilled with an exact dose of medication. It is the replaceable unit for the Tubex and Carpuject injection systems.

gauge (gāge). A standard or scale of measurement. The gauge (G) of a needle is determined by the diameter of its lumen.

hypodermic (hie"po-der'mik). Under or below the skin.

injection (in-jek'shun). The process of introducing a liquid substance into a body tissue, vein, artery, joint, or body canal.

Luer-Lok. A trademark for a type of syringe tip that is designed to facilitate the rapid and firm attachment of a needle tip to the syringe.

parenteral (par-en'ter-al). The injection of a liquid substance into the body via a route other than the alimentary canal. In standard medical practice, parenteral means by injection, such as intramuscular and subcutaneous.

sterile (ster'il). A state of being free from living microorganisms.

vial (vie'al). A small, sterile, prefilled glass bottle containing a hypodermic solution. It usually contains a multiple-dose medication.

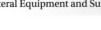

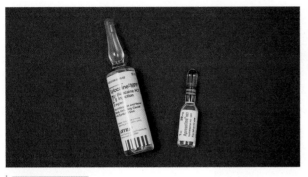

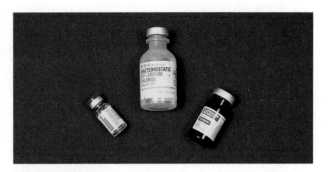

INTRODUCTION

As a medical assistant or health professional, you may be responsible for administering medications by the **parenteral** route. Thus, you must be familiar with the various types of syringes and needles and their use with **ampules** (see Figure 12-1) and **vials** (see Figure 12-2). A syringe-needle unit is an instrument that is used to inject a liquid substance into the body tissue, vein, artery, joint, or body canal of a patient. It may also be used to remove fluid from the body (aspiration, venipuncture). A *syringe alone* is used to perform an irrigation (wounds, eyes, and ears), or to administer certain oral medications. In this unit, you will become familiar with:

- The equipment (needles and syringes).
- Diseases transmitted by contaminated needles and syringes.
- The safe disposal of used equipment.

PARTS OF A SYRINGE

The component parts of a syringe consist of a barrel, a plunger, the flange, and the tip (see Figure 12-3). The *barrel* is the part that holds the medication and has graduated markings (calibrations) on its surface for use in measuring medications. The *plunger* is a movable cylinder, designed for insertion within the barrel. When inserted, the plunger forms a tight-fitting seal against the interior walls of the barrel, and provides the mechanism by which a medication (or other substance) is drawn into or pushed out of the barrel. The *flange* is at the end of the barrel where the plunger is inserted. It forms a rim around the end of the barrel and has appendages against which one places the index and middle fingers when drawing up solution for injection. The flange also prevents the syringe from rolling when laid on a flat surface. The *tip* is the end of the barrel where the needle is attached.

The parts of a syringe that *must remain* sterile during the preparation and administration of a parenteral medication are the *inside* of the barrel, the *section of the plunger that fits inside the barrel*, and the *syringe tip* to which the needle is to be attached.

CLASSIFICATION OF SYRINGES

Syringes are named according to their sizes and usages. Table 12-1 lists the types, sizes, calibrations, and uses of syringes used in the administration of parenteral medications. It is to your advantage to study this table and to memorize the information it contains.

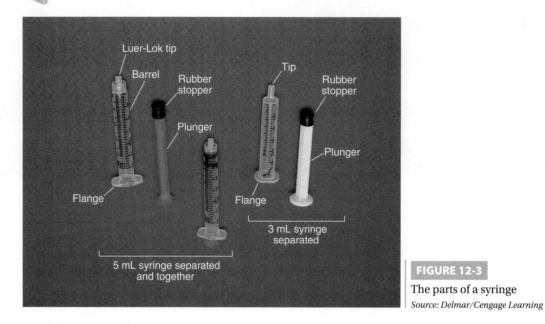

FIGURE 12-3

The parts of a syringe
Source: Delmar/Cengage Learning

TABLE 12-1 The Most Frequently Used Syringes for Parenteral Medications

TYPE OF SYRINGE	SIZE AND CALIBRATION	TYPICAL USES
Hypodermic	3 mL Calibrated 0.1 mL	Intramuscular and subcutaneous injections
Hypodermic	5 mL Calibrated 0.2 mL	Venipuncture, intramuscular
Hypodermic	Larger sizes (10 mL, 20 mL, and 60 mL)	Medical and surgical treatments, aspirations, irrigations, venipunctures, gavage (tube-to-stomach) feedings
Tuberculin	1 mL Calibrated 0.1 mL and 0.01 mL	To inject minute amounts for intradermal injections, allergy testing, allergy injections
Insulin	$\frac{3}{10}$ mL (30 units) $\frac{1}{2}$ mL (50 units) 1 mL (100 units)	Administration of insulin

Syringes are classified as disposable, as nondisposable, and as combinations of these two types. They may also be classified according to their intended use. In addition to the standard **hypodermic** syringes that are in general use, there are special-purpose syringes for irrigations or oral feedings, tuberculin syringes, and insulin syringes.

Disposable Syringes

Disposable syringes are those that are sterilized, prepackaged, nontoxic, nonpyrogenic, and ready for use. They are available as a syringe-needle unit, and are generally enclosed in individual peel-apart packages of durable paper or clear plastic. They are available in sizes from 1 milliliter to 60 cubic milliliters (see Figure 12-4). The 1-mL, 3-mL, and 5-mL syringes are the ones most often used when parenteral medications are administered.

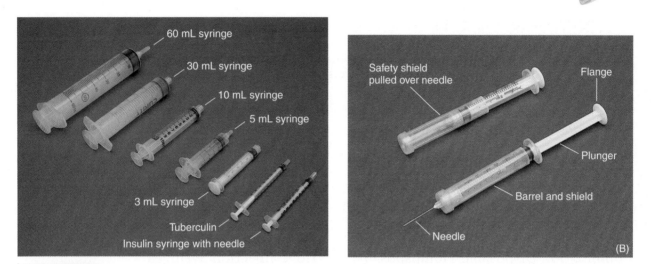

FIGURE 12-4

Various sizes of disposable syringes. (A) Syringes can range from 1 mL to 60 mL. (B) A type of safety syringe
Source: Delmar/Cengage Learning

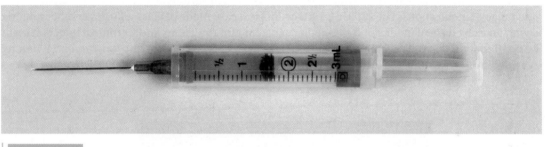

FIGURE 12-5

A disposable syringe-needle unit with 1.5 mL measurement *Source: Delmar/Cengage Learning*

A disposable syringe-needle unit consists of a syringe with an attached needle. The needle is covered by a hard plastic sheath to prevent it from accidentally penetrating the package or sticking the user. The unit may be sealed within a peel-apart package or encased in a rigid plastic container that has been heat-sealed to ensure sterility. Labeling usually includes the manufacturer's name, the type and size of the syringe, the gauge and length of the needle, and a reorder number. Packages are usually color-coded for ease of identification. Disposable syringes are generally preferred for the administration of parenteral medications (see Figure 12-5).

Advantages of Using a Disposable Syringe

1. Disposable syringe-needle units are safer for the patient and the medical assistant. The unit is guaranteed to be sterile and the needle comes attached to the syringe, minimizing the possibility of contamination.

2. A wide range of available sizes makes it convenient for the medical assistant to select a syringe-needle unit that is appropriate for the correct administration of any parenteral medication.

3. The needle in a disposable unit is made of precision-sharpened stainless steel. This allows the medical assistant to easily penetrate the patient's skin and minimizes the sense of pain that accompanies the insertion of a needle into the body.

4. The disposable syringe-needle unit saves the medical assistant time when preparing for the administration of an injection; therefore, it saves money.

5. Once used, the unit is discarded. With correct disposal technique (explained later in this unit), it is possible to lower the possibility of accidental transfer of diseases such as acquired immunodeficiency syndrome (AIDS) and hepatitis B.

Nondisposable Syringes

Nondisposable syringes are usually made of specially strengthened glass that is resistant to thermal shock. These units, consisting of round glass barrels with individually fitted plungers, are manufactured to exacting specifications.

Nondisposable glass syringes are available in sizes from 1 milliliter to 60 milliliters. These syringes are not often used for the administration of injections. They are used by physicians to perform such special procedures as paracentesis, thoracentesis, thoracotomy, and tracheotomy.

Combination Disposable/Nondisposable Cartridge-Injection Syringes

A cartridge-injection system (see Figure 12-6) such as the Tubex or Carpuject (see Figure 12-7), consists of a disposable cartridge-needle unit and a nondisposable cartridge-holder syringe. The cartridge-needle unit is factory-sealed and sterile, and contains a precisely measured unit dose of medicine. The cartridge-holder syringe may be made of durable chrome-plated brass or of plastic. These reusable syringes are designed for quick and safe loading and unloading of cartridge-needle units, which are manufactured in various sizes and dosage capacities, and contain a wide range of medications. The **cartridge** is a cylindrical case made of glass, plastic, or other material that is prefilled with an exact dose of medication. It is replaceable unit for the Tubex and Carpuject injection system.

The combination disposable/nondisposable syringe system is easy to use and convenient. When using this system, you still must be careful to read the label and compare the medication order with the label. For example,

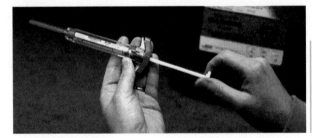

FIGURE 12-6

A prefilled syringe consists of a prefilled barrel and needle assembly placed in a reusable syringe holder. *Source: Delmar/ Cengage Learning*

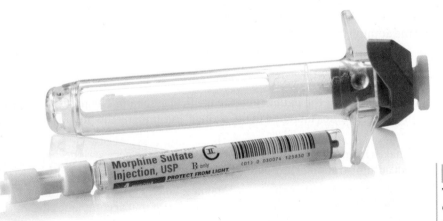

FIGURE 12-7

The Carpuject® is another kind of cartridge-injection system.
Courtesy of Hospira Inc.

the physician orders Valium 5 mg, and the cartridge is 10 mg/2mL. You would give 1mL and properly discard the other 1mL according to agency policy.

PREVENTING NEEDLESTICK INJURIES IN HEALTH CARE SETTINGS

The National Institute for Occupational Safety and Health requests assistance in preventing needlestick injuries among health care workers. These injuries are caused by needles such as hypodermic needles, blood-collection needles, intravenous stylets, and needles used to connect parts of IV delivery systems. These injuries can be avoided by eliminating the unnecessary use of needles, using devices with safety features, and promoting education and safe work practices for handling needles and related systems. These measures should be part of a comprehensive program to prevent the transmission of bloodborne pathogens.

The *Needlestick Safety and Prevention Act* became effective on March 6, 1992. It requires all employers to protect employees who may be exposed to blood or other potentially infectious material resulting from needlestick or other percutaneous injuries. This legislation covers all health care employees, such as those in physician offices, nursisng homes, and clinics, as well as in work sites that keep medical emergency kits.

✚ Safety Precautions:

Health care workers who use or may be exposed to needles are at increased risk of needlestick injury. Such injuries can lead to serious or fatal infections with bloodborne pathogens such as hepatitis B virus, hepatitis C virus, or human immunodeficiency virus (HIV).

Improved engineering controls are often among the most effective approaches to reducing occupational hazards and therefore are an important element of a needlestick prevention program. Such controls include eliminating the unnecessary use of needles and implementing devices with safety features.

Safety Device Designs

An estimated 384,000 skin puncture injuries occur in U.S. hospitals each year. A study on blood collection in physician offices and clinics showed an annual needlestick rate just as high as in hospitals. The CDC reports that up to 88 percent of needlestick injuries can be prevented by using safety-engineered needles and other devices. An increasing number and variety of needle devices with safety features are now available. Examples of safety-device designs are:

- Needleless connectors for IV delivery systems (blunt cannula for use with prepierced ports and valved connectors that accept tapered or luer ends of IV tubing).
- Protected needle IV connectors. (The IV connector needle is permanently recessed in a rigid plastic housing that fits over IV ports.)
- Needles that retract into a syringe or vacuum tube holder.
- Hinged or sliding shield attached to phlebotomy needles, winged-steel needles, and blood-gas needles.
- Protective encasements to receive an IV stylet as it is withdrawn from the catheter.
- Sliding needle shields attached to disposable syringes and vacuum tube holder.
- Self-blunting phlebotomy and winged-steel needles. (A blunt cannula seated inside the phlebotomy needle is advanced beyond the needle tip before the needle is withdrawn from the vein.)
- Retractable fingerstick and heelstick lancets.

See Figures 12-8, 12-9, and 12-10 for examples of safety syringes.

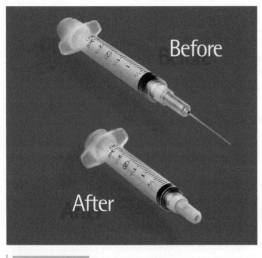

FIGURE 12-8

Retractable Technologies' VanishPoint® needle automatically retracts into the syringe barrel after injection. *Courtesy of Retractable Technologies*

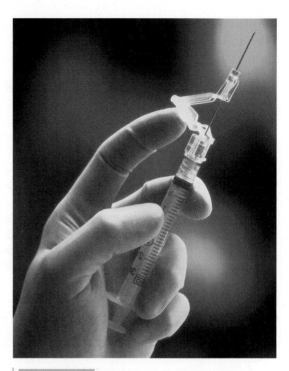

FIGURE 12-9

B-D SafetyGlide™ syringe contains a protective needle guard, which can be activated by a single finger to cover and seal the needle after injection. *Courtesy and © Becton, Dickinson and Company*

NIOSH's Recommendations for Health Care Workers

To protect themselves and their coworkers, health care workers should be aware of the hazards posed by needlestick injuries and should use safety devices and improved work practices as follows:

- Avoid the use of needles where safe and effective alternatives are available.
- Help your employer select and evaluate devices with safety features.
- Use devices with safety features provided by your employer.
- Avoid recapping needles.
- Plan safe handling and disposal before beginning any procedure using needles.
- Dispose of used needle devices promptly in appropriate sharps disposal containers.
- Report all needlestick and other sharps-related injuries promptly to ensure that you receive appropriate follow-up care.
- Tell your employer about hazards from needles that you observe in your work environment.
- Participate in bloodborne pathogen training and follow recommended infection prevention practices, including hepatitis B vaccination.

● *Note*

For additional information about needlestick injuries, call 1-800-356-4674 or visit the NIOSH web site at www.cdc.gov/niosh. ●

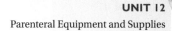

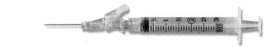

(A)

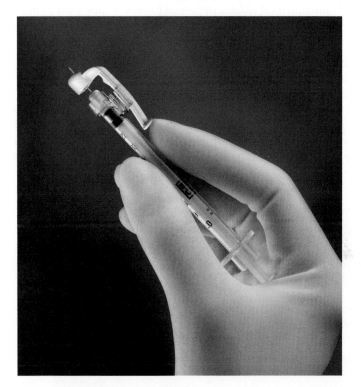

(B)

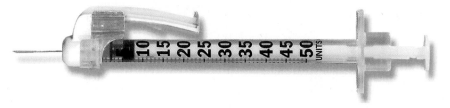

(C)

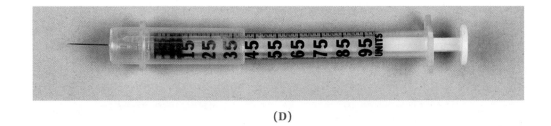

(D)

FIGURE 12-10

Safety syringes: (A) 3 mL; (B) 1 mL; (C) Lo-Dose U-100 insulin syringe; and (D) Standard U-100 insulin syringe (reverse side). *Courtesy and © Becton, Dickinson and Company*

MEASURING MEDICATION IN A SYRINGE

To precisely measure an ordered dose of medication for parenteral administration, you must know how the various syringes used for such therapy are *calibrated*.

The 3-milliliter syringe is calibrated with a single metric (mL) scale. Each small line of this scale represents 0.1 $\left(\frac{1}{10}\right)$ of a mL. The longer graduated lines represent $\frac{1}{2}$-, 1-, $1\frac{1}{2}$-, 2-, $2\frac{1}{2}$-, and 3-mL calibrations (see Figure 12-11A).

The 5-milliliter syringe is calibrated with a single metric scale. Each small line of this scale represents 0.2 $\left(\frac{2}{10}\right)$ of a mL. The longer graduated lines represent 1-, 2-, 3-, 4-, and 5-mL calibrations.

The tuberculin syringe is calibrated with a single metric scale. Each small line of this scale represents 0.01 $\left(\frac{1}{100}\right)$ of a milliliter. The longer graduated lines are used to measure tenths of a milliliter. These lines divide the scale into 10 segments ranging from 0.1 $\left(\frac{1}{10}\right)$ of a mL to a maximum of 1.0 mL (see Figure 12-12).

Insulin syringes are calibrated in *units*. The Lo-Dose insulin syringe has a scale on which each small line represents 1 unit and each longer line 5 units. The scale contains a maximum of 50 units, which is equivalent to $\frac{1}{2}$ mL.

The U-100 insulin syringe has a scale on which each small line represents 2 units and each longer line 10 units. The scale contains a maximum of 100 units, which is equivalent to 1 mL (see Figure 12-13).

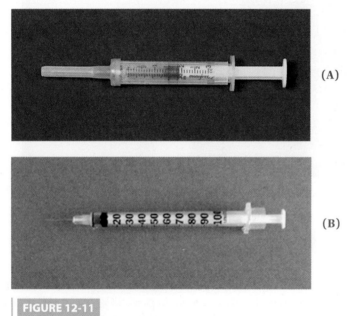

(A)

(B)

FIGURE 12-11

Types of syringes: (A) Hypodermic; and (B) Standard U-100 insulin syringe. *Source: Delmar/Cengage Learning*

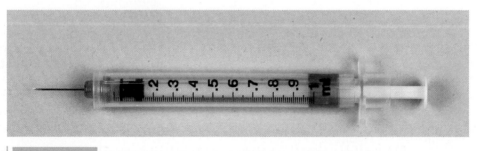

FIGURE 12-12

Tuberculin syringe *Source: Delmar/Cengage Learning*

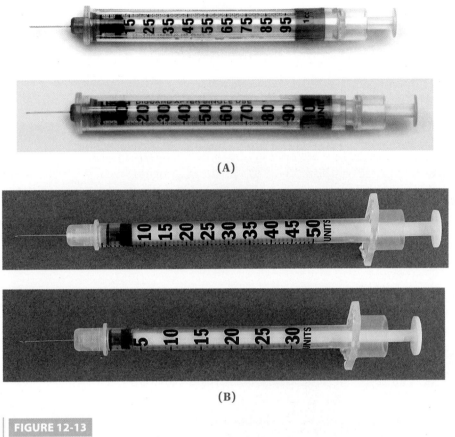

FIGURE 12-13

(A) Insulin syringes: Front and reverse of a standard U-100 insulin syringe; and
(B) Lo-Dose U-100 insulin syringes, 50 and 30 units *Source: Delmar/Cengage Learning*

Reading the Syringe

The plunger in most disposable syringes has a black rubber suction tip. The slightly pointed face of this rubber tip is designed to line up with the calibrated lines of the scale imprinted on the barrel of the syringe. The back of the rubber suction tip is flat and affixes to the plunger. When reading a syringe, one reads the calibrated scale that directly lines up with the slightly pointed edge of the black rubber tip (see Figure 12-14). Make sure you can correctly read the calibrations on syringes before proceeding to needles.

HYPODERMIC NEEDLES

Both disposable and nondisposable needles are available for use with syringes. Of these, the most frequently used are disposable needles, which are individually packaged in sterile paper or plastic containers. Disposable needles and syringe-needle units are available with a color-coded sheath. The sheath protects the needle and identifies its gauge and length. Needle **gauges** (G) range from 16 to 30, and their lengths vary from $\frac{3}{8}$ inch to 2 inches (see Figure 12-15). The needle's gauge is determined by the diameter of the *lumen* or opening at its beveled tip. The larger the gauge, the smaller is the diameter of its lumen. For example, a 30-gauge needle is much smaller than a 16-gauge needle.

Nondisposable needles are made of high-quality stainless steel. They are equipped with a mounting hub that has a cylindrical opening designed to slip over and lock onto the tip of a syringe, such as a **Luer-Lok**.

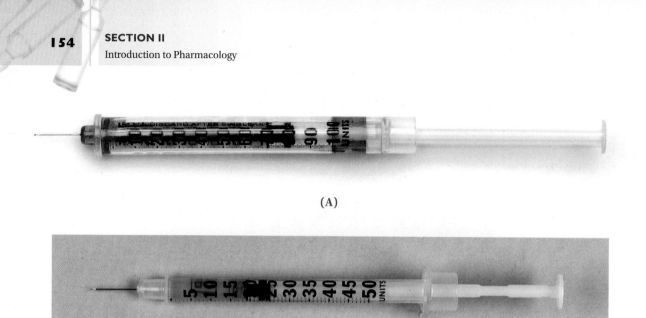

(A)

(B)

FIGURE 12-14

(A) Standard U-100 insulin syringe measuring 70 units of U-100 insulin; and (B) Lo-Dose U-100 insulin syringe measuring 19 units of U-100 insulin *Source: Delmar/Cengage Learning*

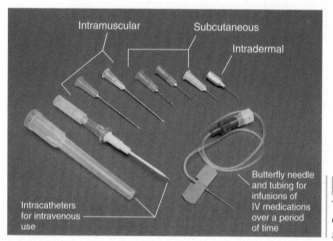

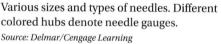

FIGURE 12-15

Various sizes and types of needles. Different colored hubs denote needle gauges.

Source: Delmar/Cengage Learning

Parts of a Needle

Figure 12-16 shows the parts of a typical needle used to administer parenteral medications. The *point* is the sharpened end of the needle. The point is formed when the end of the shaft is ground away to form a flat, slanted surface called the *bevel*. The hollow core of the needle, when exposed at the beveled point, forms an oval-shaped opening, the *lumen*. The hollow steel tube through which the medication passes is the *shaft*. The other end of the shaft attaches to the *hub*, which is that part of the needle unit that is designed to mount onto the syringe. The point at which the shaft attaches to the hub is called the *hilt*.

Selecting the Appropriate Syringe and Needle

The selection of an appropriate syringe and needle for a particular parenteral use involves a number of considerations. Two of the major factors in the selection process are the medication ordered and the age and size of the patient.

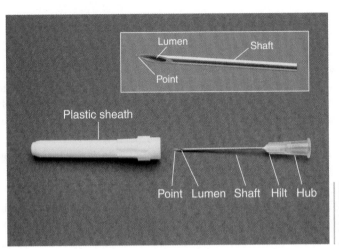

Lumen   Shaft

Point

Plastic sheath

Point Lumen Shaft Hilt Hub

FIGURE 12-16

Parts of a needle and protective cover.
Inset shows of point, lumen, and shaft.

Source: Delmar/Cengage Learning

TABLE 12-2 Syringe-Needle Combinations for Various Parenteral Routes

Subcutaneous Injection	Intramuscular Injection
3-mL syringe / 25 G, $\frac{5}{8}$-inch needle	3-mL syringe / 23 G, 1-inch needle
3-mL syringe / 26 G, $\frac{3}{8}$-inch needle	3-mL syringe / 22 G, $1\frac{1}{2}$-inch needle
3-mL syringe / 27 G, $\frac{1}{2}$-inch needle	3-mL syringe / 21 G, $1\frac{1}{2}$-inch to 2-inch needle
U-100 insulin syringe / 26 G, $\frac{1}{2}$-inch needle	
	Intradermal Injection
Intravenous Injection	1-mL syringe / 25 G, $\frac{5}{8}$-inch needle
3-mL syringe / 22 G, 1-inch needle	1-mL syringe / 26 G, $\frac{3}{8}$-inch needle
5-mL syringe / 21 G, $\frac{1}{2}$-inch needle	1-mL syringe / 27 G, $\frac{1}{2}$-inch needle

The amount and viscosity of the *medication ordered* determine the size of the syringe-needle unit to be selected. Thick, oily medications require a needle with a lumen of 21 G to 16 G that will permit the flow of such fluids. Thinner medications permit the use of higher-gauge needles. The amount of medicine that one may inject into a single site is related to the tissue area selected. For *subcutaneous tissue*, the amount should not exceed 2 mL. Injections into the *deltoid muscle* should not be greater than 2 mL. Other *intramuscular* injections should not exceed 3 mL, unless it can be determined that a larger dose can be safely administered.

Once the amount and consistency of the medication are determined, one must choose the correct site for the injection and the tissue layer into which it will be administered. Table 12-2 shows the syringe-needle combinations that are appropriate for their designated uses.

Another factor to be considered is the *age* and *size* of the patient. Geriatric and pediatric patients may have less subcutaneous or intramuscular tissue per body surface area than average adults. The size of the syringe-needle unit is related to the depth of penetration permissible in patients of different ages and sizes.

One should always choose a needle with sufficient length to reach the desired tissue level. A large person may require a longer needle to reach the correct body tissue than would be required for a smaller person. The delivery of medication to the proper tissue level is very important. A concentrated or irritating medication that is intended for deep intramuscular injection could be delivered instead into the subcutaneous tissue of an obese patient if one selects a needle that is too short. Such an inappropriate injection may cause a sterile abscess. This unnecessary complication can be avoided by considering the size of the patient when choosing the length of the needle.

The Safe Disposal of Needles and Syringes

The careless disposal of used needles and syringes may present a health risk to any person coming into contact with the used equipment. An accidental stick by a contaminated needle could transmit such diseases as hepatitis B, syphilis, Rocky Mountain spotted fever, tuberculosis, malaria, varicella zoster, and acquired immunodeficiency syndrome (AIDS). Used needles and syringes should be discarded in a rigid, puncture-proof container. Two examples of such a container are:

1. The B-D Sharps Collector Nestable is made of puncture-resistant material. It is designed for infectious waste and has a safety lock closure for an extra measure of safety (see Figure 12-17).

2. The B-D Point-of-Use Sharps Collector System eliminates the need to reshield the needle, thereby reducing the risk of an accidental needlestick. Needles are placed point downward, away from the fingers (see Figure 12-18). The disposable inner container is clearly marked and may be incinerated or autoclaved according to agency policy.

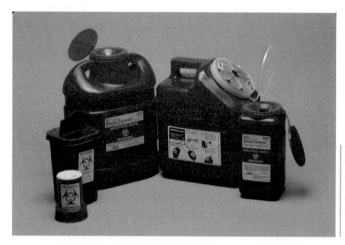

FIGURE 12-17

A few of the various sizes of biohazard puncture-proof (sharps) containers are displayed. (They are generally bright red or yellow to alert caution.) Notice the biohazardous material symbol that also alerts you to exercise caution. *Source: Delmar/Cengage Learning*

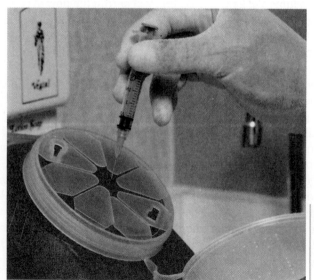

FIGURE 12-18

Discard the entire disposable syringe with used needle intact into the biohazard sharps container. The lid should be tightly affixed only when the container is three-fourths full. *Source: Delmar/Cengage Learning*

PREPARING EQUIPMENT AND SUPPLIES

An important part of giving a safe injection is preparing the equipment and supplies. This segment covers the proper procedures to follow when handling a sterile syringe-needle unit, using the Tubex injector, withdrawing medication from a vial and an ampule, mixing two medications in one syringe, and reconstituting a powder medication for administration (see Procedures 12-1, 12-2, 12-3, and 12-4).

PROCEDURE 12-1
Handling a Sterile Syringe-Needle Unit—Disposable Peel-Back Method

Standard Precautions:

Purpose:

To correctly use a sterile syringe-needle unit—disposable, peel-back method

Equipment/Supplies:

Appropriate syringe-needle package
Disposable gloves
Sharps container

Procedure Steps:

1. Verify the physician's order.

2. Work in a well-lighted, quiet, clean area.

3. Perform medical asepsis hand wash (see Figure 12-19).

4. Put on gloves.

5. Obtain a disposable, peel-back package containing a sterile syringe-needle unit.

6. Check the package label to be sure that you have selected the correct size syringe-needle unit for the ordered injection.

7. With the label facing you, open the package by slowly peeling down the outer covering until the plunger and barrel are in view.

8. Remove the unit from the package by touching *only the outside of the barrel.*

9. Hold the outside of the barrel between the thumb and index finger with the sheathed needle pointing upward.

10. Use your other hand (thumb and index finger) to touch the end of the plunger. Pull back on the flat end of the plunger to loosen it. Once loosened, push the plunger back to its original position in the barrel of the syringe. *Do not touch the plunger's stem as this could contaminate the inside of the syringe.*

11. Assure yourself that the needle is firmly attached to the syringe tip by using a clockwise motion to turn the hub of the needle on the syringe tip. Do *not* turn the hub counterclockwise as this will remove the needle from the syringe.

12. Using your thumb and index finger, loosen the sheath that protects the needle. Once loosened at the hub, turn the sheath counterclockwise, touching only that part of the sheath that is directly over the hub. Gently loosen the sheath by rocking it from side to side.

13. Remove the sheath using your thumb and index finger to slowly and carefully pull the sheath away from the hub of the needle.

14. To replace the sheath on a needle (*that has not been inserted into a patient*), lay the sheath on a clean surface, being sure that the end that the needle is going to slide into has not come in contact with any surface: then, carefully guide the needle into the sheath. Be sure that the needle does not touch the interior of the sheath (see Figure 12-20).

15. Remove gloves.

16. Wash hands.

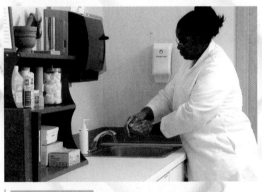

FIGURE 12-19

Medical asepsis hand wash
Source: Delmar/Cengage Learning

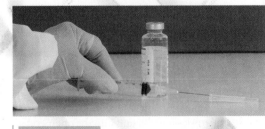

FIGURE 12-20

Replacing the sheath on the needle
Source: Delmar/Cengage Learning

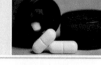

PROCEDURE 12-2
Loading and Unloading a Tubex Injector

Standard Precautions:

Purpose:

To correctly use a Tubex injector

Equipment/Supplies:

Tubex injector
Disposable gloves
Sharps container

Procedure Steps:

1. Verify the physician's order.

2. Work in a well-lighted, quiet, clean area.

3. Perform medical asepsis hand wash. Put on gloves.

4. Obtain a Tubex injector and sterile cartridge-needle unit (see Figure 12-21A).

5. Turn the ribbed collar to the "OPEN" position until it stops (see Figure 12-21B).

6. Hold the injector with the open end up, and insert the Tubex sterile cartridge-needle unit (see Figure 12-21C).

7. Tighten the ribbed collar in the direction of the "CLOSE" arrow.

8. Thread the plunger rod into the plunger of the Tubex sterile cartridge-needle unit until slight resistance is felt.

9. After use, do not recap the needle (see Figure 12-21D).

10. Disengage the plunger rod.

11. Hold the injector, needle down, over a sharps container and loosen the ribbed collar (see Figure 12-21E).

12. Discard the needle cover.

13. Remove gloves and dispose in biohazard waste container.

14. Wash hands.

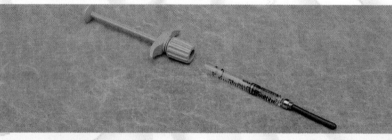

(A)

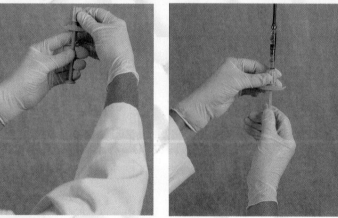

(B)   (C)

FIGURE 12-21

(A) Tubex® injector. Reusable cartridge holder with disposable sterile cartridge-needle unit. (B) Turn ribbed collar to open position. (C) Insert the sterile cartridge-needle unit into the open end of the injector.

Source: Delmar/Cengage Learning

(continues)

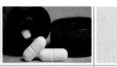

PROCEDURE 12-2 *continued*
Loading and Unloading a Tubex Injector

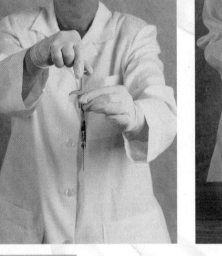

(D)

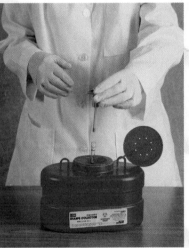

(E)

FIGURE 12-21

(D) The medical assistant prepares to dispose of the cartridge-needle unit. The needle is not recapped. The plunger rod is disengaged by unscrewing. The ribbed collar is loosened. (E) The medical assistant holds the cartridge-needle unit over a sharps container and the unit drops into the container.

Source: Delmar/Cengage Learning

PROCEDURE 12-3
Withdrawing (Aspirating) Medication from a Vial

Standard Precautions:

Purpose:

Medication is supplied in a variety of packaging. Medication from a vial must be aspirated into a syringe for parenteral injection.

Equipment/Supplies:

Medication order
Appropriate syringe and
   needle with cover
Vial of medication
Antiseptic wipes or sponges
Disposable gloves
Sharps container

Procedure Steps:

1. Read the medication order and assemble equipment. Check for the "seven rights." Read the vial label by holding it next to the medication order (first time).

2. Wash hands. Apply gloves.

3. Select the proper size needle and syringe for the medication and the route (for example, for subcutaneous injection of insulin, 100-U insulin syringe and 25 G, 5/8-inch needle). If necessary, attach the needle to the syringe.

4. Check the vial label against the mediation order (second time).

5. If the vial has not been opened, write your initials and date on the vial label. Remove the metal cap from the vial and cleanse the rubber stopper. If the vial has been opened previously, clean the rubber stopper by applying a disinfectant wipe in a circular motion (see Figure 12-22A).

(continues)

PROCEDURE 12-3 *continued*
Withdrawing (Aspirating) Medication from a Vial

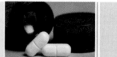

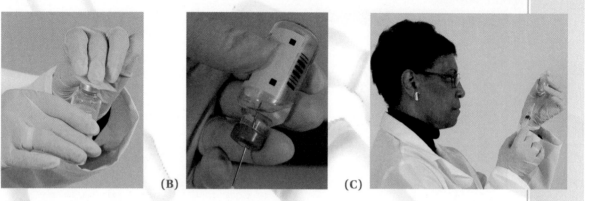

(A) (B) (C)

FIGURE 12-22

(A) Disinfect the rubber stopper on the medication vial with an alcohol swab. (B) Keeping the bevel of the needle above the fluid level, inject an amount of air equal to medication quantity to be withdrawn. (C) Hold syringe pointed upward at eye level and with the bevel of the needle in the medication. Pull back plunger and aspirate the quantity of medication ordered. *Source: Delmar/Cengage Learning*

Procedure Steps (continued):

6. Remove the needle cover—pull it straight off.
7. Inject air into the vial as follows:
   a. Hold the syringe pointed upward at eye level. Pull back the plunger to take in a quantity of air that is equal to the ordered dose of medication.
   b. Insert needle through the rubber stopper of the vial.
   c. Inject air into the air space within the vial. Injecting air into the medicine (liquid) can create more bubbles (see Figure 12-22B).
8. Withdraw the medication: Hold the vial and the syringe steady. Pull back on the plunger to withdraw the measured dose of medication. Measure accurately. Keep the tip of the needle below the surface of the liquid; otherwise, air will enter the syringe. Keep syringe at eye level (see Figure 12-22C).
9. Check the syringe for air bubbles. You may remove a large air bubble by sharply tapping on the syringe directly over the bubble. The bubble will rise to the top of the syringe and then you have to carefully remove it by pushing it out of the syringe tip into the vial. Check the syringe measurement to be sure that you have the correct dosage. If more medicine is needed, withdraw it from the vial (see Figure 12-22D).
10. Remove the needle from the vial. Replace the sterile needle cover by laying the sheath on a clean surface, being sure that the end that the

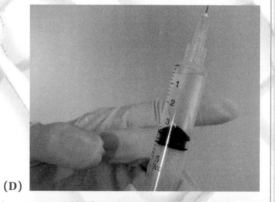

(D)

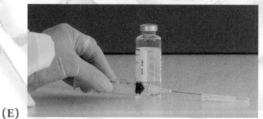

(E)

FIGURE 12-22

(D) Tap syringe to eliminate air bubbles. Hand should hold syringe while tapping it. (E) Keeping one hand behind your back, "scoop" the needle into the needle cover carefully so it does not become contaminated.
Source: Delmar/Cengage Learning

(continues)

PROCEDURE 12-3 *continued*
Withdrawing (Aspirating) Medication from a Vial

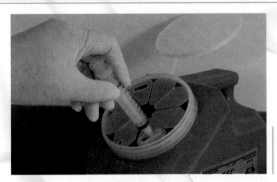

FIGURE 12-23
Dispose of used syringe-needle unit in sharps container. *Source: Delmar/Cengage Learning*

Procedure Steps (continued):

needle is going to slide into has not come in contact with any surface. Then, carefully guide the needle into the sheath, or you may "scoop" the needle into the sheath (see Figure 12-22E).

11. Check the vial label against the medication order (third time).

12. Place the filled needle and syringe on a medicine tray or cart with an antiseptic wipe and the medicine card. The dose is now ready for injection.

13. Return multiple-dose vials to the proper storage area (cabinet or refrigerator). Dispose of unused medication in a single-dose vial according to facility procedure. (Remember, disposal of a controlled substance must be witnessed and the proper forms signed.)

14. Discard used syringe-needle unit immediately after use in a sharps container (see Figure 12-23).

15. Remove gloves and dispose in biohazard waste container.

16. Wash hands.

17. Document the procedure.

PROCEDURE 12-4
Withdrawing (Aspirating) Medication from an Ampule

Standard Precautions:

Purpose:

Medication is supplied in a variety of packaging. An ampule is a sterile, glass, single-dose container of liquid medication. It is aspirated into a syringe for parenteral injection.

Equipment/Supplies:

Medicine tray
Ampule of medication
Alcohol wipes
Sterile gauze sponges
Sharps container
Sterile needle-syringe unit
Gloves

Procedure Steps:

1. Check the physician's order.

2. Wash hands and assemble equipment. Put on gloves.

3. Obtain ampule of medicine. Read label and compare to medication order for correct medication, dose, route, and time (first time). Check medication expiration date.

4. Flick ampule of medication (medication will often get "trapped" above the neck of the ampule). A sharp flick of the wrist will help force all of the medication down below the neck of the ampule into the body of the ampule (see Figure 12-24A).

RATIONALE: This step is important to ensure all medication is available in the body of the ampule to calculate the correct dose. If some of the

(continues)

PROCEDURE 12-4 *continued*
Withdrawing (Aspirating) Medication from an Ampule

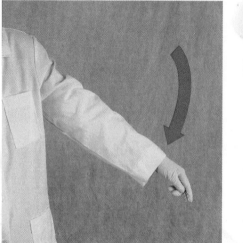

(A)

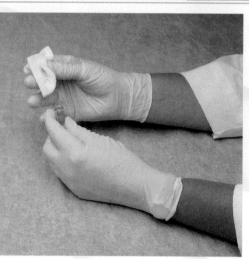

(B)

FIGURE 12-24

(A) Hold ampule by the top and force all the medication into the bottom of the ampule by a snap of the arm and wrist. (B) Remove top from ampule. Turn hand up and out simultaneously.

Source: Delmar/Cengage Learning

Procedure Steps (continued):

medication remains trapped above the neck in the top of the ampule, some medication will not be available for use and it is possible to give an incorrect dose, especially if the patient is to receive the entire contents of the ampule.

5. Thoroughly disinfect the neck with an alcohol swab. Check label (second time).

RATIONALE: The needle will enter the opening of the ampule, and wiping the neck of the ampule prior to removal of the top ensures disinfection of the neck or opening of the ampule.

6. With a sterile gauze, wipe dry the neck of the ampule. Completely surround the ampule with the gauze and forcefully snap off the top of the ampule by pushing the top away from you (see Figure 12-24B).

RATIONALE: Ensure medical assistant safety from possible injury from broken glass. Discard top in sharps container.

7. Place opened ampule down on medicine tray. Check label (third time).

8. With a prepared sterile syringe-needle unit, aspirate the required dose into the syringe (see Figure 12-24C). Cover needle with sheath and transport to patient on the medicine tray.

9. Identify the patient.

10. Administer medication.

11. Discard syringe-needle unit into sharps container. Alcohol swabs and gauze are discarded in biohazard waste container.

12. Remove gloves and dispose in biohazard waste container.

13. Wash hands.

14. Document the procedure.

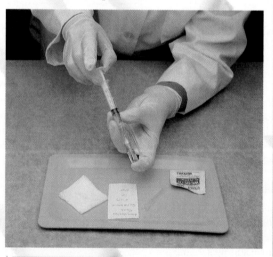

FIGURE 12-24

(C) Aspirate required dose into syringe.

Source: Delmar/Cengage Learning

Using a Filter Straw to Remove Medication from an Ampule

A filter straw is a sterile, nonpyrogenic, nontoxic device that may be used to remove medication from an ampule and is available in a peel-open package. It is designed to filter out any small particles of glass that may enter the ampule after breakage of the stem. The filter straw is for single use.

The following are the procedural steps for using a filter straw to remove medicine from an ampule.

1. Compare the medication label with the physician's order.

2. Inspect the ampule to see if any of the medicine is trapped in the stem. If necessary, tap the stem gently to cause the trapped medicine to return to the base.

3. Cover the stem portion of the ampule with a sterile gauze.

4. Exerting firm pressure over the scored portion of the stem, break off the ampule stem by pushing it away from yourself and others.

5. Place the base of the ampule on a clean surface. Discard the gauze sponge that contains the broken off stem into an appropriate container.

6. Prepare the syringe-needle unit for use. Remove the sheathed needle from the syringe. Place the sheathed needle on the inside of the peel-back syringe-needle wrapper. DO NOT CONTAMINATE.

7. Peel open the sterile filter straw package and insert the straw tip onto the syringe tip. Check to make sure that the straw tip is firmly attached to the tip of the syringe. DO NOT CONTAMINATE.

8. Slowly insert the filter straw into the opening of the ampule. Keep the tip of the straw immersed in the medication at all times.

9. Fill the barrel of the syringe with the ordered amount of medication.

10. Carefully remove the filter straw from the ampule.

11. Pull back on the plunger of the syringe to ensure that all the medication is removed from the filter straw.

12. Hold the syringe unit toward the light and make sure that there are no air bubbles. If necessary, correctly remove air bubbles.

13. Check to make sure that the amount of medicine in the syringe is the correct dose as ordered.

14. Remove the filter straw from the syringe and discard in an appropriate container.

15. Place a sterile needle onto the syringe tip.

16. Prepare to give the medication to the patient.

MIXING TWO MEDICATIONS IN ONE SYRINGE-NEEDLE UNIT

When the physician orders two medications that are to be administered by injection, you may wish to mix the medications in one syringe. First, you must check with the pharmacist to be sure that the medications are compatible and can be safely mixed in one syringe (see Procedure 12-5).

PROCEDURE 12-5
Mixing Two Medications in One Syringe-Needle Unit

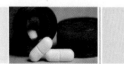

Standard Precautions:

Purpose:

To properly mix two medications in one syringe-needle unit.

Equipment/Supplies:

Medications as ordered by the physician and medicine cards
Appropriately sized syringe-needle units
Sterile needles
Antiseptic wipes

(continues)

PROCEDURE 12-5 *continued*
Mixing Two Medications in One Syringe-Needle Unit

Equipment/Supplies (continued):

Disposable gloves
Sharps container

Procedure Steps:

1. Verify the physician's order.
2. Work in a well-lighted, quiet, clean area.
3. Perform medical asepsis hand wash and put on gloves.
4. Compare the medication labels with the physician's order.
5. Prepare a syringe-needle unit for use. Check to make sure that the needle is firmly attached to the tip of the syringe.
6. Draw up an amount of air into the syringe that will be equal to the amount of medication that you plan to withdraw from the vial.
7. Cleanse the rubber-stoppered portion of the vial with an antiseptic swab.
8. Place the syringe-needle unit in your dominant hand. Remove the sheath from the needle.
9. Pick up the vial in the other hand. Invert the vial, holding it between your thumb and index finger.
10. With the bevel of the needle toward you, smoothly insert the needle straight into the rubber-stoppered portion of the inverted vial at a 90° angle.
11. Slowly inject the equal amount of air from the barrel of the syringe into the vial.
12. Keeping the needle immersed in the solution, fill the barrel with the ordered amount of medication. Be sure that you do not have any dead air space left in the barrel *before* you remove the needle from the vial.
13. To remove the needle from the vial, *pull the vial away* from the needle.
14. Replace the sheath over the needle and secure it to the hub.
15. Hold the syringe-needle unit toward the light and check for air bubbles. If necessary, remove any air bubbles before proceeding to the next step. You must make sure that you have the

exact amount of ordered medication left in the syringe *before* removing the ordered medication from the second vial or ampule.

16. Place the previously described syringe-needle unit on the medication tray or a clean, dry surface.
17. Compare the second medication label with the physician's order.
18. Open a sterile needle package and prepare to change needles.
19. Remove the needle from the filled syringe. Set the needle aside.
20. Correctly place the opened sterile needle onto the filled syringe.
21. Cleanse the rubber-stoppered portion of the second vial with an antiseptic swab.
22. Place the syringe-needle unit in your dominant hand. Remove the sheath from the needle.
23. Pick up the second vial in the other hand. Invert the vial, holding it between your thumb and index finger.
24. With the bevel of the needle toward you, smoothly insert the needle straight into the rubber-stoppered portion of the inverted vial at a 90° angle.
25. Do *not* inject air into this vial.
26. Keeping the needle immersed in the solution, fill the barrel with the ordered amount of medication.
27. To remove the needle from the vial, *pull the vial away* from the needle.
28. Replace the sheath over the needle and secure it to the hub.
29. Hold the syringe-needle unit toward the light and check for air bubbles. If you have air bubbles and have to inject any of the medications that are in the syringe, you will have to discard the filled syringe and start all over.
30. Check to be sure that the total amount of medications in the syringe is the correct total of doses as ordered.
31. Prepare to administer the medication to the patient.

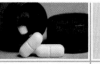

PROCEDURE 12-6
Reconstituting a Powder Medication for Administration

Standard Precautions:

Purpose:

Drugs for injection may be supplied in a powdered (dry) form and must be reconstituted to a liquid for injection. A diluent (usually sterile water) is added to the powder, mixed well, and the appropriate dose drawn up to be administered.

Equipment/Supplies:

Medication as ordered by the physician
Diluent
Two appropriately sized needles and syringe units
Antiseptic swabs
Disposable gloves
Sharps container

Procedure Steps:

1. Wash hands. Put on gloves.

2. Medical assistant prepares the needle-syringe unit in preparation for reconstituting powder medication (see Figure 12-25A).

3. Remove tops from diluent and powder medication containers and wipe with alcohol swabs (see Figure 12-25B).

4. Insert the needle of a sterile needle-syringe unit through the rubber stopper on the vial of diluent that has been cleansed with an antiseptic swab. The needle-syringe unit should have an amount of air in it equal to the amount of diluent to be withdrawn (see Figures 12-25 C and D).

5. Withdraw the appropriate amount of diluent to be added to the powder medication (see Figures 12-25E and 12-25F). Cover the sterile needle on the syringe containing appropriate amount of diluent.

6. Add this liquid to the powder medication that has been cleansed with an antiseptic swab (see Figure 12-25G).

7. Remove needle and syringe from vial with powder medication and diluent and discard into sharps container (see Figure 12-25H).

8. Roll the vial between the palms of the hands to completely mix together the powder and diluent (see Figure 12-25I). Label the multiple-dose vial with the dilution or strength of the medication prepared, the date and time, your initials, and the expiration date.

9. With a second sterile needle and syringe, withdraw the desired amount of medication (see Figure 12-25J).

10. Flick away any air bubbles that cling to side of syringe (see Figure 12-25K).

11. The medicine tray with reconstituted medication is ready for transport to the patient (Figure 12-25L).

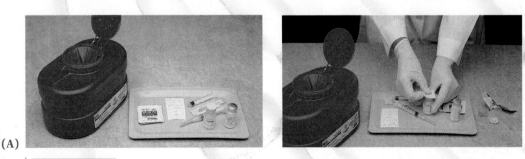

(A) (B)

FIGURE 12-25

(A) Supplies for reconstituting powder medication. (B) Remove top from diluent and powdered medication. Wipe top of each with an alcohol wipe. *Source: Delmar/Cengage Learning*

(continues)

PROCEDURE 12-6 *continued*
Reconstituting a Powder Medication for Administration

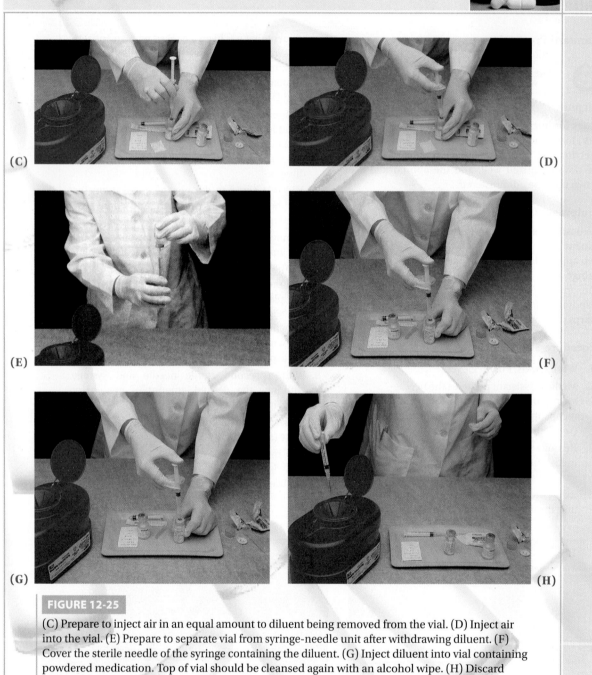

FIGURE 12-25

(C) Prepare to inject air in an equal amount to diluent being removed from the vial. (D) Inject air into the vial. (E) Prepare to separate vial from syringe-needle unit after withdrawing diluent. (F) Cover the sterile needle of the syringe containing the diluent. (G) Inject diluent into vial containing powdered medication. Top of vial should be cleansed again with an alcohol wipe. (H) Discard recapped syringe-needle unit after mixing. *Source: Delmar/Cengage Learning*

(continues)

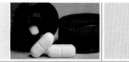

PROCEDURE 12-6 *continued*
Reconstituting a Powder Medication for Administration

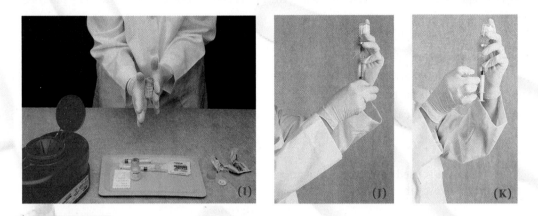

(I)   (J)   (K)

FIGURE 12-25

(I) Roll vial of powdered medication between palms of hands with the diluent to mix well. Label vial with date, amount of diluent added, strength of dilution, time mixed, and your initials. (J) Use a second sterile syringe-needle unit to draw the prescribed dose of medication ordered by the physician. (K) Flick away any air bubbles that cling to the side of the syringe.

Source: Delmar/Cengage Learning

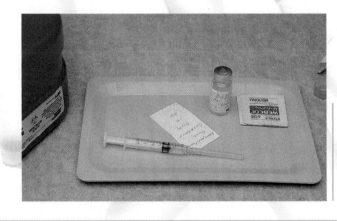

(L) Medicine tray with prepared injection is ready for transport to patient. Labeled, reconstituted medication will be placed on the shelf or in the refrigerator according to the manufacturer's instructions.

Source: Delmar/Cengage Learning

■ ■ REVIEW QUESTIONS

Directions. Select the best answer to each of the following multiple-choice question, circling the letter of your choice:

1. The component parts of a syringe consist of _____.
   a. a barrel
   b. a plunger
   c. the flange and the tip
   d. all of these

2. The parts of a typical needle are _____.
   a. the point, the lumen, the shaft
   b. the point, the shaft, the hub
   c. point, bevel, lumen, shaft, hub, and hilt
   d. point, hilt, bevel, and hub

3. Syringes are named according to _____.
   a. the manufacturer's choice
   b. the inventor's name
   c. their sizes and usages
   d. none of these

4. The parts of a syringe that *must remain sterile* during the preparation and administration of a parenteral medication are _____.
   a. the outside of the barrel, the tip, and the plunger
   b. the plunger and the tip
   c. the inside of the barrel, the plunger, and the tip
   d. the flange, the barrel, and the tip

5. A 3-mL hypodermic syringe is calibrated in _____.
   a. 0.2 mL
   b. 0.5 mL
   c. 0.1 mL
   d. 0.3 mL

6. A(An) _____ syringe is used to inject minute amounts of medication, for intradermal injections, allergy testing, and/or allergy injections.
   a. insulin
   b. tuberculin
   c. 3-mL hypodermic
   d. 5-mL hypodermic

7. Insulin syringes are calibrated in _____.
   a. cubic centimeters
   b. milliliters
   c. units
   d. minims

8. The _____ and _____ of the medication ordered determines the size of the syringe-needle unit to be selected.
   a. color and odor
   b. amount and viscosity
   c. color and amount
   d. viscosity and odor

9. When giving a subcutaneous injection, you should not inject more than _____ into subcutaneous tissue.
   a. 0.5 mL
   b. 1 mL
   c. 2 mL
   d. 3 mL

10. When selecting a syringe-needle unit for an intramuscular injection, you will _____ .
    a. consider the age and size of the patient
    b. select a needle with sufficient length to reach muscle tissue
    c. use the same size syringe-needle unit for all patients
    d. a and b

11. The _____ of a needle is determined by the diameter of its lumen.
    a. shaft
    b. hub
    c. gauge
    d. bevel

12. _____ is the injection of a liquid substance into the body via a route other than the alimentary canal.
    a. Hypodermic
    b. Parenteral
    c. Parental
    d. none of the above

13. The _____ of a syringe is the part that holds the medication, and has graduated markings on its surface.
    a. barrel
    b. plunger
    c. flange
    d. tip

14. The 5-mL syringe is calibrated with a single metric scale. Each small line of this scale represents _____ of a milliliter.
    a. 0.2
    b. 0.3
    c. 0.1
    d. 0.5

15. Each small line of the metric scale on a tuberculin syringe represents _____ of a milliliter.
    a. 0.2
    b. 0.1
    c. 0.01
    d. 0.5

16. The _____ is the sharpened end of the needle.

    a. bevel   b. lumen   c. hub   d. point

17. The point at which the shaft of the needle attaches to the hub is called the _____.

    a. flange   b. hilt   c. shaft   d. lumen

18. A 3-mL syringe, 25 G, $\frac{5}{8}$-inch needle unit may be used for a(an) _____.

    a. intravenous injection   c. subcutaneous injection

    b. intramuscular injection   d. intradermal injection

19. A 1-mL syringe, 26 G, $\frac{3}{8}$-inch needle unit may be used for a(an) _____.

    a. intravenous injection   c. subcutaneous injection

    b. intramuscular injection   d. intradermal injection

20. Used needles and syringes should be discarded in _____.

    a. a rigid, puncture-proof container   c. a plastic container

    b. a sharps collector   d. a and b

Matching. Place the correct letter from Column II on the appropriate line of Column I:

Column I	*Column II*
21. _____ AIDS	A. state of being free from living microorganisms
22. _____ hypodermic	B. a small, sterile, prefilled glass container that holds a hypodermic solution
23. _____ sterile	C. under or below the skin
24. _____ vial	D. a sterile, prefilled glass bottle containing a hypodermic solution, usually a multiple dose of medication
25. _____ ampule	E. acquired immunodeficiency syndrome
	F. above the skin

UNIT 13
Administration of Parenteral Medications

OBJECTIVES

Upon completing this unit, you should be able to:

- Define the terms listed in the vocabulary.
- Give three advantages of the parenteral routes of drug administration.
- Give eight disadvantages (possible dangers and complications) associated with the administration of parenteral medications.
- List the basic guidelines for administering an injection.
- Explain why it is important to do a patient assessment prior to the administration of an injection.
- Select the correct sites for a subcutaneous, an intramuscular, and an intradermal injection.
- Mark the correct site for an intramuscular injection.
- Prepare a patient for an injection.
- Demonstrate the proper procedure to be used when giving a subcutaneous, an intramuscular, an intradermal, and a "Z"-track intramuscular injection.
- Give the special considerations to be observed when administering insulin.
- Describe intravenous (IV) therapy and state some advantages and disadvantages of IV therapy.
- Answer the review questions correctly.

VOCABULARY

aspirate (as′pi-rāt). To remove by suction. During the injection process, aspirate means to pull back on the plunger to ascertain that the needle is not in a blood vessel.

assessment (as-sess′ment). A procedure that involves the systematic gathering and interpretation of data that relate to the patient.

hematoma (hee″ma-toe′ma). A blood tumor; collection of blood.

hemophilia (hee″mo-feel′ee-a). A hereditary blood disease.

palpate (pal′pāt). To feel; examining by means of touch.

rapport (ra-por′). A feeling of trust and understanding established between the patient and those providing health care.

taut (tot). Tight; for example, pulling a person's skin taut.

wheal (hwēl). A slight elevation of the skin that can be produced as a result of an intradermal injection.

INTRODUCTION

The parenteral route of drug administration offers an effective mode of delivering medication to a patient when a rapid and direct result is desired. Injected drugs are absorbed directly into the bloodstream; therefore, they manifest their medicinal effects within minutes. Absorption also depends upon the patient's physical state, especially his or her circulatory status, and the parenteral route of administration.

The following are the three most commonly used parenteral routes of drug administration.

- Intravenous—produces fastest effect.
- Intramuscular—produces next fastest effect.
- Subcutaneous—produces effect slower than the other two.

ADVANTAGES OF THE PARENTERAL ROUTE

There are certain situations in which the use of the parenteral route for the administration of medications is indicated because it offers definite advantages over other possible routes. The following are three major advantages offered by the parenteral route:

- It provides an effective route for the delivery of a drug when the patient's physical or mental state would make other routes (oral, sublingual, buccal, and so forth) difficult or impossible—for example, when a patient is unconscious.
- Drugs that are administered by injection are not altered by gastric acids, nor do they cause irritation to the patient's digestive system. Because parenteral medications do not enter the digestive system, there is no possibility that the drug will be lost as a result of vomiting. For example, insulin is made of amino acids and would be digested.
- The parenteral route provides a method of delivering a precise dose to a targeted area of the body. For example, a physician may give an intra-articular injection (within the joint) or an intrathecal injection (within the spinal canal) to deliver a medication to a target area.

DISADVANTAGES OF THE PARENTERAL ROUTE

A number of complications and dangers can occur when the parenteral route is used to administer medications. Medical assistants are responsible for knowing how to administer injections safely, accurately, and using the proper technique. Some of the possible disadvantages of the parenteral route are the following:

- The patient may have an allergic reaction to the injected medication. Such allergic response may range from mild to severe, and could be fatal. Allergic reactions to medications can occur immediately or manifest themselves after considerable delay.
- With the introduction of the hypodermic needle and the medication (two foreign substances) into the patient, there is the possibility for the introduction of microorganisms. This can occur as a result of incorrect preparation of equipment or the use of poor technique by the medical assistant.
- An injection can do injury to tissue, nerves, veins, and other vessels.
- The possibility of a needle breaking off from the hilt, while still in the patient, could result from defective equipment or improper injection technique.
- If you fail to **aspirate** during the injection process, a subcutaneous or an intramuscular medication could be given intravenously.
- A medication intended for intramuscular injection could be given into subcutaneous tissue, which could cause a sterile abscess.

- The needle can strike a bone in a geriatric, pediatric, or extremely thin person, as a result of improper selection of needle-syringe unit.

- Intravenous injection can traumatize a vein and cause a possible hematoma, phlebitis, or tissue damage.

PREPARING THE PATIENT FOR AN INJECTION

When explaining the injection procedure, you must take into account the patient's age, physical and mental condition, level of understanding, any hearing or visual impairments, and differences in language spoken or understood. Select an appropriate means to communicate your procedural plan. Explain the purpose of the injection and the desired effect that it should have on the patient. An informed patient will usually be more cooperative, relaxed, and agreeable.

Establish rapport with the patient by being courteous and professional (see Figure 13-1). Give the patient the opportunity to ask questions about the procedure. When possible, allow the patient to expose the intended injection site. Involving the patient in the procedure generally ensures cooperation and relieves anxiety. Drape the patient appropriately and be sure that the patient is in a comfortable position. Ask the patient to relax the site that is to be used for the injection.

When ready, inform the patient that he or she will feel a slight stick or stinging sensation when the needle is inserted. *Never* tell a patient that the injection will not hurt. This is especially true for the pediatric patient and those who have received numerous injections. An injection that is given using correct technique will cause a minimum of discomfort to the patient, and should only require a few seconds of time.

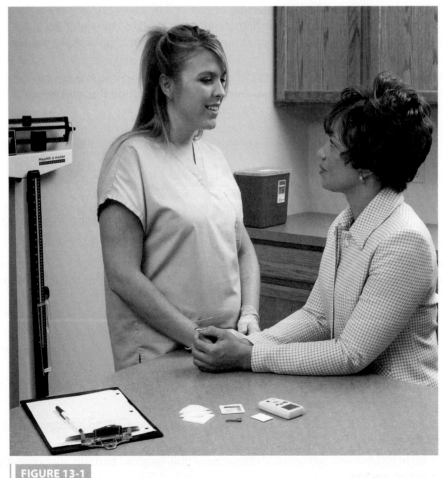

FIGURE 13-1

The medical assistant is establishing rapport with the patient. *Source: Delmar/Cengage Learning*

When administering medications that cause drowsiness, sedation, and other changes in bodily function, inform the patient of the effects, and advise the patient to report any unusual symptoms. Caution the patient about operating a motor vehicle or other machinery.

Immediately following the administration of the injection, correctly document the procedural process that was used.

PATIENT ASSESSMENT

Before administering any medication, you are to carefully assess your patient's condition. Your **assessment** should include, but is not limited to, the following conditions.

- Age: Are the medication and route suitable for the patient at a particular stage in life? The stages of life include infancy, childhood, adolescence, adulthood, and old age. During infancy, early childhood, and old age, a smaller dose of medication may be required than would be appropriate for the other stages in life.

- Physical condition: One must consider potential problems associated with the patient's physical condition. Female patients during pregnancy or while breast-feeding should not be given certain contraindicated medications. Males suffering from **hemophilia** require special considerations to counter bleeding following an injection.

- Body size: The amount of medication given and the size of the needle used are directly related to the size of the patient. Pediatric and geriatric patients usually have less subcutaneous and muscular tissue per body surface area than the average adult. Patients who are small or thin usually require less medication, and a shorter needle may be used to reach the appropriate tissue level. On the other hand, patients who are large or obese may require more medication than the average adult, and a longer needle to reach the appropriate tissue level.

- Sex: One must consider differences that are related to the sex of the patient.

  Muscular build. Male patients are generally more muscular than female patients. Always inspect and **palpate** muscle tissue with this in mind when determining the appropriate needle length to reach muscle tissue.

  Skin texture. Male patients usually have tougher skin than females. A young person's skin usually has more tone than that of an older person. Slightly more force is required to penetrate skin that is tough or lacking in tone.

- Injection site: Always inspect and palpate the skin before administering an injection. The following body areas should be *avoided* when choosing the site for an injection:
  - any type of skin lesion
  - burned areas
  - inflamed areas
  - previous injection sites
  - any traumatized area
  - scar tissue (vaccination, keloid)
  - moles, warts, birthmarks, tumors, lumps, hard nodules
  - nerves, large blood vessels, bones
  - cyanotic areas
  - edematous areas
  - paralyzed areas

SITE SELECTION

The selection of a proper site for a subcutaneous, intramuscular, or intradermal injection and the correct angle of insertion for each will ensure that the medication is delivered to the correct tissue type (see Figure 13-2).

A *subcutaneous injection* is given at an angle of 45°, just below the surface of the skin wherever there is subcutaneous tissue. The boxed areas in Figure 13-3 are usually used for subcutaneous injections of insulin because they are located away from bones, joints, nerves, and large blood vessels.

An *intramuscular injection* is given at a 90° angle (refer again to Figure 13-2), passing through the skin and subcutaneous tissue and penetrating deep into muscle tissue. Body areas normally used for intramuscular injections are the dorsogluteal area, ventrogluteal area, deltoid muscle, and vastus lateralis.

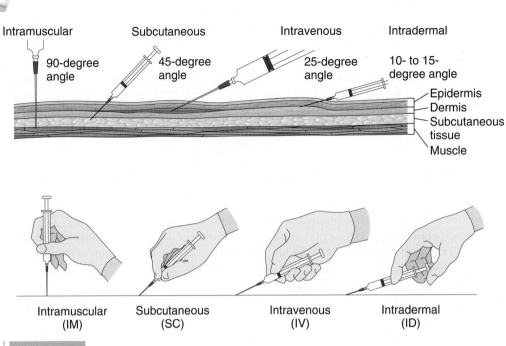

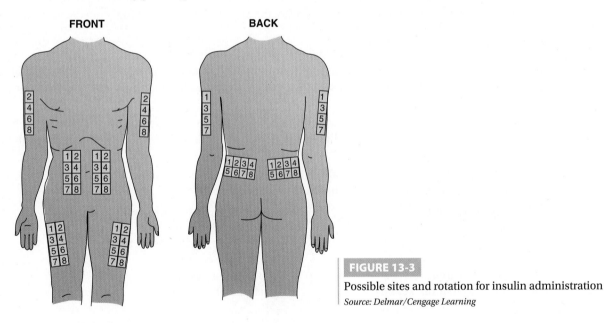

Angles of injection for intramuscular, subcutaneous, intravenous, and intradermal injections

Source: Delmar/Cengage Learning

Possible sites and rotation for insulin administration

Source: Delmar/Cengage Learning

Intradermal injections are given at an angle between 10° and 15° within the epidermal layer of the skin. The body areas used for intradermal injections are the inner forearm and the middle of the back. The reasons for the use of these two sites are that the skin is thin and there is very little hair.

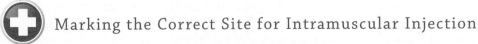 Marking the Correct Site for Intramuscular Injection

To give a safe injection, it is necessary that you become familiar with the anatomical structures associated with the injection site. With knowledge of where such structures are located, you will be able to mark injection sites that avoid bones, nerves, and large blood vessels.

The *dorsogluteal site* may be used for giving (adult) deep intramuscular injections (see Figure 13-4). Commonly referred to as the "upper outer quadrant of the buttocks," this description can be easily misinterpreted and result in an injection into an inappropriate area. To locate the correct site for a dorsogluteal injection, locate the *posterior iliac spine* and place a small X on this spot. Then locate the *greater trochanter of the femur* and mark this spot. Draw (or imagine) a diagonal line between the two locations. The area above and outside this line, but several inches below the iliac crest, is the correct location of the dorsogluteal site (see Figure 13-4).

> ### Caution:
>
> *Extreme caution should be used when giving intramuscular injections in the dorso-gluteal area. Improper site selection can result in damage to the sciatic nerve or injection into the superior gluteal artery or vein. This site is contraindicated for infants, and is used only as a site of last resort in children. The muscle mass may be degenerated in the elderly, the nonwalking, or the emaciated patient.*

The *ventrogluteal site* can generally accommodate the majority of medications ordered for intramuscular injection. It may be used for individuals from infancy to adulthood. The ventrogluteal site is relatively free of major nerves and vessels, thereby making it a choice site for IM injections. To locate the ventrogluteal injection site, palpate to find the *greater trochanter*, the *anterior superior iliac spine, and the bony ridge of the iliac crest* (see Figure 13-5). With these three locations identified, place the palm of your hand against the greater trochanter with the tip of your index finger on the anterior superior iliac spine. Then spread your middle finger as far from the index finger as possible. Place an X in the center of the triangle formed by the middle and index fingers to mark the correct injection site.

The *deltoid muscle* is a small but an adequate site for certain intramuscular injections. These IM preparations include vaccines, narcotics, sedatives, and vitamin preparations. The site should not be used for an infant. To locate the deltoid injection site, place your fingers on the shoulder and find the acromion (lateral triangular projection of the spine of the scapula forming the point of the shoulder) and the deltoid tuberosity that lies lateral to the side of the arm, opposite the axilla (see Figure 13-6). The correct injection site is 1 to 2 inches (about the width of three fingers) below the acromion.

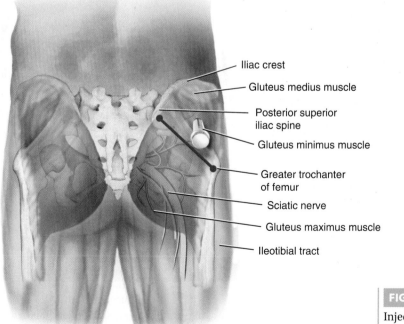

Iliac crest

Gluteus medius muscle

Posterior superior iliac spine

Gluteus minimus muscle

Greater trochanter of femur

Sciatic nerve

Gluteus maximus muscle

Ileotibial tract

FIGURE 13-4

Injection technique for dorsogluteal site, adult

Source: Delmar/Cengage Learning

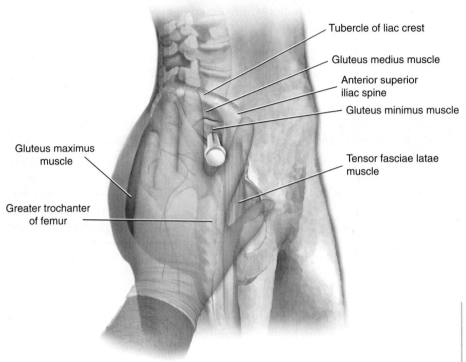

Tubercle of liac crest

Gluteus medius muscle

Anterior superior
iliac spine

Gluteus minimus muscle

Gluteus maximus
muscle

Tensor fasciae latae
muscle

Greater trochanter
of femur

FIGURE 13-5

Injection technique for
ventrogluteal site, adult

Source: Delmar/Cengage Learning

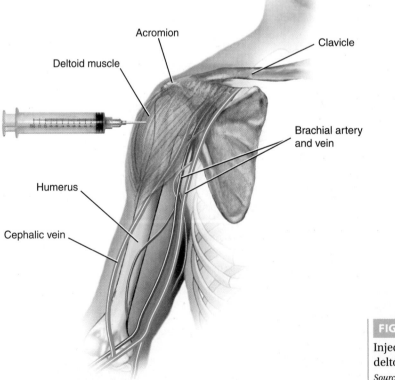

Acromion

Clavicle

Deltoid muscle

Brachial artery
and vein

Humerus

Cephalic vein

FIGURE 13-6

Injection technique for
deltoid site, adult

Source: Delmar/Cengage Learning

The *vastus lateralis* is the preferred site for intramuscular injections in most *infants and children*. It is also used for IM injections in adults. This site generally accommodates the majority of IM injections ordered, and is a relatively safe site because the nerves and vessels supplying the area are not generally endangered. The vastus lateralis is a part of the quadriceps femoris. The muscle is located on the anterolateral aspects of the thigh. The correct injection site is relative to the age of the patient. For infants and children, the site lies below the greater trochanter of the femur and within the *upper* lateral quadrant of the thigh (see Figure 13-7).

For the adult patient, the correct injection site is within the middle third of the muscle (see Figure 13-8).

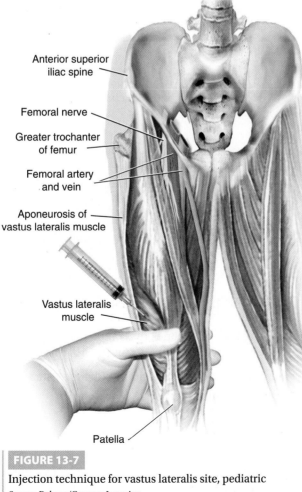

Anterior superior iliac spine

Femoral nerve

Greater trochanter of femur

Femoral artery and vein

Aponeurosis of vastus lateralis muscle

Vastus lateralis muscle

Patella

FIGURE 13-7

Injection technique for vastus lateralis site, pediatric

Source: Delmar/Cengage Learning

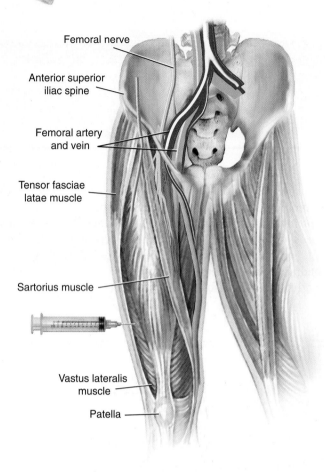

Femoral nerve

Anterior superior
iliac spine

Femoral artery
and vein

Tensor fasciae
latae muscle

Sartorius muscle

Vastus lateralis
muscle

Patella

FIGURE 13-8

Injection technique for vastus lateralis site, adult

Source: Delmar/Cengage Learning

Safety Precautions:

CAUTION: The muscle mass is likely to be degenerated in the elderly, the nonwalking, and the emaciated patient.

BASIC GUIDELINES FOR THE ADMINISTRATION OF INJECTIONS

Regardless of the type of injection, there are basic guidelines that one must follow to safeguard patients. These guidelines are given next, according to the sequence of the events to which they relate:

1. The medical assistant should follow the Essential Medication Guidelines listed in Unit 10.

2. Adhere to the "seven rights" of proper drug administration.

3. Always evaluate each patient as an individual.

4. Select a needle-syringe unit that is the appropriate size for the proper administration of a parenteral medication (see Unit 12).

5. Correctly prepare the appropriate parenteral equipment and supplies for use. Put on gloves.

6. Select the correct site for the intended injection.

7. Prepare the patient properly for the injection.

8. For subcutaneous and intramuscular injections, use a smooth, quick, dartlike motion to insert the needle into the patient's skin. Use the correct angle of insertion (45° to 90°) for the injection. Once the needle is inserted, gently pull back on the plunger (aspirate) to ensure that the needle is not in a blood vessel.

● **Note**

> **If blood appears in the syringe upon aspiration, smoothly withdraw the needle, properly discard the used unit, and prepare another injection for administration. Repeat the previously described steps. ●**

9. Inject the medication slowly into the patient.

10. With a quick, smooth motion, remove the needle from the injection site. Cover the injection site with a dry, sterile cotton swab and gently massage the site.

● **Note**

> **Do not massage the site when administering insulin, Imferon, or heparin. ●**

11. Remove the cotton swab and check for bleeding. If bruising occurs, apply ice to the injection site.

12. Observe the patient for any signs of hypersensitivity.

13. Take precautions to ensure the patient's safety.

14. Follow documentation procedures to record the administration of the medication.

15. Properly discard the used equipment and supplies. Remove gloves.

16. Before leaving the room, make sure that the patient is given proper instructions and feels all right.

See Procedures 13-1, 13-2, 13-3, and 13-4 for detailed information on administering injections.

PROCEDURE 13-1
Administration of Subcutaneous, Intramuscular, and/or Intradermal Injections

Standard Precautions:

Purpose:

To properly administer subcutaneous, intramuscular, and/or intradermal injections

Equipment/Supplies:

Medication as ordered by the physician
Appropriately sized needle-syringe unit
Antiseptic wipes
Disposable gloves
Sharps container

Procedure Steps:

1. Verify the physician's order.
2. Follow the "seven rights."
3. Perform medical asepsis hand wash. Adhere to OSHA guidelines.
4. Work in a well-lighted, quiet, clean area.
5. Obtain the appropriate syringe-needle unit and alcohol swab.
6. Obtain the correct medication.
7. Compare the medication label with the medication order (first time).
8. Check expiration date on medicine.
9. Calculate dosage, if necessary.

(*continues*)

PROCEDURE 13-1 *continued*
Administration of Subcutaneous, Intramuscular, and/or Intradermal Injections

Procedure Steps (continued):

10. Prepare syringe-needle unit for use (see Figure 13-9A through 13-9D).

11. Withdraw medication from container.

12. Compare medicine label with the medication order (second time).

13. Place filled syringe-needle unit on the medicine tray. Check the medication label with the medication order (third time).

14. Correctly transport the medicine to the patient.

15. Identify the patient. Explain the procedure.

16. Assess the patient. Put on gloves.

17. Prepare the patient for the injection (drape, position, allay apprehension).

18. Select an appropriate injection site. Follow a rotating schedule if appropriate.

19. Cleanse the injection site with a sterile antiseptic swab. Use a circular motion, working from the center out to about 2 inches beyond the planned injection site.

20. Allow the skin to dry.

21. Administer the injection (aspirate to be certain needle is not in a blood vessel). Immediately dispose of syringe-needle unit in a puncture-proof container.

22. Massage injection site unless contraindicated. Do not massage after giving insulin, iron, or heparin.

23. Observe the patient for signs of difficulty.

24. Inspect the injection site for bleeding; apply Band-Aid if necessary.

25. Properly dispose of used equipment and supplies. Remove gloves.

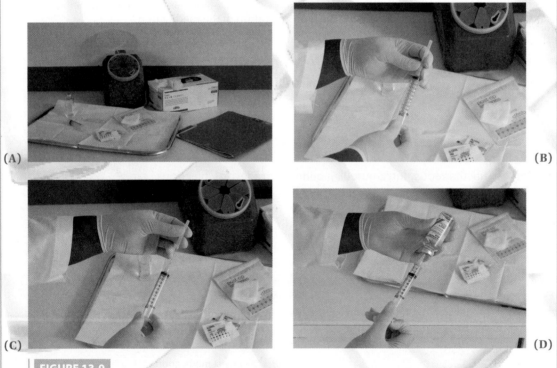

(A)   (B)   (C)   (D)

FIGURE 13-9

Preparing the syringe-needle unit for use. (A) Assemble the equipment and supplies needed to draw up medication from vial. (B) Use a clockwise motion to turn the hub of the needle on the syringe tip. (C) Remove the sheath from the needle. (D) Withdraw medication from container.

Source: Delmar/Cengage Learning

(continues)

PROCEDURE 13-1 *continued*
Administration of Subcutaneous, Intramuscular, and/or Intradermal Injections

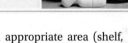

Procedure Steps (continued):

26. Perform medical asepsis hand wash.
27. Correctly document the procedure.

Procedure to follow should the medical assistant sustain an accidental needlestick after the injection:

- Thoroughly wash the site where the stick occurred with soap and water.
- Cleanse the skin with an antiseptic.
- Report the incident.
- Document the incident and retain a copy for yourself.
- Obtain medical attention. Be tested for hepatitus B virus and HIV.
- Fill out appropriate OSHA paperwork (200 form).

PROCEDURE 13-2
Administering a Subcutaneous Injection

Standard Precautions:

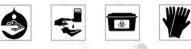

Purpose:

Correctly administer a subcutaneous injection after receiving a physician's order and assembling the necessary equipment and supplies

Equipment/Supplies:

Medication ordered by physician
Appropriately sized needle-syringe unit
Antiseptic wipe
Disposable gloves
Sharps container

Procedure Steps:

1. Verify the physician's order.
2. Follow the "seven rights."
3. Perform medical asepsis hand wash. Adhere to OSHA guidelines.
4. Work in a well-lighted, quiet, clean area.
5. Obtain the appropriate equipment and supplies.
6. Obtain the correct medication.
7. Compare the medication label with the medication order (first time).
8. Check expiration date on medicine.
9. Calculate dosage, if necessary.
10. Correctly prepare the parenteral medication.
11. Compare medication label with the medication order (second time).
12. Replace medication in appropriate area (shelf, refrigerator). Compare the medication label (third time).
13. Correctly transport the medicine to the patient.
14. Identify the patient. Explain the procedure.
15. Assess the patient. Put on gloves.
16. Prepare the patient for the injection (drape, position, allay apprehension).
17. Select an appropriate injection site.
18. Correctly cleanse the site using a circular motion starting with the injection site and moving outward to a 2-inch diameter. Allow skin to dry.
19. Remove needle guard.
20. Grasp skin to form a 1-inch fold.
21. Insert needle quickly at a 45° angle.
22. Aspirate to be certain needle is not in a blood vessel. RATIONALE: When blood appears in the needle, you are most likely in a blood vessel. If you inject the medication, it will go directly into the bloodstream (intravenous); this is not the correct route of administration. **Note: If blood appears in the syringe-needle unit upon aspiration, smoothly withdraw the needle, properly discard the used unit, and prepare another injection for administration.**
23. Slowly inject the medicine.
24. Correctly remove the needle and syringe.
25. Cover site. Massage unless contraindicated (as with insulin, iron, and heparin). RATIONALE: Massage

(*continues*)

PROCEDURE 13-2 *continued*
Administering a Subcutaneous Injection

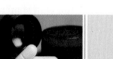

Procedure Steps (continued):

will help distribute the medication throughout the tissue.

26. Immediately dispose of needle and syringe in a sharps container.

27. Remove gloves and wash hands.
28. Provide for patient's safety.
29. Document the procedure.

PROCEDURE 13-3
Administering an Intramuscular Injection

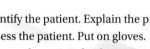

Standard Precautions:

Purpose:

Correctly administer an intramuscular injection after receiving a physician's order and assembling the necessary equipment and supplies

Equipment/Supplies:

Medication ordered by physician
Appropriately sized needle-syringe unit
Antiseptic wipe
Disposable gloves
Sharps container

Procedure Steps:

1. Verify the physician's order.
2. Follow the "seven rights."
3. Perform medical asepsis hand wash. Adhere to OSHA guidelines.
4. Work in a well-lighted, quiet, clean area.
5. Obtain the appropriate equipment and supplies.
6. Obtain the correct medication.
7. Compare the medication label with the medication order (first time).
8. Check expiration date.
9. Calculate dosage, if necessary.
10. Correctly prepare the parenteral medication.
11. Compare medicine label with the medication order (second time).
12. Replace medication on appropriate shelf and compare medication label with medication order (third time).
13. Correctly transport the medicine to the patient.

14. Identify the patient. Explain the procedure.
15. Assess the patient. Put on gloves.
16. Prepare the patient for the injection (drape, position, allay apprehension).
17. Select an appropriate injection site.
18. Correctly cleanse the site using a circular motion and covering a 2-inch diameter. Allow the skin to dry.
19. Remove needle guard.
20. Stretch the skin **taut**, pulling it tight.
21. Using a dartlike motion, insert needle to the hub at a 90° angle.
22. Release the skin.
23. Aspirate to check for blood. RATIONALE: When blood appears in the needle, you are most likely in a blood vessel. If you inject the medication, it will go directly into the bloodstream (intravenous); this is not the correct route of administration. ***Note:*** **If blood appears in the syringe-needle unit upon aspiration, smoothly withdraw the needle, properly discard the used unit, and prepare another injection for administration.**
24. Slowly inject the medicine.
25. Correctly remove the needle and syringe.
26. Cover site. Massage unless contraindicated (as with insulin, iron, and heparin). RATIONALE: Massage will help distribute the medication throughout the tissue.
27. Immediately dispose of needle and syringe in a sharps container.
28. Remove gloves.
29. Wash hands.
30. Observe the patient for signs of difficulty.
31. Provide for patient's safety.
32. Document the procedure.

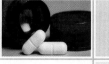

PROCEDURE 13-4
Administering an Intradermal Injection

Standard Precautions:

Purpose:

Correctly administer an intradermal injection after receiving a physician's order and assembling the necessary equipment and supplies

Equipment/Supplies:

Medication as ordered by physician
Appropriately sized needle-syringe unit
Antiseptic wipe
Disposable gloves
Sharps container

Procedure Steps:

1. Verify the physician's order.
2. Follow the "seven rights."
3. Perform medical asepsis hand wash. Adhere to OSHA guidelines.
4. Work in a well-lighted, quiet, clean area.
5. Obtain the appropriate equipment and supplies.
6. Obtain the correct medication.
7. Compare the medication label with the medication order (first time).
8. Check expiration date.
9. Calculate dosage, if necessary.
10. Correctly prepare the parenteral medication.
11. Compare medication label with the medication order (second time).
12. Replace medication on appropriate shelf and compare medication label with medication order (third time).
13. Correctly transport the medicine to the patient.
14. Identify the patient. Explain the procedure.
15. Assess the patient. Put on gloves.
16. Prepare the patient for the injection (drape, position, allay apprehension).
17. Select an appropriate injection site.
18. Correctly cleanse the site using a circular motion and covering a 2-inch diameter. Allow the skin to dry.
19. Remove needle guard.
20. Pull the skin tissue taut.
21. Carefully insert the needle at a 10° to 15° angle, bevel upward to about $\frac{1}{8}$ inch.
22. Steadily inject the medicine. Produce a **wheal**, or slight elevation of the skin.
23. Correctly remove the needle.
24. Cover site. Do not massage. Dispose of equipment. Remove gloves.
25. Wash hands.
26. Observe the patient for signs of difficulty.
27. Provide for patient's safety.
28. Document the procedure.

"Z"-TRACK METHOD OF INTRAMUSCULAR INJECTION

The "Z"-track method of injection is used for administering medications that can be irritating to or may stain subcutaneous tissue. This method may also be used to decrease pain that can be caused by certain medications and to reduce the possibility of necrosis occurring in soft tissue. Iron dextran and hydroxyzine HCl/hydroxyzine pamoate are examples of medications administered by this method.

The "Z"-track method involves pulling the skin in such a way that the needle track is sealed off after the injection. The recommended site for the injection is the dorsogluteal area.

PROCEDURE 13-5
"Z"-Track Intramuscular Injection Technique

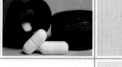

Standard Precautions:

Purpose:

Correctly administer a "Z"-track intramuscular injection after receiving a physician's order and assembling the necessary equipment and supplies

Equipment/Supplies:

Medication ordered by physician
Appropriately sized needle-syringe unit
Antiseptic wipe
Disposable gloves
Sharps container

Procedure Steps:

1. Verify the physician's order.
2. Follow the "seven rights."
3. Perform medical asepsis hand wash. Adhere to OSHA guidelines.
4. Work in a well-lighted, quiet, clean area.
5. Obtain the appropriate equipment and supplies.
6. Obtain the correct medication.
7. Compare the medication label with the medication order (first time).
8. Check expiration date.
9. Calculate dosage, if necessary.
10. Correctly prepare the parenteral medication.
11. Compare medicine label with the medication order (second time).
12. Replace medication on shelf and compare medication label with medication order (third time).
13. Correctly transport the medicine to the patient.
14. Identify the patient. Explain the procedure.
15. Assess the patient. Put on gloves.
16. Prepare the patient for the injection (drape, position, allay apprehension).
17. Select an appropriate injection site.
18. Correctly cleanse the site using a circular motion and covering a 2-inch diameter. Allow the skin to dry.
19. Remove needle guard.
20. Pull the skin laterally $1\frac{1}{2}$ inch away from the injection site.
21. Insert needle quickly, using a dartlike motion at a 90° angle. Maintain "Z" position.
22. Aspirate to check for blood.
23. Slowly inject medication.
24. Wait 10 seconds before removing needle to allow medication to begin to be absorbed.
25. Remove needle and syringe at same angle of insertion.
26. Release traction of the "Z" position to seal off the needle track. This prevents medication from reaching the subcutaneous tissues and the surface of the skin.
27. Cover site. Do not massage. RATIONALE: Because of the tissue irritating properties of the medication, do not massage the area. Dispose of equipment.
28. Remove gloves.
29. Wash hands.
30. Observe patient for signs of difficulty.
31. Provide for patient safety.
32. Document the procedure.

SPECIAL CONSIDERATIONS FOR THE ADMINISTRATION OF INSULIN

Drugs administered through the subcutaneous route are absorbed primarily by the capillaries, thus providing slower, more sustained action by the drug. Drugs recommended for subcutaneous injection should be nonirritating aqueous solutions and suspensions. Examples of drugs that are administered subcutaneously include epinephrine, certain vaccines, and insulin.

When injecting *insulin*, the following special considerations should be observed:

- Be sure that you have selected the correct insulin for administration.
- Slowly and gently roll the bottle of insulin between the palms of your hands to evenly mix the components of the drug.
- *Never* shake the bottle.

- Draw up the ordered dosage of insulin using the U-100 syringe unit.
- Using a site-rotation system, select an appropriate site. Insulin injection sites must be rotated to prevent tissue damage and the accumulation of unabsorbed medication (see Figure 13-10). Always record the site that was used.
- Do *not* massage the injection site.
- When mixing two insulins in one syringe, always make sure that they are compatible. An example of two compatible insulins that may be mixed are NPH and Regular.
- Always follow the physician's order and your institution's policy when mixing insulins.

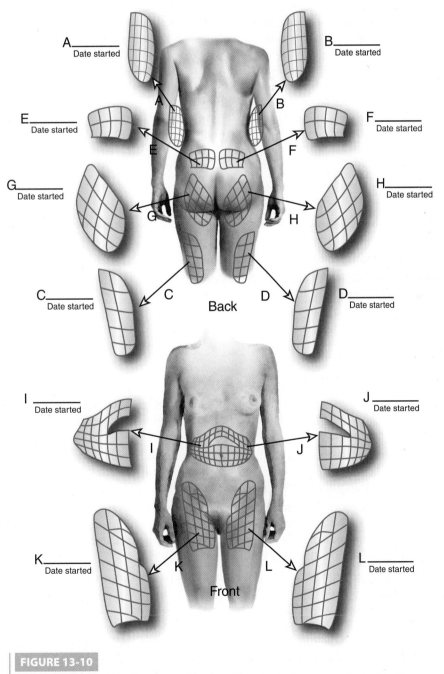

FIGURE 13-10

This injection log records sites used by date. To prevent damage to tissue, insulin injections must be rotated. *Source: Delmar/Cengage Learning*

PRINCIPLES OF INTRAVENOUS (IV) THERAPY

Intravenous therapy is the administration of fluids, solutions, electrolytes, nutrients, or medications by the venous route. A variety of fluids and solutions are used intravenously to correct fluid loss or to control imbalances that arise from disease or trauma. IV therapy is prescribed by the physician and administered by a person licensed to perform such therapy. Intravenous nursing may be defined as the utilization of the nursing process as it relates to fluids and electrolytes, infection control, oncology, pediatrics, pharmacology, quality assurance, technology, and clinical application, parenteral nutrition, and transfusion therapy. The nurse is expected to understand all aspects of such therapy—the indications, expected consequences for the patient, any anticipated side effects or adverse reactions, and all interventions needed to maintain the patient's safety and well-being.

Although in most states, a medical assistant is **not permitted** by law to administer intravenous medications or to perform intravenous therapy, it is important for the MA to be knowledgeable about the principles of such therapy. *Intravenous* means within or into a vein. An *intravenous injection* is the use of a sterile syringe-needle unit to instill a single dose of medicine into the vein of a patient. An intravenous infusion is the introduction of a solution in a larger quantity, usually 250 mL to 500 mL by means of a bottle connected to the needle by a plastic or rubber tubing. The rate of infusion may be regulated by adjusting the number of drops per minute. Flow is usually by gravity but can be given under pressure. An *infusion pump* is a special pump designed to provide constant but adjustable rate of flow of solutions given intravenously. The pump may work by applying intermittent pressure on the tubing carrying the solution so that the fluid is not actually in contact with the pump itself.

Advantages of IV Therapy

Some of the advantages of IV therapy are the following:

- It provides a direct route for immediate delivery of medication or fluid into the patient's systemic circulation.
- It is a reliable route for the unconscious or uncooperative patient, and for emergency situations.
- The absorption of the drug is directly into the bloodstream.
- It provides a route for drugs that cannot be given by other routes and for patients who are nauseated, vomiting, or having other gastrointestinal difficulties.

Disadvantages of IV Therapy

Some of the disadvantages of IV therapy are:

- *Fluid Overload.* This occurs when the circulatory system is overloaded with excessive intravenous fluids. Signs and symptoms include increased blood pressure and central venous pressure, severe dyspnea, cyanosis, cough, and puffy eyelids.
- *Air Embolism.* This is an obstruction of a blood vessel by an air bubble. Although this does not occur frequently, it is a danger of IV therapy. Signs and symptoms include sudden onset of dyspnea and cyanosis; hypotension; weak, rapid pulse; extreme anxiety; sharp chest pains; loss of consciousness.
- *Septicemia.* This may occur when aseptic technique is broken and pathogenic microorganisms are introduced into the patient's bloodstream. Signs and symptoms include abrupt elevation of temperature, backache, headache, increased pulse and respiratory rates, nausea and vomiting, diarrhea, chills and shaking, general malaise, and, if severe, vascular collapse.
- *Infection.* Infection ranges in severity from local involvement of the insertion site to systemic involvement, such as septicemia. Signs and symptoms of a local infection include redness, heat, pain or tenderness, and swelling.
- *Infiltration.* This may occur when the needle is dislodged and the fluid infiltrates into the surrounding tissue. Signs and symptoms include edema around the insertion site, discomfort, and cooling in the area of infiltration.
- *Phlebitis.* Inflammation of a vein related to both a chemical and mechanical irritation. Signs and symptoms include redness, heat, pain or tenderness, and swelling.

- *Thrombophlebitis.* The presence of a blood clot plus inflammation in the vein. Signs and symptoms include redness, heat, pain or tenderness, and swelling around the insertion site or along the path of the vein, immobility of the extremity because of discomfort and swelling, sluggish flow rate, fever, malaise, and leukocytosis.

- *Hematoma.* Occurs as a result of leakage of blood into tissues surrounding the insertion site. It can be caused by perforating the opposite vein wall during venipuncture, the needle slipping out of the vein, and insufficient pressure applied to the site after the needle or catheter is removed. Signs and symptoms include ecchymosis, immediate swelling at the site, and the leakage of blood at the site.

- *Clotting.* Clotting within the needle may occur when the IV tubing becomes kinked, there is a very slow flow rate, an empty IV bag is left hanging, or because of not flushing the tubing after intermittent medications or solutions are administered. Signs and symptoms are decreased flow rate and blood flow back into the IV tubing.

- *Pain and Discomfort.* May be described by the patient as a burning or stinging sensation; dull, aching sensation with a feeling of tightness or hardness (induration) at the site. Tenderness above the cannula insertion site. A cramping or gripping sensation (venospasm).

- *Hypersensitivity Reaction.* This is one of the most serious consequences of IV therapy. Hypersensitivity can occur to the infusate, its preservatives, or to the IV medication. The patient may be allergic to the cannula, skin antiseptic preparations, or tape. A reaction can be anything from a rash, itching, and hives to bronchial spasm and anaphylaxis. Anaphylaxis is a severe allergic reaction. Shock and death can ensue within minutes if treatment is not initiated.

Intravenous therapy requires extensive knowledge of many factors and it is not the intent of this author to present anything other than a brief overview of the subject. Intravenous therapy has changed dramatically over the past 5 years. Anyone who is involved in delivering IV therapy must be licensed to do so and must know the practice standards established by the nurse practice act of the state in which one practices.

■ ■ REVIEW QUESTIONS

Directions. Select the best answer to each of the following multiple-choice questions, circling the letter of your choice:

1. When administering a subcutaneous and/or an intramuscular injection, you would gently pull back on the plunger to _____.
   a. reduce discomfort to the patient
   b. ascertain that the needle is not in a blood vessel
   c. make sure that you are in the right site
   d. make sure that you have the right medicine

2. Before administering any medication, you are to carefully assess your patient's condition. This assessment should include _____.
   a. the patient's age and body size
   b. the patient's physical condition
   c. the muscular build and skin texture of the patient
   d. all of these

3. Body areas to avoid when choosing the site for an injection are _____.
   a. healthy muscle tissue
   b. scar tissue
   c. moles, birthmarks, warts, tumors, lumps, bones
   d. b and c

4. A subcutaneous injection is given at an angle of _____.

   a. 60°   b. 50°   c. 45°   d. 30°

5. An intramuscular injection is given at a _____.

   a. 45° angle   b. 90° angle   c. 60° angle   d. 50° angle

6. The body areas used for an intradermal injection are _____.

   a. the deltoid muscle and/or gluteal muscle

   b. the inner forearm and the middle of the back

   c. the outer forearm and the middle of the back

   d. the thigh and/or the middle of the back

7. The _____ may be used for giving (adult) deep intramuscular injections.

   a. ventrogluteal site   c. dorsogluteal site

   b. deltoid muscle   d. vastus lateralis

8. When administering an injection into the deltoid muscle, caution must be taken to avoid _____.

   a. the sciatic nerve   c. the acromion and the humerus

   b. the brachial and axillary nerves   d. b and c

9. The _____ is the preferred site for intramuscular injections in infants and children.

   a. ventrogluteal   c. dorsogluteal

   b. deltoid muscle   d. vastus lateralis

10. The following special considerations should be followed when preparing and administering insulin.

   a. *Shake* the bottle to mix evenly.

   b. Use a site-rotation system.

   c. Be sure you have the *correct* insulin for administration.

   d. b and c

11. When administering insulin, you should _____.

   a. not massage the injection site

   b. use any subcutaneous area for the injection

   c. not rotate the site of injection

   d. use a 30° angle

12. Regardless of the type of injection, there are basic guidelines that one must follow to safeguard the patient. These guidelines include _____.

   a. evaluating each patient as an individual

   b. correctly preparing parenteral equipment and supplies for use

   c. selecting the correct site for the intended injection

   d. all of these

13. What steps should be taken if blood appears in the syringe upon aspiration?

   a. Smoothly withdraw the needle   c. Prepare another injection for administration

   b. Properly discard the used unit   d. all of these

14. When cleansing the injection site with a sterile antiseptic swab, you would _____.

   a. use a circular motion

   b. work from the center out to about 2 inches beyond the planned injection site

   c. work from the outer edges of the injection site to the center

   d. a and b

15. Should an accidental stick occur after an injection, you would _____.

    a. thoroughly wash the site where the stick occurred

    b. cleanse the skin with an antiseptic

    c. report and document the incident, and obtain medical attention

    d. all of these

16. When administering an intradermal injection, the lumen of the needle should be in _____.

    a. subcutaneous tissue   c. the epidermal layer of the skin

    b. muscle tissue   d. none of these

17. Insulin injection sites must be rotated to _____.

    a. prevent tissue damage

    b. prevent accumulation of the unabsorbed medication

    c. prevent tissue hypertrophy

    d. all of these

18. A correctly administered intradermal injection will produce a _____.

    a. wen   c. wheel

    b. wheal   d. all of these

19. Examples of drugs that are administered subcutaneously are _____.

    a. antibiotics   c. certain vitamins

    b. insulin   d. b and c

Matching. Place the correct letter from Column II on the appropriate line of Column I:

Column I   *Column II*

20. _____ palpate   A. a blood tumor

21. _____ taut   B. to remove by suction

22. _____ hematoma   C. to feel

23. _____ aspirate   D. to pull or draw tight a surface, such as skin

24. _____ wheal   E. a slight elevation of the skin that can be produced as a result of an in-
                                   tradermal injection

25. _____ rapport   F. a feeling of trust and understanding established between the patient
                                   and those providing health care

                                G. to loosen a surface, such as skin

UNIT 14
Allergy: An Overview

OBJECTIVES

Upon completing this unit, you should be able to:

- Define the terms listed in the vocabulary.
- Describe the reaction between allergens and IgE antibodies.
- List the most common allergens that may cause allergy.
- State the classic symptoms of allergy.
- List factors other than allergens that may trigger symptoms of allergy.
- Describe allergic rhinitis (hay fever).
- List the most common causes of hay fever in the United States according to the American Academy of Allergy and Immunology.
- Describe how physicians determine the diagnosis of allergy.
- State the importance of the patient history.
- Describe the scratch (epicutaneous) or prick, patch, intradermal, laboratory, nasal smear, and sinus X-ray diagnostic allergy tests.
- Describe to patients with allergies the treatment regimen that may be prescribed, including the avoidance of allergens, drug therapy, and immunotherapy.
- Describe the medical assistant's responsibilities with regard to the administration of allergenic extracts.
- Answer the review questions correctly.

VOCABULARY

allergen (al'er-jen). Any substance that causes allergy.

allergy (al-er-gee). An individual hypersensitivity to a substance, usually an antibody-allergen reaction.

anaphylaxis (an"a-fi-lak'sis). An allergic hypersensitivity reaction of the body to a foreign substance, usually to a protein substance or a drug. Anaphylactic shock usually occurs suddenly and can be life threatening.

atopy (at'o-pee). An allergy for which there is a genetic predisposition. There is an inherited tendency to develop a certain type of allergy, but not the allergy itself. The principal *atopic* manifestations are vasomotor rhinitis, bronchial asthma, and chronic urticaria.

colic (kol'ik). Pertaining to spasm in any hollow soft organ accompanied by pain.

desensitize (de-sĕn'si-tize). To lessen the sensitivity of an individual by administration of the specific antigen or antigens (in minute dosage).

immunoglobulin gamma E (IgE) (im"u-no-glob'u-lin gam'ma). A protein produced by the lining of the respiratory and intestinal tracts. It is important in forming reagin.

reagin (re'a-jin). A type of immunoglobulin gamma E (IgE) that is present in the serum of atopic individuals. It is deposited in cutaneous tissue and may enter the bloodstream, causing the primary reaction that appears as edema in allergic rhinitis.

INTRODUCTION

Approximately 50 million Americans are allergic to certain substances. Individuals with allergies have an inherited defect in their immune system. They are likely to suffer from an abnormality of a Y-shaped blood molecule **immunoglobulin gamma E (IgE)**. IgE is produced by cells of the lining of the respiratory and intestinal tracts. It is called the **reaginic** antibody and is present in the serum of individuals with **atopy**. These individuals have a tendency to develop **allergies** to substances that are generally harmless to others.

The most common allergies are due to **allergens** such as pollens, animal danders, house dust, house dust mites, molds, certain drugs, insect stings, and many foods. Many other substances may act as allergens. Some of these substances are dyes, perfumes, cosmetics, soaps, detergents, tobacco, feathers, fabrics, smoke, chemicals, vapors, gases, fumes, metals, and latex.

⚠️ Latex Allergy:

The incidence of latex allergy has increased with the expanded use of gloves in hospitals and other health care settings.

Question each patient about any allergic reactions to latex products. If an allergic reaction occurred, this should be noted in red on the patient's chart. Health care workers should not wear latex gloves while performing any type of procedure on this patient.

Health care workers who are sensitive to latex should use nonlatex gloves. For copies of the guidelines to help prevent and manage latex allergy, you can call the American College of Allergy and Immunology at 708-359-2800 or write the ACAI at 800 E. Northwest Highway, Suite 1080, Palatine, IL 60067.

An allergic condition may manifest itself as hay fever, asthma, eczema, conjunctivitis, dermatitis, urticaria or hives, food allergy, occupational allergy, and anaphylaxis. In this unit, emphasis is placed on allergic rhinitis (hay fever).

Hay fever, an allergic reaction to trees, grass, and weed pollens, is America's Number 1 chronic illness. This condition can be brought on by hundreds of different kinds of pollens and molds. Approximately 500 pollens are distributed by the wind and may wind up in a person's nose, eyes, and respiratory tract. When such a pollen lands on a susceptible individual's mucous membrane, the reaction between allergens and IgE antibodies causes the release of chemical substances such as *histamine, leukotrienes,* and *prostaglandins*. These chemicals cause the classic symptoms of allergy: sneezing, congestion, rhinorrhea, postnasal drip, scratchy throat, itchy eyes and nose, pressure under and behind the eyes, and a feeling of general discomfort.

According to the National Institute of Allergy and Infectious Diseases, more people miss school and work because of seasonal allergies than from any other single cause. An estimate $500 million is spent on over-the-counter (OTC) and prescription antihistamines, decongestants, and nasal sprays to alleviate the symptoms of *allergic rhinitis* (hay fever).

APPEARANCE OF SYMPTOMS

Allergy symptoms can occur at any age. However, the most frequent appearance of symptoms occurs during childhood. The infant who has **colic**, is irritable and restless, and has difficulty taking formula, is most likely suffering from an allergy. The child who is restless, irritable, disruptive, and has one cold after another may be suffering from a new condition called "allergic irritability syndrome." The American College of Allergists says that this condition may affect as many as 10 percent of American children.

Other signs and symptoms that may indicate allergy are dark circles under the eyes, sneezing, wheezing, cough, redness of the eyes and nose, tearing, nausea, vomiting, diarrhea, skin rash, noisy breathing, malaise, fatigue, and pain in the forehead, cheeks, and teeth. When these or other symptoms are present, allergy should be suspected. Allergy symptoms can be relieved by proper diagnosis and treatment.

Factors other than allergens that may trigger symptoms of allergy are fatigue, stress, overexertion, changes in temperature, cold air, changes in atmospheric pressure, and changes in humidity. These factors, plus exposure to the offending allergen, cause the majority of symptoms in individuals with allergies.

ALLERGIC RHINITIS

Allergic rhinitis (IgE-mediated) may be seasonal or perennial or both. Both forms have the characteristic symptoms of sneezing, rhinorrhea, congestion, and so forth. The following are the most common seasonal causes of hay fever in the United States, according to the American Academy of Allergy and Immunology:

- *Early spring:* Trees produce most of the pollen.

Elm	Hickory	Cypress
Birch	Sycamore	Walnut
Ash	Maple	Poplar

- *Late spring and summer:* Grasses produce most of the pollen.

Timothy grass	Sweet vernal grass	Bluegrass
Bermuda grass	Redtop grass	Johnson grass
Orchard grass		

- *Fall:* Weeds produce most of the pollen.

Ragweed	Cockle weed	Tumbleweed
Goldenrod	Russian thistle	Sagebrush
Pigweed		

DIAGNOSIS

To determine the cause and nature of an individual's illness, the physician will carefully evaluate the history of the disease process and the signs and symptoms exhibited, and, when indicated, order special tests or procedures.

Patient History

One of the key ingredients in determining a diagnosis is the patient's history, past and present. The physician who specializes in otolaryngology, immunology, or allergy usually has a special history form for the patient to fill out before the initial examination. This form asks questions that are specifically related to allergies. By carefully evaluating the patient's answers to the questions, the physician can determine the possible cause of the patient's illness, and decide whether to order a series of tests that will help establish a diagnosis.

Diagnostic Allergy Tests

It is most important for the physician to determine the specific allergens that are responsible for a patient's symptoms. To arrive at a diagnosis, the physician can employ several tests or procedures. Skin tests, patch tests, laboratory tests, nasal smears, and sinus X-rays are some of the diagnostic tests or procedures utilized in testing for an allergy.

It is of vital importance that the patient be given specific written instructions to follow before the initiation of allergy testing. The patient must understand that *all* antihistamine drugs must be stopped one week prior to the scheduled tests. This includes all over-the-counter cold and allergy medications (tablets, capsules, caplets, nose drops and sprays, cough drops, and so forth), and any prescription antihistamine. Steroids should be discontinued for at least 30 days prior to the tests.

Skin Testing:

When an individual presents sufficient factors that indicate the cause of illness is directly related to an allergy, the physician most likely will order a series of skin tests. The three basic types of skin tests are the scratch (epicutaneous) or prick, patch, and intradermal tests. These tests involve the introduction of a suspected allergen on or into the patient's skin. The degree of the reaction to the allergen usually indicates a patient's allergic state. Many times an allergic individual is susceptible to more than one allergen. It is prudent to have the patient sign a consent form prior to the testing procedure.

Precautions:

When testing a patient for hypersensitivity to certain substances, such as allergens, be sure that you have the drug epinephrine and an antihistamine such as Benadryl available for emergency use. See Unit 10 for a more detailed description of emergency supplies and medications that should be available when administering any drug.

Basic Types of Skin Tests

- Scratch (epicutaneous) or Prick Tests. The *scratch* test involves the placement of a suspected allergen in the uppermost layers of the epidermis. The method by which this is accomplished depends upon the physician. One technique is to place a drop of the allergen on the skin of the forearm or back. Pass a sterile lancet or needle through the drop, and prick the skin no deeper than the uppermost layers of the epidermis.

  Another technique is to make the scratch in the skin, and then drop the allergen into the scratch. When multiple allergens are to be introduced by the scratch method, a systematic approach must be employed. The skin site and allergen must be identified. For example, the skin site is marked with washable ink, indicating the type of allergen applied. This may involve a number system or letter system, depending upon the labeling of the allergen extract bottles.

  Allergen extracts may be labeled as 1 (ragweed), 2 (animal dander), 3 (house dust), or A (ragweed), B (animal dander), C (house dust), and so forth. When the physician orders scratch tests, it is most important that you understand which allergens he or she wishes to be tested. You should follow the basic procedure for the administration of parenteral medications. See Unit 13 if you need to review this process.

  After you have followed the basic procedure, identified the patient, checked for allegies, explained the procedure, positioned the patient, washed your hands, and put on gloves, you should:

1. Prepare the skin sites. First, use sterile alcohol swabs to cleanse the skin. Second, mark the sites with the appropriate labeling (allow $1\frac{1}{2}$ to 2 inches between sites).

2. Prepare the sterile lancet or needle for use. You will need additional sterile lancets or needles for each allergen extract that is to be tested.

3. Perform the skin tests. Make a small ($\frac{1}{8}$ inch) scratch in the selected site and then drop the allergen extract in the scratched area. Discard the used lancet or needle. Using another sterile lancet or needle, repeat the same process, until all ordered allergen extracts have been applied.

4. Ask the patient to remain relatively still for 20 minutes.

5. Read the reaction or reactions according to the guide provided by your physician or the one that comes with the tests. Most skin reactions are read according to the degree of redness or the size of the wheal.

> The following is an example of a guide for recording skin tests reactions:
>
> 0 = No reaction
> +1 = Reaction up to 5 mm in diameter
> +2 = Reaction greater than 5 mm, and up to 10 mm in diameter
> +3 = Reaction greater than 10 mm, and up to 15 mm in diameter
> +4 = Reaction greater than 15 mm in diameter

6. Record the patient's skin reaction or reactions on an appropriate form.

7. Give specific instructions to the patient. This will depend upon the physician's orders. Some physicians like the patient to return for a follow-up check in 24 hours.

8. Care for used equipment and supplies.

9. Remove gloves and then wash your hands.

- Patch Tests. The *patch* test involves the placement of a suspected allergen onto the skin. This is usually accomplished by saturating a gauze square with the suspected allergen, and placing it onto the patient's skin. The gauze is secured in place by using nonallergenic tape. The skin test reaction or reactions are read at 24-hour and again at 48-hour time periods. Reading of the skin reactions is the same as for the scratch tests.

- Intradermal Tests. *Intradermal* tests involve the injection of a minute amount of suspected allergen into the epidermal layer, thus producing a wheal. In testing for allergy, there are two types of intradermal tests that may be employed:

1. *A single dilution procedure* generally involves the injection of 0.01 mL to 0.02 mL of the allergen extract into the epidermis of the selected site (upper arm or forearm), and producing a wheal about 3 mm or 4 mm in diameter.

2. *A serial dilution end-point titration procedure* involves a series of fivefold dilutions to determine a patient's sensitivity to suspected allergens. Atopic individuals usually show sensitivity at intermediate or weak dilutions. Individuals with an end point at the strongest dilution are usually not allergic. This type of intradermal test determines not only what the person is allergic to, but also the person's degree of sensitivity.

- Laboratory Tests. Today, certain blood tests may be used to ascertain an individual's sensitivity to allergens. Radioimmunoassay (RIA) technology has made it possible to detect and measure the amounts of immunoglobulin gamma E (IgE) that are present in human serum. Atopic individuals usually have an elevated total IgE serum level.

  The *radioallergosorbent test* (RAST) is one of the blood tests that may be used to determine an individual's IgE serum level. It is capable of measuring minute quantities of IgE in blood serum. Individuals who are allergic to certain substances will develop antibodies that can be detected by using this test.

  The *paper radioimmunosorbent test* (PRIST) is another blood test used to determine an individual's sensitivity to allergens. It employs a highly specific antibody that will bind only to IgE.

- Nasal Smears. Microscopic analysis of nasal smears can provide the physician with diagnostic information. The presence of bacteria and neutrophils may indicate a bacterial infection. An increased number of eosinophils, goblet cells, and a few mast cells are characteristic of IgE-mediated allergic rhinitis.

- Sinus X-Rays. Sinus X-rays are often taken when the patient has chronic sinusitis. The physician will order the X-ray views and then study the developed film for abnormalities. A thickened sinus mucosa, a significant opacity, or an air fluid level is consistent with sinusitis.

TREATMENT

Once the physician has determined the diagnosis, a treatment regimen is prescribed for the patient. This treatment regimen may include avoidance of allergens, drug therapy, immunotherapy, or some combination of these.

Avoidance of Allergens

Allergic reactions occur when the body comes into contact with the allergens. Allergens may enter the body by several modes of entry. These modes of entry are inhalation, ingestion, direct contact, injection, and insect stings. The allergic individual needs to be aware of these modes of entry, and to try to avoid them.

Complimentary patient education booklets that provide comprehensive allergen avoidance information can be ordered from Pharmacia Diagnostics Division of Pharmacia Inc., 800 Centennial Avenue, Piscataway, NJ 08854.

Drug Therapy

Antihistamines, decongestants, corticosteroids, and cromolyn are the major drug agents that are used to treat allergic disease. These agents are prescribed to alleviate the symptoms or prevent the symptoms from occurring. In addition to the major drug agents, other medications that may be used to treat allergic disease include antileukotrienes-leukotrienes receptor antagonists (blockers), bronchodilators, and a monoclonal antibody-omalizumab (Xolair). The physician evaluates each patient, and then determines the best type of drug therapy for that patient.

- *Antihistamines* are structurally related to histamine and act to counter its effects. They inhibit the interaction between histamine and cellular histamine receptor sites. They are effective in relieving the classic symptoms of allergic rhinitis and are used in the treatment of urticaria and pruritus occurring as a result of histamine. See Unit 24, Table 24-1, for selected antihistamines.

- *Decongestants* are commonly used for symptomatic relief of nasal congestion. They act by stimulating alpha-adrenergic receptors of vascular smooth muscle. As a result, dilated arterioles (small blood vessels) in the nasal mucosa are constricted. This reduces blood flow to the affected area, slows the formation of mucus, improves drainage, and opens obstructed nasal passages. See Unit 24, Table 24-2, for selected decongestants.

- *Corticosteroids* are anti-inflammatory agents that are chemically related to the naturally occurring hormone *cortisone*. Their exact mechanism of action is unknown. Corticosteroids are used in the treatment of seasonal or perennial allergic rhinitis when conventional forms of treatment are not effective. They may also be used to prevent the symptoms from occurring. Corticosteroids are available for inhalation, topical, oral, and parenteral administration. Recent studies have determined that when inhaled via metered-dose inhaler, anti-inflammatory steroids are more effective in treating allergic rhinitis than systemic steroids. Examples of inhalation via metered-dose inhaler steroids are beclomethasone dipropionate (Qvar), and flunisolide (Areobid).

- *Cromolyn sodium* inhibits the degranulation of sensitized mast cells that occurs after exposure to specific antigens. Cromolyn sodium inhibits the release of histamine and SRS-A (the slow-reacting substance of anaphylaxis, that is, leukotrienes). Nasalcrom Nasal Solution is an example of cromolyn sodium. It is indicated for the prevention and treatment of the symptoms of allergic rhinitis.

- *Antileukotrienes-Leukotrienes Receptor Antagonists* (Blockers) are medications that help fight allergic inflammation by blocking leukotrienes and leukotriene receptor occupation. Many of the cells involved in causing airway inflammation are known to produce potent chemicals within the body called leukotrienes. Leukotrienes are responsible for increasing inflammation within the body, causing contraction of the airway muscle, and increasing leakage of fluid from blood vessels in the airways, which are associated with the signs and symptoms of asthma. Examples include zafirlukast (Accolate), and montelukast sodium (Singulair).

- *Bronchodilators* are medications used to dilate the bronchi and to improve pulmonary airflow. There are several classes of bronchodilators available; they are mainly used to treat asthma and chronic obstructive pulmonary disease. See Unit 24, Tables 24-5 and 24-6, for selected bronchodilators.

- *Monoclonal antibody-omalizumab* (Xolair) is a genetically engineered protein that blocks IgE. IgE is an antibody that is present in the body and is responsible for causing allergic problems in certain people. The body forms antibodies in response to the allergen, and this immune system reaction prompts inflammation, causing airway narrowing and other symptoms. Xolair blocks this immune response. It is indicated for patients with moderate to severe persistent allergic asthma. Only patients who have asthma caused by allergies can benefit from this treatment. Therefore, the product's labeling states that this type of asthma should be established by skin or blood test before treatment. The product is given as an injection under the skin. It is a second-line treatment, recommended only after first-line treatments have failed; it is not approved for children under the age of 12; and it is known to work and is approved only for patients with moderate to severe, allergy-related asthma.

Immunotherapy

Immunotherapy is the treatment of a disease process by stimulating the body's immune system. It may be the treatment of choice for allergic rhinitis when:

1. It has been determined that the allergy is IgE-mediated.
2. The patient is unable to avoid the offending allergen/allergens.
3. The patient does not adequately respond to other types of treatment.
4. The symptoms interfere with one's lifestyle (school, work, social).
5. The patient is ready to accept immunotherapy and adhere to its regimen.

Immunotherapy for allergic rhinitis involves the injection of minute allergen or allergens into the patient's subcutaneous tissue. The initial injections are of minute amounts of allergen extract, and are then gradually increased until a maintenance dose is reached. This maintenance dose is usually taken for several years, unless there are complications or the allergic symptoms do not improve.

The aim of immunotherapy is to desensitize the individual with allergies. The physician prescribes the specific desensitizing program for each patient with allergies. Allergenic extracts are to be given per the written order of the prescribing physician. It is essential that anyone giving these extracts follow the written instructions, the doses ordered, and the dosage schedule very carefully. Only individuals who have had adequate preparation in the preparation and administration of parenteral medications should give allergenic extracts.

ADMINISTRATION OF ALLERGENIC EXTRACTS

As a medical assistant, you may be responsible for administering allergenic extracts. In addition to the information that has already been provided, you will need to know the following:

- The ordered dosage of extract must be verified and administered correctly.
- Allergenic extracts are always given in subcutaneous tissue, never in the muscle.
- Use a tuberculin syringe with a 25 G, $\frac{5}{8}$-inch needle, or a 26 G, $\frac{3}{8}$-inch needle, or a 27 G, $\frac{1}{2}$-inch needle. See Figure 14–1.

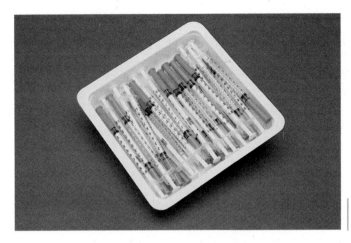

FIGURE 14-1

Allergist syringes *Source: Delmar/Cengage Learning*

- Use a site-rotation system for each injected extract.
- Correctly document the procedure (see the following example).

EXAMPLE

Patient's Name _____

Date	Dose	Site
6/24/xx	1st 0.05 mL subq.	Lt. arm
6/27/xx	2nd 0.10 mL subq.	Rt. arm
6/30/xx	3rd 0.15 mL subq.	Lt. arm

- Allergenic extracts are to be refrigerated. They should retain their potency for 10 to 12 weeks.
- *Adverse reactions* such as itching, swelling, and redness should be reported to the physician stat.
- Severe reactions have occurred; therefore, emergency equipment and supplies *must* be available for use.
- Allergy testing can only be done when a physician is present.

> The patient should be observed for 15 to 30 minutes following the injection of an allergenic extract.

Remember, susceptible individuals can develop allergic reactions to many foreign substances. It is prudent that the person allergies be totally aware of those substances and known allergens.

During summer, one should be especially careful to avoid insect stings. Honeybees', wasps', and yellow jackets' stings can be fatal for susceptible individuals. The allergic reaction to such a sting can occur as a rash, hives, severe pain, difficulty in breathing, nausea, vomiting, dizziness, weakness, shock, and cardiovascular collapse. If the person does not seek medical attention *immediately*, death can occur. An estimated 25 percent of all deaths caused by envenomation are caused by honeybees.

Experts in the field of stinging insects give the following *safety tips* to help prevent getting stung:

1. If you come into contact with stinging insects, move away slowly. Don't beat the air with your hands or slap at the insect. This may trigger an attack.

2. Wear close-fitting clothes that won't trap insects in the folds. Long sleeves and pants provide further protection.

3. Be especially careful after a rainstorm. Pollen is scarce then and insects are easily provoked.

4. Don't look or smell like a flower. Light, bright-colored clothing and sweet-smelling perfume, cologne, aftershave lotion, and suntan lotion will attract insects.

5. If you get stung, scrape the stinger out (with your fingernail or a knife blade). Apply ice to reduce swelling. Pulling stingers out with your fingers or tweezers squeezes more venom into your skin.

6. Seek medical help *immediately* if you experience any swelling away from the sting site, any nausea or vomiting, difficulty breathing, dizziness, weakness, or hives.

■ ■ REVIEW QUESTIONS

Directions. Select the best answer to each of the following multiple-choice questions, circling the letter of your choice:

1. _____ is an allergy for which there is a genetic predisposition.

    a. Allergen   b. Colic   c. Atopy   d. Antibody

2. The most common allergens that may cause allergy are _____.

    a. dyes, perfumes, cosmetics, and soaps

    b. detergents, tobacco, feathers, and fabrics

    c. smoke, chemicals, vapors, gases, and fumes

    d. pollens, animal danders, house dust, molds, and certain drugs

3. The reaction between allergens and IgE antibodies causes the release of chemical substances such as _____.

    a. histamine, leukotrienes, and prostaglandins

    b. histamine, leukocytes, and prostaglandins

    c. histamine, reagin, and prostaglandins

    d. histamine, basophils, and neutrophils

4. The classic symptoms of allergy are _____.

    a. pain, fever, and sore throat

    b. sneezing, congestion, rhinorrhea, postnasal drip, and scratchy throat

    c. nausea, vomiting, and diarrhea

    d. headache, fever, and nausea

5. The most common causes of hay fever in the United States according to the American Academy of Allergy and Immunology are _____.

    a. in the early spring (grasses)   c. in the fall (weeds)

    b. in the late spring and summer (trees)   d. none of these

6. In determining the diagnosis of allergy, the physician may _____.

    a. evaluate the history of the disease process   c. order diagnostic allergy tests

    b. evaluate the patient's signs and symptoms   d. all of these

7. Before the initiation of allergy testing, the patient is _____.

    a. given written instructions about medications to stop taking

    b. to sign a consent form

    c. carefully evaluated by the physician

    d. all of these

8. When testing a patient for hypersensitivity to certain substances, such as allergens, one should have the following drugs available for emergency use: _____

   a. epinephrine and Tigan
   b. epinephrine and Benadryl
   c. epinephrine and heparin
   d. epinephrine and insulin

9. The _____ skin tests involve the placement of a suspected allergen in the uppermost layers of the epidermis.

   a. patch   b. scratch   c. intradermal   d. none of these

10. A skin test reaction of +2 indicates a reaction _____.

    a. up to 5 mm in diameter
    b. greater than 5 mm, and up to 10 mm in diameter
    c. greater than 10 mm, and up to 15 mm in diameter
    d. greater than 15 mm in diameter

11. Two laboratory blood tests that may be used to ascertain an individual's sensitivity to allergens are _____.

    a. hemoglobin and hematocrit
    b. WBC and RBC
    c. RAST and PRIST
    d. all of these

12. The treatment of allergy may include _____.

    a. avoidance of allergens
    b. drug therapy
    c. immunotherapy
    d. all of these

13. It is vitally important that the patient be given specific written instructions to follow *before* the initiation of allergy testing. These instructions should include _____.

    a. that *all* antihistamine drugs must be stopped one week prior to the scheduled tests
    b. that steroids should be discontinued for at least 30 days prior to the tests
    c. that it is not necessary to stop over-the-counter cold medications
    d. a and b

14. The _____ tests involve the injection of a minute amount of suspected allergen into the epidermal layer, thus producing a wheal.

    a. patch   b. intradermal   c. scratch   d. none of these

15. The presence of bacteria and neutrophils in a nasal smear may indicate _____.

    a. bacterial infection
    b. IgE-mediated allergic rhinitis
    c. viral infection
    d. all of these

16. Major drug agents that are used to treat allergic disease are _____.

    a. antihistamines
    b. decongestants
    c. corticosteroids and cromolyn
    d. all of these

17. _____ is the treatment of a disease process by stimulating the body's immune system.

    a. Immunotherapy
    b. Chemotherapy
    c. Diet therapy
    d. none of these

18. When administering allergenic extracts, you will _____.

    a. *always* give the extract in subcutaneous tissue
    b. use a tuberculin syringe with a 25 G, 26 G, or 27 G needle
    c. use a site-rotation system
    d. all of these

Matching. Place the correct letter from Column II on the appropriate line of Column I:

Column I	Column II
19. _____ allergen	A. a type of immunoglobulin gamma E (IgE) that is present in the serum of atopic individuals
20. _____ atopy	B. a protein produced by the lining of the respiratory and intestinal tracts
21. _____ colic	C. any substance that causes allergy
22. _____ desensitize	D. an allergy for which there is a genetic predisposition
23. _____ immunoglobulin gamma E (IgE)	E. pertaining to spasm in any hollow soft organ accompanied by pain
24. _____ reagin	F. to lessen the sensitivity of an individual by administering the specific antigen or antigens
25. _____ hay fever	G. an allergic reaction to foods
	H. an allergic reaction to trees, grass, and weed pollens

SECTION THREE

Medications, Supplements, and Drug Abuse

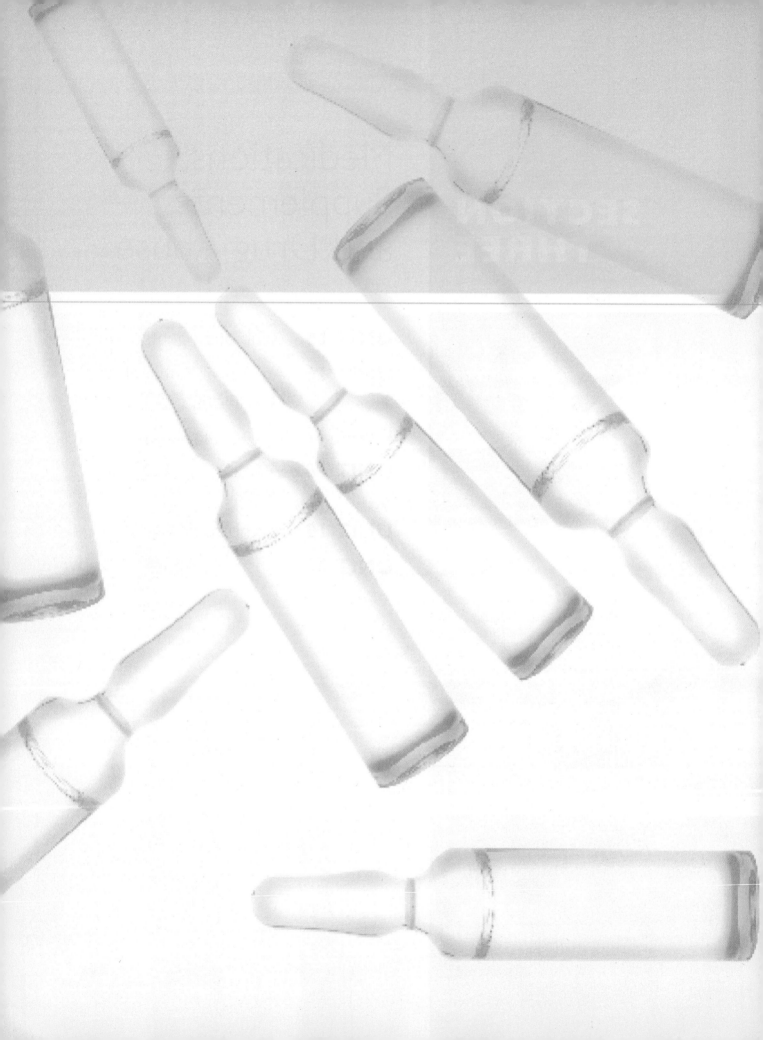

UNIT 15
Antibiotic Agents

OBJECTIVES

Upon completing this unit, you should be able to:

- Define the terms listed in the vocabulary.
- Describe infection.
- List the danger signs of a serious infection.
- Describe ways people may minimize their risk of developing a serious infection.
- State why infections are generally more serious in older adults.
- List possible reasons why children who attend a day care center are more likely to contract ear infections, pneumonia, and meningitis.
- Complete the critical thinking questions and activities presented in this unit.
- List the characteristics of an effective antibiotic.
- Describe four adverse reactions that may occur with the administration of an antibiotic.
- Explain how the overuse of antibiotics has helped cause drug-resistant strains of bacteria.
- State the actions, uses, contraindications, adverse reactions, dosages, and routes for selected antibiotics.
- Give the implications for patient care with regard to selected antibiotics.
- Complete the Spot Check on major antibiotic groupings.
- Describe antiseptics and disinfectants.
- State the substance, strength, action, and comments for selected antiseptics and disinfectants.
- Answer the review questions correctly.

VOCABULARY

antiseptic (an"ti-sep'tik). A substance that prevents or inhibits the growth of microorganisms, especially bacteria.

bacteria (bak-te're-a). Any microorganism of the Schizomycetes class.

bactericidal (bak"ter-i-si"dal). Pertaining to the killing or destruction of bacteria.

bacteriostatic (bak-te-re-o-stat'ik). Pertaining to inhibiting or retarding bacterial growth.

beta-lactamase (bay'tah-lack"tah-mayce). An enzyme produced by certain microorganisms that has the ability to resist the action of certain types of antibiotics.

disinfectant (dis-in-fekt'ant). A chemical agent that kills vegetative forms of bacteria.

infection (in-fek'shun). The process or state whereby a pathogenic agent invades the body or a body part, multiplies, and produces injury.

microorganism (mi-kro-or'gan-izm). Any living body not visible to the naked eye. It may be pathogenic (disease-producing) or nonpathogenic.

pathogenic (path"o-jen'ik). Pertaining to a microorganism or substance that is capable of producing disease.

INTRODUCTION

We live in a virtual "sea" of microorganisms, organisms so tiny that they cannot be seen with the naked eye. Many of these organisms are not harmful to humans, whereas others are agents of disease. Infectious diseases are the fourth largest cause of death in human beings. Approximately 50 percent of all infectious diseases are virus-related. Other agents that cause infectious diseases are bacteria, fungi, protozoa, rickettsia, and helminths.

Infection is the process or state whereby a pathogenic agent invades the body or a body part, multiplies, and produces injury. Infection occurs when certain factors or conditions exist. The conditions that determine whether a pathogenic agent enters the body, multiplies, and produces disease may vary with the type of invading organism and the susceptibility of the individual.

The invading organism has to be of sufficient number, and have the power and degree of pathogenicity, to produce disease. Next, the environment has to have certain conditions that favor growth. These conditions are moisture, darkness, warmth, organic material (food), oxygen, and a slightly alkaline environment. Last, but not least, there must be a portal of exit from the host. This portal of exit may be via the blood, body secretions, body fluids, mucous membranes, feces, or urine.

A pathogenic agent has to have a mode of transmission from one source to another. The more common modes of transmission are by:

- airborne droplets (produced, for example, by sneezing, coughing, and laughing).
- direct contact of one person with another.
- direct, indirect, or intermediary animal contact.
- vectors (insects).
- contaminated food.
- contaminated water.
- fomites (inanimate objects).
- soil-borne spore-forming organisms.
- contaminated blood.
- transplacentally, or via maternal membranes.
- human carriers.

The average, healthy body is equipped with a natural defense that functions to protect it from microorganisms and their harmful effects. These natural defenses are intact skin, cleansing action of the body's secretions, white blood cells, body chemicals, and antibodies.

The immune system is the body's defense mechanism against invading foreign substances. Scientists have learned how immunity works and how the body fights invading organisms. Through their discoveries, new advances have been made in the treatment of infectious diseases.

Infectious Diseases

According to a recent World Health Organization report, heart ailments, infectious disease, and cancer remain the world's top three killers. Heart attacks and related problems are the top killer, claiming 29 percent of people who die each year. In second place, infectious diseases lead to 16.2 percent of worldwide deaths. Scientists have identified 335 emerging infectious diseases in people. Some of the factors that contribute to the emergence and reemergence of deadly microorganism are:

- Increased international travel and shipment of food.
- Unprecedented population growth cramming people together in unsanitary conditions.
- Changes in how food is grown and handled.
- Decaying public health infrastructure in many areas.

- More people living with immune systems suppressed by AIDS, cancer, diabetes, and organ transplants.

- Increased use of antibiotics in people and livestock, which contributes to the growing resistance of microorganisms to antibiotics.

- Infections (such as potentially deadly staph infections) becoming resistant to even the antibiotic of choice.

Methicillin-resistant *Staphylococcus aurens* (MRSA) is a type of bacteria that is resistant to certain antibiotics. These antibiotics include methicillin and other more common antibiotics such as oxacillin, penicillin, and amoxicillin. Staph infections, including MRSA, occur most frequently among people who have weakened immune systems in hosipitals and health care facilities (such as nursing homes and dialysis centers).

MRSA infections that occur in otherwise healthy people who have not been recently (within the past year) hospitalized or had a medical procedure (such as dialysis, surgery, catheters) are known as community-associated (CA)-MRSA infections. These infections are usually skin infections, such as abscesses, boils, and other pus-filled lesions. A person can get MRSA through direct contact with an infected person or by sharing personal items, such as towels or razors that have touched infected skin.

MRSA skin infections can occur anywhere. Some meetings have factors that make it easier for MRSA to be transmitted. These factors, referred to as the five Cs are as follows: crowding, frequent skin-to-skin contact, compromised skin (i.e., cuts or abrasions), contaminated items and surfaces, and lack of cleanliness. Locations where the five Cs are common include schools, dormitories, military barracks, households, correctional facilities, and day care centers.

Clostridium difficile, often called *C. difficile* or "*C. diff*," is a bacterium that can cause symptoms ranging from diarrhea to life-threatening inflammation of the colon. The majority of *C. difficile* cases occur in health care settings, where germs spread easily, antibiotic use is common, and people are especially vulnerable to infection. The antibiotics that most often lead to *C. difficile* infections include fluoroquinolones, cephalosporins, clindamycin, and penicillins.

Once established, *C. difficile* can produce toxins that attack the lining of the intestine. The toxins destroy cells and produce patches (plaques) of inflammatory cells and decaying cellular debris inside the colon.

An aggressive strain of C. difficile has emerged that produces far more deadly toxins than other strains do. The new strain is more resistant to certain medications and has shown up in people who haven't been in the hospital or taken antibiotics.

The first step in treating *C. difficile* is to stop taking the antibiotic that triggered the infection. This may be enough to relieve symptoms of mild illness, but many people require further treatment. In an ironic twist, the standard treatment for *C. difficile* is another antibiotic. Physicians usually prescribe metronidazole (Flagyl) for mild to moderate illness. Vancomycin (Vancocin) may be prescribed for more severe symptoms. These antibiotics keep *C. difficile* from growing, which allows normal bacteria to flourish again in the intestine.

Escherichia coli is a common gram-negative bacterium found in normal human bacterial flora; however, some strains can cause severe and life-threatening diarrhea. Recently, there has been an increase in disease caused by strain 0157:H7, both worldwide and in the United States. Contaminated ground beef has been incriminated as the major mode of transmission. The most common way of getting the infection is by eating rare or inadequately cooked meat. Fresh fruits and vegetables may also become contaminated with *E. coli*. Person-to-person transmission can occur if infected people do not wash their hands after using the bathroom. When a fecal accident occurs, usually by an infant or a child with diarrhea, a swimming pool, hot tub, or other water facility can become contaminated with *E. coli*.

Infection with this strain usually results in diarrhea, but it can cause hemorrhagic colitis and hemolytic uremic syndrome (HUS), which is the leading cause of acute renal failure in children under the age of 4. People developing HUS have a mortality rate of 3 to 10 percent.

Salmonellosis is a common bacterial infection caused by any of more than 2,000 strains of Salmonella. These bacteria infect the intestinal tract and occasionally the blood. Salmonellosis is typically a food-borne illness acquired from contaminated raw poultry, eggs, and unpasteurized milk and cheese products, but all foods including vegetables may become contaminated. Food may also become contaminated by the hands of an infected food handler. Salmonella may also be found in the feces of some pets, especially those with diarrhea, and people can become infected if they do not wash their hands after contact with these pets. Reptiles (turtles, iguanas, other lizards, snakes) are particularly likely to harbor Salmonella, and so people should wash their hands after handling a reptile.

Most people infected with Salmonella develop diarrhea, fever, and abdominal cramps 12 to 72 hours after infection. The illness usually lasts four to seven days, and most people recover without treatment. However, in some people the diarrhea may be so severe that the patient needs to be hospitalized. The elderly, infants, and those with impaired immune systems are more likely to have a severe illness.

Every year approximately 40,000 cases of salmonellosis are reported in the United States. Because many milder cases are not diagnosed or reported, the actual number of infections may be 20 or more times greater. Salmonellosis is more common in the summer than winter. Children are the most likely to get salmonellosis. It is estimated that approximately one thousand people die each year with acute salmonellosis.

Campylobacteriosis is an infectious disease caused by bacteria of the genus *Campylobacter*. It is the most common bacterial cause of diarrheal illness in the United States. *Campylobacter* occurs widely as part of the normal flora of many warm-blooded animals, including chickens and turkeys. In addition, the organism occurs in raw water and raw milk. In man, transmission is via contaminated food, water, or milk. The main route is thought to be either undercooking of poultry or cross-contamination from raw to ready-to-eat food. Over 10,000 cases are reported to the Centers for Disease Control and Prevention (CDC) each year. Many more cases go undiagnosed or unreported, and campylobacteriosis is estimated to affect over 2 million people every year, or 1 percent of the population. It occurs more frequently in the summer months than in the winter.

Most people who become ill with campylobacteriosis get diarrhea, cramping, abdominal pain, and fever within two to five days after exposure to the organism. The diarrhea may be bloody and can be accompanied by nausea and vomiting. The illness typically lasts one week. Some people who are infected may not have any symptoms at all. In people with compromised immune systems, Campylobacter occasionally spreads to the bloodstream and causes a serious life-threatening infection.

Group B streptococcus (GBS) is a type of bacterium that causes illness in newborn babies, pregnant women, the elderly, and adults with other illnesses such as diabetes or liver disease. GBS is the most common cause of life-threatening infections in newborns. It is the most common cause of sepsis and meningitis in newborns. It is a frequent cause of newborn pneumonia and is more common than other, better known, newborn problems such as rubella, congenital syphilis, and spina bifida.

Approximately one of every 100 to 200 babies whose mothers carry GBS develop signs and symptoms of GBS disease. Three-fourths of the cases of GBS disease among newborns occur in the first week of life, and most of these cases are apparent a few hours after birth. Sepsis, pneumonia, and meningitis are the most common complications.

Most GBS disease in newborns can be prevented by giving certain pregnant women antibiotics intravenously during labor. In fact, any pregnant woman who previously had a baby with GBS disease or who has a urinary tract infection caused by GBS should receive antibiotics during labor. Penicillin is very effective at preventing GBS disease in the newborn and is generally safe.

Severe acute respiratory syndrome (SARS) is a viral respiratory illness caused by a coronavirus, called SARS-associated coronavirus (SARS-CoV). SARS was first reported in Asia in February 2003. Over the next few months, the illness spread to more than two dozen countries. According to the World Health Organization (WHO), a total of 8,098 people worldwide became sick with SARS during the 2003 outbreak and of these, 744 died. In the United States, only eight people had laboratory evidence of SARS-CoV infection. All of these people had traveled to other parts of the world known to be associated with SARS.

SARS seems to spread primarily by close person-to-person contact. The virus is thought to be transmitted most readily by respiratory droplets (droplet spread) produced when an infected person coughs or sneezes. The virus also can spread when a person touches a surface or object contaminated with infectious droplets and then touches his or her mouth, nose, or eye(s). In addition, it is possible that the SARS virus might spread more broadly through the air (airborne spread) or by other means that are not now known. In general, SARS begins with a high fever (temperature greater than 100.4°F). Other symptoms may include headache, an overall feeling of discomfort, body aches, dry cough, and diarrhea. Most patients develop pneumonia.

Spotlight

Group A Streptococcal (GAS) Disease
(strep throat, necrotizing fasciitis, impetigo)

Group A streptococcus is a bacterium often found in the throat and on the skin. People may carry group A streptococci in the throat or on the skin and have no symptoms of illness. Most GAS infections are relatively mild illnesses such as "strep throat" or impetigo. On rare occasions, these bacteria can cause other severe and even life-threatening disease.

These bacteria are spread through direct contact with mucus from the nose or throat of people who are infected or through contact with infected wounds or sores on the skin. Ill people, such as those who have strep throat or skin infections, are most likely to spread the infection. People who carry the bacteria but have no symptoms are much less contagious. Treating an infected person with an antibiotic for 24 hours or longer generally eliminates their ability to spread the bacteria. However, it is important to complete the entire course of antibiotics as prescribed. It is not likely that household items like plates, cups, or toys spread these bacteria.

Infection with GAS can result in a range of symptoms:

- No illness
- Mild illness (strep throat or a skin infection such as impetigo)
- Severe illness (necrotizing faciitis, streptococcal toxic shock syndrome)

Severe, sometimes life-threatening, GAS disease may occur when bacteria get into parts of the body where bacteria usually are not found, such as the blood, muscle, or the lungs. These infections are termed *invasive GAS disease*. Two of the most severe, but least common, forms of invasive GAS disease are necrotizing fasciitis and streptococcal toxic shock syndrome. Necrotizing fasciitis (occasionally described by the media as "the flesh-eating bacteria") destroys muscles, fat, and skin tissue. Streptococcal toxic shock syndrome (STSS) causes blood pressure to drop rapidly and organs (such as kidney, liver, and lungs) to fail. STSS is not the same as the "toxic shock syndrome" frequently associated with tampon usage. About 20 percent of patients with necrotizing fasciitis and more than half with STSS die. About 10 percent to 15 percent of patients with other forms of invasive group A streptococcal disease die.

Invasive GAS infections occur when the bacteria get past the defenses of the person who is infected. This may occur when a person has sores or other breaks in the skin that allow the bacteria to get into the tissue, or when the person's ability to fight off the infection is decreased because of chronic illness or an illness that affects the immune system. Also, some virulent strains of GAS are more likely to cause severe disease than others.

Few people who come in contact with GAS will develop invasive GAS disease. Most people will have a throat or skin infection, and some may have no symptoms at all. Although healthy people can get invasive GAS disease, people with chronic illnesses like cancer, diabetes, and kidney failure requiring dialysis, and those who use medications such as steroids have a higher risk.

Early signs and symptoms of necrotizing fasciitis include the following:

- Fever
- Severe pain and swelling
- Redness at the wound site

Early signs and symptoms of STSS include the following:

- Fever
- Dizziness
- Confusion
- A flat red rash over large areas of the body

GAS infections can be treated with many different antibiotics. Early treatment may reduce the risk of death from invasive group A streptococcal disease. However, even the best medical care does not prevent death in every case. For those with very severe illness, supportive care in an intensive care unit may be needed. For people with necrotizing fasciitis, surgery often is needed to remove damaged tissue.

The spread of all types of GAS infection can be reduced by good hand washing, especially after coughing and sneezing and before preparing foods or eating. People with sore throats should be seen by a doctor who can perform tests to find out whether the illness is strep throat. If the test result shows strep throat, the person should stay home from work, school, or day care until 24 hours after taking an antibiotic. All wounds should be kept clean and watched for possible signs of infection such as redness, swelling, drainage, and pain at the wound site. A person with signs of an infected wound, especially if fever occurs, should seek medical care. It is not necessary for all people exposed to someone with an invasive group A strep infection (such as necrotizing fasciitis or strep toxic shock syndrome) to receive antibiotic therapy to prevent infection. However, in certain circumstances, antibiotic therapy may be appropriate. That decision should be made after consulting with your doctor.

Minimize Your Risk of Developing a Serious Infection

- Have at least five servings of fruits and vegetables daily.
- Don't smoke.
- Reduce stress.
- Exercise regularly.
- Get a proper amount of sleep. This is usually 6 to 8 hours in a given 24-hour time period.
- Eat garlic or take a garlic supplement.
- Make sure you stay up-to-date on your immunizations.
- Drink at least eight glasses of water daily.
- Keep a positive attitude.
- Practice good hygiene: Wash your hands (scrub out germs). Clean hands don't spread germs.
- Don't share food or drink with another person.
- Keep your fingers away from your mouth, nose, and eyes.

Danger Signs; Seek Medical Attention Immediately . . .

- A sudden onset of high fever (in an adult, a fever of 102 degrees or higher), violent chills, or confusion
- An infection that seems to be spreading
- An injury that becomes extremely painful
- An injury that rapidly enlarges, especially if there is a high fever
- Redness and blistering of the skin
- Pain in muscles
- Enlarged lymph nodes under the arm
- Increasing pain in the incision after a surgical procedure
- For a patient with chicken pox (on or beyond the fourth day of pox eruption): fever of 101 degrees or higher, vomiting, lethargy, and painful or swollen areas of the body; inflammation that has spread beyond the area of the chicken pox sores
- Pregnant women with flulike symptoms

■ Special Considerations: **OLDER ADULTS**

Infections are generally more serious in the older adult because of:

- The normal aging process.
- Diminished functioning of the immune system.
- Disruption of normal defense mechanisms.
- Decreased cough reflex.
- Thin, atrophic skin.
- Poor circulation, especially of the hands and feet.
- Decreased gastric acid production.
- Decreased vaginal secretions.
- Preexisting chronic disease.
- Lifestyle choices such as smoking and drinking alcoholic beverages.
- Lack of exercise.
- Fixed income.
- Failure to follow the complete drug regimen or therapy.
- Exposure to pathogenic organisms in health care facilities.

■ Special Considerations: **CHILDREN**

Children age 2 and younger who attend day care centers are 36 times more likely to contract ear infections, pneumonia, and meningitis than kids that stay at home. Kids in day care also put their siblings at greater risk of infection.

Possible causes are that children:

- Don't wash their hands very often.
- Don't cover their nose when they sneeze.
- Don't cover their mouth when they cough.
- Share toys.
- Share food and drink.
- Put just about anything in their mouths.
- Drop their bottles and pacifiers on the floor and put them right back in their mouths.

To help prevent the spread of infection, teach children and day care workers to:

- Wash their hands often.
- Cough and sneeze into disposable tissues.
- Dispose of tissues in a proper container, then wash their hands.
- Not eat or drink after anyone.
- Not share cups, glasses, or eating utensils with others.
- Wash toys often with warm, soapy water, then rinse with clear water.
- Wash bottles and pacifiers often with warm, soapy water, then rinse with clear water.

■■ Critical Thinking **QUESTIONS AND ACTIVITIES**

Make arrangements to present a program on infection control at a local day care center. Using the information in Special Considerations: Children, ask yourself:

- Why are children who attend day care centers more likely to contract ear infections, pneumonia, and meningitis than kids who stay at home? How could I go about explaining this to a group of children in day care?
- What could I teach the children and day care workers about ways to prevent the spread of infection?
- What are some hands-on activities that I can use to demonstrate infection control?
- What could I use to teach the children about sneezing and coughing, so that they would not spread infection?
- How could I teach the children not to drink and eat after anyone?

TREATMENT OF INFECTIOUS DISEASES

Antibiotics are used to treat infectious diseases in plants, animals, and man. Antibiotics may be natural or synthetic substances that inhibit the growth of or destroy microorganisms, especially bacteria.

Bacteria may be described as gram-positive, gram-negative, or acid-fast. These types of bacteria cause a variety of infectious diseases. Gonorrhea, syphilis, tuberculosis, pneumonia, chlamydia, rheumatic fever, scarlet fever, meningitis, strep throat, and salmonellosis are some of the diseases caused by bacteria.

Today, there are many antibiotics produced by various pharmaceutical companies. These antibiotics may be effective against gram-positive bacteria, gram-negative bacteria, or both.

Antibiotics may be classified as broad-spectrum, narrow-spectrum, or extended-spectrum.

Classification of Antibiotics

- *Broad-spectrum* antibiotics are those effective against many different kinds of microorganisms. Amoxil (amoxicillin) is an example of a broad-spectrum antibiotic.
- *Narrow-spectrum* antibiotics are those effective against limited types of microorganisms. Penicillin V is an example of a narrow-spectrum antibiotic.
- *Extended-spectrum* antibiotics are those for which the antimicrobial activity is extended to include *Pseudomonas*, *Enterobacter*, and *Proteus* species. Ciprofloxacin (Cipro) is an example of an extended-spectrum antibiotic.

Administering Antibiotics

Before administering any antibiotic, ask the patient if he or she is allergic to any drug. If the patient has an allergy or sensitivity to any antibiotic or other drug, this information is reported to the physician and recorded in *red* on the patient's permanent record. An antibiotic is *never* administered to a patient when there is an allergy to the drug.

To determine the type of invading organism, the physician orders a culture and sensitivity test. This test should be performed as soon as possible to guarantee that the appropriate antibiotic is prescribed for the patient.

Characteristics of an Effective Antibiotic

The characteristics of an effective antibiotic are: (1) It must be harmless to the blood, the liver, the bone marrow, and the kidneys; (2) its possibility of causing toxicity to the body must be low; (3) it must be effective against the invading microorganism; and (4) it must be more beneficial than harmful.

ADVERSE REACTIONS

Antibiotics may cause certain harmful effects to occur within the bodies of some patients. The adverse effect of an antibiotic may manifest itself in the following ways.

Hypersensitivity

Reactions may range from an allergic response to anaphylactic shock. The symptoms of an allergic response may include urticaria, skin eruptions (especially rash), fever, headache, nausea, vomiting, and diarrhea.

Anaphylactic shock is a severe allergic reaction, usually to a substance to which the person has become sensitized. The symptoms of anaphylaxis are facial or laryngeal edema, dyspnea, cyanosis, circulatory collapse, and convulsions. *Death may occur if emergency treatment is not initiated.* Such treatment consists of the administration of a vasopressor agent (epinephrine), corticosteroids, oxygen, diphenhydramine (Benadryl), and dopamine.

● ***Note***

> **If there is any question about a person's hypersensitivity to an antibiotic, especially penicillins and cephalosporins, an appropriate skin test should be performed before initiating drug therapy.** ●

Organ Toxicity

This condition may occur when high doses of an antibiotic are used for an extended length of time, or when the patient has impaired liver or renal function. The symptoms of liver dysfunction may include pain in the right upper quadrant, fever, nausea, vomiting, and jaundice. Changes in liver function tests are indicative of dysfunction. The symptoms of renal dysfunction are oliguria and proteinuria. These may be detected through changes in renal function tests.

Superinfection

This condition may occur when there is overgrowth of a resistant strain of bacteria, fungi, or yeast. The symptoms may include black tongue, sore mouth, perianal infection and itching, foul-smelling vaginal discharge, loose stools, sudden fever, and cough.

Clostridium difficile Associated Diarrhea (CDAD)

Clostridium difficile associated diarrhea (CDAD) has been reported with use of nearly all antibacterial agents and may range in severity from mild diarrhea to fatal colitis. Treatment with antibacterial agents alters the normal flora of the colon, leading to overgrowth of *C. difficile.*

C. difficile produces toxins A and B, which contribute to the development of CDAD. Hypertoxin-producing strains of *C. difficile* cause increased morbidity and mortality, as these infections can be refractory to antimicorbial therapy and may require colectomy. CDAD must be considered in all patients who present with diarrhea following antibiotic use. Careful medical history is necessary because CDAD has been reported to occur over two months after the administration of antibacterial agents.

If CDAD is suspected or confirmed, ongoing antibiotic use not directed against *C. difficile* may need to be discontinued. Appropriate fluid and electrolyte management, protein supplementation, antibiotic treatment of *C. difficile*, and surgical evaluation should be instituted as clinically indicated.

Overuse of Antibiotics

Drug-Resistant Strains of Bacteria

In recent years, certain strains of bacteria have become increasingly resistant to drugs such as penicillin, erythromycin, vancomycin, and tetracycline. Experts blame the problem on the overuse of antibiotics that kill the weakest bacteria and leave the strongest to become more powerful. Drug-resistant organisms develop when a genetic mutation enables one or two bacteria to survive out of the millions in an infected person. The new strain multiplies and spreads, eventually replacing the older, less lethal type. It is noted that all organisms have what are called "survival-of-the-fittest" type mechanisms. The emergence of drug-resistant strains of bacteria could become a public health threat. Drug-resistant bacteria can be spread from one person to another by human contact.

The World Health Organization warns that increasingly drug-resistant infections in rich and developing nations alike are threatening to make once-treatable diseases incurable. Scientists have been urging action for years to fight the growing problem of infections becoming impervious to treatment.

Bacteria, parasites, and viruses all naturally evolve to fight treatment. Organisms exposed to drugs that do not kill them become stronger, able to withstand subsequent treatment attempts, and pass on that drug resistance to their next generation.

The widespread use of antibiotics to treat common viral illnesses such as colds, the flu, and viral sinusitis is one of the primary causes of antibiotic resistance. Antibiotics kill bacteria, not viruses, and therefore should not be used for viral illnesses. In developed countries, people often overuse antibiotics, demanding them for illnesses like colds and the flu. The body harbors germs, so each unneeded antibiotic dose is an opportunity for germs to evolve. It is estimated that antibiotics are overprescribed by 50 percent in the United States and Canada.

Another problem is half the world's antibiotics are used on the farm, sometimes to treat illness, but mostly to help healthy animals grow bigger. That encourages drug-resistant germs that cause food poisoning.

Dangers of Antibiotic Resistance

Antibiotic resistance has been called one of the world's most pressing public health problems. It can cause significant danger and distress for people who have common infections that once were easily treatable with antibiotics. When antibiotics fail to work, the consequences are longer-lasting illnesses; more doctor visits or extended hospital stays; and the need for more expensive and toxic medications.

Points to Remember

- Taking antibiotics for viral infections will increase the risk of antibiotic resistance.
- Tens of millions of antibiotics prescribed in doctors' offices each year are for viral infections, which cannot effectively be treated with antibiotics. Doctors cite diagnostic uncertainty, time pressure on physicians, and patient demand as the primary reasons why antibiotics are overprescribed.
- The spread of viral infections can be reduced through frequent hand washing and by avoiding close contact with others.
- The following are the CDC's Get Smart recommendations for the use of antibiotics.

What To Do

☑ Talk with your health care provider about antibiotic resistance.

☑ When you are prescribed an antibiotic,

1. Take it exactly as the doctor tells you. Complete the prescribed course even if you are feeling better. If treatment stops too soon, some bacteria may survive and reinfect you.

2. This goes for children, too. Make sure your children take all medication as prescribed, even if they feel better.

3. Throw away any leftover medication once you have completed your prescription.

What Not To Do

☑ Do not take an antibiotic for a viral infection like a cold, a cough, or the flu.

☑ Do not demand antibiotics when a doctor says they are not needed. They will not help treat your infection.

☑ When you are prescribed an antibiotic,

1. Do not skip doses.

2. Do not save any antibiotics for the next time you get sick.

3. Do not take antibiotics prescribed for someone else. The antibiotic may not be appropriate for your illness. Taking the wrong medicine may delay correct treatment and allow bacteria to multiply.

MAJOR ANTIBIOTIC GROUPINGS

Antibiotics may be grouped when they have a similar action and usage. The major antibiotic groupings described in this section are penicillins, cephalosporins, carbapenems, tetracyclines, aminoglycosides, macrolides and fluoroquinolones.

The beta-lactam antibiotics include the penicillins, cephalosporins, and carbapenems. The FDA has recently approved a number of new agents and new dosage forms of some older agents. In the cephalosporin category, a new oral third-generation cephalosporin, cefditoren pivoxil (Spectracef), has been recently released. With a spectrum of activity that includes typical community respiratory pathogens, various streptococci, and methicillin-susceptible *Staphylococcus aureus*, this agent is approved for the treatment of adults and children older than age 12 who have acute bacterial exacerbation of chronic bronchitis (400 mg twice a day), pharyngitis/tonsillitis (200 mg twice a day), or uncomplicated skin and skin structure infections (200 mg twice a day). Spectracef is available in a 200-mg tablet (no liquid dosage form is available).

Penicillins

Penicillin was discovered in 1928, by Sir Alexander Fleming, a British bacteriologist. Today, the penicillins consist of a group of natural and semisynthetic agents that are highly active against gram-positive and gram-negative cocci and bacilli. Penicillin may be either the natural product of such molds as *Penicillium notatum* and *Penicillium chrysogenum*, or a semisynthetic derivative of the *Penicillium* molds.

Actions

The penicillins act by interfering with bacterial cell wall synthesis among newly formed bacterial cells. Unable to develop rigid cell walls when affected by penicillin, the rapidly developing cells die as a result of an increase in the flow of fluid into the cell.

Uses

There are a number of penicillins, each with a similar effect on bacterial cells, yet differing in stability and absorption rate when introduced into the body. Physicians, after an analysis of the factors associated with a disease, choose among the types of penicillins for the variety most effective against the invading microorganisms.

Some of the diseases for which a physician might prescribe a penicillin are pneumonia, gonorrhea, syphilis, meningitis, diphtheria, sinusitis, bronchitis, acute osteomyelitis, otitis media, and infections caused by *staphylococci, streptococci, Escherichia coli*, and *Salmonella bacteria*.

Contraindications

Penicillins are contraindicated in patients who are known to be allergic or hypersensitive to any of its varieties, or to any of the cephalosporins. People known to be sensitive to either of these groups of drugs should wear a Medic Alert bracelet or other identification warning of this condition.

A patient's drug allergy must be noted in *red* ink on the chart.

Adverse Reactions

The most common adverse reaction to penicillins is an allergic one. This reaction may be an immediate anaphylactic response requiring emergency treatment, or a delayed response whereupon the patient must discontinue the medication and seek medical attention. Other adverse reactions may include nausea, vomiting, diarrhea, fever, chills, rash, itching, and signs of superinfection.

With intramuscular administration, there may be pain at the site of injection, inflammation, sterile abscess, phlebitis, and thrombophlebitis.

Dosage and Route

The dosage and route of administration are determined by the physician and will vary with the type of penicillin prescribed. Table 15-1 lists some of the frequently used penicillins, the average adult and children's dosages, and the usual route of administration.

TABLE 15-1 Selected Penicillins, Routes, and Dosages

GENERIC NAME	TRADE NAME	ROUTE		USUAL DOSAGE
amoxicillin	Amoxil	Oral:	*Adults:*	250 to 500 mg every 8 hours
			Children:	(Under 20 kg) 20 to 40 mg/kg daily in divided doses every 8 hours
ampicillin		Oral:	*Adults:*	250 to 500 mg every 6 hours
			Children:	50 to 100 mg/kg daily in divided doses every 6 hours
penicillin G benzathine	Bicillin L-A	IM:	*Adults:*	1.2 million units as a single dose
			Children:	300,000 to 1.2 million units as a single dose
			Neonates:	50,000 units/kg as a single dose
penicillin V potassium		Oral:	*Adults:*	125 to 500 mg q.i.d
			Children under 12:	25 to 50 mg/kg/day in 3–4 divided doses
piperacillin sodium	Zosyn	IM:	*Adults:*	2 to 8 g daily in 2 to 4 divided doses

Implications for Patient Care

Medical assistants should treat each patient as an individual and take a careful history of allergies. It is very important to determine if the patient has an allergy to penicillins or cephalosporins before either of these groups of drugs is prescribed.

It is recommended that certain emergency supplies and medications be readily available when administering any drug to a patient, especially penicillins or cephalosporins. See Unit 10 for the recommended emergency supplies and medications.

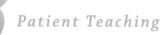

Patient Teaching

Instruct patients to report any signs of an adverse reaction, and to take their medication as prescribed until all of the drug has been taken. It is most important that the patient understand this instruction, as many times once patients start to feel better, they may discontinue taking the antibiotic, and a relapse can occur. Caution patients against taking any medication, unless it is prescribed for them. Instruct patients that the prescribed medication is for them, and they should not allow anyone else to take their medication. ■

Special Considerations

- Oral doses should be taken on an empty stomach, one hour before or two hours after a meal.
- It is best to take with 8 ounces of water and should not be taken with soft drinks, fruit juices, or wine, as the acid in these products can destroy the drug.
- Administration with erythromycin or a tetracycline may diminish effectiveness.

Penicillinase-Resistant Penicillin

Penicillinase-resistant penicillin makes up a group of penicillins that was developed because some organisms are resistant to penicillin. These drugs are effective against most gram-positive and gram-negative aerobes and a few gram-positive and gram-negative anaerobic bacteria (see Table 15-2).

TABLE 15-2 Selected Penicillinase-Resistant Penicillins

GENERIC NAME	TRADE NAME	ROUTE (S)	USUAL DOSAGE (S)	
cloxacillin	Cloxapen	Oral:	*Adults:*	250 to 500 mg every 6 hours
			Children:	(Up to 20 kg) 12.5 to 25 mg/kg every 6 hours
				(Under 20 kg) 50 to 100 mg/kg/day in 4 divided doses every 6 hours
dicloxacillin sodium		Oral:	*Adults:*	125 to 250 mg every 6 hours
			Children:	(Up to 40 kg) 12.5 to 25 mg/kg/day in divided doses every 6 hours
mezlocillin sodium		IM:	*Adults:*	200 to 300 mg/kg/day in 4 to 6 divided doses
			Children:	150 to 300 mg/kg/day in 2 to 6 divided doses
nafcillin sodium		Oral:	*Adults:*	250 mg: 1 g every 4 to 6 hours
			Children:	Neonates: 10 mg/kg every 6 to 8 hours
			Older Children:	25 to 50 mg/kg/day in 4 divided doses every 6 hours
oxacillin	Bactocill	Oral:	*Adults:*	500 mg: 1 g every 4 to 6 hours
			Children:	(Under 40 kg) 50 to 100 mg/kg/day in 4 equally divided doses

Cephalosporins

The cephalosporins are semisynthetic, broad-spectrum antibiotics that are derivatives of *cephalosporin C*, which is obtained from the fungus *Cephalosporium*. They are chemically and pharmacologically related to the penicillins.
Cephalosporins are classified into three generations:

- First-generation cephalosporins tend to have the greatest bacteriostatic or bactericidal activity against gram-positive and several gram-negative organisms, and are generally susceptible to being inactivated by beta-lactamase enzymes produced by some bacteria.

  EXAMPLE   cefadroxil (Duricef)   cefazolin (Ancef, Zolicef)

  cephalexin (C-Lexin, Keflex, Keftab)   cephalothin

- Second-generation cephalosporins have a broader spectrum of activity against gram-negative organisms and a slightly more diminished activity against gram-positive organisms than first-generation cephalosporins. *Haemophilus influenzae* is especially sensitive to second-generation cephalosporins.

  EXAMPLE   cefonicid   cefprozil (Cefzil)

  cefoxitin   cefuroxime (Ceftin, Zinacef)

- Third-generation cephalosporins have an even broader spectrum of activity against such gram-negative organisms as *Escherichia coli* (*E. coli*), *Klebsiella* species, *Proteus mirabilis* and possibly *Proteus vulgaris*, *Providencia rettgeri* and *Morganella morganii*, *streptococcus*, *staphylococcus*, *Neisseria gonorrhoeae*, and *Haemophilus*. The third-generation drugs are resistant to the defensive beta-lactamase enzymes that some bacteria secrete.

  EXAMPLE   cefepime (Maxipime)   ceftazidime (Fortaz, Tazicef)

  cefotaxime (Claforan)   ceftibuten (Cedax)

  cefpodoxime (Vantin)   ceftriaxone (Rocephin)

  cefditoren pivoxil (Spectracef)

Actions

The cephalosporins, like penicillins, act by inhibiting bacterial cell wall synthesis, thereby promoting the death of developing microorganisms.

Uses

Cephalosporins are indicated in the treatment of mild to severe infections of the respiratory tract, especially those caused by *Haemophilus influenzae* organisms that have developed a resistance to penicillins. They may also be prescribed for otitis media, skin and soft tissue infections, septicemia, gastrointestinal infections, genitourinary tract infections, meningitis, and bone and joint infections.

Contraindications

Hypersensitivity to cephalosporins or penicillins may result in an allergic reaction. Use caution in patients with impaired renal function and a history of colitis.

Adverse Reactions

Reactions include allergic, anaphylaxis, drug fever, Stevens-Johnson syndrome, serum sickness-like reaction, erythema multiforme, toxic epidermal necrolysis, colitis, renal dysfunction, toxic nephropathy, reversible hyperactivity, hypertonia, hepatic dysfunction including cholestasis, aplastic anemia, hemolytic anemia, hemorrhage, and superinfection.

Several cephalosporins have been implicated in triggering seizures, particulary in patients with renal impairment when the dosage was not reduced. If seizures associated with drug therapy occur, the drug should be discontinued. Anticonvulsant therapy can be given if clinically indicated.

Dosage and Route

The dosage and route of administration are determined by the physician. See Table 15-3 for selected cephalosporins.

Implications for Patient Care

Take a careful history of allergies. Patients who are allergic to penicillins are likely to be allergic to cephalosporins. Keep emergency drugs on hand.

 Patient Teaching

Advise the patient to report any signs of hypersensitivity. Instruct the patient to continue the medication as prescribed until all of the drug has been taken.

Instruct the patient to avoid the use of alcohol and that over-the-counter medications such as certain mouthwashes and cough preparations may contain alcohol. ■

Special Considerations

- Oral doses may be taken on a full or empty stomach.
- Administration with erythromycin or tetracycline may interfere with cephalosporin's bactericidal action.
- For diabetics—This medicine may cause false test results with some urine sugar tests. Patients should check with their physicians before changing their diet or dosage of diabetes medicine.

TABLE 15-3 Selected Cephalosporins, Routes, and Dosages

GENERIC NAME	TRADE NAME	ROUTE	USUAL DOSAGE	
cefaclor	Ceclor	Oral	*Adults:*	250 to 500 mg every 8 hours, not to exceed 4 g daily
			Children:	(1 month and older) 20 to 40 mg/kg daily in divided doses every 8 hours, not to exceed 1 g daily
cefadroxil	Duricef	Oral	*Adults:*	500 mg capsules or 1 g tablets once or twice a day every 12 hours
			Children:	30 mg/kg per day in divided doses every 12 hours
cefazolin sodium	Ancef	IM	*Adults:*	250 mg to 1 g every 6, 8, or 12 hours
			Children:	25 to 50 mg/kg/day divided into 3 to 4 equal doses
cefonicid		IM	*Adults:*	1 g once a day every 24 hours
cefotaxime	Claforan	IM	*Adults:*	1 to 2 g every 8 to 12 hours
			Children:	50 to 180 mg/kg divided into 4 to 6 equal doses
cefoxitin sodium		IM	*Adults:*	1 to 2 g every 6 to 8 hours
			Children:	(3 months and older) 80 to 160 mg/kg/day divided into 4 to 6 doses
cefpodoxime proxetil	Vantin	Oral	*Adults:*	200 to 400 mg every 12 hours
			Children:	100 mg/kg/day; maximum 400 mg/day
ceftazidime	Fortaz	IM	*Adults:*	250 mg to 2 g every 8 to 12 hours
			Children:	30 to 50 mg/kg every 8 hours
ceftriaxone sodium	Rocephin	IM	*Adults:*	1 to 2 g once a day
			Children:	50 to 100 mg/kg in divided doses every 12 hours (not to exceed 4 g)
cefuroxime	Ceftin	Oral	*Adults:*	250 to 500 mg twice a day
			Children:	20 to 30 mg/kg/day twice a day
cephalexin		Oral	*Adults:*	250 mg to 500 mg every 6 hours
			Children:	25 to 50 mg/kg in 4 divided doses
cefditoren pivoxil	Spectracef	Oral	*Adults and Adolescents:*	200 to 400 mg twice a day

- Avoid alcohol consumption during the use of certain cephalosporins. Cephalosporins may interact with acute alcohol consumption and produce a disulfiram-like (Antabuse-like) reaction, which is a severe hypersensitivity to alcohol. Symptoms that may occur are flushing, chest pain, palpitations, tachycardia, hypotension, syncope (fainting), and arrhythmias.

Carbapenems

The carbapenems are a class of beta-lactam antibiotics with a broad spectrum of antibacterial activity, and have a structure that renders them highly resistant to beta-lactamases. Carbapenem antibiotics were originally developed from thienamycin, a naturally derived product of *Streptomyces cattleya*. Carbapenems exhibit bacteriocidal activity by binding to the penicillin-binding proteins (PBP), thus preventing linking of the peptidoglycan strands and further synthesis of the bacterial cell wall. The carbapenem class provides the most broad-spectrum coverage of all the anti-infectives marketed. Their broadest activity is against gram-positive and gram-negative, aerobic, and anaerobic microorganisms.

Imipenem/cilastatin (Primaxin by Merck), meropenem (Merrem by AstraZeneca), ertapenem (Invanz by Merck) and doripenem (Doribax by Ortho-McNeil) are the four beta-lactam antibiotics of the carbapenem class. Imipenem/cilastatin was approved first in 1987, followed by meropenem in 1996, ertapenem in 2001, and then, most recently, doripenem in 2007.

Actions

The carbapenems are structurally very similar to the penicillins, but the sulfur atom in position 1 of the structure has been replaced with a carbon atom, and hence the name of the group, the carbapenems. Carbapenems exhibit bacteriocidal activity by binding to the penicillin-binding proteins, thus preventing linking of the peptidoglycan strands and further synthesis of the bacterial cell wall. They exert their action by penetrating bacterial cells readily and interfering with the synthesis of vital cell wall components, which leads to cell death.

Uses

Indicated for the treatment of patients with moderate to severe infections caused by susceptible isolates of aerobic gram-positive, aerobic gram-negative, and anaerobic microorganisms. These agents have the broadest antibacterial spectrum compared to other beta-lactam classes such as penicillins and cephalosporins. Additionally they are generally resistant to the typical bacterial beta-lactamase enzymes that are one of the principal resistance mechanisms of bacteria.

Contraindications

Contraindicated in patients with known hypersensitivity to any of the drugs in the same class or in patients who have demonstrated anaphylactic reactions to beta-lactams.

Adverse Reactions

The carbapenems have overall safe adverse effect profiles. The most commonly reported adverse effects include local irritation at injection site, diarrhea, rash, nausea, vomiting, and pruritis.

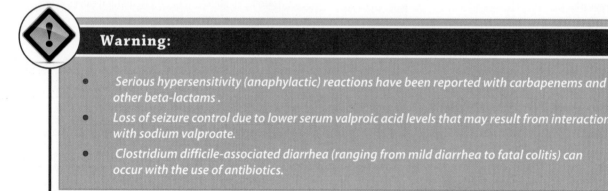

Warning:

- *Serious hypersensitivity (anaphylactic) reactions have been reported with carbapenems and other beta-lactams.*
- *Loss of seizure control due to lower serum valproic acid levels that may result from interaction with sodium valproate.*
- *Clostridium difficile-associated diarrhea (ranging from mild diarrhea to fatal colitis) can occur with the use of antibiotics.*

Dosage and Route

The dosage and route of administration are determined by the physician and varies with the drug prescribed. Each of the carbapenems are formulated as parenteral agents. Imipenem/cilastatin (Primaxin) IM or IV and meropenem (Merrem) IV are administered as either a 500 mg or 1 g dose every six to eight hours. Ertapenem (Invanz) is unique in the fact that it is administered once daily as a 1 g dose IM or IV. Doripenem (Doribax) is approved for a dose of 500 mg IV every six to eight hours.

Implications for Patient Care

Take a careful history of allergies. Patients who are allergic to penicillins and/or cephalosporins are likely to be allergic to carbapenems.

Patient Teaching

Patients should be counseled that antibacterial drugs should only be used to treat bacterial infections. They should be told that although it is common to feel better early in the course of therapy, the medication should be taken exactly as directed. Skipping doses or not completing the full course of therapy may (1) decrease the effectiveness of the immediate treatment, and (2) increase the likelihood that bacteria will develop resistance and will not be treatable in the future. Diarrhea is a common problem caused by antibiotics, which usually ends when the antibiotic is discontinued. Sometimes after starting treatment with antibiotics, patients can develop watery and bloody stools (with or without stomach cramps and fever) even as late as two or more months after having taken the last dose of the antibiotic. If this occurs, patients should contact their physician as soon as possible. ■

Tetracyclines

Tetracyclines are primarily *bacteriostatic*, and are active against a wide range of gram-negative and gram-positive microorganisms. There are both natural and semisynthetic tetracyclines, which are derived from various species of *streptomyces*. The tetracycline drugs exhibit similarities in their range of antimicrobial activity.

Actions

The tetracyclines are thought to exert their effect on microorganisms by inhibiting protein synthesis in the bacterial cell.

Uses

Tetracyclines are indicated in the treatment of rickettsial disease, respiratory infections, venereal diseases, acne, and amebiasis.

Contraindications

Tetracyclines are contraindicated in patients with renal and liver impairment, during pregnancy and lactation, and with children 8 years of age and younger. These drugs cause *permanent discoloration of tooth enamel* and a predisposition to cavities among children with developing teeth.

Adverse Reactions

Nausea, vomiting, diarrhea, colitis, anorexia, photosensitivity, permanent discoloration of deciduous teeth, and overgrowth of fungi (candidiasis or moniliasis).

Dosage and Route

The dosage and route of administration are determined by the physician (see Table 15-4).

Implications for Patient Care

Medical assistants should be familiar with the signs of hypersensitivity and superinfection. It may be your responsibility to advise the patient about such signs. Instruct the patient to report any signs of hypersensitivity or superinfection to the physician.

Tetracyclines should be given on an empty stomach (one hour before meals or two hours after meals) with a full glass of water. The drug expiration date should always be checked before administration, as renal injury (Fanconi-like syndrome) and other problems may result from the use of outdated tetracyclines.

TABLE 15-4   Selected Tetracyclines, Routes, and Dosages

GENERIC NAME	TRADE NAME	ROUTE	USUAL DOSAGE	
demeclocycline hydrochloride	Declomycin DMCT	Oral:	*Adults:*	150 mg every 6 hours
			Children:	3 to 6 mg/lb daily in 2 to 4 divided doses
doxycycline hyclate	Doryx-Caps Vibramycin Vibra-Tabs	Oral:	*Adults:*	100 mg every 12 hours on 1st day, then 100 mg once daily
			Children:	2 mg/kg for 2 doses every 12 hours, then 2.3 to 4.4 mg/kg once daily
minocycline hydrochloride	Minocin	Oral:	*Adults:*	200 mg initially followed by 100 mg every 12 hours
			Children:	Above 8 years of age, 4 mg/kg initially followed by 2 mg/kg every 12 hours

Patient Teaching

Advise patients to avoid direct or artificial sunlight, as they are more sensitive to it and may suffer a sunburn. Instruct patients to not eat dairy products or take antacids, laxatives, or iron supplements within one to two hours of taking tetracycline. ▪

Special Considerations

- Oral doses should be taken on an empty stomach, one hour before or two hours after a meal.
- It is best to take with 8 ounces of water and should not be taken with milk or any dairy product. Alkaline products can interact with tetracycline and make it less effective.
- Administration with calcium supplements, antacids, or iron may reduce tetracycline absorption.
- Concurrent use with oral contraceptives may render oral contraceptives less effective.

Aminoglycosides

The aminoglycosides include any of a group of *bactericidal* antibiotics derived from various species of microbes from the genus *Streptomyces*. The aminoglycosides are broad-spectrum antibiotics, the best known of which is streptomycin.

Actions

The aminoglycosides act by interfering with the synthesis of bacterial cell protein, thereby promoting the death of the affected microorganism.

Uses

Aminoglycosides are indicated in the treatment of diseases caused by gram-negative microorganisms. They may be used to treat active tuberculosis, plague, subacute bacterial endocarditis, *Haemophilus influenzae*, pneumonia, peritonitis, respiratory tract infections, urinary tract infections, and infections caused by *Escherichia coli*.

● *Note*

Bacterial cultures should be obtained prior to and during treatment to isolate and identify etiologic organisms and to test their susceptibility to the prescribed aminoglycoside. ●

Contraindications

Do not prescribe for those with hypersensitivity to drugs of the aminoglycosides. These drugs are contraindicated in patients with labyrinthine disease or myasthenia gravis, and those who are pregnant and/or lactating. Use cautiou in patients with impaired renal function, the elderly, infants, and children. Aminoglycosides should not be given concurrently with potent diuretics, such as ethacrynic acid and furosemide. Ototoxicity may be enhanced by these diuretics.

Adverse Reactions

Aminoglycosides can cause *irreversible damage to the auditory branch of the eighth cranial nerve* (*acoustic*). Factors contributing to this side effect include the drug, the patient's condition, the dose, the length of therapy, and the patient's renal function. Other adverse reactions may include skin rashes, pruritus, stomatitis, headache, muscular weakness, and *nephrotoxicity* with signs of oliguria and proteinuria. Patients may experience vertigo, tinnitus, dizziness, ataxia, nausea, and vomiting.

Dosage and Route

The dosage and route of administration are prescribed by the physician (see Table 15-5).

Implications for Patient Care

Observe for signs of ototoxicity (nausea, vomiting, vertigo, and acute loss of hearing). Monitor patients with impaired renal function for signs of oliguria and proteinuria by recording the intake and output volume, and by urinalysis.

TABLE 15-5   Selected Aminoglycosides

GENERIC NAME	TRADE NAME	ROUTE	USUAL DOSAGE	
amikacin sulfate	Amikin	IM	*Adults:*	15 mg/kg/day divided into 2 to 3 equal doses
gentamicin sulfate		IM	*Adults:*	3 mg/kg/day in 3 divided doses every 8 hours
			Children:	6 to 7.5 mg/kg/day (2 to 2.5 mg/kg every 8 hours)
kanamycin		Oral	*Adults:*	1 to 8 g daily in 4 divided doses.
			Children:	50 mg/kg daily in 4 to 6 divided doses every 6 hours
		IM	*Adults and Children:*	15 mg/kg in 2 to 4 divided doses
netilmicin		IM	*Adults:*	With normal renal function: complicated urinary tract infections: 3.0 to 4.0 mg/kg/day serious systemic infections: 4.0 to 6.5 mg/kg/day dosage for patients with impaired renal function must be individualized
streptomycin sulfate	Streptomycin	IM	*Adults:*	1 to 2 g daily (15 to 25 mg/kg) 500 mg to 1 g every 12 hours
			Children:	20 to 40 mg/kg daily in 2 divided doses
tobramycin sulfate	Tobrex	IM	*Adults:*	3 mg/kg daily in 3 equal doses every 8 hours
			Children:	2 to 2.5 mg/kg every 8 hours

Patient Teaching

Advise the patient to drink plenty of fluids. Instruct the patient to report any signs of hypersensitivity. Patients with tuberculosis should be advised that drug therapy is only a part of their long-term treatment, in combination with proper diet and adequate rest. ■

Special Considerations

- Because of the potential toxicity associated with aminoglycosides, patients should be under close clinical observation. The major toxic effects are the action on the auditory and vestibular branches of the eighth nerve and the renal tubules. Patients should be instructed to observe for signs of ototoxicity or nephrotoxicity.

- Watch for signs of ototoxicity: nausea, vomiting, tinnitus (ringing sound in the ear), vertigo, acute loss of hearing.

- Watch for signs of nephrotoxicity: oliguria (decreased amount of urine formation) and proteinuria (presence of protein [albumin] in the urine).

- Patients should be encouraged to drink plenty of liquids (eight glasses of water a day) to reduce the development of nephrotoxicity.

- Administration with anesthetics, muscle relaxants, or both could cause neuromuscular blockade and respiratory paralysis.

- Avoid Administering with other drugs that could cause ototoxicity or nephrotoxicity. This is particularly true of polymyxin B, bacitracin, colistin, amphotericin B, cisplatin, vancomycin, potent diuretics, and all other aminoglycosides.

Macrolides

Macrolide antibiotics include the erythromycins and azithromycin (Zithromax) and clarithromycin (Biaxin).These drugs exert their antimicrobial action by binding to the bacterial 50S ribosomal subunit, thereby inhibiting protein synthesis. Numerous erythromycin preparations exist today; see Table 15-6. Azithromycin (Zithromax) and clarithromycin (Biaxin) are also described in this section.

Ketolides

Ketolides are a new class of macrolides designed particularly to combat respiratory tract pathogens that have acquired resistance to macrolides. The ketolides are semisynthetic derivatives of the 14-membered macrolide

TABLE 15-6 Selected Erythromycins

GENERIC NAME	TRADE NAME	ROUTE	USUAL DOSAGE	
erythromycin base	E-Mycin Ery-Tab	Oral	*Adults:*	250 to 500 mg every 6 hours
			Children:	30 to 50 mg/kg/day in 3 to 4 divided doses
erythromycin estolate		Oral	*Adults:*	250 to 500 mg every 6 hours
			Children:	30 to 50 mg/kg/day in 3 to 4 divided doses
erythromycin ethylsuccinate	EES Ery-Ped	Oral	*Adults:*	250 mg every 6 hours
			Children:	30 to 50 mg/kg/day in 3 to 4 divided doses
erythromycin stearate	Erythrocin	Oral	*Adults:*	250 to 500 mg every 6 hours
			Children:	30 to 50 mg/kg/day in 3 to 4 divided doses

erythromycin A, and they retain the erythromycin macrolactone ring structure as well as the D-desosamine sugar attached at position 5. Ketolides potently inhibit protein synthesis by interacting close to the peptidyl transferase site of the bacterial 50S ribosomal subunit. They bind to ribosomes with higher affinity than macrolides. They exhibit good activity against gram-positive aerobes and some gram-negative aerobes, and they have excellent activity against drug-resistant *Streptococcus pneumoniae*.

Telithromycin (Ketek) is the first member of this new class to be approved for clinical use. It is given at a dose of 800 mg once daily, for 5 to 10 days. Food does not affect absorption. Gastrointestinal intolerance appears to be the main adverse effect.

Erythromycin

Erythromycin is produced by a strain of the actinomycete Saccharopolyspora erythraea (*Streptomyces erythraecus*), and belongs to the *macrolide* group of antibiotics. Depending upon the concentration of the drug and the nature of the microorganism against which it is used, erythromycin can be bacteriostatic or bactericidal.

Actions

Erythromycin works by inhibiting protein synthesis in susceptible bacteria.

Uses

Erythromycin is a broad-spectrum antibiotic, similar to penicillin, and is often used against penicillin-resistant microorganisms. It is also indicated for patients who are allergic to penicillin. Infections for which erythromycin might be prescribed include pneumococcal and diplococcal pneumonia, pelvic inflammatory disease, *Neisseria gonorrhoeae*, Legionnaires' disease, upper and lower respiratory tract infections, and infections of the skin and soft tissues.

Contraindications

Caution should be used when administering this drug to patients with liver dysfunction. Its safe use in pregnancy has not been established.

Adverse Reactions

Erythromycin may cause nausea, vomiting, diarrhea, and abdominal discomfort when given orally. Hypersensitivity reactions include urticaria, skin eruptions, and fever. Superinfection by nonsusceptible bacteria, yeasts, or fungi may occur. When applied topically, burning, tenderness, dryness or oiliness, pruritus, and erythema may occur.

Dosage and Route

Dosage and route are prescribed by the physician (see Table 15-6).

Implications for Patient Care

Observe the patient for signs of hypersensitivity. Monitor liver function tests. Give on an empty stomach (one hour before or two hours after meals). Enteric-coated tablets may be given without regard to meals.

Patient Teaching

Patients should be instructed to follow the complete course of therapy, to avoid taking the drug with fruit juices, and to report signs of *hepatotoxicity* such as jaundice and abdominal cramps. ■

Grapefruit juice seems to decrease how quickly the body breaks down certain medications. Drinking grapefruit juice while taking certain medications may increase the effects and side effects of the drug.

It is important to instruct patients to tell the doctor or pharmacist of all prescription and nonprescription and herbal products used. Instruct patients not to use with drugs that may affect heart rhythm, such as cisapride and pimozide. Inform that erythromycin may decrease the effectiveness of combination-type birth control pills, which could result in pregnancy.

Azithromycin (Zithromax)

Actions

Zithromax is an azalide, a subclass of a macrolide antibiotic. It acts by binding to the 50S ribosomal subunit of susceptible microorganisms and thus interferes with microbial protein synthesis.

Uses

Indicated for the treatment of individuals 16 years of age and older with mild to moderate infections caused by susceptible strains of the designated microorganisms in lower respiratory infections due to *Haemophilus influenzae, Moraxella catarrhalis,* or *Streptococcus pneumoniae.* As an alternative to first-line drug therapy in the treatment of upper respiratory infections such as streptococcal pharyngitis/tonsillitis, Zithromax is often effective in the eradication of susceptible strains of *Streptococcus pyogenes* from the nasopharynx. It is also used in the treatment of uncomplicated skin and skin structure infections due to *Staphylococcus aureus, Streptococcus pyogenes,* or *Streptococcus agalactiae.* It may be used in the treatment of nongonococcal urethritis and cervicitis due to *Chlamydia trachomatis.*

Contraindications

Zithromax is contraindicated in patients with known hypersensitivity to azithromycin, erythromycin, or any macrolide antibiotic.

Adverse Reactions

In clinical trials, most of the reported side effects were mild to moderate in severity and were reversible upon discontinuation of the drug. Most of the side effects were related to the gastrointestinal tract: nausea, vomiting, diarrhea, or abdominal pain. Rare, but potentially serious side effects, were angioedema and cholestatic jaundice.

Dosage and Route

Zithromax is given orally in capsules or in an oral suspension. Dosage is 500 mg as a single dose on the first day, then 250 mg once daily on days 2 through 5 for a total dose of 1.5 grams.

Implications for Patient Care

Observe the patient for signs of hypersensitivity. Medication should be administered at least one hour before a meal or at least two hours after a meal. Because some strains of bacteria are resistant to Zithromax, susceptibility tests should be performed before and during treatment. Zithromax, at the recommended dose, should not be relied upon to treat gonorrhea or syphilis.

 Patient Teaching

Patients should be instructed to follow the complete course of therapy, and to avoid the use of aluminum- or magnesium-containing antacids when taking Zithromax. ▪

Clarithromycin (Biaxin)

Actions

Clarithromycin inhibits protein synthesis at the level of the 50S bacterial ribosome and exerts bacteriostatic action against susceptible bacteria.

Uses

It is used to treat upper respiratory tract infections including streptococcal pharyngitis and sinusitis, and lower respiratory tract infections including bronchitis and pneumonia; treatment (with ethambutol) and prevention of disseminated mycobacterium avium complex (MAC); and treatment of the following infections in children: otitis media, sinusitis, pharyngitis, skin and skin structure infections. It is part of a combination regimen (with a gastric-acid pump inhibitor and amoxicillin or with ranitidine bismuth citrate) for ulcer disease due to *Helicobacter pylori*. Clarithromycin can also be used to treat endocarditis prophylaxis.

Contraindications

Avoid prescribing to those with hypersensitivity to clarithromycin, erythromycin, or other macrolide anti-infective. Avoid using when a patient is pregnant and lactating unless no alternatives available. Also, use cautiously in severe liver or renal impairment.

Adverse Reactions

Headache, pseudomembranous colitis, abdominal pain or discomfort, abnormal taste, diarrhea, dyspepsia, and nausea are some of the reactions.

Dosage and Route

The following are oral dosages of clarithromycin for adults: 250 mg every 12 hours for bronchitis, pneumonia, skin and soft tissue infections; 500 mg every 12 hours for bronchitis, sinusitis, disseminated MAC/*H. pylori*; and 500 mg 1 hour before procedure for endocarditis prophylaxis.

The following are oral dosages of clarithromycin for children: 7.5 mg/kg every 12 hours for most infections (up to 500 mg/dose for MAC); and 15 mg/kg 1 hour before procedure for endocarditis prophylaxis.

Implications for Patient Care

Assess patient for infection at beginning of and throughout therapy. Obtain specimens for culture and sensitivity prior to initiating therapy. First dose may be given before receiving results. Administer around the clock, without regard to meals. Food slows but does not decrease the extent of absorption. Shake suspension well before administration. Do not administer within 4 hours of zidovudine.

 Patient Teaching

Instruct the patient to take the medication around the clock and to finish the drug completely as directed, even if feeling better. Missed doses should be taken as soon as possible, unless it is almost time for the next dose. Do not double doses. Do not share medication with anyone. Advise patients to report signs of superinfections, fever and diarrhea to a health care provider. Caution patients taking zidovudine that clarithromycin and zidovudine must be taken at least 4 hours apart. Advise patients to notify a health care provider if symptoms do not improve within a few days. ■

Fluoroquinolones

Fluoroquinolones are synthetic, broad-spectrum antibiotics/anti-infectives that have a rapid bactericidal action against most gram-negative and many gram-positive bacteria. They alter deoxyribonucleic acid (DNA) by interfering with DNA gyrase, an enzyme that is necessary for the duplication, transcription, and repair of bacterial DNA. Because humans do not have this enzyme, their cells are not affected.

These drugs are indicated for treatment of susceptible strains of designated microorganisms that cause a wide range of mild to moderate gentiourinary tract infections, including cystitis, urinary tract infection, prostatits, and sexually transmitted diseases such as gonorrhea and chlamydia, upper respiratory infections, infectious diarrhea, ophthalmic infections, bone and joint infections, for dental work, gum and tooth infections.

Examples of fluoroquinolones are ciprofloxacin (Cipro), enoxacin, levofloxacin (Levaquin), lomefloxacin, moxifloxacin (Avelox), norfloxacin (Noroxin), and ofloxacin (Floxin).

Certain adverse reactions are common to the fluoroquinolones and others are drug-specific. For dosage, route, and selected adverse reactions, see Table 15-7.

> **Warning:**
>
> *Fluoroquinolones are associated with an increased risk of tendonitis and tendon rupture. This risk is further increased in those over age 60, in recipients of kidney, heart, and lung transplant, and with use of concomitant steroid therapy. Physicians should advise patients, at the first sign of tendon pain, swelling, or inflammation, to stop taking the fluoroquinolone, to avoid exercise and use of the affected area, and to promptly contact their doctor about changing to a nonfluoroquinolone antimicrobial drug.*

TABLE 15-7 Selected Fluoroquinolones

MEDICATION	USUAL DOSAGE			ADVERSE REACTIONS
ciprofloxacin (Cipro)	*Oral*	*Adults:*	500 to 700 mg every 12 hours for 1 to 2 weeks	Nausea, diarrhea, vomiting, rash, headache, tremors, abdominal pain, dry or painful mouth, Stevens-Johnson syndrome
enoxacin	*Oral*	*Adults:*	200 to 400 mg every 12 hours for 1 to 2 weeks	Anorexia, bloody stools, gastritis, stomatitis, anxiety, tremors, Stevens-Johnson syndrome
levofloxacin (Levaquin)	*Oral*	*Adults:*	250 to 500 mg every 24 hours	Nausea, vomiting, diarrhea, dry or painful mouth, headache, dizziness, photosensitivity, CV collapse
lomefloxacin	*Oral*	*Adults:*	400 mg daily for 10 to 14 days	Confusion, tremor, vertigo, anxiety, anorexia, coma, bad taste in mouth, dysphagia, tongue discoloration
moxifloxacin (Avelox)	*Oral*	*Adults:*	400 mg every 24 hours for 10 days	Anaphylaxis after the first dose, CV collapse, loss of consciousness, vertigo, dysphagia
norfloxacin (Noroxin)	*Oral*	*Adults:*	400 mg every 12 hours for 72 hours	Nausea, vomiting, diarrhea, dry or painful mouth, headache, dizziness
ofloxacin (Floxin)	*Oral*	*Adults:*	300 to 400 mg every 12 hours for 10 days	Photosensitivity, CV collapse

Monobactams

Monobactams are synthetic antibiotics that contain a cyclic beta-lactam structure. They are bactericidal against gram-negative aerobic pathogens. Aztreonam (Azactam) is the most widely known representative of the monobactam family. It acts by inhibiting cell-wall synthesis due to a high affinity of the drug for penicillin-binding protein 3; this results in cell lysis and death.

Aztreonam (Azactam)

Actions

Azactam is the first member of a new class of antibiotics classified as *monobactams*. It is a totally synthetic bactericidal antibiotic with activity against a wide spectrum of gram-negative aerobic pathogens.

Uses

Indicated for the treatment of infections caused by susceptible gram-negative microorganisms; urinary tract, lower respiratory tract, skin and skin structure, intra-abdominal, gynecologic infections, and septicemia.

Contraindications

Azactam is contraindicated in patients with known allergy to this antibiotic.

Adverse Reactions

Discomfort/swelling at the injection site can occur following IM administration. Other reactions can include diarrhea, nausea and/or vomiting, skin rash, anaphylaxis, pancytopenia, abdominal cramps, purpura, hypotension, weakness, headache, fever, and malaise.

Dosage and Route

Dosage adjustments are recommended for patients with impaired renal function. In elderly patients, estimates of creatinine clearance should be obtained and appropriate dosage modifications made if necessary. The dosage and route of administration are determined by the physician. Azactam is available in single-dose, 15-mL vials containing 500 mg, 1 g, or 2 g per vial for IM injection.

Implications for Patient Care

Medical assistants should obtain a history of hypersensitivity to any antibiotic or other drug. It is important to relay this information to the physician. Antibiotics should be given with caution to any patient who has had some form of allergy to drugs.

Oxazolidinones

Oxazolidinones are a new class of antibiotics that act by inhibiting the formation of the ribosomal initiation complex, a unique site not overlapping other ribosomally active antimicrobials. Linezolid (Zyvox) is the first of this class and the first entirely new type of antibiotic in 35 years. It attacks bacteria by stopping protein production at an early point in the process that is different from any other antibiotic. Without protein production, bacteria cannot multiply, and bacteria die.

Linezolid (Zyvox) has primary activity against all gram-positive organisms. It is approved for the treatment of adult patients with vancomycin-resistant *Enterococcus faecium* (VREF) infections by indicated bacteria, nosocomial pneumonia, complicated and uncomplicated skin and skin structure infections, and community-acquired pneumonia. It is mainly intended for hospital or institutional care settings. Due to concerns about inappropriate use of antibiotics leading to an increase in resistant organisms, prescribers should carefully consider alternatives before initiating treatment with Zyvox in the outpatient setting.

The most common adverse reactions to the drug are diarrhea, headache, nausea, and vomiting. The most important laboratory test change was a decrease in platelet counts. It is available in 400 mg and 600 mg tablets, oral suspension of 100 mg/5mL, and intravenous bags of 200 mg/100 mL, 400 mg/200 mL, and 600 mg/300 mL. Interactions of Zyvox with other drugs include "over-the-counter cold remedies that contain pseudoephedrine or phenylpropanolamine" with a risk of increasing blood pressure. Patients receiving Zyvox should inform their physicians if they are taking such medications.

Streptogramins

Streptogramins are a distinct class of antibacterials. Synercid (quinupristin/dalfopristin) IV is the first injectable antibiotic approved by the U.S. Food and Drug Administration (FDA) to treat bloodstream infections due to vancomycin-resistant *Enterococcus faecium* and skin and skin structure infections (SSSI) caused by methicillin-susceptible *Staphylococcus aureus* or *Streptococcus pyogenes.*

The two distinct antibiotic agents that form Synercid, quinupristin, and dalfopristin work synergistically to inhibit or destroy susceptible bacteria through a two-pronged attack on protein synthesis in bacterial cells, which are inactivated or die. The most common adverse reactions are inflammation and at the infusion site and pain at the infusion site. Other adverse reactions are arthralgia, myalgia, nausea, vomiting, diarrhea, constipation, dyspepsia, oral moniliasis, pancreatitis, stomatitis, headache, anxiety, confusion, dizziness, insomnia, thrombophlebitis, palpitation, rash, pruritus, urticaria, hematuria, dyspnea, allergic reaction, chest pain, fever, infection, superinfection, and pseudomembranous colitis (antibiotic-associated colitis).

ADDITIONAL ANTIBIOTICS

Table 15-8 lists additional antibiotics. Only the basic drug information is provided. Before administering any of these drugs, you should refer to a *Physicians' Desk Reference* or some other drug reference book for more detailed information.

Table 15-9 lists **antiseptics** and **disinfectants** that are in general use. Note that the brand or trade names for these products are shown in parentheses.

TABLE 15-8   Additional Antibiotics and Antibacterials

MEDICATION	USUAL DOSAGE			ADVERSE REACTIONS
chloramphenicol (Ak chlor)	*Oral*	50 mg/kg/day every 6 hours in divided doses		Bone marrow depression, blood dyscrasias, headache, confusion, nausea, vomiting, diarrhea, stomatitis, hypersensitivity, superinfection
clindamycin HCl (Cleocin)	*Oral*	*Adults:*	150 to 450 mg every 6 hours with 8 ounces of water	Diarrhea, rash, GI upset, jaundice, renal dysfunction
		Children:	8 to 20 mg/kg/day in 3–4 divided doses	
	IM	*Adults:*	1.2 to 2.7 g/day in 2 to 4 equal divided doses.	
		Children:	20 to 40 mg/kg/day in 3 to 4 equal divided doses	

(continues)

TABLE 15-8 *(continued)*

MEDICATION	USUAL DOSAGE			ADVERSE REACTIONS
lincomycin HCl (Lincocin)	Oral	Adults:	500 mg every 6 to 8 hours	Nausea, vomiting, diarrhea, hypersensitivity, superinfection, hematopoietic changes
		Children:	(Over 1 month old) 3 to 60 mg/kg/day in 3 to 4 divided doses	
	IM	Adults:	600 mg once or twice daily	
		Children:	(Over 1 month old) 10 mg/kg once or twice daily	
metronidazole HCl (Flagyl)	Oral		7.5 mg/kg every 6 hours	Nausea, vomiting, diarrhea, skin rash, seizures, peripheral neuropathy
polymyxin B-bacitracin neomycin (Neosporin)	Ointment or Cream		Apply a thin layer to the area 2 to 5 times a day	Ototoxicity, nephrotoxicity, hypersensitivity to neomycin
spectinomycin HCl (Trobicin)	IM	Adults:	2 g	Urticaria, dizziness, nausea, chills, fever, insomnia
vancomycin HCl (Vancocin HCl)	Oral	Adults:	500 mg every 6 hours or 1000 mg every 12 hours	Nausea, chills, fever, urticaria, macular rashes, eosinophilia, hypersensitivity
		Children:	44 mg/kg/day in divided doses	

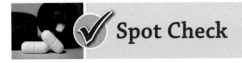

Spot Check

For each of the antibiotic groupings given, list several aspects of patient teaching and several special considerations.

MAJOR ANTIBIOTIC GROUPING	PATIENT TEACHING	SPECIAL CONSIDERATIONS
penicillins		
cephalosporins		
tetracyclines		
aminoglycosides		

ANTISEPTICS AND DISINFECTANTS

Antiseptics are substances that prevent or inhibit the growth of microorganisms. The process by which growth is inhibited is called *bacteriostatic* action. Antiseptics are generally applied to the surface of living tissue. Due to their lack of potency, they do little or no damage to surrounding tissue.

Disinfectants are substances, usually of chemical origin, that kill vegetative forms of microorganisms. They are described as having a *bactericidal* action due to their destruction of bacteria. Sometimes referred to as *germicides*, these agents are of sufficient strength to cause harm to living tissue; therefore, they are usually applied to inanimate objects. Disinfectants rapidly kill microorganisms on the surfaces to which they are applied, and are used on walls, floors, bed linens, furniture, and bathroom fixtures. *Fungicides* are closely related agents and have the ability to kill fungi and their spores.

Phenol was the first antiseptic. Other antiseptics are compared with phenol to measure their effectiveness; this measure is known as the phenol coefficient (P/C). Many antiseptics contain phenol and related compounds (see Table 15-9).

Alcohol may be used as an antiseptic or as a germicide depending upon the type used and its strength. Ethyl alcohol (70% solution) is often used as an antiseptic for minor injuries, and to prepare the skin for injections. Used full strength, isopropyl alcohol is a germicide for the disinfection of instruments. It may also be used in a 70% solution for the disinfection of oral thermometers.

Tincture of iodine contains 2% iodine and 2.4% sodium iodide diluted in 50% ethyl alcohol. It may be used as a disinfectant for the skin, and as a germicide. Adding three drops of tincture of iodine to a quart of water will kill amoebas and bacteria within 30 minutes, and the water will still be potable (see Table 15-9).

The effectiveness of an antiseptic or a disinfectant depends upon the following factors.

- Strength of the solution
- Temperature of the solution
- Time of exposure
- The ionization rate of the substance used

Change Bleach Solutions Often

OSHA recommends bleach more than any other disinfection solution in medical and dental practices. Bleach solutions have a short potency span, however, and they usually need to be replaced every two or three days.

TABLE 15-9 Antiseptics and Disinfectants

SUBSTANCE	STRENGTH	ACTION	COMMENTS
alcohol Ethyl Isopropyl (rubbing)	70% solution full strength	antiseptic germicide	For external use only; used to prepare the skin for injections, venipuncture, and IV therapy; flammable
benzalkonium chloride (Zephiran)	1 : 750 1 : 2000–1 : 5000 1 : 5000 1 : 5000–1 : 10,000 1 : 2000–1 : 20,000	antiseptic	On intact skin, mucous membranes, superficial injury Vaginal douching Wet dressings Irrigations of the eye, body cavities Infected wounds

(continues)

TABLE 15-9 *(continued)*

SUBSTANCE	STRENGTH	ACTION	COMMENTS
chlorhexidine gluconate (Hibiclens)	4%	antiseptic antimicrobial	Skin cleanser; surgical scrub, health care personnel hand wash. For patients preoperative showering and bathing, patient preoperative skin preparation, skin wound cleanser, and general skin cleanser
chlorhexidine gluconate (Hibistat Towelette)	0.5%	germicidal hand wipe	Germicidal hand rinse; used in those situations where hands are physically clean, but in need of degerming, when routine hand washing is not convenient or desirable
formalin (Cidex)	0.5 to 0.9% 6 to 12 hours	disinfectant	Effective against viruses, spores; irritates tissues
gentian violet	1 : 100–1 : 1000	antiseptic, fungicide, dye	Used on skin and mucous membrane for fungus infections (thrush, impetigo)
green soap (solution or tincture)	1 : 10	antiseptic	Hand wash; used to wash thermometers
hexachlorophene (pHisoHex) (WescoHex) (Septi-Soft) (Septisol)	3% topical emulsion, liquid soap, lotions, ointments, and shampoos	bacteriostatic against gram-positive bacteria on the skin	Not used for bathing infants. Rinse skin after use. May produce erythema, dryness, and scaling on patients with sensitive skin
hydrogen peroxide	3% (diluted with 1 to 4 parts water)	antiseptic	Cleans wounds of pus, dead tissue; deteriorates upon standing. Store in a cool, dark place
iodine (solution or tincture) (Wescodyne) (Betadine)	2% 1 to $1\frac{1}{2}$% iodine and detergent	antiseptic germicide fungicide	Used on small wounds and abrasions. *Check for allergies* Hand rinse; kills organisms sensitive to iodine
phenolics (Cresol) (Lysol) (Amphyl) (Staphene)	2% to 5% $\frac{1}{2}$% $2\frac{1}{2}$%	disinfectant antiseptic disinfectant	On contaminated objects: linens, basins, bedpans; action not affected by organic material As a footbath for athlete's foot. Prolonged use may be injurious to tissues
sodium hypochlorite (household bleach)	1 : 10 1 : 100	germicide germicide	HIV (AIDS) inactivator. Used on contaminated surfaces

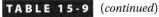

REVIEW QUESTIONS

Directions. Select the best answer to each of the following multiple-choice question, circling the letter of your choice.

1. An individual hypersensitivity to a substance, usually an antibody-antigen reaction, is known as _____.

   a. anaphylaxis   b. allergy   c. superinfection   d. toxicity

2. _____ is the process whereby a pathogenic agent invades the body, multiplies, and produces injury.

   a. Inflammation   b. Allergy   c. Infection   d. Disease

3. _____ may be natural or synthetic substances that inhibit the growth of or destroy microorganisms, especially bacteria.

   a. Disinfectants   b. Antiseptics   c. Antibiotics   d. Antineoplastics

4. _____ may occur when there is overgrowth of a resistant strain of bacteria, fungi, or yeast.

   a. Hypersensitivity   c. Superinfection

   b. Organ toxicity   d. Renal impairment

5. The most common adverse reaction to penicillins is _____.

   a. an allergic one   c. fever

   b. nausea   d. diarrhea

6. _____ antibiotics include the erythromycins and azithromycin (Zithromax) and clarithromycin (Biaxin).

   a. Ketolide   b. Fluoroquinolone   c. Macrolide   d. Monobactam

7. The cephalosporins are chemically and pharmacologically related to _____.

   a. tetracyclines   c. aminoglycosides

   b. penicillins   d. erythromycin

8. _____ are synthetic antibiotics that contain a cyclic beta-lactam structure. They are bactericidal against gram-negative aerobic pathogens.

   a. Ketolides   c. Macrolides

   b. Quinolones   d. Monobactams

9. Tetracyclines are contraindicated in _____.

   a. patients with renal and liver impairment

   b. pregnant and lactating patients

   c. children 8 years of age and younger

   d. all of these

10. _____ can cause irreversible damage to the auditory branch of the eighth cranial nerve (acoustic).

   a. Penicillins   c. Tetracyclines

   b. Aminoglycosides   d. Cephalosporins

11. Signs of ototoxicity are _____.

   a. diarrhea, fever, and sweating   c. pruritus, stomatitis, and headache

   b. nausea, vomiting, and vertigo   d. oliguria and proteinuria

12. A broad-spectrum antibiotic, similar to penicillins, and one which is often used against penicillin-resistant microorganisms is _____.

   a. erythromycin   c. chloromycetin

   b. neosporin   d. metronidazole

13. Before administering any drug, you should _____.

   a. check the drug's expiration date

   b. verify the order

   c. refer to a drug reference book for detailed information

   d. all of these

14. Zyvox (linezolid) is the first of a/an _____ class of antibiotic. It attacks bacteria by stopping protein production at an early point in the process. Without protein production, bacteria cannot multiply and bacteria die.

   a. ketolide   c. oxazolidinone

   b. Fluoroquinolone   d. monobactam

15. Emergency medications that should be readily available when administering any drug should include _____.

    a. epinephrine   c. dopamine and steroids

    b. diphenhydramine   d. all of these

16. Cefotetan (Cefotan) is classified as a _____.

    a. penicillin   c. cephalosporin

    b. tetracycline   d. erythromycin

17. Signs of hepatotoxicity are _____.

    a. jaundice, headache, and dizziness

    b. jaundice, diarrhea, and constipation

    c. jaundice and abdominal cramps

    d. nausea, vomiting, and diarrhea

Matching. Place the correct letter from Column II on the appropriate line of Column I:

Column I		*Column II*
18. ___D___ bactericidal		A. a microorganism or substance that is capable of producing disease
19. ___E___ bacteriostatic		
20. ___F___ disinfectant		B. a minute living body that is not visible to the naked eye
21. ___G___ infection		C. a substance that prevents or inhibits the growth of microorganisms, especially bacteria
22. ___A___ pathogen		
23. ___C___ antiseptic		D. pertaining to the killing or destruction of bacteria
24. ___H___ bacteria		E. pertaining to inhibiting or retarding bacterial growth
25. ___B___ microorganism		F. a chemical agent that kills vegetative forms of bacteria
		G. the process or state whereby a pathogenic agent invades the body or a body part, multiplies, and produces injury
		H. any microorganism of the Schizomycetes class
		I. a chemical substance that destroys fungi

UNIT 16
Antifungal, Antiviral, and Immunizing Agents

OBJECTIVES

Upon completing this unit, you should be able to:

- Define the terms listed in the vocabulary.
- State the actions, uses, contraindications, adverse reactions, dosages, routes, and implications for patient care of selected antifungal and antiviral agents.
- Describe the four general classes of antiretroviral agents.
- Describe highly active antiretroviral therapy (HAART).
- Describe zidovudine's role in the reduction of perinatal transmission of HIV.
- Describe the treatment regimen for AIDS in the older adult.
- Complete the critical thinking questions and activities presented in this unit.
- Differentiate between active and passive immunization.
- State the general recommendations of immunization.
- Describe the conditions when a live, attenuated virus vaccine should not be given.
- Define *vaccine*, *toxoid*, *immune globulin*, *specific immune globulin*, and *antitoxin*.
- State who should be immunized against vaccine-preventable diseases.
- Become familiar with the immunization schedule given in this unit and influenza A (H1N1) vaccines usage, administration, and storage.
- Complete the Spot Check on immunizations.
- Answer the review questions correctly.

VOCABULARY

adenovirus (ad'e-no-vi'rus). One of a group of closely related viruses that can cause infections of the upper respiratory tract.

antibody (an'ti-bod"e). A protein substance that is developed in response to an antigen.

antigen (an'ti-jen). Substances such as bacteria, toxins, or certain allergens that induce the formation of antibodies that specifically interact with the antigen.

antigenic (an-ti-jen'ik). Capable of causing the production of an antibody.

Candida (kan'di-da). A genus of yeastlike fungi. It is a part of the normal flora of the mouth, skin, intestinal tract, and vagina. *Candida* is one of the most common causes of vaginitis in women during the reproductive years. Formerly called *Monilia*.

cryptococcosis (krip"to-kok-o'sis). A systemic fungus infection that may involve any organ of the body, especially the lungs, the skin, and the brain and its meninges.

cytomegalovirus (si"to-meg"a-lo-vi'rus). One of a group of species-specific herpes viruses.

epidemiology (ep"i-de-me-ol'o-je). The study of the science concerned with defining and explaining the interrelationship of factors that determine the frequency and distribution of disease.

(continues)

histoplasmosis (his″to-plaz-mo″sis). A systemic, fungal respiratory disease.

human immunodeficiency virus (HIV). The appropriate name for the retrovirus that has been implied as the causative agent of AIDS (acquired immunodeficiency syndrome).

immunocompetence (im″u-no-kom′pe-tens). Being capable of developing an antibody (antigenic response) to stimulation by an antigen.

immunodeficiency (im″u-no-de-fish′en-se). A decreased ability or inability to respond to antigenic stimuli, this suppressing or altering the body's natural immune response.

phagocytosis (fag″o-si-to′sis). The ingestion and digestion of bacteria and particles by cells of the reticuloendothelial system and white blood cells.

retrovirus (ret″ro-vi′rus). Ribonucleic acid (RNA)-containing virus.

varicella (var″i-sel′a). A benign, highly contagious disease caused by varicella-zoster (V-Z) virus. *Chickenpox.*

volar (vo′lar). Refers to the palm of the hand or the palmar surface.

INTRODUCTION

Viruses are parasitic, minute organisms that may invade normal cells and cause disease. They depend upon the invaded cells for nutrition, metabolism, and reproduction. To date, over 300 viruses have been isolated from animal hosts. Many of these viruses are considered to be harmless, yet others are the cause of approximately half of all infectious diseases. The common cold (coryza), smallpox, yellow fever, most childhood diseases, herpes, influenza, Epstein-Barr syndrome, rabies, hepatitis B, HIV (human immunodeficiency virus) and AIDS (acquired *immunodeficiency* syndrome) are virus-related infections.

In 2009, a new strain of influenza virus A was identified as H1N1 influenza (also called swine flu). This virus was orginally referred to as "swine flu" because laboratory testing showed that many of the genes in this new virus were very similar to influenza viruses that normally occur in pigs (swine) in North America. Further study showed that this new virus was very different from what normally circulates in North American pigs. It has two genes from flu viruses that normally circulate in pigs in Europe and Asia and bird (avian) genes and human genes.

Like othe flu viruses, H1N1 spreads from person to person through coughing, sneezing, and sometimes through touching objects contaminated with the virus. Signs of infection include fatigue, fever, sore throat, muscle aches, chills, coughing, and sneezing. Some people also have diarrhea and vomitting. The H1N1 flu is very different from seasonal flu viruses. Most people have little or no immunity to this virus. On June 11, 2009, the World Health Organization (WHO) signaled that a pandemic of H1N1 flu was underway. In October 2009, vaccines for H1N1 became available in the United States.

Fungi are plantlike organisms that also depend upon a host for their existence. These organisms, which include molds and yeasts, may be parasitic, or grow in dead and decaying organic matter. Many forms of fungi are pathogenic to plants and animals, causing such diseases as histoplasmosis, Candida infections, cryptococcosis, athlete's foot, and tinea.

As mentioned in Unit 15, the immune system is the body's defense mechanism against viruses, fungi, bacteria, and other foreign substances. Known collectively as antigens, these foreign substances, when detected, are the targets of a number of specialized cells that are activated in response to their presence. Simply stated, there are four general phases associated with the body's immune response to a foreign substance:

1. The recognition of the enemy or foreign substance.

2. Amplification of the body's defenses—white blood cells:

    Phagocytes—the "cell eater," especially macrophages

    Lymphocytes—T cells and B cells

    > *Helper T cells* are the commander in chief. The identify the enemy and rush to the spleen and lymph nodes, where they stimulate the production of other cells to aid in the fight of the infection.

    > *Killer T cells* specialize in killing cells of the body that have been invaded by foreign substances. They also fights cells that have turned cancerous.

    > *B cells* are the biologic arms factory. They resides in the spleen or lymph nodes and produce antibodies.

3. The attack phase, during which these defenders of the body seek to kill and remove the foreign invader.

4. The slowdown phase, during which the number of defenders return to normal following victory over the foreign invader.

ANTIFUNGAL AGENTS

Antifungal agents are synthetic drugs that destroy or inhibit the growth of fungi. They are also effective against yeast.

Characteristics and Uses

Actions

Antifungal agents act by exerting *fungistatic* or *fungicidal* action on both resting and growing cells. They bind to certain sterols of the cell membrane, thus allowing leakage of essential intracellular compounds, which results in death of the cell. They are not effective against bacteria, *rickettsiae*, or viruses.

Uses

Antifungal agents are used for systemic, skin, and mucous membrane fungal infections. Some diseases for which a physician may prescribe an antifungal agent are *histoplasmosis*; **Candida** infections of the skin, mucous membrane, intestines, and vagina; *cryptococcosis*; athlete's foot; and tinea (ringworm) infections.

Contraindications

Patients with hypersensitivity to antifungal agents should avoid them. They are also contraindicated in patients with bone marrow depression or renal function impairment. Safe use of some agents during pregnancy and lactation has not been established.

Adverse Reactions

Reactions include nausea, vomiting, diarrhea, headache, vertigo, muscle pain, tinnitus, anemia, leukopenia, and hypersensitive reactions such as pruritus, urticaria, rash, fever, and anaphylaxis.

Dosage and Route

The dosage and route of administration are determined by the physician. See Table 16-1 for selected antifungal agents.

Implications for Patient Care

Observe the patient for any signs of hypersensitivity. Care should be exercised when inserting an antifungal agent intravaginally. To prevent possible spread of the disease, one must wear gloves. When applying a cream, lotion, or ointment to the candidal lesions, one must wear gloves, use an appropriate applicator, and not contaminate the medication container.

Patient Teaching

Instruct patients in the importance of following the prescribed medication regimen. Patients with vaginal infections should be advised that fungus or yeast infections are easily spread. Some physicians prefer that patients refrain from sexual intercourse while the infection is being treated. Inform patients that their infection

TABLE 16-1   Selected Antifungal Agents

MEDICATION	USUAL DOSAGE		ADVERSE REACTIONS
amphotericin B (Fungizone)	*Cream, lotion, ointment*: Applied liberally to the Candidal lesions 2 to 4 times a day		No evidence of systemic toxicity; may have a "drying" effect on some skin, local irritation, erythema, pruritus, or burning
clotrimazole (Lotrimin) (Mycelex)	*Cream, lotion, ointment*: Gently massage sufficient medicine into the affected and surrounding skin areas twice a day, in the morning and evening		Erythema, stinging, blistering, peeling, edema, pruritus, urticaria, burning, and general irritation of the skin
fluconazole (Diflucan)	*Oral:*	200 mg on the first day, then 100 mg once a day for 2 to 4 weeks *Children:* 3 mg/kg = 100 mg adult dose 6 mg/kg = 200 mg adult dose	Nausea, headache, skin rash, vomiting, abdominal pain, diarrhea
flucytosine (Ancobon)	*Oral:*	50 to 150 mg/kg/day at 6-hour intervals	Nausea, vomiting, diarrhea, rash, anemia, leukopenia, thrombopenia, elevated hepatic enzymes
griseofulvin (Grifulvin V)	*Oral:* *Adults:* *Children:*	500 mg daily dose 5 mg/lb body weight per day 30 to 50 lbs 125 to 250 mg over 50 lbs 250 to 500 mg	Hypersensitivity, skin rashes, urticaria, oral thrush, nausea, vomiting, epigastric distress, diarrhea, headache, fatigue, dizziness
ketoconazole (Nizoral)	*Oral:* *Adults:* *Children:*	200 mg (1 tab) to 400 mg (2 tabs) once daily Over 2 years of age 3.3 to 6.6 mg/kg daily dose	Anaphylaxis (rare cases), hypersensitivity, nausea, vomiting, abdominal pain, pruritus, headache, fever, diarrhea, gynecomastia, impotence, oligospermia
miconazole nitrate (Monistat-3)	*Vaginal suppository:* One 100 mg suppository is inserted intravaginally once daily at bedtime for 7 nights *Vaginal cream:* 1 applicatorful intravaginally once daily at bedtime for 7 days		Vulvovaginal burning, itching or irritation, cramping, headache, hives, skin rash
nystatin (Mycostatin)	*Oral:* 500,000 to 1,000,000 units (1–2 tabs) t.i.d. *Suspension:* *Adults and Children:* 4–6 ml q.i.d. (400,000 to 600,000 units) *Infants:* 2 ml q.i.d. (200,000 units) *Vaginal tabs:* 100,000 units (1 tab) daily for 2 weeks		Virtually nontoxic—large oral doses have occasionally produced diarrhea, nausea, vomiting *having few adverse effects*
terbinafine (Lamisil)	*Oral:* For fingernail onychomycosis: one 250 mg tab, once daily for 6 weeks. Toenail onychomycosis: one 250 mg tab, once daily for 12 weeks		Diarrhea, dyspepsia, abdominal pain, liver test abnormalities, rash, urticaria, pruritus, taste disturbances
terconazole (Terazol)	*Vaginal suppository:* 1 suppository (80 mg) at bedtime for 3 days *Vaginal cream:* 1 applicatorful (5 g) of 0.4% cream at bedtime for 7 days		Headache, local irritation, sensitization, vulvovaginal burning, hypersensitivity reactions, body pain

can be spread through sexual intercourse, that their partner could become infected, and then possibly reinfect them. It is highly recommended that a protective device, such as a condom, be utilized during sexual intercourse.

Patients with *Candida* infections should be instructed in correct hand washing procedure, proper personal hygiene (drying the genital area after bathing, showering, or swimming; wiping from front to back after a bowel movement, so that the organisms from the rectum will not be spread to the vagina), and wearing cotton underclothes. They should also avoid using heavily fragranced products such as soaps, bubble baths, toilet paper, and feminine hygiene sprays, as these products contain ingredients that can worsen any local irritation. ■

To improve the safety and effectiveness of over-the-counter antifungal products, the U.S. Food and Drug Administration (FDA) has released guidelines on topical products used to treat tinea infections—athlete's foot, jock itch, and ringworm. These guidelines include the following:

- Product may contain only one active ingredient—limited to clioquinol, haloprogin, miconazole nitrate, povidone-iodine, tolnaftate, or undecylenic acid and its salts.
- Ingredients banned because of their ineffectiveness as antifungal agents are alcloxa, aluminum sulfate, basic fuchsin, boric acid, camphor, chloroxylenol, menthol, and salicylic acid.
- Antifungal products must carry a label that reads, "This product is not effective on the scalp or nails," and a warning against use in children under 2 years of age unless directed by a physician and, then, only using the product externally.

ANTIVIRAL AGENTS

Antiviral agents are synthetic drugs that have been developed to combat specific viral diseases. Viruses are responsible for many diseases, such as the common cold (coryza), influenza, genital herpes, herpes zoster, and AIDS. In the United States, several antiviral drugs are employed in the treatment of specific viral diseases. Details on selected antiviral drugs follow. (*Note:* The generic drug name is listed first, followed by the trade name, in parentheses.)

Acyclovir (Zovirax)

Actions

Acyclovir has in vitro inhibitory activity against *herpes simplex virus* types 1 and 2 (HSV-1 and HSV-2), varicella-zoster, Epstein-Barr, and cytomegalovirus.

Uses

It is used for treatment for initial episodes and the management of recurrent episodes of genital herpes in certain patients. *It is not a cure for genital herpes.*

Contraindications

It is not to be used in patients who develop hypersensitivity or intolerance to the components of the formulation. It is not to be used during pregnancy. Use cautious during lactation.

Adverse Reactions

Nausea, vomiting, diarrhea, dizziness, anorexia, fatigue, edema, skin rash, leg pain, inguinal adenopathy, confusion, and headache are possible reactions.

Dosage and Route

Oral: Initial: 200 mg cap every 4 hours for total of 5 caps daily for 10 days (total of 50 caps)

Recurrent disease: one 200 mg cap t.i.d. for up to 6 months

Ointment: Apply sufficient quantity to adequately cover all lesions every 3 hours, 6 times a day for 7 days

> A finger cot or glove should be used when applying Zovirax to prevent autoinoculation of other body sites and transmission of infection to other people.

Implications for Patient Care

Medical assistants should observe a patient for any signs of hypersensitivity, nausea, and vomiting. Care should be exercised when applying Zovirax to lesions. To prevent possible spread of the disease, one *must* wear a finger cot or gloves.

Patient Teaching

Patients should be informed that genital herpes is a sexually transmitted disease, and that intercourse should be avoided when lesions are visible because of the risk of infecting one's sexual partner. Advise patients to contact their physician if sufficient relief is not obtained, if there are any adverse reactions, if they become pregnant or plan to become pregnant, or if they have any questions. ■

Amantadine hydrochloride (Symmetrel)

Actions

Antiviral activity against influenza A is not completely understood. The mode of action appears to be prevention of the release of infectious viral nucleic acid into the host cell.

Uses

Use for influenza A virus respiratory tract illness prevention and treatment. Also use in Parkinson's disease/syndrome and drug-induced extrapyramidal reactions.

Contraindications

Do not use in patients with known hypersensitivity to the drug, or during pregnancy. Use caution during lactation.

Adverse Reactions

These can include depression, congestive heart failure, orthostatic hypotensive episodes, psychosis, urinary retention, drowsiness, and dizziness.

Dosage and Route

Oral: Adults: 200 mg daily dose (two 100 mg caps) or 4 tsp of syrup

Children: 1 to 9 years of age

100 mg twice a day (one 100 mg cap) or 2 tsp b.i.d.

Implications for Patient Care

Medication should be taken after meals. Patient assessment includes observing for signs of hypersensitivity and adverse reactions.

Patient Teaching

Instruct the patient not to stand or to change positions too quickly, as orthostatic hypotensive episodes may occur. With these episodes, the patient would feel faint, as the blood pressure drops suddenly. Inform the patient to take the drug for the full course of therapy as prescribed and to notify the physician if confusion, dizziness, insomnia, irritability, slurred speech, swelling (especially of feet and legs), persistent or severe GI symptoms, increased frequency of urination, or changes in vision occur. Advise the patient to avoid alcoholic beverages while taking amantadine. ■

Trifluridine (Viroptic ophthalmic solution 1%)

Actions

Antiviral activity against herpes simplex virus, types 1 and 2 and vaccinia virus. Some strains of adenovirus are also inhibited in vitro.

Uses

Use for topical treatment of epithelial keratitis caused by herpes simplex virus, types 1 and 2, and treatment of primary keratoconjunctivitis.

Contraindications

Do not use in patients who develop hypersensitivity reactions or chemical intolerance to trifluridine, or during pregnancy or lactation.

Adverse Reactions

Mild burning or stinging upon instillation, or hypersensitivity may occur.

Dosage and Route

Ophthalmic: Instill 1 drop onto cornea of affected eye every 2 hours. Maximum daily dose is 9 drops until corneal ulcer has completely reepithelialized.

Implications for Patient Care

Use aseptic technique when instilling drops.

Patient Teaching

Instruct the patient to follow the recommended dosage and not to exceed the number of drops prescribed. Aseptic technique should be used when instilling eye drops. Instruct the patient in the proper instillation of eye drops:

- Wash hands.
- Do not touch the dropper tip directly to eye.

- Draw up the correct amount of medication into the eye dropper.
- Tilt the head back.
- Place the hand in which the eye dropper is held directly over the eye to be medicated.
- Pull lower eyelid down to form a small pouch.
- Gently drop the prescribed number of drops into the middle of the pouch.
- Do not instill eye drops directly onto the eyeball.
- Keep eyes closed for a few minutes, trying not to blink and not to rub the eyes. ■

Famciclovir (Famvir)

Actions

It prevents viral replication by inhibition of DNA synthesis.

Uses

The medication is indicated for the management of acute herpes zoster (shingles) and recurrent herpes genitalis in patients with **immunocompetent**.

Contraindications

Do not use in patients with known hypersensitivity to the product.

Adverse Reactions

Headache, nausea, diarrhea, and fatigue are possible reactions.

Dosage and Route

For herpes zoster: give 500 mg every 8 hours for 7 days; for herpes genitalis, give 125 mg twice daily for 5 days.

Implications for Patient Care

For best results, treatment should begin as soon as herpes zoster is diagnosed. Treatment is most effective if started within 48 hours of rash onset. In patients with reduced renal function, dosage reduction is recommended.

 Patient Teaching

Famvir may be taken without regard to meals. Advise patients to report any adverse reactions to their physician. ■

Rimantadine (Flumadine)

Actions

This medication has antiviral activity against influenza A virus.

Uses

In adults, rimantadine is indicated for the prevention and treatment of illness caused by various strains of influenza A virus. In children, it is only approved for prevention.

Contraindications

Do not use when patients have a known hypersensitivity to rimantadine or other drugs of the adamantane class such as amatadine (Symadine, Symmetrel).

Adverse Reactions

Reactions include nausea, vomiting, nervousness, insomnia, and dizziness.

Dosage and Route

Oral: Adults: 100 mg twice a day

For geriatric patients or anyone with kidney failure or severe liver problems, the dose is reduced to 100 mg once a day.

Children: 10 years or older 100 mg twice a day

1 to 9 years 5 mg/kg, but not exceeding 150 mg

Implications for Patient Care

For prevention, one should start on medication as early as possible after a community outbreak of influenza A. For additional prophylaxis after one has been vaccinated, medication may be taken for two to four weeks.

 Patient Teaching

Advise patients to report any adverse reactions to their physician. Inform geriatric patients that they may experience gastrointestinal problems, insomnia, and nervousness. ▪

Penciclovir (Denavir)

Actions

With antiviral activity against herpes viruses types 1 (HSV-1) and types 2 (HSV-2), Penciclovir penetrates into the infected cells to block the multiplying of the virus that causes the cold sore.

Uses

In adults, penciclovir cream is indicated for the treatment of recurrent herpes labialis (cold sores).

Contraindications

This medicine is contraindicated in patients with known hypersensitivity to any of the components of the product.

Adverse Reactions

Reactions include headache, application site reaction, hypesthesia or local anesthesia, taste perversion, pruritus, pain, rash, allergic reaction.

Dosage and Route

Apply every 2 hours during waking hours for a period of 4 days. Treatment should be started as early as possible (during the prodrome or when lesions appear).

Implications for Patient Care

Denavir should only be used on herpes labialis on the lips and face. It is not indicated for internal use on mucous membranes inside the mouth, nose, genital, or rectal areas.

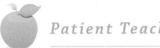 *Patient Teaching*

Instruct patient to wash hands thoroughly before application and to avoid application in or near the eyes because it may cause irritation. ▓

Oseltamivir Phosphate (Tamiflu)

Actions

This medicine has antiviral activity against influenza viruses Types A and B.

Uses

In adults, oseltamivir is indicated for the treatment of uncomplicated acute illness due to influenza infection, for patients who have been symptomatic for no more than 2 days.

Contraindications

Contraindicated in patients with known hypersensitivity to any of the components of the product.

Adverse Reactions

Reactions include nausea and vomiting.

Dosage and Route

The recommended oral dose is 75 mg twice daily for 5 days. Treatment should begin within 12 to 48 hours from the onset of symptoms of influenza. It may be taken with or without food. However, when taken with food, tolerability may be enhanced in some patients.

Implications for Patient Care

Tamiflu is not a substitute for a flu shot. Patients should continue receiving an annual flu shot according to guidelines on immunization practices.

Patient Teaching

Instruct patient to begin treatment with Tamiflu as soon as the first appearance of flu symptoms appear. Inform the patient to take any missed doses as soon as one remembers, except if it is within 2 hours of the next scheduled dose, and then continue to take Tamiflu at the prescribed times. ▓

Zanamivir (Relenza)

Actions

This medicine has antiviral activity against influenza A and B viruses.

Uses

In adults and adolescents aged 12 years and older, zanamivir is indicated for the treatment of uncomplicated acute illness due to influenza infection, who have been symptomatic for no more than 2 days.

Contraindications

Contraindicated in patients with known hypersensitivity to any of the components of the product.

Adverse Reactions

The most common adverse events reported in less than 1.5% of patients treated with Relenza and more commonly than in patients treated with placebo are:

- Sinusitis and dizziness (in treatment studies).
- Fever and/or chills, arthrlgia, and articular rheumatism (in prophylaxis studies).

> **Warning:**
>
> - Serious, sometimes fatal, cases of **brochospasm** have occured. Not recommended in individuals with underlying airways disease. Discontinue Relenza if bronchospam or decline in respiratory function develops.
> - Discontinue Relenza and initate appropriate treatment if an **allergic reaction** occurs or is suspected.
> - Patients with influenza, particularly pediatric patients, may be at an increased risk of **neuropsychiatric events**: seizures, confusion, or abnormal behavior early in their illness. Monitor for signs of abnormal behavior.

Dosage and Route

Taken 10 mg twice daily for five days. Patients inhale Relenza orally using a handheld, breath-activated device called a Diskhaler. When the patient takes a breath, Relenza is delivered directly to the surface of the respiratory tract, the primary site of infection where the influenza virus replicates.

Implications for Patient Care

Relenza is not a substitute for a flu shot. Patients should continue receiving an annual flu shot according to guidelines on immunization practices.

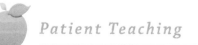 *Patient Teaching*

Instruct patient to begin treatment with Relenza as soon as possible from the first appearance of flu symptoms. Instruct the patient in the proper use of the inhaler, including a demonstration whenever possible. Patients should also read and carefully follow the Patient Instructions for Use included with the drug. ■

ANTIRETROVIRAL AGENTS

Antiretroviral agents consist of a group of drugs used to treat HIV infection. There are four general classes: nucleoside reverse transcriptase inhibitors (NRTIs), non-nucleoside reverse transcriptase inhibitors (NNRTIs), protease inhibitors (PIs), and fusion (entry) inhibitors (FIs).

- Intravenous drug use is a high risk factor in the older adult.
- Older adults may have contracted AIDS from a blood transfusion. Screening of donated blood began in 1985, and has reduced the risk of contracting AIDS from a blood transfusion.

Possible Signs and Symptoms of AIDS in Older Adults

- HIV/AIDS dementia (usually has a rapid onset)
- Extrapyramidal symptoms resembling parkinsonism without resting tremors
- Ataxia, leg tremors
- Peripheral neuropathy progressing to weakness and abnormal reflexes, such as a positive Babinski
- Confusion
- Opportunistic infections
- Tuberculosis
- Esophageal or recurrent genital candidiasis, toxoplasmosis
- Non-Hodgkin's lymphoma
- Kaposi's sarcoma
- *Pneumocystis carinii* pneumonia (PCP)
- Human papilloma virus infection

Differential Diagnosis

In addition to a general medical history, a social history should be taken and include questions relating to a person's sexual activities. Also, a medication history should be taken and one should ask about use of any drugs, especially those not prescribed by a physician. Laboratory and diagnostic tests should be used to detect or rule out possible causes of any abnormal condition presented by the patient.

Diagnosis

ELISA (enzyme-linked immunosorbent assay) test result—positive

Western blot test—positive

CD4 lymphocyte count of less than 200 cells/mm^3 (normal is 1,000 to 1,300 cells/mm^3)

The diagnosis of AIDS can be devastating to any individual, especially older adults who have to tell their family about the diagnosis. Professional assistance may be necessary to help older adults with this task. A list of agencies with addresses and phone numbers should be made available to older adults who wishes them. Information on services available for older adults with HIV infection and AIDS may be obtained by calling the CDC's AIDS Hotline at 1-800 342 AIDS or the Georgia Department of Human Resources at 1-706-724-8802.

Treatment

The treatment regimen includes treating any associated condition with proper medical intervention, and starting the patient on an antiretroviral drug or a combination of antiretroviral drugs. Drug therapy should be carefully evaluated for older adults because of preexisting conditions, such as cardiac disease or renal insufficiency, that can make them less tolerant of drugs. Also, they are generally more prone to adverse drug effects than younger individuals; therefore they will need clinical evaluation and laboratory monitoring every 3 to 6 months and more frequently if indicated.

Teaching the Older Adult About AIDS

It would be very helpful to provide brochures and any other written materials that you could on any or all of the following subjects, so that older adults may better understand his or her condition.

- Explain how HIV infection can and cannot be transmitted.
- Explain universal precautions and when they should be used.
- Explain the general effects of HIV infection and how AIDS is diagnosed.
- Explain the general effects of AIDS on the body.
- Instruct the patient on how to prevent the spread of AIDS and what precautions should be used during sexual acts.
- Go over the patient's medication regimen, making sure that he or she understands all aspects of drug therapy and any adverse effects that should be reported to the physician.
- Inform the patient about available home health agencies and visiting nurses associations.
- Inform the patient about other community resources such as "Meals on Wheels" and hospice care.
- Instruct patients on how to prevent infections and ways to improve their immune system.
- Explain the importance of good nutrition.
- Advise the patient not to smoke.
- Inform the patient on how to reduce stress.
- Explain the importance of regular exercise.
- Explain the importance of getting the proper amount of sleep. This is usually 6 to 8 hours in a given 24-hour time period.
- Advise the patient to drink at least 8 glasses of water daily.
- Talk about how to develop and keep a positive attitude.
- Teach the patient how to practice good personal hygiene. Instruct patients on how to wash their hands and when.
- Advise the patient to stay away from individuals who have contagious diseases.

◼ Critical Thinking **QUESTIONS AND ACTIVITIES**

Your patient is a 62-year-old female who has been diagnosed with AIDS. As you are talking with her, she says, "I didn't know that 'old' people could get AIDS. I know so little about the disease and I am sure that my friends don't know very much either. We need to be educated. I often go to the local senior citizen's center where they have guest speakers who present programs on all sorts of topics. Would you be willing to present a program on AIDS for our group? It would help me to explain my disease to my friends and maybe make someone else aware that he or she could get AIDS."

With the assistance of your patient, make arrangements to present a program on AIDS to a local group of senior citizens. To assist you in formulating a program, use the information in Special Considerations: Older Adults. Ask yourself:

- How do older adults become infected with HIV? How can I go about explaining this to a group of senior citizens?
- What could I teach older adults about possible signs and symptoms of AIDS?
- How can I explain the diagnosis of AIDS?
- What information could I provide the group about HIV infection and AIDS and about services available to older adults?
- How could I explain the treatment regimen for AIDS?
- In teaching the older adult about AIDS:
  What materials could I leave with the group, so that they could better understand AIDS?
  What are some points and facts that I would like to emphasize about preventing the spread of AIDS?

IMMUNIZATION

Immunity is the state of being protected from or resistant to a particular disease due to the development of antibodies. The mechanisms of immunity involve an *antigen-antibody* response. When an *antigen* enters the body, complex activities are set into motion. These activities involve chemical and mechanical forces that defend and protect the body's cells and tissues. *Antibodies* are formed and released from plasma cells, after which they enter the body fluids where they react with the invading antigen.

The mechanisms of immunity are based on the body's ability to:

- protect itself against specific infectious microorganisms
- defend body cells and tissues that are invaded by foreign substances
- accept or reject another's blood or organ (blood transfusion or organ transplant)
- protect itself against cancer and immunodeficiency disease

● *Note*

The following portion of this unit is adapted from materials printed by the U.S. Department of Health and Human Services, Public Health Service, Centers for Disease Control and Prevention, Atlanta, GA 30333. ●

Immunization is a term denoting the process of inducing or providing immunity artificially by administering an immunobiologic (immunizing agent). Immunization can be active or passive:

- *Active immunization* denotes the production of antibody or antitoxin in response to the administration of a vaccine or toxoid.
- *Passive immunization* denotes the provision of temporary immunity by the administration of preformed antitoxins or antibodies. Three types of immunobiologics are used for passive immunization:
  1. pooled human immune globulin (Ig)
  2. specific Ig preparations
  3. antitoxin

General Recommendation for Immunization

Recommendations for immunization of infants, children, and adults are based on facts about immuno-biologics and scientific knowledge about the principles of active and passive immunization, and on judgments by public health officials and specialists in clinical and preventive medicine. Benefits and risks are associated with the use of all products—no vaccine is completely safe or completely effective. The benefits range from partial to complete protection from the consequences of disease, and the risks range from common, trivial, and inconvenient side effects to rare, severe, and life-threatening conditions.

Thus, recommendations on immunization practices balance scientific evidence of benefits, costs, and risks to achieve optimal levels of protection against infectious or communicable diseases. These recommendations may apply only in the United States, as epidemiological circumstances and vaccines may differ in other countries.

Immunobiologics

The specific nature and content of immunobiologics may differ. When immunobiologics against the same infectious agents are produced by different manufacturers, active and inert ingredients among the various products may differ. Practitioners are urged to become familiar with the constituents of the products they use. The constituents of immunobiologics include the following:

Suspending Fluid

This frequently is as simple as sterile water or saline, but it may be a complex fluid containing small amounts of proteins or other constituents derived from the medium or biologic system in which the vaccine is produced (serum proteins, egg antigens, cell culture–derived antigens).

Preservatives, Stabilizers, Antibiotics

These components of vaccines are used to inhibit or prevent bacterial growth in viral culture or the final product, or to stabilize the antigen. They include such material as mercurials and specific anti-biotics. Allergic reactions may occur if the recipient is sensitive to one of these additives.

Adjuvants

An aluminum compound is used in some vaccines to enhance the immune response to vaccines containing inactivated microorganisms or their products—for example, toxoids and hepatitis B virus vaccine. Vaccines with such adjuvants must be injected deeply in muscle masses, because subcutaneous or intracutaneous administration may cause local irritation, inflammation, granuloma formation, or necrosis.

Immunizing Agents

Immunobiologics include vaccines, toxoids, and antibody-containing preparations from human or animal donors, including globulins and antitoxins.

Vaccine

A suspension of attenuated live or killed microorganisms (bacteria, viruses, or *rickettsiae*), or fractions thereof, administered to induce immunity and thereby prevent infectious disease.

Toxoid

A modified bacterial toxin that has been rendered nontoxic, but that retains the ability to stimulate the formation of antitoxin.

Immune Globulin (IG)

A sterile solution containing antibody from human blood. It is a 15 to 18 percent protein obtained by cold ethanol fractionation of large pools of blood plasma. It is primarily indicated for routine maintenance of certain immunodeficient people, and for passive immunization against measles and hepatitis A.

Specific Immune Globulin

Special preparations obtained from donor pools preselected for a high antibody content against a specific disease (for example, hepatitis B immune globulin (Hbig), varicella zoster immune globulin (VZIG), rabies immune globulin (RIG), and tetanus immune globulin (TIG).

Antitoxin

A solution of antibodies derived from the serum of animals immunized with specific antigens (diphtheria, tetanus) used to achieve passive immunity or to effect a treatment.

Route and Site Selection

Route

There is a recommended route of administration for each immunobiologic. To avoid unnecessary local or systemic effects and to ensure optimal efficacy, the practitioner should not deviate from the recommended route of administration.

Site

Injectable immunobiologics should be administered in an area where there is minimal opportunity for local, neural, vascular, or tissue injury. Subcutaneous injections are usually administered into the thigh of infants and in the deltoid area of older children and adults. Intradermal injections are generally given on the volar surface of the forearms, except for human diploid cell rabies vaccine, with which reactions are less severe when given in the deltoid area.

Intramuscular Injections

Preferred sites for intramuscular injections are the anterolateral aspect of the upper thigh and the deltoid muscle of the upper arm. In most infants, the anterolateral aspect of the thigh provides the largest muscle mass and, therefore, is the preferred site. In older children, the deltoid mass is of sufficient size for intramuscular injection. An individual decision must be made for each child, based on the volume of the injected material and the size of the muscle into which it is to be injected. In adults, the deltoid is generally used for routine intramuscular vaccine administration.

The upper, outer quadrant of the gluteal region should be used only for the largest volumes of injection or when multiple doses need to be given, such as when large doses of IG must be administered. The site selected should be well into the upper, outer mass of the gluteus maximus and away from the central region of the buttocks.

Hypersensitivity to Vaccine Components

Vaccine antigens produced in systems or with substrates containing allergenic substances (for example, antigens derived from growing microorganisms in embryonated chicken eggs) may cause hypersensitivity reactions. These reactions may include anaphylaxis when the final vaccine contains a substantial amount of the allergen. Yellow fever vaccine is such an antigen. Vaccines with such characteristics should *not* be given to people with known hypersensitivity to components of the substrates.

Screening people by history of ability or inability to eat eggs without adverse effects is a reasonable way to identify those possibly at risk from receiving measles, mumps, and influenza vaccine. Individuals with anaphylactic hypersensitivity to eggs (hives, swelling of the mouth and throat, difficulty breathing, hypotension, or shock) should *not* be given these vaccines.

Those administering vaccines should carefully review the information provided with the package insert and ascertain whether the patient is hypersensitive to any of its components. The physician must carefully evaluate each patient with known hypersensitivity before administering the vaccine.

Altered Immunocompetence

Virus replication after administration of live, attenuated virus vaccines may be enhanced in people with immunodeficiency diseases, and in those with suppressed capability for immune response, as occurs with leukemia, lymphoma, generalized malignancy, or therapy with corticosteroids, alkylating agents, antimetabolites, or radiation. Patients with such conditions should *not* be given live, attenuated virus vaccines. Also, because of the possibility of familial immunodeficiency, live, attenuated virus vaccines should *not* be given to a member of a household in which there is a family history of congenital or hereditary immunodeficiency, until the immune competence of the potential recipient is known.

Severe Febrile Illnesses

Minor illnesses, such as mild upper respiratory infections, should not cause postponement of vaccine administration. However, immunization of people with severe febrile illnesses should generally be deferred until they have recovered.

Immunization During Pregnancy

On the grounds of a theoretical risk to the developing fetus, live, attenuated virus vaccines are not generally given to pregnant women or to those likely to become pregnant within three months after receiving vaccine(s). With some of these vaccines, particularly rubella, measles, and mumps, pregnancy is a contraindication.

There is no convincing evidence of risk to the fetus from immunization of pregnant women using inactivated virus vaccines, bacterial vaccines, or toxoids. Tetanus and diphtheria toxoid (Td) should be given to inadequately immunized pregnant women because it affords protection against neonatal tetanus.

Adverse Events Following Immunization

Modern vaccines are extremely safe and effective, but not completely so. Adverse events following immunization have been reported with all vaccines. To improve knowledge about adverse reactions, all temporarily associated events severe enough to require the recipient to seek medical attention should be evaluated and reported in detail to local or state health officials and to the vaccine manufacturer.

Sources of Vaccine Information

Official Package Circular

Manufacturers provide product-specific information along with each vaccine; some of these are reproduced in their entirety in the *Physicians' Desk Reference* (PDR) and dated.

Health Information for International Travel

Published annually by the Centers for Disease Control and Prevention (CDC) as a guide to requirements and recommendations for specific immunizations and health practices for travel to various countries. It can be obtained for $5 from the Superintendent of Documents, U.S. Government Printing Office, Washington, DC 20402.

Additional Information

CDC-INFO Contact Center Monday–Friday 8 a.m.–11 p.m. (Eastern Time): 1-800-232-4636.

Antigen(s)

Antigens are substances inducing the formation of antibodies. In some vaccines, the antigen is highly defined—for example, in vaccines for pneumococcal polysaccharide, hepatitis B surface antigen, tetanus, or diphtheria toxoids. In other vaccines, it is complex or incompletely defined—for example, in vaccines for killed pertussis bacteria, live, attenuated viruses.

Immunization Schedules

In general, immunization policies have been directed toward vaccinating infants, children, and adolescents. Although immunization is a routine measure in pediatric practice, it is not usually routine in the practice of physicians who treat adults.

The widespread and successful implementation of childhood immunization programs has greatly reduced the occurrence of many vaccine-preventable diseases. However, successful childhood immunization alone will not necessarily eliminate specific disease problems. A substantial proportion of the remaining morbidity and mortality from vaccine-preventable disease now occurs in older adolescents and adults. People who escaped natural infection or were not immunized with vaccines and toxoids against diphtheria, tetanus, measles, mumps, rubella, and poliomyelitis may be at risk of these diseases and their complications.

To reduce further the unnecessary occurrence of these vaccine-preventable diseases, all those who provide health care to older adolescents and adults should provide immunizations as a routine part of their practice. In addition, the epidemiology of other vaccine-preventable diseases (for example, hepatitis B, rabies, influenza, and pneumococcal disease) indicates that individuals who have special health problems are at increased risk of these illnesses and should be immunized. Travelers to some countries may be at increased risk of exposure to vaccine-preventable illnesses. Foreign students, immigrants, and refugees also may be susceptible to these diseases.

A systematic approach to immunization is necessary to ensure that all individuals are appropriately protected against vaccine-preventable diseases. Several factors need to be considered before any patient is vaccinated. These include:

- The susceptibility of the patient.
- The risk of exposure to the disease.
- The risk from the disease.
- The benefits and risks from the immunizing agent.

Physicians should maintain detailed information about previous vaccinations received by each individual, including type of vaccination, date of receipt, and adverse events, if any, following vaccination. Information should also include the person's history of vaccine-preventable illness, occupation, and lifestyle. After the administration of any immunobiologic, the patient should be given written documentation of its receipt and information on which vaccines or toxoids will be needed in the future.

For more detailed information on immunobiologics, and before administering any immunizing agent, refer to an appropriate source of information regarding indications, side effects, adverse reactions, precautions, contraindications, dosages, and route of administration. Vaccination is recommended in people of all ages, especially those who are or will be at increased risk of infection with hepatitis B virus. Those who should be vaccinated include:

- Health care personnel.
- Selected patients and patient contacts.
- Infants born to hepatitis B positive mothers.
- Population with high incidence of the disease.
- Military personnel identified as being at increased risk.
- Morticians and embalmers.
- Blood bank and plasma fractionation workers.
- People at increased risk due to sexual practices.
- Prisoners.
- Users of illicit injectable drugs.

An immunization schedule for children and adults is presented in Table 16-5. Immunization schedules are recommended by the CDC's Advisory Committee on Immunization Practices (ACIP), the American Academy of Pediatrics (AAP), and the American Academy of Family Physicians (AAFP). These schedules are updated on a regular basis and recommendations for an immunization may change yearly. Detailed recommendations about the use of vaccines are available from the manufacturers' package inserts, the current Red Book, or ACIP statements on specific vaccines.

● *Note*

When giving vaccines to infants and children, the medical assistant must get a signed consent from the parent or guardian. The medical assistant must also document on the patient's record the lot number of the vaccine used. ●

TABLE 16-5 Immunizations for Children and Adults

VACCINE (BRAND NAME)	DOSAGE AND ROUTE	SCHEDULE
Diphtheria, Tetanus Toxoids, and Acellular Pertussis Adsorbed (DTaP) Vaccine	*IM:* 0.5 mL	Given at 2, 4, 6, and 15 to 18 months. Booster: 4 to 6 years.
Haemophilus b Conjugate (Meningococcal Protein Conjugate) Liquid Vaccine	*IM:* 0.5 mL	Given in a two-dose primary regimen before 12 months of age, usually at 2 and 4 months. Booster: 12 to 15 months of age, but not earlier than 2 months after the second dose.
Haemophilus b Conjugate (Meningococcal Protein Conjugate) and Hepatitis B (Recombinant) Vaccine	*IM:* 0.5 mL	Given at 2, 4, and 12 to 15 months of age.
Hepatitis A Vaccine (Inactivated) (VAQTA)	*Pediatric/Adolescent:* *IM:* 25 U (0.5 mL) *Adult:* *IM:* 50 U (1 mL)	Single dose at elected date. Booster: 6 to 18 months later. Single dose at elected date. Booster: 6 months later.
Hepatitis A Vaccine (HAVRIX)	*Children/Adolescent:* 2 to 18 yrs *IM:* 360 EL. U (0.5 mL) *Adult:* IM: 1440 EL. U (1 mL)	Regimen consists of two doses: Second dose is given 1 month after the primary dose. Booster: 6 to 12 months after the primary dose. Regimen consists of one dose. Booster: 6 to 12 months after the primary dose.
Hepatitis B Vaccine (Recombinant) (Recombivax HB)	*Infants, Children, and Adolescents 0 to 19 yrs:* *IM:* 5 mcg (0.5 mL) *Adults 20 years +:* *IM:* 10 mcg (1 mL) *Adolescents 11 to 15 yrs:* *IM:* 10 mcg (1 mL) *Predialysis and Dialysis Patients:* *IM:* 40 mcg (1 mL)	Regimen consists of three doses: initial dose, then 1 month later, and then 6 months from initial dose. Regimen consists of two doses: initial dose, then second dose 4 to 6 months later. Regimen consists of three doses: initial dose, then 1 month later, and then 6 months from initial dose.
Hepatitis B Vaccine (Recombinant)	*Pediatric/Adolescent:* *IM:* 10 mcg (0.5 mL) *Adult:* *IM:* 20 mcg (1 mL)	Regimen consists of three doses: initial dose, then 1 month later, and then 6 months from initial dose.
Influenza Type A and Type B	*Children 6 months or older and Adults:* *IM:* 0.5 mL	Given during the fall of the year, usually in early October. Single dose given to adults and children with chronic heart or lung disorders; patients in nursing homes or chronic care facilities; individuals with diabetes, kidney disease, and other chronic diseases. May be given as a preventive measure to those who wish to receive the vaccine.

(*continues*)

TABLE 16-5   (*continued*)

VACCINE (BRAND NAME)	DOSAGE AND ROUTE	SCHEDULE
Pneumococcal Vaccine Polyvalent (PNEUMOVAX 23)	*Children/Adults:* IM: 0.5 mL	Single dose given to high-risk children over 2 years of age, all high-risk adults, and adults at age 50 and again at age 65.
Pneumococcal 7-valent Conjugate Vaccine (Prevnar)	*Infants and Toddlers:* IM: 0.5 mL	Regimen consists of three doses given at approximately 2-month intervals, followed by a fourth dose at 12 to15 months of age. The customary age for the first dose is 2 months of age, but it can be given as young as 6 weeks of age.
Poliovirus-IPV (inactivated poliovirus) Vaccine	SC: 0.5 mL	Given at 2, 4, 6, and 15 to 18 months. Booster: 4 to 6 years.
Measles, Mumps, and Rubella Virus Vaccine Live (MMR)	SC: 0.5 mL	Primary: 12 to 15 months. Booster: 4 to 6 years.
Varicella Virus Vaccine Live (VARIVAX)	*Children 12 months to 12 years:* SC: 0.5 mL — *Adolescent and Adult:* SC: 0.5 mL	Single dose of 0.5 ml. — Regimen consists of two doses: primary dose and a second dose 4 to 8 weeks later.
Human Papillomavirus (HPV) Recombinant Vaccine (Gardasil)	*Girls 11 to 12 yrs; can be given to girls as young as 9:* IM: 0.5 mL	Regimen consists of three doses: initial dose, then 2 months later, and then 6 months from initial dose.
Live, Attenuated Influenza Vaccine (LAIV) Nasal Spray (FluMist)	*Children, Adolescents, and Adults 2 to 49 years:* *Intranasal:* 0.2 mL premeasured dosage (0.1 mL per nostril)	Given during the fall of the year, usually in early October. Children 2 to 8 yrs, not previously vaccinated 2 doses (0.1 mL per nostril) at least 1 month apart.
Meningococcal Polysaccharide Vaccine, Groups A, C, Y and W-135 combined (Menomune-A/C/Y/W-135)	*Children 2 to 10 yrs and Adults older than 55 years:* SC: 0.5 mL	People 2 years and older should get 1 dose.
Meningococcal Polysaccharide (Serogroups A, C, Y and W-135) Diphtheria Toxoid Conjugate Vaccine (Menactra)	*Children and adolescents 11 through 18 years:* IM: 0.5 mL	One dose is recommended. *Preferred vaccine for people 2 through 55 years who are at increased risk for meningococcal disease.*
Rotavirus Vaccine (RotaTeq)	*Infants:* Oral: 2 mL	Series of three ready-to-use liquid doses administered starting at 6 to 12 weeks of age, with the subsequent doses administered at 4- to 10-week intervals. The third dose should not be given after 32 weeks of age.

(continues)

TABLE 16-5 *(continued)*

VACCINE (BRAND NAME)	DOSAGE AND ROUTE	SCHEDULE
Zoster (Shingles) Vaccine (Zostavax)	*Adults 60 yrs of age and older: SC:* 0.65 mL	Administered in the deltoid region of the upper arm. Zostavax is stored frozen and should be reconstituted immediately upon removal from the freezer. The diluent should be stored separately at room temperature or in the refrigerator. The vaccine is administered immediately after reconstitution, to minimize loss of potency.
Haemophilus influenzae Type B Conjugate Vaccine (Hib)	*Infants minimum age 6 weeks: IM:* 0.5 mL	4 doses by age of 15 months. Given at 2, 4, and 6* months, with a booster dose between 12 and 15 months. *Depending on which Hib vaccine is used, an infant may not need the dose at 6 months of age.
Tetanus, diphtheria, and acellular Pertussis (Tdap)	*Adults 19 to 64 yrs of age and adolescents 11 to 18 years of age IM:* 0.5 mL	A single dose of Tdap in place of the Td (tetanus, diphtheria) booster previously recommended for all adults and adolescents.

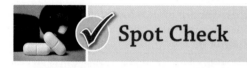

Spot Check

For immunizations, there are routinely recommended ages and a range of acceptable ages for each vaccine. For each of the selected vaccines, give the recommended schedule for immunization.

VACCINE	RECOMMENDED IMMUNIZATION SCHEDULE
Hepatitis B (Recombinant)	
Diphtheria, Tetanus, Pertussis (DTaP)	
Haemophilus influenza Type B Conjugate Vaccine (Hib)	
Poliovirus vaccine (IPV)	
Measles, Mumps, Rubella (MMR)	

Influenza A (H1N1) 2009 Monovalent Influenza Vaccine Dosage, Administration, and Storage

Inactivated Vaccine: Dosage, Administration, and Storage

The composition of the influenza A (H1N1) 2009 monovalent inactivated influenza vaccine varies according to manufacturer, and package inserts should be consulted. Inactivated vaccine formulations in multidose vials contain the vaccine preservative thimerosal; preservative-free, single-dose preparations also are available. Inactivated vaccine should be stored at 35°F to 46°F (2°C to 8°C) and should not be frozen. Inactivated vaccine that has been frozen should be discarded. Dosage recommendations and schedules vary according to age group. Children through 9 years of age should receive two doses of vaccine, about a month apart. Older children and adults need only one dose.

The intramuscular route is recommended for administering the influenza A (H1N1) 2009 monovalent inactivated vaccine. Adults and older children should be vaccinated in the deltoid muscle. A needle length of 1 inch or longer (25 mm or longer) should be considered for people in these age groups because needles of less than 1 inch might be of insufficient length to penetrate muscle tissue in certain adults and older children. When injecting into the deltoid muscle in children with adequate deltoid muscle mass, a needle length of 7/8" to 1.25 inches is recommended. Infants and young children should be vaccinated in the anterolateral aspect of the thigh. A needle length of 7/8" to 1 inch should be used for children younger than 12 months of age.

Live Attenuated Influenza Vaccine (LAIV): Dosage, Administration, and Storage

Each dose of 2009 monovalent LAIV contains the same vaccine antigen used in the inactivated vaccine. However, the antigen is constituted as a live, attenuated, cold-adapted, temperature-sensitive vaccine virus. Providers should refer to the package insert, which contains additional information about the formulation of this vaccine and other vaccine components. LAIV is intended for intranasal administration only and should not be administered by the intramuscular, intradermal, or intravenous route. LAIV is not licensed for vaccination of children younger than 2 years or adults older than 49 years of age. LAIV is supplied in a prefilled, single-use sprayer containing 0.2 mL of vaccine. Approximately 0.1 mL (that is half of the total sprayer contents) is sprayed into the first nostril while the recipient is in the upright position. An attached dose-divider clip is removed from the sprayer to administer the second half of the dose into the other nostril while the recipient is in the upright position. LAIV is shipped at 35°F to 46°F (2°C to 8°;C). LAIV should be stored at 35°F to 46°F (2°C to 8°C) on receipt and can remain at that temperature until the expiration date is reached. To learn more about H1N1 vaccines, contact the Centers for Disease Control and Prevention (CDC) at 1-800-CDC-INFO (232-4636) or visit CDC's websites at www.cdc.gov/h1n1flu, or www.cdc.gov/flu, or www.flu.gov.

● *Note*

> The U.S. Food and Drug Administration Advisory Committee recommends that protection against the 2009 H1N1 virus, which was first identified in 2009, be included in the 2010-2011 seasonal influenza vaccine starting in the fall of 2010. Most Americans will be able to return to the traditional routine of having one flu vaccine to protect them against the major circulating flu viruses. Younger children who have never had a seasonal vaccine will still need two doses. This recommendation includes protection against the 2009 H1N1 flu strain in the flu vaccine. The World Health Organization has made the same recommendation. ●

■ ■ REVIEW QUESTIONS

Directions. Select the best answer to each of the following multiple-choice question, circle the letter of your choice:

1. The ingestion and digestion of bacteria and particles by white blood cells is known as _____.

    a. histoplasmosis   b. phagocytosis   c. cryptococcosis   d. lymphokines

2. Some diseases for which a physician may prescribe an antifungal agent are _____.
   a. pneumonia, genital herpes, influenza
   b. coryza, acquired immunodeficiency syndrome, herpes zoster
   c. histoplasmosis, *Candida* infections, tinea
   d. hepatitis, yellow fever, diphtheria

3. Patients with *Candida* infections should be given instructions about _____.
   a. correct hand-washing procedure
   c. the wearing of cotton underclothes
   b. proper personal hygiene
   d. all of these

4. _____ agents consist of a group of drugs used to treat HIV infection.
   a. Antiviral
   b. Antifungal
   c. Antiretroviral
   d. Antibiotic

5. Genital herpes is _____.
   a. a sexually transmitted disease
   c. not an infectious disease
   b. spread by casual contact
   d. a disease that is easily cured

6. An antiviral agent that has in vitro inhibitory activity against herpes simplex types 1 and 2, varicella zoster, Epstein-Barr, and cytomegalovirus is _____.
   a. amantadine hydrochloride (Symmetrel)
   b. acyclovir (Zovirax)
   c. zidovudine (Retrovir)
   d. famciclovir (Famvir)

7. _____ is the medical term for the common cold.
   a. Pertussis   b. Candida   c. Coryza   d. Cozrya

8. _____ is the state of being protected from or resistant to a particular disease due to the development of antibodies.
   a. Immunization
   c. Immunity
   b. Vaccination
   d. Immunobiologic

9. Injectable immunobiologics should be administered _____.
   a. in the recommended route of administration for each immunizing agent
   b. in an area free of nerves and vessels
   c. in the lower quadrant of the gluteal muscle
   d. a and b

10. Patients who should not receive live, attenuated virus vaccines include _____.
    a. people with normal immune response
    b. people with immunodeficiency disease
    c. people with leukemia
    d. b and c

11. _____ are parasitic, minute organisms that may invade normal cells, and cause disease.
    a. Bacteria   b. Fungi   c. Viruses   d. Protozoa

12. _____ include molds and yeasts.
    a. Bacteria   b. Fungi   c. Viruses   d. Protozoa

13. _____ is one of the most common causes of vaginitis in women during the reproductive years.

   a. Crytococcosis   b. Cytomegalovirus   c. Candida   d. Varicella

14. _____ agents act by exerting fungistatic or fungicidal action on both resting and growing cells.

   a. Antifungal   b. Antiviral   c. Antibiotic   d. Immunizing

15. Monistat is an example of an _____.

   a. antifungal agent   c. antibiotic

   b. antiviral agent   d. immunizing agent

16. Herpes simplex virus type 2 (HSV-2) causes _____.

   a. AIDS   c. fever blisters

   b. cold sores   d. genital herpes

Matching. Place the correct letter from Column II on the appropriate line of Column I:

Column I

17. ___E___ adenovirus
18. ___D___ antigen
19. ___B___ cytomegalovirus
20. ___A___ antibody
21. ___F___ antigenic
22. ___C___ herpes simplex virus type 1
23. ___H___ varicella
24. ___G___ volar
25. ___J___ human immunodeficiency virus (HIV)

Column II

A. a protein substance that is developed in response to an antigen

B. one of a group of species-specific herpes viruses

C. causes cold sores or fever blisters

D. a substance that induces the formation of antibodies

E. one of a group of closely related viruses that can cause infections of the upper respiratory tract

F. capable of causing the production of an antibody

G. refers to the palm of the hand

H. chicken pox

I. causative agent of genital herpes

J. causative agent of AIDS

UNIT 17
Antineoplastic Agents

OBJECTIVES

Upon completing this unit, you should be able to:

- Define the terms listed in the vocabulary.
- List the signs and symptoms of breast cancer.
- List the symptoms of benign prostatic hyperplasia (BPH).
- Describe prostate cancer.
- List the possible symptoms of prostate cancer.
- List the guidelines for care of the older adult with cancer.
- List the cancer screening test or procedure that an individual 50 or older should have.
- Give the suggested ways that one may communicate with a child about a parent's serious illness.
- Complete the critical thinking questions and activities presented in this unit.
- State when chemotherapy is the treatment of choice for cancer.
- List the normal cells that have the greatest sensitivity to destruction from antineoplastic agents.
- State the aim of chemotherapy.
- State who should prepare and administer antineoplastic agents.
- Describe examples of adverse reactions associated with antineoplastic agents.
- List and give the normal ranges of certain laboratory tests that are performed to establish a patient's baseline data before initiation of chemotherapy.
- Explain the care of chemotherapy patients.
- Describe the classifications of antineoplastic agents.
- Describe other forms of treatment for cancer.
- Complete the Spot Check on the classifications of antineoplastic agents.
- Answer the review questions correctly.

VOCABULARY

adjuvant chemotherapy (ad'ju-vant kem"o-ther'a-pe). In cancer therapy, the use of chemotherapy in addition with other treatments. For example, patients who had surgery as their primary therapy are often given drugs to kill unseen cancer cells that can remain after surgery. The goal of adjuvant therapy is to kill any hidden cells.

alopecia (al"o-pe'shi-a). Pertaining to hair loss.

anorexia (an"o-rek'si-a). A loss of appetite.

carcinogenic (kar"si-no-jen'ik). Pertaining to producing cancer.

cytotoxic (si"to-toks'ik). Destructive to cells.

dedifferentiation (de-dif"er-en"she-a'shun). The process whereby normal cells lose their specialization and become malignant.

deoxyribonucleic acid; DNA (de-ok" si-ri"bo-nu-kle'ik as'id). A complex protein that is found in the nucleus of every cell.

differentiation (dif"er-en"she-a'shun). The process whereby normal cells have a distinct appearance and specialized function.

exacerbation (eks-as"er-ba'shun). The time when the symptoms of a disease process are most severe.

extravasation (eks-trav"a-sa'shun). The process whereby fluids (especially IV) escape into surrounding tissues.

(continues)

laminar airflow. Filtered air flowing along separate planes or layers. This method of airflow helps to prevent bacterial contamination and collection of hazardous chemical fumes in areas where pollution of the work environment could be detrimental to one's health. The use of a laminar airflow hood in the preparation of antineoplastic agents is recommended.

local therapy (lo'kal ther'a-pe). Type of treatment that is intended to treat a tumor at the site without affecting the rest of the body. Surgery and radiation therapy are examples of local therapies.

malignant (ma-lig'nant). Tending to metastasize; cancerous.

metastasis (me-tas'ta-sis). The spreading process of cancer cells from one part of the body to another.

neoadjuvant chemotherapy (ne″o- ad'ju-vant kem″o-ther 'a-pe). In cancer therapy, this is when chemotherapy is given before the main cancer treatment (such as surgery or radiation).

oncologist (ong-kol'o-jist). One who specializes in tumors, especially neoplasms (new growths).

proliferation (pro-lif″er-a'shun). The process of rapid reproduction.

remission (re-mish'un). The time when the symptoms of a disease process are lessened.

ribonucleic acid; RNA (ri″bo-nu-kle'ik as'id). A nucleic acid, found in all living cells, which is responsible for protein synthesis.

stomatitis (sto″ma-ti' tis). Inflammation of the mouth.

systemic therapy (sis- tem'ik ther'a-pe). Type of treatment in which drugs can be given by mouth or directly into the bloodstream to reach cancer cells anywhere in the body. Chemotherapy, hormone therapy, and targeted therapy are systemic therapies.

teratogenic (ter″a-to-jen'ik). Pertaining to producing or forming a severely malformed fetus.

INTRODUCTION

The incidence of cancer is five times greater now than it was 100 years ago. Cancer will strike one out of every four Americans, according to recent statistics from the American Cancer Society. With early detection, followed by immediate treatment, the cure rate for cancer is now one in every two.

Oncologists have identified numerous factors that play a role in the development of cancer. These factors are environmental, hereditary, and biological. Over 200 forms of cancer have been identified.

The treatment of cancer may be any one or a combination of surgery, chemotherapy, radiation therapy, and immunotherapy. The treatment of choice depends upon the type of cancer, its location, its invasive process, and the patient's state of health.

Treatments can be classified into broad groups, based on how they work and when they are used. Local therapy is intended to treat a tumor at the site without affecting the rest of the body. Surgery and radiation therapy are examples of local therapies. Systemic therapy refers to drugs that can be given by mouth or directly into the bloodstream to reach cancer cells anywhere in the body. Chemotherapy, hormone therapy, and targeted therapy are systemic therapies. Today, more than 100 drugs are used for chemotherapy, either alone or in combination with other drugs or treatments.

For some people, chemotherapy is the only treatment that is used for their cancer. In other cases, chemotherapy may be given in addition with other treatments. It may be used as adjuvant therapy (after surgery or radiation) or neoadjuvant therapy (before surgery or radiation).

- Adjuvant chemotherapy is the use of chemotherapy in addition with other treatments in cancer therapy. For example, patients who had surgery as their primary therapy are often given drugs to kill unseen cancer cells that can remain after surgery. The goal of adjuvant therapy is to kill any hidden cells. Adjuvant treatment can also be given after using radiation to kill the cancer, such as adjuvant hormone therapy after radiation for prostate cancer.

- Neoadjuvant chemotherapy is when chemotherapy is given before the main cancer treatment (such as surgery or radiation). Giving chemotherapy first can shrink a large tumor, making it easier to remove with surgery. Shrinking the tumor may also allow it to be treated more easily with radiation. Neoadjuvant chemotherapy also kills small deposits of cancer cells that cannot be seen on scans or X-rays.

Spotlight

Breast Cancer

Approximately 186,772 women and approximately 1,815 men may be diagnosed with breast cancer in a given year. It kills about 40,954 women a year and is the leading cause of death in women between the ages of 32 and 52. Two genes have been linked to familial breast and ovarian cancer: BRCA-1 and BRCA-2. These genes may encourage breast cancer to develop. The genes tell cells how to produce a protein called cyclin D, one of several proteins that tell cells to produce an extra set of genetic material to be passed along when the cell divides. If further research supports the theory, scientists may be able to develop a test that could distinguish microscopic noncancerous breast abnormalities from cancerous ones. They may also be able to develop drugs for women at high risk that would slow the overactive genes.

In cancer, there is an abnormal process wherein a cell or group of cells undergoes changes and no longer carries on normal cell functions. The process whereby normal cells have a distinct appearance and specialized function is called **differentiation**. The failure of immature cells to develop specialized functions is called **dedifferentiation** It is believed that this process involves a disturbance in the DNA of the affected cells. Malignant cells usually multiply rapidly, forming a mass of abnormal cells that enlarges, ulcerates, and sheds malignant cells to surrounding tissues. This process destroys the normal cells, with malignant cells taking their places, and often results in the formation of a tumor.

If cancer is not detected and treated early, it will continue to grow, invade and destroy adjacent tissue, and spread into surrounding lymph nodes. It can be carried by the lymph or blood or both to other areas of the body and, once this process (known as **metastasis**) has occurred, the cancer is usually advanced and/or disseminated and the five-year survival rate is low. Early detection of breast cancer is extremely important. Until recently, surgical biopsy offered the only means for accurate diagnosis of breast cancer. Now, a new technique called stereotactic breast biopsy is helping reduce the need for surgical biopsy. The procedure is designed to sample millimeter-size breast lumps for malignancy with little intrusion into the body. With stereotactic breast biopsy, the physician works from a computer image of the breast that shows the lump's exact location. A small sampling needle is then placed inside the breast to draw out a sample of tissue to be tested.

The stereotactic breast biopsy is usually done in less than an hour and leaves the woman with little more than a temporary mark resembling a pinprick. Researchers state that this procedure is not for all women, as there are circumstances that would still require the traditional surgical biopsy. For example, if a woman had a large area or she could feel the lump, she would not be a candidate for stereotactic biopsy. The five-year survival rate for women with localized and properly treated breast cancer is 92 percent.

Approximately 50 percent of malignant tumors of the breast appear in the upper, outer quadrant and extend into the armpit. Eighteen percent of breast cancers occur in the nipple area, 11 percent in the lower outer quadrant, and 6 percent in the inner quadrant.

Signs and Symptoms

Signs and symptoms of breast cancer are generally insidious and may include:

- A new lump in the breast.
- A lump that has changed.
- A change in the size or shape of the breast.
- Pain in the breast or nipple that does not go away.
- Flaky, red, or swollen skin anywhere on the breast.

Your Breast

Being informed could save your life
Risk factors in order of importance:

1. Family history—Increased risk when breast cancer occurs before menopause in mother, sister, or daughter, especially if cancer occurs in both breasts.
2. Over age 50 and nullipara.
3. Having a first baby after age 30.

(continues)   *(continues)*

Signs and Symptoms (*continued*)

- A nipple that is very tender or that suddenly turns inward.
- Blood or any other type of fluid coming from the nipple that is not milk when nursing a baby.

Your Breast (*continued*)

4. History of chronic breast disease, especially epithelial hyperplasia.
5. Exposure to ionizing radiation of more than 50 rad during adolescence.
6. Obesity.
7. Early menarche, late menopause.

Examine your breasts every month
Appearance
Size, shape, symmetry
Tenderness, thickening, texture changes

Know Your Breast and Your Risk Factors

More than 90 percent of all breast lumps are discovered by women themselves. The majority of these lumps are benign (noncancerous) but of those that are not, early detection and treatment are essential.

Spotlight

Abnormal Conditions of the Prostate Gland

The prostate gland is about 4 centimeters wide and weighs about 20 grams. It is composed of glandular, connective, and muscular tissue and lies behind the urinary bladder. It surrounds the first 2.5 centimeters of the urethra and secretes an alkaline fluid that aids in maintaining the viability of spermatozoa. The prostate gland produces semen, the thick fluid that carries sperm from the testicles. Normal functioning of the prostate gland depends on the male hormone testosterone, which is made by the testicles. Male hormones, such as testosterone, are believed to stimulate prostate cancer growth.

Benign Prostatic Hyperplasia (BPH)

Enlargement of the prostate gland may occur in men who are 50 years of age and older. As the prostate enlarges, it compresses the urethra, thereby restricting the normal flow of urine. This restriction generally causes a number of symptoms and can be referred to as *prostatism*. Prostatism is any condition of the prostate gland that interferes with the flow of urine from the bladder.

Benign Prostatic Hyperplasia (BPH)

Symptoms usually include:

- A weak or hard-to-start urine stream.
- A feeling that the bladder is not empty.
- A need to urinate often, especially at night.
- A feeling of urgency (a sudden need to urinate).

- Abdominal straining, a decrease in size and force of the urinary stream.
- Interruption of the stream.
- Acute urinary retention.
- Recurrent urinary infections.

Treatment for Benign Prostatic Hyperplasia

Surgery. Transurethral resection of the prostate (TURP or TUR) is the most common form of surgery used for benign prostatic hyperplasia. During this procedure, an endoscopic instrument that has ocular and surgical capabilities is introduced directly through the urethra to the prostate, and small pieces of the prostate gland are removed by using an electrical cutting loop.

Medication. Proscar (finasteride), an oral medication, may be prescribed by a physician to help relieve the symptoms of BPH. It lowers the levels of dihydrotestosterone (DHT), which is a major factor in enlargement of the prostate. Lowering of DHT leads to shrinkage of the enlarged prostate gland in most men. Although this can lead to gradual improvement in urine flow and symptoms, it does not work for all cases. Sometimes the prostate may shrink without improvement in symptoms and it may take 6 months or more to determine if it is working for an individual. Side effects may include impotence and less desire for sex. Proscar can alter the prostate-specific antigen test (PSA) that is used to screen for prostate cancer.

Balloon Dilation. During this procedure a balloon catheter is placed in the distal urethra and is inflated by injecting a dilute contrast media at high pressure. The balloon is left in place for approximately 10 minutes and then the pressure is released and the catheter is removed.

Prostate Cancer

By age 60, four out of five men may have an enlarged prostate and suffer urinary difficulties. By age 75, one in ten men may develop prostate cancer. Approximately 230,000 new cases of prostate cancer occur each year, with a death toll of 38,000 lives.

A malignant neoplasm that affects the prostate tissue is known as prostatic cancer. It tends to spread to other parts of the body, often spreading to the bones of the spine or pelvis. The majority of these neoplasms are classified as adenocarcinomas. This disease is rare before the age of 50; however, it is the second leading cause of cancer deaths in men.

The exact cause of prostate cancer is not known. It has been reported that researchers have found a genetic defect they think might trigger prostate cancer by robbing cells of an enzyme that fights the disease. The enzyme glutathione S-transferase is part of a group of chemicals produced in the body that fights cancer. A genetic change, which apparently alters the body's natural cancer-fighting mechanisms, appeared in 91 prostate victims that were studied, and was not found in the tissues of healthy men. If continued research confirms this hypothesis, tests might be developed that could identify future prostate cancer patients before the disease progresses.

It is recommended that men aged 40 and over should have a digital rectal exam each year, and that men aged 50 and over should have a prostate-specific antigen (PSA) blood test each year. Those men who are at high risk should have the exam and blood test at an earlier age.

A rectal examination will help in diagnosing a tumor, but a biopsy is essential for a positive diagnosis. To localize and gauge the extent of the tumor, a computed tomography scan or ultrasonography may be used. The PSA blood test can detect prostate cancer by measuring the concentration in the blood of a protein made in the prostate.

Although prostate cancer frequently develops with no noticeable signs, possible symptoms may include:

- Inability to urinate.
- Frequent urination especially at night.

- Pain or burning sensation when urinating or ejaculating.
- Blood or pus in the urine or semen.
- Persistent pain in the back, hip, and pelvis.
- Fatigue and anemia.

These symptoms may also be caused by benign prostate conditions. Benign conditions including infections, prostate stones, and BPH are common as men age.

Treatment for Prostate Cancer

Doctors have varying opinions on which treatment, if any, is best for patients with prostate cancer. The *New England Journal of Medicine* published a study concluding that, for many men, observation may be just as effective as surgery or radiation. Surgery can have serious side effects, such as impotency and incontinence. And men in their 70s and 80s are likely to die from other causes before their prostate cancer becomes deadly, some doctors argue. It is not easy, however, for men to live with a potentially fatal disease. It is recommended that the best thing that a man who has been diagnosed with prostate cancer can do is to become educated about the options that are available. The most common treatments are the following:

Radical prostatectomy. The total removal of the prostate gland that involves surgery under general anesthesia, followed by a several-day hospital stay. Surgery leaves 1 to 2 percent of men incontinent, and 15 to 20 percent sexually impotent.

Radiation. Regular doses of high-energy X-rays are targeted to the prostate area. The risk of incontinency and impotency is the same as with surgery.

Interstitial implantation therapy. Using needles, radioactive seeds are implanted in the prostate to kill cancerous tissue. Impotency rate is about 10 percent, and incontinence is rare.

Hormones. Often used in conjunction with radiation or surgery, hormones reduce the levels of testosterone, the male hormone that promotes the growth of prostate cancer. Hormone treatment causes impotence in a small number of men.

Cryosurgery. This is an outpatient procedure that freezes cancerous tissue, andthat carries the risk of impotence and incontinence.

Watchful waiting. This is the decision to delay treatment of prostate cancer in favor of careful monitoring of the cancerous cells. The theory behind watchful waiting is that most prostate cancerous cells usually grow slowly. If a patient can reasonably expect to benefit from a more aggressive treatment for a period of 10 years or more, physicians usually recommend pursuing other treatment options. Patients who are older or who wish to avoid the side effects of other treatments, such as incontinence and impotence, may choose watchful waiting. Also, patients who have low Gleason scores, other medical complications, or low-grade tumors may wish to postpone treatment of their cancer.

● *Note*

The Gleason grading system produces the Gleason score, which is the classifying of the stage and grade of prostate cancer. The pathologist studies the patterns of cancerous cells underneath a microscope. If the cancerous cells look very similar to the healthy cells, the cancerous cells are called well differentiated. If the cancerous cells are very different from the healthy cells, however, they are called poorly differentiated. Based on the most common pattern of differentiation, the pathologist will assign a number 1 through 5. Then based on the second most common pattern of cell differentiation, the pathologist assigns a second number of 1 through 5. **The sum of these two numbers is the Gleason score.** The Gleason score can range from 2 to 10. Most of the prostate cancer cases diagnosed today have Gleason scores of 5, 6, or 7. The more aggressive forms of prostate cancer have scores of 8, 9, or 10. ●

About one in 10 American men will develop prostate cancer by the age of 85. Age is a risk factor of developing prostate cancer. More than 80 percent of all prostate cancers are diagnosed in men older than 65. It is unclear whether family history, environment, or diet plays a role in developing prostate cancer. Black individuals contract the disease at a rate almost twice that of white individuals.

Almost 60 percent of all prostate cancers are discovered while they are still confined to the prostate. The five-year survival rate for patients at this stage is 92 percent. The survival rate for all stages of prostate cancer is 78 percent. For more information about cancer, one may call the National Cancer Institute's toll-free number: 1-800-422-6237.

■ Special Considerations: **OLDER ADULTS**

Guidelines for Care of the Older Adult with Cancer

Explain the probable course of the disease, including the diagnosis, hospital stay, treatment regimen, and follow-up care. Provide information about support groups and hospice care. Other considerations are the following:

- Modification of chemotherapy should be employed.
- Anxiety and depression should be anticipated and treated.
- Fatigue that can be debilitating should be recognized.
- Bone marrow function should be evaluated.
- Skin changes should be noted:
  Xerosis (dry skin) is common.
  Skin moisture is lost.
  The aging skin is more prone to developing skin cancers.
  Carcinomas appear on the nose, eyelid, or cheek from sun exposure.
- Modifications in lifestyle will be hard to accomplish, and assistance should be provided when applicable.
- Anorexia, nausea, vomiting, and alopecia may be intensified.
- Fear of death may be present and understanding should be provided.

Early Diagnosis and Prompt Treatment

Early diagnosis and prompt treatment of cancer could save more than 50 percent of all cancer patients. The five-year survival rate for women with localized and properly treated breast cancer is 92 percent. Almost 60 percent of all prostate cancers are discovered while they are still confined to the prostate. The five-year survival rate for patients at this stage is 92 percent. The American Cancer Society recommends that individuals who are 50 and older should have the following cancer screening test or procedure performed on a regular basis:

TEST OR PROCEDURE	GENDER	FREQUENCY
Digital rectal exam (DRE)	Men and women	Every year
Prostate-specific antigen (PSA) test	Men	Every year
Stool guaiac slide test	Men and women	Every year
Sigmoidoscopy	Men and women	Every 3 to 5 years
Pap test	Women	Every year
Breast self-exam	Women	Every month
Breast physical exam	Women	Every year
Mammogram	Women	Every year

◼️ Special Considerations: **CHILDREN**

A diagnosis of cancer has a great impact on patients, their families, and especially the patient's children. Researchers at the University of Washington who have studied the responses of children to their mothers' breast cancer found that an almost universal reaction among children is that they do not want to add to their mother's burden, so they try to hide their fears.

Based upon the age of the child and his or her level of understanding, the following are suggested ways that may help encourage communication about a parent's serious illness: Each should be based upon the age of the child and his or her level of understanding.

- Create a comfortable environment. Sitting around a kitchen table or on a sofa, ask open-ended questions. Share information about the disease process, treatment, and possible outcome. Spread the sharing of this information over a given time period. Do not overload the child with too much information at one time.
- Draw pictures to illustrate the disease. Encourage the child to ask questions. Answer the questions openly and honestly.
- Plan ahead how to answer the question, "Are you going to die?". One may explain that all living things die sooner or later and then talk about death.
- Many times a child is going to feel guilty because he or she cannot understand what is happening and may think that he or she caused the illness. When this occurs, the parent should reassure the child and provide any additional information about the condition that would help alleviate feelings of guilt.
- Involve the child in daily living activities. Let the child help out around the house. Simple tasks such as picking up toys, clothes, and so on may foster a sense of security for the child.
- The parent should provide extra time for "hugs and kisses."
- The parent should plan for time spent away from the family, such as hospitalization. Tape-recorded bedtime stories and songs can be a big help to a child when a parent is away. Hearing a mother's or father's voice can often quiet distressing feelings.
- The other parent or another adult should be involved in all phases of communicating with the child or children regarding a serious illness. By being present and involved, this individual may provide additional support to all concerned.
- Household routines should be kept as close to normal as possible, as this provides stability to the family.
- One should be informed about support groups and seek professional assistance when applicable. For information on cancer, one may call 1-800-4CANCER (1-800-422-6237) or 1-800-ACS-2345.

◼️ Critical Thinking **QUESTIONS AND ACTIVITIES**

Your patient is a 32-year-old mother of two who has been diagnosed with advanced breast cancer. She is very upset and nervous, and says, "How am I going to tell my children about this?". Formulate your response by using the information provided in Special Considerations: Children. Ask yourself:

- What are the ages of the children, and why is this so important for me to know?
- What information on cancer can I provide for my patient, so that she can explain this disease to her children?
- What suggestions can I give that will help her illustrate this disease process to her children?
- How can I find out more information on death, so that I can help my patient talk about it?
- How can I help my patient plan for time that she is going to have to spend away from her family? What can I recommend that she do?
- How can I help her learn about support groups?
- What professional assistance is available for this patient?

CHEMOTHERAPY WITH ANTINEOPLASTIC AGENTS

Chemotherapy (the use of chemical agents, such as cancer drugs, to destroy cancer cells) may be the treatment of choice when the cancer is disseminated and cannot be removed surgically. It is also used when a tumor fails to respond to radiation therapy, and is used in combination with other forms of therapy.

	ANTINEOPLASTIC
A	anticancer drugs cause
N	nausea and vomiting
T	treatment regimen must be carefully planned, followed, and evaluated
I	individualized dosage
N	new drugs appear on the market, and new forms of treatment are being studied
E	exposure time should be kept to a minimum
O	only a physician or those qualified with special certification or education should prepare or administer antineoplastic agents
P	protect yourself
L	look, listen, and learn
A	assessment of laboratory tests is very important
S	safe dosage based on or kilogram of body weight
T	toxicities such as bone marrow depression, alopecia, stomatitis can occur
I	inform and teach patient essentials of chemotherapy
C	classification of antineoplastic agents essential for understanding

Antineoplastic, anticancer agents do injury to individual cells, interfere with their vital functions, and kill or destroy malignant cells. In rendering cancerous cells harmless, certain normal cells may also be destroyed. The normal cells with the greatest sensitivity to destruction are the hematopoietic cells, epithelial cells, and hair follicles.

The plan of treatment for patients undergoing chemotherapy is individualized. The aim of chemotherapy is to put the patient in **remission** so that life may continue without **exacerbation** of symptoms.

Antineoplastic agents are potentially hazardous, and fatal complications can occur. Most are **cytotoxic**, *mutagenic*, and **carcinogenic**.

The following are key concepts about antineoplastic agents.

- Only physicians or those qualified with special certification or education should prepare and administer antineoplastic agents.

- Antineoplastic drugs are curative agents in choriocarcinoma, acute lymphocyctic leukemia, some cases of Hodgkin's disease, Burkitt's lymphoma, diffuse histiocytic lymphoma, certain testicular tumors, and perhaps osteogenic sarcoma.

- They accomplish tumor regression and enhance survival in acute myelocytic leukemia, non-Hodgkin's lymphoma, multiple myeloma, chronic leukemias, and adenocarcinomas of the breast and ovary.

- They are used in conjunction with surgery and radiation, and are effective in Wilms' tumor, embryonal rhabdomyosarcoma, and Ewing's sarcoma.

- They are used as an adjuvant therapy in breast cancer and other cancerous tumors.

How Chemotherapy Works

There are five phases in the cell cycle. Because cell reproduction happens over and over, the cell cycle is as a circle. All the steps lead back to the resting phase (G0), which is the starting point.

After a cell reproduces, the two new cells are identical. Each of the two cells that are made from the first cell can go through this cell cycle again when new cells are needed.

The Cell Cycle

- **G0 phase (resting stage):** The cell has not yet started to divide. Cells spend much of their lives in this phase. Depending on the type of cell, G0 can last for a few hours to a few years. When the cell is signaled to reproduce, it moves into the G1 phase.

- **G1 phase:** During this phase, the cell starts making more proteins and growing larger, so the new cells will be of normal size. This phase lasts about 18 to 30 hours.

- **S phase:** In the S phase, the chromosomes containing the genetic code (DNA) are copied so that both of the new cells formed will have matching strands of DNA. This phase lasts about 18 to 20 hours.

- **G2 phase:** In the G2 phase, the cell checks the DNA and prepares to start splitting into two cells. It lasts from 2 to 10 hours.

- **M phase (mitosis):** In this phase, which lasts only 30 to 60 minutes, the cell actually splits into two new cells.

This cell cycle is important to oncologists because many chemotherapy drugs work only on cells that are actively reproducing (not on cells in the resting phase, G0). Some drugs specifically attack cells in a particular phase of the cell cycle (the M or S phases, for example). Understanding how these drugs work helps oncologists predict which drugs are likely to work well together. Doctors can also plan how often doses of each drug should be given based on the timing of the cell phases.

When chemotherapy drugs attack reproducing cells, they cannot tell the difference between reproducing cells of normal tissues (that are replacing worn-out normal cells) and cancer cells. The damage to normal cells can cause side effects. Each time chemotherapy is given, it involves trying to find a balance between destroying the cancer cells (to cure or control the disease) and sparing the normal cells (to lessen unwanted side effects).

Toxicities and Adverse Reactions

Toxicities and adverse reactions may vary with the antineoplastic agent and with each individual patient. Some examples of adverse reactions are the following:

Gastrointestinal

Anorexia, nausea, vomiting, mucositis, stomatitis, colitis, and liver dysfunction.

Hematopoietic

Bone marrow depression or suppression, anemia, leukopenia, thrombocytopenia, and pancytopenia.

Secondary Neoplasia

May increase incidence of a second malignant tumor.

Gentiourinary

Sterile hemorrhagic cystitis, hyperuricemia, and renal failure.

Gonadal Suppression

Amenorrhea, azoospermia.

Integument

Alopecia, skin and fingernails may become darker, rash, maculopapular skin eruption.

Pulmonary

Interstitial pulmonary fibrosis.

Cardiac

Acute left ventricular failure, arrhythmias, cardiomyopathy.

Respiratory

Dyspnea.

Immunosuppressive Activity

May predispose patient to bacterial, viral (herpes zoster), or fungal infection.

Chromosomal Abnormalities

Mutagenic.

Teratogenic Effects

May produce or cause Teratogenic formation of a severely malformed fetus. Women of childbearing potential should be advised to avoid becoming pregnant.

Extravasation

May result when IV fluids escape into subcutaneous tissues, resulting in a painful inflammation. The area usually becomes indurated and sloughing of tissue may occur.

Patient Evaluation

The physician carefully evaluates each patient, and determines an exact diagnosis. A plan of treatment is prescribed. When chemotherapy is the treatment regimen or part of the treatment regimen, certain laboratory tests are performed to determine the patient's baseline data before the initiation of therapy.

Tests	*Normal Ranges*
• Platelet count	There are approximately 150,000–450,000 thrombocytes per cubic millimeter of blood.
• White blood cell count (WBC)	There are approximately 5,000–10,000 leukocytes per cubic millimeter of blood.
• Hemoglobin	Adult female: 12–16 g/100 milliliter of blood Adult male: 14–18 g/100 milliliter of blood Children: varies with age
• Hematocrit	Adult female: 37–47% Adult male: 40–54% Children: varies with age from 35–49% Newborn: 49–54%

- Differential
  Neutrophils 40–60%
  Eosinophils 1–3%
  Basophils 0.5–1%
  Lymphocytes 20–40%
  Monocytes 4–8%

- Liver function and kidney function
  Tests determine these vital organ's functioning abilities.

During chemotherapy, these laboratory tests must be evaluated very carefully. When there is a deviation from normal, the physician is notified. At this time, the physician will evaluate the results of the test and determine the course of action to take.

● *Note*

Those who prepare or administer antineoplastic agents should have the same laboratory tests performed before and during their contact with these agents. Any deviation from normal should be carefully assessed by a physician. ●

Dosage

The dosage of antineoplastic agents is individualized for each patient. The dosage is based upon body surface area or kilogram of body weight. The physician will order the chemotherapy regimen, giving the patient's name, the agent or agents to use, the dose, route, rate, and time for administration. Those preparing and administering these agents should have a second qualified person check and verify the order and their preparation of the drug or drugs.

Protecting Yourself

Remember, only those qualified with special certification or education should prepare and administer antineoplastic agents. Ideally, the pharmacy department of a hospital should prepare antineoplastic agents under a vertical laminar airflow hood.

The National Institutes of Health (NIH) and the National Study Commission on Cytotoxic Exposure have prepared recommended guidelines for safely handling chemotherapeutic agents. The American Society of Hospital Pharmacists (ASHP) has also developed guidelines and procedures for handling cytotoxic agents.

CARE OF CHEMOTHERAPY PATIENTS

Patients who are receiving chemotherapy need special consideration, physical and emotional support, encouragement, education about their disease process, education about support groups, and ways in which they can lessen the severity of the disease. The following are some general suggestions that you may use to care for patients receiving chemotherapy:

- Encourage patients to express their emotional feelings about the disease process. Take time to listen to each patient.

- Encourage patients to ask questions, and if you cannot answer the questions, find someone who can.

- Be sure the patients understand their chemotherapy regimen.

- Be sure the patients understand about possible adverse reactions and what to do if they occur.

- If a patient experiences nausea and vomiting, the physician should be informed so appropriate antiemetics may be prescribed.

To lessen the severity of nausea and vomiting, you may want to advise the patient to:

- Avoid hot, spicy, greasy, and acidic foods and beverages.
- Avoid unpleasant odors.
- Eat small frequent meals.
- Take a prescribed antiemetic before chemotherapy.
- Suck on ice chips and/or sugarless hard candy.
- Refrain from smoking.

Protect patients from infection by maintaining a clean environment, using sterile equipment and supplies when appropriate, and washing your hands as indicated. Educate patients and their families about the spread of infectious diseases. Teach patient to be alert for the following signs of infection, and to report such signs to the attending physician:

- An elevated body temperature
- Sneezing, coughing, and malaise, usual indications of a viral upper respiratory infection
- Signs of inflammation, such as pain, heat, redness, swelling, and impaired function

Teach the patient to be consciously alert for the following signs of bleeding, and to report such signs to the attending physician:

- Excessive bruising
- Nosebleed (epistaxis), rectal bleeding, abnormal vaginal bleeding, and bleeding gums
- Small, purplish, hemorrhagic spots on the skin (petechiae), possible indications of abnormality in blood clotting

One of the most dreaded adverse reactions to chemotherapy is *alopecia*, the loss of hair. You may want to suggest that the patient temporarily wear a wig or some other form of scalp cover. Usually, the hair will begin to grow back after the effects of chemotherapy are eliminated from the patient's body. The new hair may be even darker than the hair that was lost.

Inform patients to notify the physician's office if the analgesic that is prescribed for pain does not provide relief. Many times the dose has to be adjusted or another type of analgesic needs to be prescribed.

Provide patients with information on support groups that are available in the community for cancer patients. You may wish to contact the American Cancer Society, in-service departments of local hospitals, and the local health department for information that you can give to your patients.

Nausea and vomiting may be controlled with the use of Zofran (ondansetron), or Kytril (granisetron) or together with Anzemet (dolasetron) administered at the time of chemotherapy. The dose of these medications will be different for different patients. The following information includes only the average oral doses of medications that may be used to prevent the nausea and vomiting associated with chemotherapy.

Ondansetron (Zofran)

Uses

To prevent the nausea and vomiting that may occur after treatment with chemotherapy or radiation, or after surgery.

Dosage and Route

For prevention of nausea and vomiting after anticancer medicine. For adults and children 12 years of age and older—Oral dosage (tablets): At first, the dose is 8 mg taken 30 minutes before the anticancer medicine is given. The 8-mg dose is taken again eight hours after the first dose. Then, the dose is 8 mg every 12 hours for one to two days. For children 4 to 12 years—At first, the dose is 4 mg taken 30 minutes before the anticancer medicine is given. The 4-mg dose is taken again 4 to 8 hours after the first dose. Then, the dose is 4 mg every eight hours for one to two days. For children up to 4 years, the dose must be determined by the patient's physician.

● *Note*

Instruct the patient that if vomiting starts within 30 minutes after taking this medicine, the same amount of medicine should be taken again. If vomiting continues, the patient should check with his or her physician for further instructions. If the patient misses a dose of this medicine and does not feel nauseous, skip the missed dose and go back to the regular dosing schedule. If the patient misses a dose of this medicine and feels nauseous or vomits, the missed dose should be taken as soon as possible. ●

Granisetron (Kytril)

Uses

To prevent the nausea and vomiting that may occur after treatment with chemotherapy.

Dosage and Route

For prevention of nausea and vomiting after anticancer medicine. For adults and teenagers—Oral dosage (tablets): dose is usually 1 mg taken up to one hour before the anticancer medicine. The 1-mg dose is taken again 12 hours after the first dose.

Dolasetron (Anzemet)

Uses

To prevent and treat the nausea and vomiting that may occur after treatment with anticancer medicines or after surgery.

Dosage and Route

For prevention of nausea and vomiting after anticancer medicine. For adults—Oral dosage (tablets): 100 mg given within one hour before the anticancer medicine is given. For children 2 to 16 years of age—1.8 mg/kg of body weight given within one hour before the anticancer medicine is given. The dose generally is not greater than 100 mg.

CLASSIFICATIONS OF ANTINEOPLASTIC AGENTS

Antineoplastic agents prevent the development, growth, or proliferation of malignant cells. The following are the primary classifications of antineoplastic agents:

Alkylating Agents

Alkylating agents are chemical compounds that cause chromosome breakage and prevent the formation of new DNA (deoxyribonucleic acid), thereby interfering with cell division. They affect all rapidly proliferating cells, and often cause toxicity to the hematopoietic system. Bone marrow depression or suppression, anemia, leukopenia, thrombocytopenia, and pancytopenia may occur. Most alkylating agents disrupt cells within the gastrointestinal tract, thereby producing nausea and vomiting.

EXAMPLE

busulfan (Myleran)	mechlorethamine HCl (Mustargen)
chlorambucil (Leukeran)	melphalan (Alkeran)
cisplatin (Platinol)	thiotepa

Nitrosoureas

Nitrosoureas act in a similar way to alkylating agents. They inhibit enzymes that are needed for DNA repair. These agents are able to travel to the brain so they are used to treat brain tumors, as well as non-Hodgkin's lymphomas, multiple myeloma, and malignant melanoma.

> **EXAMPLE**   carmustine (BICNU)
>
>   lomustine (CEENU)

Antimetabolites

Antimetabolites are substances that interfere with the metabolic process of the cell, thus preventing cell reproduction. They act only on dividing cells, and are most effective in treating rapid proliferation of malignant cells. These agents often cause toxicity to the hematopoietic system. Bone marrow depression/suppression, anemia, leukopenia, thrombocytopenia, and pancytopenia may occur. They also cause nausea and vomiting.

> **EXAMPLE**   cytarabine (Cytosar)   mercaptopurine (Purinethol)
>
>   fluorouracil (5-FU)   methotrexate (Rheumatrex)

Antitumor Antibiotics

Certain *antibiotics* have an antineoplastic effect. These antibiotics are derived from species of microorganisms, and are not to be confused with antibiotics that are used in the treatment of infections. Their action is not known, but it appears they act by interfering with one or more stages of RNA (ribonucleic acid) and DNA synthesis. They interfere with the malignant cell's ability to grow and reproduce. These antibiotics do cause toxicity.

> **EXAMPLE**   bleomycin sulfate (Blenoxane)   daunorubicin HCl (Cerubidine)
>
>   dactinomycin (Cosmegen)   mitomycin (Mutamycin)

Mitotic Inhibitors

Mitotic inhibitors are plant alkaloids and natural products that can inhibit mitosis or inhibit enzymes that prevent protein synthesis needed for reproduction of the cell. These are phase-cycle specific and work during the M (mitosis) phase.

> **EXAMPLE**   docetaxel (Taxotere)   vinblastine sulfate
>
>   etoposide (VePesid)   vincristine (Oncovin)
>
>   paclitaxel (Taxol)   vinorelbine (Navelbine)

COMBINATION CHEMOTHERAPY

The combination of certain antineoplastic agents has proven to be effective in treating acute leukemia; Hodgkin's disease; non-Hodgkin's lymphoma; carcinoma of the breast, testis, and ovary; childhood neuroblastoma; Wilms' tumor; and osteogenic sarcoma. The physician who prescribes combination chemotherapy weighs the anticipated benefits against the possible additive toxic effects of the drugs.

Additional Types of Cancer Drugs

The following are some additional drugs and biological treatments that are used to treat cancer. They often have less serious side effects than chemotherapy drugs because they are targeted to work mainly on cancer cells, not normal, healthy cells. Many are used along with chemotherapy.

Targeted Therapies

As researchers have learned more about the inner workings of cancer cells, they have begun to create new drugs that attack cancer cells more specifically than traditional chemotherapy drugs can. Most attack cells with mutant versions or certain genes, or cells that express too many copies of a particular gene. These drugs can be used as part of primary treatment or after treatment to maintain remission or decrease recurrence.

EXAMPLE imatinib (Gleevec), gefitinib (Iressa), erlotinib (Tarceva), bortezomib (Velcade)

Differentiating Agents

Differentiating agents act on the cancer cells to make them mature into normal cells.

EXAMPLE tretinoin (ATRA, Atralin), bexarotene (Targretin), arsenic trioxide

Hormone Therapy

Drugs in this category are sex hormones, or hormonelike drugs, that alter the action or production of female or male hormones. They are used to slow the growth of breast, prostate, and endometrial (uterine) cancers, which normally grow in response to natural hormones in the body. These cancer treatment hormones do not work in the same ways as standard chemotherapy drugs, but rather by preventing the cancer cell from using the hormone it needs to grow, or by preventing the body from making the hormones.

EXAMPLE

- antiestrogens fulvestrant (Faslodex), tamoxifen citrate (Nolvadex, Soltamox), toremifene citrate (Fareston)
- aromatase inhibitors, such as anastrozole (Arimidex), exemestane (Aromasin), letrozole (Femara)
- progestins such as megestrol acetate (Megace)
- estrogens, such as estramustine phosphate sodium (EMCYT)
- antiandrogens, such as bicalutamide (Casodex), flutamide, nilutamde (Nilandron)
- gonadotropin-releasing hormone (GnRH) agonists, such as leuprolide (Lupron), goserelin (Zoladex).

OTHER FORMS OF TREATMENT FOR CANCER

Treatment for cancer may be any one or a combination of chemotherapy, surgery, radiation therapy, immunotherapy, and other forms of treatment that have emerged from scientific investigation and the advent of genetic engineering.

Surgery

Surgery may be the treatment of choice when the tumor is small and localized and the surrounding tissue is accessible for removal. The aim of surgery is the removal of all cancerous tissue plus some of the surrounding normal tissue. Surgery may also be used to alleviate some of the complications of cancer, such as the obstruction of an area caused by the enlargement of a tumor.

Radiation Therapy

Radiation therapy is the treatment of disease by the use of ionizing radiation. The aim of this treatment is to deliver a precise, calculated dose of radiation to diseased tissue, such as a tumor, causing the least possible damage to surrounding normal tissue. Malignant cells are more sensitive to radiation than are normal cells. They seem less able to repair themselves; therefore, radiation is frequently used in the treatment of patients with cancer, as either a curative or a palliative mode of therapy.

Immunotherapy

Immunotherapy is the treatment of disease by stimulation of the body's immune system. It may be used as an adjuvant to other types of treatment. Immunotherapy, sometimes called biological therapy, biotherapy, or biological response modifier therapy, uses the body's own immune defense system to attack cancer. Once the body's immune system has recognized cancer cells by their foreign substances (antigens), it can send immune cells to destroy the cancer. It can also manufacture antibodies that attach themselves to the cancer cells' antigens and help the immune system destroy the targeted invader.

CANCER TREATMENT OF THE FUTURE

Over the years, the development and use of chemotherapy drugs have resulted in the successful treatment of many individuals with cancer. Yet, some cancers still recur. There are several innovative uses of chemotherapy and other agents that hold even more promise for controlling cancer. These include new chemotherapy medications, novel approaches to targeting drugs more specifically at the cancer cells (like attaching drugs to monoclonal antibodies or packaging them inside liposomes) to produce fewer adverse reactions, drugs to reduce adverse reactions like colony-stimulating factors and chemoprotective agents, hematopoietic stem-cell transplantation, and agents that overcome multidrug resistance.

With the identification of gene sequencing and the announcement of the mapping of the human genome, the future of cancer therapy will be focused at the chromosomal level. Therapies will be targeted at preventing disease, identifying genetic abnormalities, and developing agents that will trick tumor cells into self-destruction without causing any toxicity for the patient.

New and expected advances in chemotherapy include the following:

- New classes of chemotherapy medicines and combinations of medicines are being developed.

- New ways to give the drugs are being studied, such as using smaller amounts over longer periods of time or giving them continuously with special pumps.

- Some new medicines, called targeted therapies, are specifically developed to attack a particular target on cancer cells. These drugs may have fewer side effects than standard chemotherapy drugs and may eventually be used along with them. Several are now under study. Some are already in use; for instance, lapatinib ditosylate (Tykerb) can be used along with other drugs to treat women whose breast cancer is positive for HER2/neu.

- Other approaches to targeting drugs more specifically at the cancer cells such as attaching drugs to monoclonal antibodies may make them more effective and cause fewer side effects. Monoclonal antibodies, which are special types of proteins made in the lab, can be designed to guide chemotherapy medicines directly to the tumor. Mylotarg (gemtuzumab ozogamicin) is a chemotherapy agent composed of a recombinant humanized IgG4, kappa antibody conjugated with a cytotoxic antitumor antibiotic, calicheamicin, isolated from fermentation of a bacterium, Micromonospora echinospora, subspecies calichensis. This drug is used to treat acute myelogenous leukemia. Monoclonal antibodies (without attached chemotherapy) can also be used as immunotherapy drugs, to strengthen the body's immune response against cancer cells. For instance, rituximab (Rituxan) and alemtuzumab (Campath) are directed at certain lymphoma cells, and are used to treat some types of non-Hodgkin's lymphoma. More of these types of drugs are being developed.

- Liposomal therapy involves using chemotherapy drugs that have been packaged inside liposomes (synthetic fat globules). The liposome helps the drug penetrate the cancer cells more selectively and decreases possible side effects (such as hair loss, nausea and vomiting). Examples of liposomal medicines already in use are doxorubicin hydrochloride (Doxil) and daunorubicin citrate (Daunoxome).

- Chemoprotective agents are being developed to protect against specific side effects of certain chemotherapy drugs. For example, dexrazoxane hydrochloride (Totect, Zinecard) helps prevent heart damage, amifostine (Ethyol) helps protect the kidneys, and mesna protects the bladder.

Cancer cells often become resistant to chemotherapy by developing the ability to pump the drugs out of the cells. Some new agents may be given along with chemotherapy to help overcome drug resistance. These new agents inactivate the pumps, allowing the chemotherapy to remain in the cancer cells longer and hopefully making it more effective.

✓ Spot Check

For each of the classifications of antineoplastic agents given, list several examples of drugs and their action. Give the major toxicity of each classification.

CLASSIFICATION	ACTION	MAJOR TOXICITY
alkylating agents		
antimetabolites		
antitumor antibiotics		
mitotic inhibitors		

▆▆ REVIEW QUESTIONS

Directions. Select the best answer to each of the following multiple-choice questions, circling the letter of your choice:

1. The process whereby normal cells have a distinct appearance and specialized function is known as _____.

    a. dedifferentiation   b. remission

    c. differentiation   d. exacerbation

2. The medical term for loss of appetite is _____.

    a. anorexia   b. alopecia   c. stomatitis   d. cytotoxic

3. Chemotherapy is the treatment of choice when the cancer is _____.

    a. disseminated   c. localized

    b. surgically inoperable   d. a and b

4. The normal cells that are most sensitive to chemotherapy are _____.

    a. hematopoietic cells   c. hair follicles

    b. epithelial cells   d. all of these

5. Antineoplastic agents may be prepared and administered by _____.

    a. any nurse or health professional

    b. physicians only, who are qualified to do so

    c. those qualified with special certification or education

    d. b and c

6. Adverse reactions to antineoplastic agents include _____.

    a. nausea and vomiting   c. alopecia

    b. bone marrow depression   d. all of these

7. The normal range of thrombocytes per cubic millimeter of blood is _____.

    a. 100,000 to 300,000   c. 200,000 to 400,000

    b. 150,000 to 450,000   d. 150,000 to 600,000

8. Patients who are receiving chemotherapy need _____.

    a. special consideration

    b. physical and emotional support

    c. education about their disease, support groups, and ways to lessen the severity of the disease

    d. all of these

9. When the patient's nausea, vomiting, and pain are not controlled by the prescribed antiemetic dose, you should _____.

    a. notify the physician   c. a and b

    b. seek a more satisfactory regimen   d. none of these

10. To lessen the severity of nausea and vomiting, the patient should _____.

    a. avoid unpleasant odors   c. eat small frequent meals

    b. avoid hot, spicy, greasy foods   d. all of these

11. You should teach your patient to be alert for signs of bleeding and to report such signs to the physician. Signs of bleeding include _____.

    a. epistaxis   c. excessive bruising

    b. petechiae   d. all of these

12. Antineoplastic agents may be classified as _____.

    a. alkylating agents   b. antimetabolites   c. antibiotics   d. all of these

13. _____ is the time when the symptoms of a disease process are most severe.

    a. Extravasation   b. Exacerbation   c. Malignant   d. Remission

14. _____ is the time when the symptoms of a disease process are lessened.

    a. Extravasation   b. Exacerbation   c. Malignant   d. Remission

15. The spreading process of cancer cells from one area of the body to another area is called _____.

    a. extravasation   b. metastasis   c. proliferation   d. exacerbation

16. The treatment of cancer may be one or a combination of _____.

    a. surgery
    b. chemotherapy
    c. radiation therapy and/or immunotherapy
    d. all of these

17. There are approximately _____ leukocytes per cubic millimeter of blood.

    a. 150,000 to 450,000
    b. 12,000 to 15,000
    c. 5,000 to 10,000
    d. 1 to 2 million

18. Recommended guidelines for safely handling chemotherapeutic agents have been prepared by _____.

    a. the National Institutes of Health (NIH)
    b. the National Study Commission on Cytotoxic Exposure
    c. the American Society of Hospital Pharmacists (ASHP)
    d. all of these

Matching. Place the correct letter from Column II on the appropriate line of Column I:

Column I	*Column II*
19. _____ alopecia	A. loss of appetite
20. _____ cytotoxic	B. producing cancer
21. _____ teratogenic	C. loss of hair
22. _____ carcinogenic	D. inflammation of the mouth
23. _____ proliferation	E. producing or forming a severely malformed fetus
24. _____ stomatitis	F. the process of rapid reproduction
25. _____ malignant	G. destructive to cells
	H. tending to metastasize; cancerous

UNIT 18
Vitamins, Minerals and Herbals

OBJECTIVES

Upon completing this unit, you should be able to:

- Define the terms listed in the vocabulary.
- Describe how many health problems could be prevented by proper nutrition.
- Describe the five major food groups.
- Give four examples of when a body may require additional nutrients.
- Describe "5 A Day for Better Health" as recommended by the National Institutes of Health and the Centers for Disease Control and Prevention.
- Select fruits and vegetables by color.
- Describe factors that may affect an older adult's dietary regimen.
- Describe the surgeon general's call to action to prevent and decrease obesity in children and adolescents.
- State what is being done to promote physical activity and healthy weight in children and adolescents.
- Complete the critical thinking questions and activities presented in this unit.
- Differentiate between fat-soluble and water-soluble vitamins.
- Give the functions, food sources, USRDA, and indications of deficiency of selected vitamins and minerals.
- State the symptoms of hypervitaminosis for vitamins A, D, and E.
- Describe the importance of cations and anions in electrolyte balance.
- Complete the Spot Check on selected vitamins and minerals.
- Describe selected herbal preparations, possible uses, side effects/adverse reactions, and drug interactions as described in Table 18-4.
- Answer the review questions correctly.

VOCABULARY

anion (an'i-on). An ion with a negative charge of electricity.

antioxidants (an"te-ok 'si-dants). Plant substances that protect the body by neutralizing free radicals, or unstable oxygen molecules, which can damage cells and lead to poor health.

avitaminosis (a-vi"ta-mi-no'sis). A deficiency disease that is due to a lack of vitamins in the diet.

cation (kat'i-on). An ion with a positive charge of electricity.

dietary supplement (di-e-tary-sup'la-ment). A product taken by mouth that contains a "dietary ingredient" intended to supplement the diet.

electrolytes (e-lek'tro-lits). Particles that result from disintegration of compounds.

herbal (herb'al). A plant with a soft stem containing little wood, especially an aromatic plant used in medicines or seasoning.

homeostasis (ho"me-o-sta'sis). The normal fluid state in which positive and negative ions are in balance.

hypervitaminosis (hi"per-vi"ta-min-o'sis). A condition caused by an excessive amount of vitamins, especially from taking too many vitamin pills.

hypovitaminosis (hi"po-vi"ta-min-o'sis). A condition due to a lack of vitamins, especially from an inadequate diet. The signs of hypovitaminosis may include fatigue and pain and aches throughout the body. It can be corrected by a well-balanced diet.

(continues)

macrominerals (mak″ro-min′er-als). Minerals that are required in large amounts.

microminerals (mi″kro-min′er-als). Minerals that are required in small amounts.

minerals (min′er-als). Nonorganic substances that are essential constituents of all body cells.

obesity (o-be′si-te). An excessively high amount of body fat or adipose tissue in relation to lean body mass.

phytochemical (fi″to-kem′i-kal). Any one of a hundred natural chemical substances present in plants.

RDA. The recommended daily allowance. The nutrient level of intake that is considered by the National Research Council (NRC) and Nutrition Board to be adequate for most healthy individuals.

supplement (sup′la-ment). Something added to fill a need, or to reinforce.

USRDA. The United States recommended daily allowance.

vitamins (vi′ta-mins). Organic substances that are essential for normal metabolism, growth, and development of the human body.

INTRODUCTION

Carbohydrates, fats, proteins, water, electrolytes, vitamins, and minerals are nutrients that are essential for life. Carbohydrates and fats furnish heat and energy. Proteins provide energy and build and repair body tissues. Water and electrolytes are essential for maintaining the body's acid-base balance. Vitamins, minerals, and water help regulate such body processes as circulation, respiration, digestion, and elimination.

At least four of the ten leading causes of death in the United States (heart disease, cancer, stroke, and diabetes) are directly related to a person's eating habits. It is now noted that many health problems could be prevented by proper nutrition. For example, atherosclerosis can begin in early childhood, and this process can be halted if healthy changes in diet and lifestyle are initiated and followed. The gradual bone thinning that results in osteoporosis may be prevented if enough calcium is consumed throughout life.

The U.S. Food and Drug Administration ordered that most breads, flour, pasta and other food from grains be fortified with folic acid. It is recommended that women of childbearing age and children over 4 years of age consume 0.4 mg of folic acid daily. There is strong evidence that folic acid reduces a chemical, homocysteine, that is associated with high risk of heart attacks and strokes. When pregnant women consume too little folic acid, infants may have malformations of the spinal cord such as spina bifida or anencephaly.

Diabetes in the United States has risen to almost an epidemic state. The rise is blamed largely on obesity. Obesity is defined as an excessively high amount of body fat or adipose tissue in relation to lean body mass. The concern about the amount of body fat (or adiposity) is for both the distribution of fat throughout the body and the size of the adipose tissue deposits. Body fat distribution can be estimated by skin fold measures, waist-to-hip circumference ratios, or techniques such as ultrasound, computed tomography, or magnetic resonance imaging.

It is estimated that 64 percent of U.S. adults are either overweight or obese, defined as having a body mass index (BMI) of 25 or more. The obesity rate has increased to nearly one in five Americans. Nearly 30 percent of patients diagnosed as overweight in the past years have been 35 years of age or younger. The number of overweight children between 6 and 17 years of age has risen 22 percent since the 1960s. Less than 30 percent of American children eat the recommended five servings of fruits and vegetables per day, and many young people do not get enough physical exercise to burn the calories that they consume. Obesity is associated with increased risks of high blood pressure, heart disease, high cholesterol, stroke, diabetes, cancer, gallbladder disease, arthritis, sleep disturbances, complications in pregnancy, and early death.

Good nutrition involves balance, variety, and moderation. High-fat foods can be balanced with low-fat foods and calorie intake can be offset by enough activity to maintain normal weight. Good nutrition should be a part of an overall healthy lifestyle (see Figure 18-1).

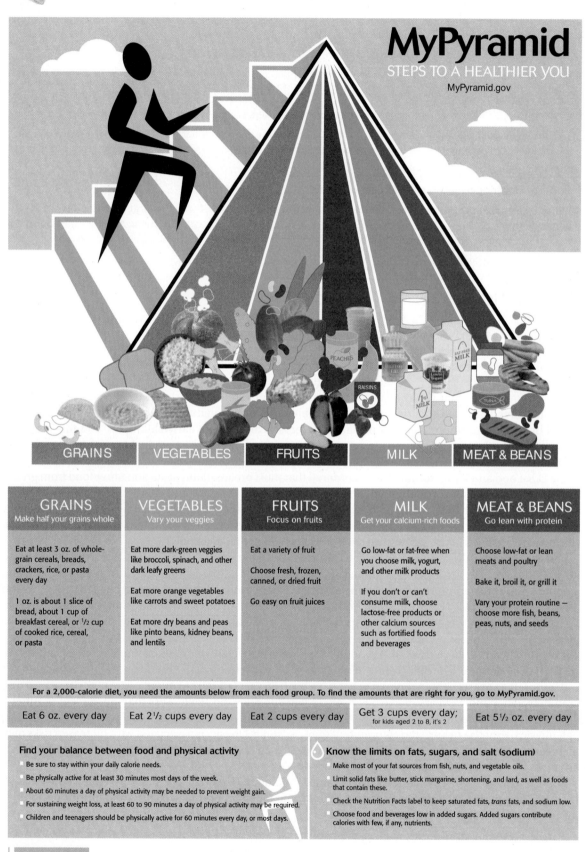

FIGURE 18-1

MyPyramid food guidance system. *(Courtesy of U.S. Department of Agriculture and the U.S. Department of Health and Human Services.)*

FIVE MAJOR FOOD GROUPS

1. **Bread, Cereal, Rice, and Pasta**

    Consume 3 or more ounce-equivalents of whole-grain products per day, with the rest of the recommended grains coming from enriched or whole-grain products. In general, at least half the grains should come from whole grains.

2. **Fruit**

3. **Vegetables**

    Consume a sufficient amount of fruits and vegetables while staying within energy needs. Two cups of fruit and $2\frac{1}{2}$ cups of vegetables per day are recommended for a reference 2,000-calorie intake, with higher or lower amounts depending on the calorie level. Choose a variety of fruits and vegetables each day. In particular, select from all five vegetable subgroups (dark green, orange, legumes, starchy vegetables, and other vegetables) several times a week.

4. **Milk, Yogurt, and Cheese**

    Consume 3 cups per day of fat-free or low-fat milk or equivalent milk products.

5. **Meat, Poultry, Fish, Dry Beans, Eggs, and Nuts**

    Consume two to three servings per day. In particular, select from nonfat, lean foods.

Fats

Consume less than 10 percent of calories from saturated fatty acids and less than 300 mg/day of cholesterol, and keep trans-fatty acid consumption as low as possible.

Keep total fat intake between 20 to 35 percent of calories, with most fats coming from sources of polyunsaturated and monounsaturated fatty acids, such as fish, nuts, and vegetable oils. When selecting and preparing meat, poultry, dry beans, and milk or milk products, make choices that are lean, low-fat, or fat-free. Limit intake of fats and oils high in saturated and/or trans-fatty acids, and choose products low in such fats and oils.

Carbohydrates

Choose fiber-rich fruits, vegetables, and whole grains often.

Choose and prepare foods and beverages with little added sugars or caloric sweeteners, such as amounts suggested by the USDA Food Guide and the DASH Eating Plan.

Reduce the incidence of dental caries by practicing good oral hygiene and consuming sugar- and starch-containing foods and beverages less frequently.

Sodium and Potassium

Consume less than 2,300 mg of sodium (approximately 1 teaspoon of salt) per day.

Choose and prepare foods with little salt. At the same time, consume potassium-rich foods, such as fruits and vegetables.

Some basic principles to follow for healthy eating are:

- Eat a variety of foods.
- Control calorie intake to manage body weight.
- Eat more fruits, vegetables, and whole grains.
- Reduce saturated fat and cholesterol.
- Use low-fat or nonfat milk products or yogurt.
- Limit sugar and salt.

- Drink alcoholic beverages in moderation, if at all.
- Eat moderate-sized portions. This is most important when trying to lose weight.

   One serving size for fruits and vegetables:

   1 medium-size fruit

   $\frac{3}{4}$ cup (6 oz.) of 100 percent fruit or vegetable juice

   $\frac{1}{2}$ cup fresh, frozen, or canned fruit (in 100 percent juice) or vegetables

   1 cup raw leafy vegetables

   $\frac{1}{2}$ cup cooked dry peas or beans

   $\frac{1}{4}$ cup dried fruit

- Include physical activity in your daily routine.

Through proper selection of foods, most healthy adults can receive the nutrients essential for life. There are times that a body may require additional nutrients such as during the various stages of growth and development, pregnancy, breast-feeding, surgery, disease processes, and aging. Also, teenagers with irregular eating habits, vegetarians, dieters, and people who avoid entire food groups may need a multivitamin and mineral supplement. Smokers may have lower vitamin C levels in their blood than nonsmokers and may benefit from supplementation of up to 500 mg of vitamin C a day.

People with deficiency diseases or absorption disorders may need therapeutic doses prescribed by a physician of nutrients that may be two to ten times the **RDA** (recommended daily allowance). The RDA is the nutrient level of intake that is considered by the National Research Council (NRC) and Nutrition Board to be adequate for most healthy individuals. People who take prescription medications that interfere with nutrients or who abuse alcohol or other drugs may also need a supplement. Women may need to supplement calcium to help prevent osteoporosis, and those who bleed excessively during menstruation may need to take a multivitamin and mineral supplement that contains iron.

Additional nutrients are generally prescribed as a vitamin or mineral supplement (or combination supplement) by a physician. It is important for the patient to understand that the prescribed nutrient is a drug and should be used as such.

Spotlight

Proper Nutrition—A Plan to Improve Health

You have heard the saying, "You are what you eat." The correlation between dietary habits and health has become a much-researched topic. Much has been learned about fat intake and heart disease; calcium intake and osteoporosis; sodium and hypertension; and fiber-containing grain products, fruits, and vegetables and cancer.

The National Institutes of Health and the Centers for Disease Control recommend the program "5 A Day for Better Health." To assist in this endeavor, "5 A Day The Color Way" provides an array of information on the web at www.5aday.org.

Eating five or more servings of colorful fruits and vegetables a day is part of an important plan for healthier living. Deeply hued fruits and vegetables provide the wide range of vitamins, minerals, fiber, and phytochemicals the body needs to maintain good health and energy levels, protect against the effects of aging, and reduce the risk of cancer and heart disease. See Table 18-1 and Figure 18-2.

Vitamins and minerals are natural substances contained in a wide variety of foods that have long been recognized as essential to maintaining healthy body systems. Scientists have defined specific daily amounts of vitamins and minerals that are necessary for good health.

TABLE 18-1		Fruits and Vegetables by Color Category		
BLUE/PURPLE	**GREEN**	**WHITE**	**YELLOW/ORANGE**	**RED**
Purple asparagus	Green apples	Bananas	Yellow apples	Red apples
Purple belgian endive	Artichokes	Cauliflower	Apricots	Beets
Blackberries	Arugula	Dates	Yellow beets	Blood oranges
Black currants	Asparagus	Garlic	Butternut squash	Red cabbage
Black salsify	Avocados	Ginger	Cantaloupe	Cherries
Blueberries	Green beans	Jicama	Carrots	Cranberries
Purple carrots	Broccoli	Mushrooms	Yellow figs	Pink/Red grapefruit
Dried plums	Broccoli rabe	White nectarines	Grapefruit	Red grapes
Eggplant	Brussels sprouts	Onions	Golden kiwifruit	Red onions
Elderberries	Green cabbage	Parsnips	Lemon	Red pears
Purple figs	Celery	White peaches	Mangoes	Red peppers
Purple grapes	Chayote squash	Pears	Nectarines	Pomegranates
Purple peppers	Chinese cabbage	White potatoes	Oranges	Red potatoes
Plums	Cucumbers	Shallots	Papayas	Radicchio
Purple potatoes	Green grapes	Turnips	Peaches	Radishes
Raisins	Honeydew melon		Yellow pears	Raspberries
Kiwifruit		Yellow peppers	Rhubarb	
	Leafy greens		Persimmons	Strawberries
	Leeks		Pineapples	Tomatoes
	Lettuce		Yellow potatoes	Pink/Red watermelon
	Limes		Pumpkin	
	Okra		Rutabagas	
	Grean onion		Yellow summer squash	
	Peas		Sweet corn	
	Green pears		Sweet potatoes	
	Green pepper		Tangerines	
	Spinach		Yellow Tomatoes	
	Zucchini		Yellow watermelon	
			Yellow winter squash	

A **phytochemical** is any one of a hundred natural chemical substances present in plants. Many of the bright colors in fruits and vegetables come from phytochemicals. Many have nutritional value; others are protective (antioxidants) or cause cell damage (free radicals). Garlic, soybeans, licorice root, broccoli, carrots, and tomatoes are just a few of the many foods that have been analyzed by scientists, who are exploring how phytochemicals might help prevent cancer and other diseases. It is believed that some may keep cancer cells from forming or attaching to healthy cells. They may also help offset some of the damage that cause cancers

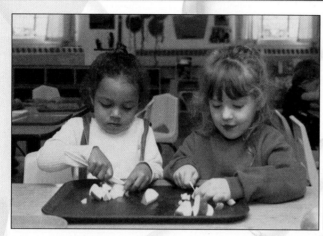

FIGURE 18-2

Eating apples as part of the
"5 A Day for Better Health" program
Source: Delmar/Cengage Learning

by toxins, such as cigarette smoke and pollutants. Some of the phytochemicals that have been linked with disease prevention include:

- *Capsaicin* found in peppers.
- *Coumarins* in citrus fruit and tomatoes.
- *Flavonoids* in citrus fruit and tomatoes, as well as berries, peppers, and carrots.
- *Indoles* in broccoli and cabbage.
- *Isothiocyanates* in broccoli and cabbage, as well as in mustard and horseradish.
- *lycopene* in tomatoes and red grapefruit.
- *S-allycsteine* in garlic, onions, and chives.
- *Triterpenoids* in licorice root and citrus fruit.

Antioxidants are plant substances that protect the body by neutralizing free radicals, or unstable oxygen molecules, which can damage cells and lead to poor health. The body makes antioxidants, and antioxidants are found in various foods, herbs, and nutritional supplements. Vitamins C and E and beta-carotene are known as antioxidant vitamins.

Antioxidants help to protect the body's cells. The billions of cells in the body are continually exposed to free radicals that are produced through normal bodily processes, as well as external sources such as air pollution and tobacco smoke. It is believed that this cellular damage, along with other factors, may lead to aging and the development of chronic diseases such as cancer, cataracts, and heart disease.

The positive benefits of proper nutrition are many. It is believed that if one eats a variety of foods, maintains desirable weight, avoids too much fat, sugar, and sodium, eats high-fiber foods, and consumes beverages and foods containing antioxidants, the quality of life will be improved, and certain diseases may be prevented.

Special Considerations: **OLDER ADULTS**

Carbohydrates, fats, proteins, vitamins, minerals, and water are essential ingredients that are needed for the proper functioning of the human body. Because of reduced physical activity and a decline in metabolic processes, older adults generally need fewer calories than when they were younger. It is suggested that calories should be reduced by 7 to 8 percent every 10 years after a person has reached age 25. Although older adults need to reduce calories, the intake of salt, cholesterol, and saturated fats, a balanced diet still needs to include the five basic food groups:

- Bread, cereal, rice, and pasta
- Fruits

- Vegetables
- Milk, yogurt, and cheese
- Meat, poultry, fish, dry beans, eggs, and nuts

It is estimated that 25 percent of U.S. households do not have nutritionally balanced diets. There are many reasons for this, among which are lack of knowledge about nutrients and the proper amount of nutrients to make up a balanced diet and food sources rich in these nutrients; too little time to prepare balanced meals; loss of vitamin content during food preparation; taste preference for less nutritious foods; and lack of knowledge about their individual nutrient needs. In addition to these, older adults may have other factors affecting their dietary regimen, such as:

- Reduced income that limits the purchase of nutritional foods
- Lack of adequate cooking facilities
- Loneliness and having to eat alone
- Physical inability to prepare meals
- Loss of teeth or poorly fitting dentures
- Lack of means to go grocery shopping
- Loss of interest in food
- Depression
- A lack of tase for food or desire to eat due to medications that affect these
- Disease or multiple disease processes that affect the older adult's desire to eat

Older adults who is able needs to continue to participate in food selection and preparation. Likes and dislikes need to be discussed and a meal plan should be formulated that covers all the essential nutrients that the body needs. For those individuals who need assistance with meals, "Meals on Wheels" is a good program. For those individuals who can attend a community senior citizens center, daily lunches can be enjoyed at a minimal cost. In addition to a good meal, older adults may enjoy the socialization and recreational activities that are provided at these centers.

▪▪ Special Considerations: **CHILDREN**

The Surgeon General's Call to Action to Prevent and Decrease Overweight and Obesity

The Problem of Overweight in Children and Adolescents

- In 1999, 13 percent of children aged 6 to 11 and 14 percent of adolescents aged 12 to 19 in the United States were overweight. This prevalence has nearly tripled for adolescents in the past two decades.
- Risk factors for heart disease, such as high cholesterol and high blood pressure, occur with increased frequency in overweight children and adolescents compared to children with a healthy weight.
- Type 2 diabetes, previously considered an adult disease, has increased dramatically in children and adolescents. Overweight and obesity are closely linked to Type 2 diabetes.
- Overweight adolescents have a 70 percent chance of becoming overweight or obese adults. This increases to 80 percent if one or more parent is overweight or obese. Overweight or obese adults are at risk for a number of health problems, including heart disease, Type 2 diabetes, high blood pressure, and some forms of cancer.
- The most immediate consequence of overweight as perceived by the children themselves is social discrimination. This is associated with poor self-esteem and depression.

The Causes of Overweight in Children and Adolescents

- Overweight in children and adolescents is generally caused by lack of physical activity, unhealthy eating patterns, or a combination of the two, with genetics and lifestyle both playing important roles in determining a child's weight.
- Our society has become very sedentary. Television, the computer, and video games contribute to children's inactive lifestyles.
- Of adolescents, 43 percent watch more than 2 hours of television each day.
- Children, especially girls, become less active as they move through adolescence.

Determination of Overweight in Children and Adolescents

- Doctors and other health care professionals are the best people to determine whether your child's or adolescent's weight is healthy, and they can help rule out rare medical problems as the cause of unhealthy weight.
- A body mass index can be calculated from measurements of height and weight. Health professionals often use a BMI "growth chart" to help them assess whether a child or adolescent is overweight.
- A physician will also consider your child's or adolescent's age and growth patterns to determine whether his or her weight is healthy.

General Suggestions

- Let your child know he or she is loved and appreciated whatever his or her weight. An overweight child probably knows better than anyone else that he or she has a weight problem. Overweight children need support, acceptance, and encouragement from their parents.
- Focus on your child's health and positive qualities, not your child's weight.
- Try not to make your child feel different if he or she is overweight but focus on gradually changing your family's physical activity and eating habits.
- Be a good role model for your child. If your child sees you enjoying healthy foods and physical activity, he or she is more likely to do the same now and in the future.
- Realize that an appropriate goal for many overweight children is to maintain their current weight while growing normally in height.

Physical Activity Suggestions

- Be physically active. It is recommended that Americans accumulate at least 30 minutes (adults) or 60 minutes (children) of moderate physical activity most days of the week. Even greater amounts of physical activity may be necessary for the prevention of weight gain, for weight loss, or for sustaining weight loss.
- Plan family activities that provide everyone with exercise and enjoyment.
- Provide a safe environment for your children and their friends to play actively; encourage swimming, biking, skating, ball sports, and other fun activities.
- Reduce the amount of time you and your family spend in sedentary activities, such as watching TV or playing video games. Limit TV time to less than 2 hours a day.

Healthy Eating Suggestions

- Follow the Dietary Guidelines for healthy eating (www.health.gov/dietaryguidelines).
- Guide your family's choices rather than dictate foods.
- Encourage your child to eat when hungry and to eat slowly.
- Eat meals together as a family as often as possible.
- Carefully cut down on the amount of fat and calories in your family's diet.
- Don't place your child on a restrictive diet.

- Avoid the use of food as a reward.
- Avoid withholding food as punishment.
- Even with extremely overweight children, weight loss should be gradual.
- Crash diets and diet pills can compromise growth and are not recommended by many health care professionals.
- Weight lost during a diet is frequently regained unless children are motivated to change their eating habits and activity levels for a lifetime.
- Weight control must be considered a lifelong effort.
- Any weight management program for children should be supervised by a physician.

What's Being Done to Promote Physical Activity and Healthy Weight

Widespread efforts are underway throughout the public and private sectors to develop effective means of combating inactivity and excessive weight in young people.

Excessive weight in this age group has reached epidemic levels. The health consequences for our children, both now and in the future, as well as the health costs of this epidemic are staggering.

Shaping America's Youth is a nationwide initiative to identify and centralize information on what is being done throughout all sectors of American society to reverse the rapidly increasing prevalence of overweight and inactivity among children and adolescents.

To date, Shaping America's Youth has obtained data from over 1,200 parties through a cross-sector survey designed to identify current programs addressing the problem of sedentary lifestyles and unhealthy diets of America's children. This information will be included in a summary report and in a national database. Availability of this information in a single registry will help enable all interested parties—including, but not limited to, health professionals, government agencies, educators, corporations, foundations, and the general public—to focus funding, research, and interventions where they are most needed, most promising, and most effective.

With the support of Nike, McNeil Nutritionals, Campbell Soup Company, and Gerber Products Company, and the involvement of the Office of the United States Surgeon General, the American Academy of Pediatrics, American Diabetes Association, American Obesity Association, and Kaiser Permanente, Shaping America's Youth is creating a comprehensive registry of funding sources, ongoing research, and intervention programs to increase physical activity and healthy eating among children and adolescents. The registry will encompass the efforts of federal and state governments, health and education organizations, and the private sector, including both for-profit and nonprofit entities.

■■ Critical Thinking **QUESTIONS AND ACTIVITIES**

Analyze your own eating habits by charting what you actually eat and drink for 5 days. You may use the following chart to assist you.

	BREAD, CEREAL, RICE, AND PASTA	FRUIT	VEGETABLES	MILK, YOGURT, CHEESE	MEAT, POULTRY, FISH, DRY BEANS, EGGS, NUTS
Day 1					
Day 2					
Day 3					
Day 4					
Day 5					

Ask yourself:

- How many servings of bread, cereal, rice, and pasta did I have each day?
- How many servings of fruit did I have each day?
- How many servings of vegetables did I have each day?
- How many servings of milk, yogurt, and cheese did I have each day?
- How many servings of meat, poultry, fish, dry beans, eggs, and nuts did I have each day?
- How well did I choose the proper foods that I should eat on a daily basis?
- How can I improve my eating habits?

VITAMINS

Vitamins are organic substances that are essential for normal metabolism, growth, and development of the human body. They are complex chemical substances that may be obtained naturally from plants, animals, and sunshine, or they may be made commercially.

Vitamins may be classified as fat-soluble and water-soluble (see Table 18-2). The fat-soluble vitamins are A, D, E, and K. The water-soluble vitamins are thiamine (B_1), riboflavin (B_2), niacin (nicotinic acid), pyridoxin (B_6), folic acid, cyanocobalamin (B_{12}), biotin, and C (ascorbic acid).

The fat-soluble vitamins are stored in adipose tissue and the liver. The water-soluble vitamins are not stored in the body. They are essential to health and need to be replaced on a daily basis. The *United States recommended daily allowance* (USRDA) for each vitamin is given in Table 18-2. When an individual follows these recommended allowances, conditions such as avitaminosis, hypovitaminosis, and hypervitaminosis can be prevented.

Some of the commonly prescribed vitamin products are Theragram, Centrum, Citracal, B–C–Bid, Therabid, Vicon-C, Vicon Forte, Vita-plus H, Nico-400, Os-Cal Forte, cyanocobalamin—vitamin B_{12} (Redisol, Rubramin), folic acid (Folvite), folinic acid (Leucovorin), and vitamin K (AquaMEPHYTON).

MINERALS

Minerals are nonorganic substances that are essential constituents of all body cells. Minerals play an important role in maintaining the water balance of the body (see Table 18-3).

Electrolytes

The body's weight is 60 to 70 percent water. All cells are bathed by an aqueous solution that brings nourishment to the cells and removes wastes. Electrolytes (acids, bases, and salts) are suspended in this solution. Electrolytes are particles that result from disintegration of compounds. They are found dissolved in body fluids as *ions* that carry electrical charges. A cation is an ion with a positive charge of electricity. An anion is an ion with a negative charge of electricity. Cations and anions are involved in metabolic activities, and are essential to the normal function of all cells. The normal fluid state in which positive and negative ions are in balance is called homeostasis.

The chief cations and anions are:

Cations		*Anions*	
NA^+	Sodium	Cl^-	Chloride
K^+	Potassium	HCO_2^-	Carbonate
Ca^{++}	Calcium	HPO_4^-	Phosphate
Mg^{++}	Magnesium	SO_4^-	Sulfate

Selected minerals and their functions, food sources, RDAs, indications of deficiency, and toxicity are described in Table 18-2 in this unit. Minerals are excreted daily from the body; therefore, it is most important to replace them through a well-balanced diet.

Minerals may be grouped as macrominerals and microminerals. Macrominerals are minerals that are required in large amounts. This group includes calcium, phosphorus, magnesium, sodium, potassium, chlorine, and sulfur. Microminerals are minerals that are required in small amounts. They are also known as trace elements. This group includes iron, copper, iodine, manganese, zinc, fluorine, cobalt, chromium, tin, selenium, vanadium, silicon, nickel, and molybdenum.

Spot Check

Vitamins and minerals are very important nutrients that are needed for proper functioning of the human body. For each selected vitamin and mineral, provide the function, and USRDA.

VITAMIN/MINERAL	FUNCTION	USRDA
vitamin A		
vitamin D		
vitamin E		
vitamin C		
folic acid		
sodium		
potassium		

TABLE 18-2 Vitamins

	VITAMIN AND FUNCTION	FOOD SOURCES	USRDA	INDICATIONS OF DEFICIENCY	HYPERVITAMINOSIS
A	Important for healthy mucous membranes, skin, epithelial cells, development of bones and teeth, and for vision in dim light.	Dairy products, fish, liver oils, animal liver, and green and yellow vegetables.	5,000 I.U.	Retarded growth, susceptibility to disease, skin lesions, and night blindness.	Anorexia, loss of hair, pain in long bones, fragility of bones, dry skin, pruritus, and enlarged liver and spleen.
D	Aids in the proper use of calcium and phosphorus in the body.	Ultraviolet rays, dairy products and commercial foods that contain supplemental vitamin D (milk and cereals), and fish liver oils.	400 I.U.	*Childhood:* Rickets. *Adults:* Osteomalacia, muscle spasms, and spontaneous fractures.	Demineralization (softening) of bone, hypercalcemia, calcium deposits in soft tissue, hypertension, diarrhea, and deafness.
E	May promote normal reproduction, and helps in the formation of muscles and red blood cells.	Leafy green vegetables, wheat germ, and margarine.	30 I.U.	Edema, ataxia, and absence of reflexes.	Not definitely known. Large doses may destroy vitamin K in the intestine.
K	Essential in the formation of prothrombin in the liver, which is necessary for normal blood clotting.	Dairy products, leafy green vegetables, cauliflower, soybeans, liver, peas, potatoes, and tomatoes.		Poor blood clotting, even hemorrhage.	
C	Important for maintenance of bones, teeth, and small blood vessels. Prevents scurvy and promotes healing of wounds and formation of protein collagen. Aids in the absorption of calcium. *May* help in preventing the common cold.	Citrus fruits, tomatoes, melons, fresh berries, raw vegetables, and sweet potatoes.	60 mg	Fatigue, irritability, fleeting joint pain, tendency to bruise, and small petechiae under the tongue.	
B_1	Essential for the release of energy from carbohydrates and nerve conduction.	Yeast, wheat germ, lean meats, pork, dried beans and peas, dairy products, poultry, eggs, dark-green vegetables, and whole-grain enriched foods.	1.5 mg	Beriberi, malaise, polyneuritis, and numbness and tingling in the extremities.	
B_2	Essential for cellular oxidation and the storage of energy. Helps maintain the skin and mucous membranes.	Organ meats, lean meats, milk, green vegetables, eggs, poultry, and yeast.	1.7 mg	Skin and lip lesions, seborrheic dermatitis, inflamed tongue, lack of vigor, and ocular changes.	

(continues)

TABLE 18-2 (continued)

VITAMIN AND FUNCTION		FOOD SOURCES	USRDA	INDICATIONS OF DEFICIENCY	HYPERVITAMINOSIS
Niacin	Important for cellular respiration, glycolysis, and lipid synthesis.	Liver, lean meats, fish, poultry, whole grain, and enriched flour and cereals.	20 mg	Pellagra, dermatitis, irritability, dizziness, and skin and mucous membrane lesions.	
B₅	Aids in the metabolism of foods. Also helps the work of certain hormones, and chemicals in the nervous system.	Whole and enriched grain products, dried beans and peas, legumes, dairy products, eggs, organ meats, lean meats, poultry, dark-green vegetables, and fish.	10 mg	Not known.	
B₆	Necessary for the metabolism of amino acids and fatty acids. Also aids in the production of red blood cells.	Muscle meats, liver, yeast, molasses, and whole-grain cereals.	2 mg	Skin lesions, anemia, hypochromic anemia, insomnia, and numbness in extremities.	
B₁₂	Vital for the production of red blood cells and genetic material. Helps the nervous system function properly.	Liver, kidney, milk, fish, and muscle meats.	6 mcg		
Folic Acid	Necessary for the synthesis of amino acids, DNA, and formation of red blood cells.	Liver, yeast, green leafy vegetables, and most food groups.	0.4 mg	Fatigue, sore tongue, low RBC count, and macrocytic anemia.	
Biotin	Regulates amino acid and fatty acid metabolism.	Liver, kidney, egg yolk, yeast, nuts, legumes, and cauliflower.	0.3 mg	Dermatitis, glossitis, anorexia, and muscle pain.	

TABLE 18-3 Minerals

MINERAL AND FUNCTION	FOOD SOURCES	RDA	INDICATIONS OF DEFICIENCY	TOXICITY
Sodium (Na) Chief *cation* in the extracellular fluid. Important for maintaining acid-base balance, regulating osmotic pressure in cells and body fluids, controlling fluid volume in the body. Helps in maintaining normal heart action, regulating muscle, and nerve irritability.	Meats, sardines, cheese, green olives, table salt, baking soda, baking powder, milk, eggs, beets, spinach, and is added to many foods such as nuts, potato chips, soups, butter, breads, cakes, sauces, salad dressings, and cereals.	100–3300 mg/daily	Hyponatremia, loss of weight, weakness, cramps, "salt hunger," and nervous disorders.	Hypernatremia, confusion, and coma.
Potassium (K) Chief *cation* in the intracellular fluid. Helps maintain the acid-base balance. Important in nerve impulse conduction, and muscle tissue excitability.	Cereals, dried peas and beans, fresh vegetables, fresh or dried fruits (especially bananas, prunes, and raisins), sunflower seeds, nuts, meats, molasses, oranges, and orange juice.	50–150 mEq/daily	Hypokalemia, muscle weakness, thirst, dizziness, mental confusion, and arrhythmias.	Hyperkalemia, confusion, and coma.
Calcium (Ca) Plays a key role in blood clotting and lactation. Helps in maintaining acid-base balance. Activates enzymes. Needed for proper functioning of the nerves and muscles. Maintains cell membrane permeability. In combination with phosphorus helps form strong bones and teeth.	Dairy products, beans, cauliflower, egg yolk, molasses, leafy green vegetables, tofu, sardines, clams, and oysters.	800–1200 mEq/daily	Hypocalcemia, brittle bones, poor development of bones and teeth, rickets, tetany, excessive bleeding, and irritability.	Hypercalcemia, gastrointestinal atony, renal stones or failure, psychosis, drowsiness, and lethargy.
Magnesium (Mg) Important in maintaining muscle and nerve irritability. Helps regulate body temperature, and aids in bone and tooth development. Activates certain enzymes.	Widely distributed in foods, especially whole grains, fruits, milk, nuts, vegetables, seafoods, and meats.	400 mg daily	Hypomagnesemia, tetany, muscle tremor and weakness, mental confusion, depression, and ataxia.	Hypermagnesemia, respiratory failure, and cardiac disturbances.

(continues)

TABLE 18-3 (continued)

MINERAL AND FUNCTION	FOOD SOURCES	RDA	INDICATIONS OF DEFICIENCY	TOXICITY
Phosphorus (P) Needed for metabolism of fats, carbohydrates, and proteins. Helps the body extract energy from foods. Important for healthy bones, teeth, and tissues. Helps maintain acid-base balance.	Dairy products, eggs, fish, poultry, meats, dried peas and beans, whole grain cereals, and nuts.	800–1200 mg/daily	Hypophosphatemia, irritability, weakness, retarded growth, poor tooth and bone development, rickets, anorexia, malaise, and pain in bones.	Hyperphosphatemia.
Iron (Fe) Essential to hemoglobin formation. Component of proteins in the blood and muscle.	Liver, soybean flour, muscle meats, dried fruits, egg yolk, enriched breads and cereals, potatoes, and dark-green leafy vegetables.	18 mg/daily	Anemia, dizziness, weakness, fatigue, loss of weight, pallor; spoon-shaped nails, poor resistance to infection, and anorexia.	Hemochromatosis.
Iodine (I) Important in the development and functioning of the thyroid gland, formation of thyroxine (T_4) and triiodothyronine (T_3). Aids in the prevention of goiter.	Seafood and iodized salt.	150 mg/daily	Simple goiter and cretinism.	Occasional myxedema.
Copper (Cu) Helps iron form blood cells and aids to enzyme activity. Helps the central nervous system function properly.	Liver, nuts, shellfish, kidney, fruits, and dried peas and beans.	2 mg/daily	Anemia.	Hepatolenticular degeneration.
Zinc (Zn) Aids in enzyme activity, wound healing, and growth.	Meats, liver, eggs, and seafood.	15 mg/daily	Retarded growth, hypogonadism, anorexia, impaired wound healing, night blindness, and white spots on nails.	

HERBALS AND SUPPLEMENTS

Under the Dietary Supplement Health and Education Act of 1994 (DSHEA), Congress defined the term **dietary supplement** as a product taken by mouth that contains a *dietary ingredient* intended to **supplement** the diet. The dietary ingredients in these products may include vitamins, minerals, herbs or other botanicals, amino acids, and substances such as enzymes, organ tissues, glandulars, and metabolites.

Dietary supplements can also be extracts or concentrates, and may be found in many forms such as tablets, capsules, softgels, gelcaps, liquids, or powders. Under DSHEA, a company is responsible for determining that the dietary supplements it manufactures or distributes are safe and that any representations or claims made about them are substantiated by adequate evidence to show that they are not false or misleading. This means that dietary supplements do not need approval from the Food and Drug Administration (FDA) before they are marketed. Under DSHEA, once the product is marketed, the FDA has the responsibility for showing that a dietary supplement is "unsafe" before it can take action to restrict the product's use or removal from the marketplace.

Herbals and supplements are marketed and used by people interested in more "natural" ways of treating disease. They are available, without a prescription, and sold in a variety of stores. They are frequently viewed as harmless and safer than prescribed drugs. However, most herbs and supplements are not tested by the FDA for safety or effectiveness. Many are not regulated for content, so different products with similar names may be quite different. Because of this, the USP Verification Program for dietary supplements was developed in response to the increasing concerns expressed about dietary supplements in the marketplace. Through compliance testing and document review, adherence to good manufacturing practices (GMPs), and post-marketing surveillance, the USP Verification Program is designed to help ensure that dietary supplement products contain the declared ingredients in the declared quantities. Further information about the USP Verification Program is at www.uspverified.org.

If taking supplements, one should look for the mark earned by dietary supplements that have passed USP's five important quality tests. This mark on a label tells that USP has tested and verified the ingredients, the product, and the manufacturing process. Products that earn the mark undergo a comprehensive testing and evaluation process, backed by USP's 180-year history of scientific leadership. This assures users that the supplement passed the following five important quality tests and that the product:

1. Contains the ingredients stated on the label.
2. Has the declared amount of ingredients.
3. Will disintegrate or dissolve effectively to release nutrients for absorption into your body.
4. Has been screened for harmful contaminants such as pesticides, bacteria, and heavy metals.
5. Has been manufactured using safe, sanitary, and well-controlled procedures.

Any medication, including herbs, can cause allergic reactions and produce side effects. Many herbal supplements contain active ingredients that can be harmful to a patient, especially if taken with certain prescription or over-the-counter drugs. All supplements that contain alcohol could interact with metronidazole (Flagyl) or disulfiram (Antabuse).

Patients should be advised to inform their physician about any herb or supplement they are taking or plan to take, as it could interact adversely with other medications or cause other health changes. A patient pregnant or breast-feeding should talk with her physician *before* taking any herbal product.

It is very important that one should be aware of certain medical situations that could increase the risk of adverse effects of herbal products. Some of these conditions are:

- high blood pressure
- thyroid problems
- depression
- psychiatric problems
- Parkinson's disease
- enlarged prostate gland
- blood-clotting problems
- diabetes

- heart disease
- epilepsy
- glaucoma
- history of stroke
- organ transplant

All patients should be questioned regarding their use of herbal medicines and other alternative therapies when recording or reviewing their medication history. It is important to be aware of the potentially significant adverse effects and drug interactions that may arise due to the use of such therapies (see Table 18-4).

TABLE 18-4 Selected Herbal Preparations, Possible Uses, Side Effects/Adverse Reactions, and Drug Interactions

NAME	POSSIBLE USES	POSSIBLE SIDE EFFECTS/ ADVERSE REACTIONS	POSSIBLE DRUG INTERACTIONS
Echinacea	Stimulate the immune system	Nausea, vomiting, diarrhea, nervous stimulation Hepatotoxic effects with prolonged use	Avoid taking with known hepatotoxic drugs, anabolic steroids, amiodarone, methotrexate, ketoconazole; anticoagulants. Should not be combined with drugs that cause liver damage. May elevate the levels of HIV protease inhibitors, calcium channel blockers, and antianxiety drugs, and may interfere with immunosuppresants.
Feverfew	Prophylaxis of migraines. Comfort and pain relief. Treatment of fever, menstrual problems, asthma, dermatitis, and arthritis	Gastrointestinal discomfort. Discontinuation may produce muscle and joint stiffness and nervous system reactions such as rebound migraine symptoms, anxiety, and poor sleep patterns.	Avoid taking with anticoagulants (may increase risk of bleeding) or aspirin (increases antiplatelet effect).
Garlic	Antiplatelet, antibacterial, antifungal, antihypertensive, antihyperlipidemic, and anti-inflammatory properties. Stimulate the immune system	Gastrointestinal effects, heartburn, flatulence (gas), sweating, light-headedness, allergic reactions, menorrhagia	Avoid taking with anticoagulants (may increase risk of bleeding). May decrease the effectiveness of immunosuppressants and HIV protease inhibitors.
Ginger	Antinauseant, antispasmodic	None noted	Avoid taking with aspirin, ticlopidine (Ticlid), clopidogrel (Plavix), warfarin (Coumadin), H_2 blockers, and proton pump inhibitors. May increase the effect of anticoagulants, which may cause excessive bleeding. May also increase the production of stomach acid, which could counteract the effects of antacid medications. May lower blood pressure or blood sugar levels.

(*continues*)

TABLE 18-4   (*continued*)

NAME	POSSIBLE USES	POSSIBLE SIDE EFFECTS/ ADVERSE REACTIONS	POSSIBLE DRUG INTERACTIONS
Gingko	Increase blood flow. Improve memory. Relieve depression, anxiety, dizziness, headaches	Mild gastrointestinal upset, diarrhea Headache Dizziness, vertigo, fainting	Avoid taking with aspirin, ticlopidine (Ticlid), clopidogrel (Plavix), warfarin (Coumadin), antidepressants, antipsychotic medications, and insulin. May increase the anticoagulant effect of these drugs and has the potential to cause spontaneous and excessive bleeding when used in conjunction with these medications. Can also increase the amount of antidepressant medication in the blood. When combined with antipsychotic medications, gingko may cause seizures. Also affects insulin levels.
Ginseng	Increase endurance and stamina, strengthen mental performance, and boost immune system	Headache, nervousness, agitation, insomnia, diarrhea, fast or irregular heartbeat, skin rash, unusual vaginal bleeding	Avoid taking with warfarin (Coumadin), phenelzine (Nardil), digoxin (Lanoxicaps, Lanoxin), insulin, and oral hypoglycemic agents. Can reduce the blood-thinning effects of Coumadin. May cause headache, trembling, and manic behavior when taken with Nardil. May interfere with digoxin's pharmacologic action or the ability to monitor digoxin's activity. Can reduce blood sugar levels in people with Type 2 diabetes.
Goldenseal	Treat infections of the mouth, lungs, traveler's diarrhea, urinary infections, inflammation, indigestion, cold and flu symptoms	Nausea, vomiting, diarrhea, nervous stimulation	Shown to have coagulant activity. May oppose the action of heparin. May decrease vitamin B absorption.
Kava	Reduce anxiety, stress, restlessness	Tolerance may develop Dry, flaking, discolored skin and reddened eyes with long-term use of high doses Weight loss, muscle weakness, ataxia, liver toxicity	Avoid taking with sedatives, sleeping pills, antipsychotics, alcohol, and drugs used to treat anxiety and Parkinson's disease. Combined with these drugs, kava can produce sleep sedation and, in some cases, even coma.
Melatonin	Improve sleep	Concentration difficulties, dizziness, fatigue, headache, irritability	May not be safe with other drugs that cause drowsiness. May reduce nifedipine's (Adalat, Procardia) ability to lower blood pressure.
Saint John's Wort	Reduce anxiety, depression	May induce photosensitivity, including cataracts Gastrointestinal irritations Allergic reactions Tiredness, restlessness	Avoid taking with any prescription medications. Has been shown to affect the body's metabolism and the metabolism of pharmaceutical medications.

(*continues*)

TABLE 18-4 (*continued*)

NAME	POSSIBLE USES	POSSIBLE SIDE EFFECTS/ ADVERSE REACTIONS	POSSIBLE DRUG INTERACTIONS
Saw palmetto	Treat benign prostatic hyperplasia. Act as diuretic, urinary antiseptic	Gastrointestinal upset	None noted
Valerian	Reduce restlessness and nervous disturbances of sleep, anxiety, gastrointestinal spasm	Sedation Headaches, hangover, excitability, insomnia, uneasiness, cardiac disturbances, ataxia, decreased consciousness of sensation, hypothermia, hallucinations, and increased muscle relaxation	May increase sedative affects of barbiturates, benzodiazepines, opiates, and alcohol.

■ ■ REVIEW QUESTIONS

Directions. Select the best answer to each of the following multiple-choice questions, circling the letter of your choice.

1. A deficiency disease that is due to a lack of vitamins in the diet is known as _____.
    a. hypervitaminosis   b. megadose   c. avitaminosis   d. none of these

2. Nutrients that help regulate body processes such as circulation, respiration, digestion, and elimination are _____.
    a. carbohydrates, fats, and proteins   c. sugars, starch, and fats
    b. vitamins, minerals, and water   d. proteins, vegetables, and fruit

3. A serving size for fruits and vegetables include _____.
    a. $\frac{1}{2}$ cup cooked dry peas or beans
    b. $\frac{1}{2}$ cup dried fruit
    c. 1 cup fruit or vegetable juice
    d. $\frac{1}{4}$ cup canned fruit

4. Plant substances that protect the body by neutralizing free radicals or unstable oxygen molecules are called _____.
    a. anions
    b. phytochemicals
    c. antioxidants
    d. macrominerals

5. Vitamin _____ is important for healthy mucous membranes, skin, epithelial cells, development of bones and teeth, and vision in dim light.
    a. C   b. A   c. D   d. K

6. An indication of vitamin D deficiency is _____.
    a. poor blood clotting   c. rickets
    b. beriberi   d. pellagra

7. Vitamin _____ is important for maintenance of bones, teeth, and small blood vessels. It prevents scurvy and promotes healing of wounds.

    a. B_1 b. E c. D d. C

8. Vitamin _____ is vital for the production of red blood cells and genetic material.

    a. biotin b. niacin c. B_5 d. B_{12}

9. The chief *cations* are _____.

    a. sodium, chloride, calcium, sulfate

    b. sodium, carbonate, magnesium, chloride

    c. sodium, potassium, phosphate, sulfate

    d. sodium, potassium, calcium, magnesium

10. Cereals, dried peas and beans, fresh vegetables, fresh or dried fruits, sunflower seeds, nuts, meats, molasses, oranges, and orange juice are food sources of _____.

    a. sodium b. potassium c. calcium d. iodine

11. Indications of iron deficiency are _____.

    a. simple goiter b. anemia c. hyponatremia d. hypokalemia

12. A(n) _____ is any one of a hundred natural chemical substances present in plants.

    a. physiochemical c. cation

    b. anion d. phytochemical

14. Obesity, diabetes, diseases of the heart and blood vessels, and some forms of cancer are linked to _____.

    a. excercise b. rest c. diet d. sleep

14. _____ are organic substances that are essential for normal metabolism, growth, and development of the human body.

    a. Minerals b. Vitamins c. Electrolytes d. Cations

15. _____ are particles (acids, bases, and salts) that result from disintegration of compounds.

    a. Minerals b. Vitamins c. Electrolytes d. Cations

16. Conditions that could increase the risk of adverse effects of herbal products include _____.

    a. high blood pressure c. thyroid problems

    b. diabetes d. all of these

Matching. Place the correct letter from Column II on the appropriate line of Column I:

Column I		*Column II*
17. _____ USRDA		A. minerals required in large amounts
18. _____ RDA		B. an excessively high amount of body fat in relation to lean body mass
19. _____ minerals		C. U. S. recommended daily allowance
20. _____ obesity		D. an ion with a positive charge of electricity
21. _____ phytochemical		E. an ion with a negative charge of electricity
22. _____ anion		F. any one of a hundred natural chemical substances present in plants
23. _____ cation		G. nonorganic substances that are essential constituents of all body cells
24. _____ macrominerals		H. minerals required in small amounts
25. _____ microminerals		I. the recommended daily allowance.
		J. minerals required in excessive amounts

OBJECTIVES

Upon completing this unit, you should be able to:

- Define the terms listed in the vocabulary.
- Describe the four classifications of psychotropic drugs.
- Define stress.
- State five diseases or conditions that may be implicated in stress.
- Describe symptoms of anxiety.
- List possible stressors for older adults.
- Explain how stress, anxiety, or depression could affect a child.
- Complete the critical thinking questions and activities presented in this unit.
- State the actions, uses, contraindications, adverse reactions, dosages, routes, and implications for patient care of selected antianxiety, antidepressive, antipsychotic, and antimanic agents.
- List the symptoms of marked elevation of blood pressure.
- List the foods and beverages a person should *avoid* when taking monoamine oxidase inhibitors.
- Complete the Spot Check on psychotropic agents.
- Answer the review questions correctly.

VOCABULARY

adrenergic (ad-ren-er′jik). Pertaining to nerve fibers that, when stimulated, release norepinephrine or epinephrine at synapses.

affective (a-fek′tiv). Pertaining to an emotion or mental state; feeling, mood, emotional response.

anticholinergic (an″ti-ko″lin-er′jik). An agent that blocks parasympathetic nerve impulses.

anxiolytic (ang″zi-o-lit′ik). Literally means a dissolution of anxiety.

bioavailability (bi″o-a-val″a-bil′i-te). The rate and extent to which an active agent, drug, or metabolite enters the general circulation. Bioavailability of such a substance is determined either by measuring the concentration of the drug in body fluids (blood) or by the magnitude of the pharmacologic response.

catecholamine (kat″e-kol′a-men). Biochemical substances, epinephrine, norepinephrine, and dopamine, that have a marked effect on the nervous system, cardiovascular system, metabolic rate, temperature, and smooth muscle.

dopamine (do′pa-men). A catecholamine synthesized in adrenergic nerve terminals, the adrenal gland, and other sites in the central nervous system. It acts to increase the force of contraction of the heart and blood pressure, especially the systolic phase. It also increases urinary output.

endogenous (en-doj′e-nus). Pertaining to being produced or arising from within a cell or organism.

extrapyramidal (eks′tra-pi-ram′i-dal). Pertaining to outside the pyramidal tracts of the central nervous system. The extrapyramidal system is involved in body movement and posture.

limbic (lim′bik) **system**. A group of brain structures that is activated by motivated behavior and arousal. The endocrine and autonomic motor nervous systems are influenced by the limbic system.

norepinephrine (nor-ep″i-nef′rin). A hormone produced by the adrenal medulla. It is chiefly a vasoconstrictor.

(continues)

303

orthostatic hypotension (or'tho-stat'ik). A condition in which there is a decrease of systolic and diastolic blood pressure below normal. It is due to a sudden change in body position, especially when arising from a lying position to a standing position.

serotonin (se"ro-ton'in). A chemical present in gastrointestinal mucosa, platelets, mast cells, and carcinoid tumors. It is a vasoconstrictor and affects sleep and sensory perception.

tyramine (ti'ra-men). Intermediate product in the conversion of tyrosine to epinephrine. Tyramine is found in most cheeses, beer, and protein foods that are aged.

INTRODUCTION

Health is defined by the World Health Organization as a state of complete physical, mental, and social well-being. When a deviation from normal occurs in any of these states, a process known as disease, illness, or disorder generally appears.

Mental health may be defined as a state of well-being of the mind. When there is a disturbance in the functioning of the mind, a state of emotional or mental disorder may appear. The exact cause of mental illness is not known. Contributing factors may include genetics, environment, biochemical changes occurring in the brain, and certain drugs.

The treatment of emotional and mental disorders encompasses a wide scope of factors. In this unit, emphasis is given to four classifications of drugs that are prescribed to reduce and control symptoms of emotional disturbances.

The physician determines a diagnosis, and then prescribes a plan of treatment. This plan has to be carefully monitored on a continuous basis to determine the effectiveness of the program. Psychotropic drugs are usually only a part of the prescribed treatment plan. The dosage is individualized for each patient and is carefully evaluated for maximum effectiveness.

Drugs that affect psychic function, behavior, or experience are called *psychotropic*. These drugs may be classified as:

- *Antianxiety agents*. Drugs that counteract or diminish anxiety are called *anxiolytic*.
- *Antidepressant agents*. Drugs that elevate a person's mood.
- *Antimanic agents*. Drugs used to treat the manic episode of bipolar disorder or manic-depressive illness.
- *Antipsychotic agents*. Drugs that modify psychotic behavior are called *neuroleptic*.

Psychotropic drugs are among the most frequently prescribed medications in the United States. It should be noted that these drugs when misused can cause physical and psychological dependence.

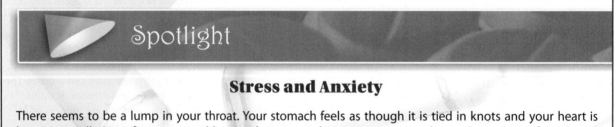

Spotlight

Stress and Anxiety

There seems to be a lump in your throat. Your stomach feels as though it is tied in knots and your heart is beating rapidly. Your fingers are cold as ice, but your palms are sweaty. You know these signs of stress and anxiety, because you have had them before. Stress may be defined as the physical or psychological forces that are experienced by an individual. According to the *Occupational Health and Safety News*, U.S. Chamber of Commerce, U.S. Department of Human Services, and the National Institute on Drug Abuse, an estimated 14 percent of all occupational disease claims were stress-related and carried a cost of approximately $34 billion dollars.

Stress is implicated in immune system dysfunction, cancer, hypertension, heart disease, and ulcers. An agent or condition that is capable of causing stress is called a stressor. Many conditions can be stressors and these will vary with each individual. Finances, health problems, birth, death of a loved one, school, peer pressure, relationships, crime, and things beyond one's control are only a few conditions that may be stressors. It is believed that a certain amount of stress helps the body maintain homeostasis, a state of balance. When stress becomes more powerful than an individual can handle, certain physical symptoms appear.

The body responds to stressful situations the same way it responds to physical danger. It automatically prepares one for combat or retreat. This is known as the "fight-or-flight" response that is produced when the hypothalamus flashes signals through the nervous and endocrine systems. The anterior pituitary gland secretes the hormone adrenocorticotropic (ACTH) into the bloodstream, thereby stimulating the adrenal glands. During this alarm reaction, the adrenal medulla releases epinephrine (adrenaline; Adrenalin) and norepinephrine directly into the bloodstream.

Epinephrine elevates the systolic blood pressure; increases the heart rate and cardiac output; and increases glycogenolysis, thereby hastening the release of glucose from the liver. Through this action, the blood sugar level is elevated and the body is supplied with a "spurt of energy"; it also dilates the bronchial tubes and the pupils. Norepinephrine acts as a vasoconstrictor and elevates the systolic blood pressure.

As stress continues, perspiration increases and the palms become moist. Blood flow is slowed to the extremities and the fingers and toes feel "cold." The digestive process is slowed down, and under prolonged stress, hydrochloric acid within the stomach begins to eat away at the stomach lining. Muscles tense up and breathing may become rapid and then shallow.

Anxiety may be defined as a feeling of uneasiness, apprehension, worry, or dread. It is an involuntary or reflex reaction of the body to stress. When its negative effects cause a change in one's behavior or performance and it continues for a long period of time, persistent underlying anxiety may be diagnosed.

It is important to recognize the symptoms of stress and anxiety, and to find out what is causing the symptoms. Once this is done, the stressor or stressors may be eliminated. If not, the individual must learn to cope with the situation. Developing coping skills is a technique that one can learn. Find out what works for you, such as taking a warm bath or shower, talking to a friend, taking a walk, reading a book, and so on.

You have heard the saying "laughter is the best medicine". As a way to relieve stress and anxiety, laughter certainly can work wonders. Try it. Just laugh out loud and see how you feel.

Symptoms of Anxiety

Physical:

fast heart rate	nausea
palpitations	dyspepsia
shortness of breath	diarrhea
hot flashes	cold, sweaty, tremulous hands
chills	smothering sensation
dry mouth	frequent urination
dizziness	lump in throat
light-headedness	band-like pressure about the head

Emotional:

irritability	extreme feeling of worry
keyed-up feeling	inability to concentrate
problems with sleeping	

Tension:

restlessness	trembling, twitching, or feeling shaky
fatigue	

■■ Special Considerations: **OLDER ADULTS**

For older adults, stress is many times just a part of daily life. With the increase in health care cost and the cost of just about everything, the "worries" of how one is going to pay the bills on a fixed income can be a major stressor of daily living. Other stressors that may affect older adults are related to health problems, loss of physical and mental abilities, death of a spouse, and loneliness. How older adults adjust to stress is an individual process and depends upon many factors. When one cannot control stress or adapt to it, overload can occur and certain symptoms signal that it is time for one to say, "I must do something about this."

The Symptoms of Stress Overload

- headache
- stomachache
- sleeplessness

- backache
- irritability (snapping at others)
- forgetfulness

What can older adults do about reducing stress? Naturally, this is going to depend on the cause of the stress and the individual.

General Guidelines for Reducing Stress

- Analyze your financial situation. Make a budget that works for you. Plan for unexpected expenses.
- Take control. When one has control over situations in his/her life, then stress is reduced and the harmful effects of stress can be lessened.
- Reach out to others. Sharing feelings and concerns often lessens the burden and stress is reduced. Try to do something nice for someone else each day.
- Develop healthy habits. A good diet, rest, and exercise help to control stress. Avoid heavy use of alcohol, tobacco, caffeine, and self-medication.
- Strive for balance. Include time for yourself each day. Work hard, but also learn to play hard. Do work that you are capable of doing, that you really enjoy.
- Avoid negative thoughts. Learn to think positively.
- Be realistic—don't expect too much of yourself. Take things one at a time.
- Keep fit emotionally. Know your own strengths and weaknesses. Get involved in things that you are comfortable doing. Avoid things that are unpleasant for you.
- Find out where to go for help if and when you need assistance. The local mental health center or hospital(s) may offer services for reducing stress. In addition to your physician, there are many professionals who deal with stress such as psychiatrists, psychologists, clergy, social workers, nurses, mental health counselors, or state or local health associations. Do not be afraid to get help when help is needed.
- It has been shown that having a pet reduces stress. There are programs that have adopted this theory and place pets in nursing homes and other long-term care facilities. Pets give love and seek very little in return. They can provide comfort and companionship. It has been shown that they may lower blood pressure, reduce feelings of loneliness, and provide older adults with a purpose in life.

Older adults should have a complete physical examination regularly. There is more evidence that mental health plays a role in physical health: A study found that skin wounds heal more slowly in people suffering chronic stress. The findings suggest that stress reduction might speed healing in people who are recovering from accidents or surgery, according to researchers at Ohio State University in Columbus. The study involved 13 women age 47 to 81 who were caring for relatives with dementia and who scored high on tests of psychological stress, and 13 women who were not caregivers and who scored low on stress tests. Researchers removed a tiny piece of skin from their forearms. The women in the no-stress group healed after 39 days and the stressed group took 10 days longer. It is unclear how stress may slow healing, but researchers noted that the women under stress had lower levels of an immune system compound called interleukin-1 beta, which is known to play a role in wound repair.

◼ Special Considerations: **CHILDREN**

At some time in life, almost every individual experiences stress and/or depression. Experts have known that adolescents are as prone to depression as adults. Recently they have begun to realize that children as young as 3 and 4 can experience the blues. Clinical depression affects roughly 2.5 percent of school-age children. When a child generally behaves well and then suddenly becomes irritable or disrespectful, one should suspect a medical or psychological problem. Children who are depressed will typically "act up" and undergo a total behavior change. The usual calm child may turn demonstrably angry; the happy-go-lucky child may become sullen and hide in a corner, closet, basement, or some other part of the house.

Symptoms of Depression in the Child

- *Toddlers:* sadness; inactivity; stomachaches; and in rare cases, self-destructive behavior.
- *Elementary school-age children:* unhappiness; poor school performance; irritability; refusal to take part in activities one used to enjoy; occasional thoughts of suicide.
- *Adolescents:* sadness; withdrawal; feelings of hopelessness or guilt; changes in sleeping or eating habits; frequent thoughts of suicide.

Children do not understand feelings of stress, anxiety, or depression. They do not know how to ask for help, so when children exhibit dramatic mood or behavior shifts, a physician should be consulted immediately. A physician may recommend psychotherapy or prescribe an antidepressant for children who are at least 5 years of age or older.

◼ Critical Thinking **QUESTIONS/ACTIVITIES**

Your patient is a 66-year-old female who has been admitted with pneumonia. You recognize her as being one of your former instructors from college. She seems to be irritable and complains of a headache and stomachache. She states, "I just can't get a good night's sleep anymore. I wake up around 3 o'clock in the morning, and I just can't go back to sleep. This is wearing me out." You recall that it had been about three months since the death of her husband. Using the information in Special Considerations: Older Adults, ask yourself:

- What do the symptoms—headache, stomachache, irritability, and sleeplessness—signal?
- What are some of the factors that cause this condition in older adults?
- Which of the guidelines for reducing stress would benefit my patient?
- How am I going to discuss these guidelines with my patient? What approach should I use?
- What are some available community resources that deal with stress? Should I provide the addresses and telephone numbers for such resources?

ANTIANXIETY AGENTS

Antianxiety agents are chemical substances that relieve anxiety and muscle tension. They are indicated when anxiety interferes with a person's ability to function properly. *Anxiety* may be defined as a feeling of uneasiness, apprehension, worry, or dread. It is an involuntary or reflex reaction of the body to stress. The signs and symptoms of anxiety vary with the cause and an individual's response to the distressing situation. The physiologic signs may include palpitation, heart pain, nausea, anorexia, dyspepsia, constriction of the throat, muscle tension, pressure about the head, and cold, sweaty, tremulous hands. The psychological symptoms may include feelings of nervousness, apprehension, tension, inadequacy, indecisiveness, and insomnia.

Benzodiazepines

Benzodiazepines are a group of drugs with similar chemical structures and pharmaceutical activities. They are the most widely prescribed drugs for the treatment of anxiety.

Actions

The precise mechanism of action of the benzodiazepines is not known. They appear to exert their primary action on the limbic system (a group of brain structures, including the hippocampus that is activated by motivated behavior and arousal). The benzodiazepines suppress the response to conflict or aggression in animals; they produce muscle relaxation and control induced seizures in experimental test models.

Uses

Benzodiazepines are used for the management of anxiety disorders, for the short-term relief of symptoms of anxiety, withdrawal symptoms of acute alcoholism, and preoperative apprehension and anxiety.

Contraindications

Hypersensitivity to benzodiazepines.

Adverse Reactions

Drowsiness, daytime sedation, ataxia, dizziness, fatigue, muscle weakness, dryness of the mouth, nausea, vomiting, increased irritability, insomnia, hyperactivity, and blood dyscrasia.

Dosage and Route

The dosage and route of administration are determined by the physician. The dosage is individualized for each patient and regulated according to the effectiveness of the medication. See Table 19-1 for selected benzodiazepines.

Implications for Patient Care

Observe the patient for any signs of hypersensitivity. Note the effectiveness of the drug. Are the signs and symptoms improved? Observe for adverse reactions. Be especially aware of possible signs of blood dyscrasia such as a sore throat, fever, purpura, jaundice, or excessive and progressive weakness. Report any adverse reactions to the proper authority or to the physician. In geriatric or debilitated patients, be especially aware of signs of confusion, drowsiness, and ataxia. Provide adequate protection.

 Patient Teaching

Inform the patient that benzodiazepines may impair mental or physical abilities; therefore, one should not operate machinery or drive a motor vehicle while on these medications. Teach the patient that alcohol and other central nervous system depressants have an additive effect and should not be used while on these medications. Teach the patient that smoking may enhance the metabolism of benzodiazepines and larger doses may be needed to maintain a sedative effect. Advise patients who smokes to discuss this matter with their physician.

Inform the patient that physical dependence may occur. Withdrawal symptoms will be similar to those produced by dependence on alcohol or barbiturates. Insomnia, anxiety, irritability, headache, muscle tremor, weakness, anorexia, nausea, and vomiting are symptoms of withdrawal from an addictive substance. Instruct the

TABLE 19-1 Selected Benzodiazepines

GENERIC NAME	TRADE NAME	ROUTE	USUAL DOSAGE		
alprazolam	Xanax	Oral:	*Adults:*	0.25 to 2 mg t.i.d.	
			Pediatrics or debilitated patients:		
				0.25 mg b.i.d. or t.i.d.	
clonazepam	Klonopin	Oral:	*Adults:*	0.5 mg t.i.d.; may increase by 0.5 to 1 mg every 3rd day. Total daily maintenance dose not to exceed 20 mg	
				Panic disorder:	
				0.125 mg b.i.d.; increase after 3 days toward target dose of 1 mg/day	
			Children:	Up to 10 yrs old or 30 kg:	
				Initial dose of 0.01 to 0.03 mg/kg/day (not to exceed 0.05 mg/kg/day) given in 2 to 3 equally divided doses; increase by no more than 0.25 to 0.5 mg every 3rd day until therapeutic blood levels are reached (not to exceed 0.2 mg/kg/day)	
clorazepate	Tranxene	Oral:	*Adults:*	15 to 60 mg daily in divided doses	
				For elderly or debilitated:	
				7.5 to 15 mg daily in divided doses	
chlordiazepoxide HCl	Librium	Oral:	*Adults:*	Mild and moderate anxiety:	
				5 to 10 mg t.i.d. or q.i.d.	
				Severe anxiety:	
				20 to 25 mg t.i.d. or q.i.d.	
			Pediatrics or debilitated patients:		
				5 mg 2 to 4 times daily	
			Children:	6 to 12 years old:	
				5 mg 2 to 4 times daily	
				May be increased in some children to 10 mg 2 to 3 times daily	
diazepam	Valium	Oral:	*Adults:*	2 to 10 mg 2 to 4 times daily	
			Pediatrics or debilitated patients:		
				2 to 2.5 mg 1 to 2 times daily	
			Children:	6 months and older:	
				1 to 2.5 mg 3 to 4 times daily	
lorazepam	Ativan	Oral:	*Adults:*	2 to 6 mg daily in 2 to 3 divided doses	
			Pediatrics or debilitated patients:		
				1 to 2 mg/day in divided doses	
oxazepam	Serax	Oral:	*Adults:*	Mild and moderate anxiety:	
				10 to 15 mg t.i.d. or q.i.d.	
				Severe anxiety:	
				15 to 30 mg t.i.d.	
			Pediatrics or debilitated patients:		
				10 mg t.i.d.	

patient to take the medication as ordered. If the prescribed dosage does not produce the desired results, the patient should notify his or her physician. One should not stop taking the drug abruptly.

Benzodiazepines should be kept out of the reach of children or those who may have a tendency to abuse drugs. ■

Warning:

Benzodiazepines have been used in suicide attempts. When taken in large amounts, and mixed with alcohol or other central nervous system depressants, the effects may be fatal.

Preexisting depression may emerge or worsen during the use of benzodiazephines.

Use of benozodiazepines alone and in combination with other central nervous system (CNS) depressants may lead to potentially fatal respiratory depression.

Use of benzodiapines may lead to physical and psychological dependence.

Patients should be advised to inform their physician about:

- All over-the-counter drugs being taken.
- Any plans to become pregnant.
- Being pregnant.
- Presently breast-feeding.
- All other prescription medications being taken.
- Consumption of alcohol.

ANTIDEPRESSANT AGENTS

Antidepressant agents are chemical substances that relieve the symptoms of depression. They are indicated when depression interferes with a person's ability to function properly. The signs and symptoms of depression vary with the cause and each individual. Most individuals experience some form of depression during their lifetime. When the feelings of depression occur every day and persist for weeks, then a severe depressive illness may be present. This form of depression is called an affective disorder.

An **affective** *disorder* is characterized by a disturbance of mood, accompanied by a manic or depressive syndrome. This syndrome is not caused by any other physical or mental disorder. *Mood* is a pervasive and sustained emotion that may play a key role in an individual's perception of the world. With depression, there is generally a loss of interest in food, sex, work, family, friends, and hobbies. Feelings of helplessness, worthlessness, and guilt prevail in a person with this form of depression. Suicide is often contemplated or attempted.

There are various forms of depression. Depression is one of the most common illnesses in America today. It is estimated that 18 million Americans are affected by clinical depression every year. Twenty-five percent of all women and 13 percent of men suffer at least one episode of serious depression during their lifetimes. It is estimated that 20 percent to 40 percent of older adults experience depressive symptoms, with the highest rates of depression found among those who are medically ill or in long-term care. Depression is not something that occurs normally as a result of aging or illness. In three out of ten older adults with depression, the depression is related to treatable physical illness, or adverse effects of medications. For others, it is a recurring and disabling illness that is unrelated to any other health problem or medications.

When depression lasts more than a few weeks and gets in the way of living, it is more than a mood. It is an illness that needs to be treated by a professional. The symptoms of clinical depression include a deep sense of sadness, a noticeable change in appetite or sleep patterns, a loss of interest in pleasurable activities, fatigue or loss of energy, a feeling of worthlessness, recurrent thoughts of death or suicide, as well as other possible symptoms.

Clinical Depression Test

If one answers yes to five or more of the following questions and if the symptoms described have been present nearly every day for 2 weeks or more, one should seek professional assistance:

- Are there persistent feelings of sadness, emptiness, pessimism, or anxiety?
- Are there feelings of helplessness, hopelessness, guilt, or worthlessness?
- Is it difficult to make decisions, concentrate, or remember?
- Is there loss of interest or pleasure in everyday activities?
- Is there loss of drive or energy?
- Is there a significant change in sleep patterns (insomnia, early-morning waking, oversleeping)?
- Is there a significant change in appetite or weight change when not dieting?
- Are there symptoms such as headache, stomachache, backache, or chronic aches and pains of the joints and muscles? Sometimes depressive disorders masquerade as chronic physical symptoms that do not respond to treatment.
- Are there feelings of restlessness or irritability?
- Is there a significant change in smoking and drinking habits?
- Are there thoughts about death or suicide?

For more information on depression, you can call The National Institutes of Mental Health's hotline at 1-800-421-4211.

The physician who diagnoses and prescribes treatment for depression carefully evaluates each individual. After an accurate diagnosis is made, the physician may prescribe antidepressant agents as part of the patient's treatment regimen.

Classification of Antidepressant Agents

Antidepressant agents may be grouped as selective serotonin reuptake inhibitors (SSRIs), serotonin-norepinephrine reuptake inhibitor (SNRI), tricyclic antidepressants (TCAs), monamine oxidase inhibitors (MAOIs), lithium carbonate, atypical antipsychotics, and miscellaneous drugs.

- *Selective serotonin reuptake inhibitors.* Drugs in this group specifically block reabsorption of serotonin. The most widely known are fluoxetine (Prozac), sertraline (Zoloft), paroxetine (Paxil), and fluvoxamine (Luvox).
- *Serotonin-norepinephrine reuptake inhibitor.* Venlafaxine (Effexor) is an antidepressant that inhibits the reuptake of both serotonin and norepinephrine.
- *Tricyclic antidepressants.* Drugs in this group raise the level of norepinephrine and serotonin in the brain by slowing the rate at which they are reabsorbed by nerve cells. There are many drugs in this group, and examples are imipramine (Tofranil) and nortriptyline (Pamelor).
- *Monoamine oxidase inhibitors.* Drugs in this group work by blocking the breakdown of two potent neurotransmitters—norepinephrine and serotonin—and by allowing them to bathe the nerve endings for an extended length of time. There are many drugs in this group, and examples are phenelzine (Nardil) and tranylcypromine (Parnate).
- *Lithium carbonate.* Although this is not a group of drugs, various lithium medications control mood disorders by directly affecting internal nerve cell processes in all the neurotransmitter systems. Lithium is best known as an antimanic drug used in the treatment of bipolar disorder.

- *Atypical antipsychotics.* Drugs in this group affect serotonin and dopamine. The most commonly prescribed are risperidone (Risperdal), clozapine, and olanzapine (Zyprexa).

- *Miscellaneous drugs.* There are many newly created drugs for treating depression. Some of these drugs are used for other illnesses and are being tested for treating depression; then there are those that do not fit into any of the described groups. Examples are pramipexole (Mirapex), bupropion (Wellbutrin), and mirtazapine (Remeron).

  Pramipexole (Mirapex) is a drug used to treat Parkinson's disease. It is currently being tested as an antidepressant. It is believed that the drug affects the D-3 dopamine receptor and elevates mood.

  Bupropion (Wellburtin) is a monocyclic aminoketone used for the treatment of major depression, bipolar depression, chronic fatigue syndrome, cocaine addiction, nicotine addiction, and ADHD (attention deficit/hyperactivity disorder). It increases the supply of norepinephrine and dopamine to the brain and is a stimulant to brain activity. It is contraindicated in patients with a seizure disorder, in patients being treated with Syban, and in patients with a current or prior diagnosis of bulimia or anorexia nervosa because of a higher incidence of seizures noted in these types of patients.

  Mirtazapine (Remeron) stimulates norepinephrine and serotonin release while also blocking two specific serotonin receptors (5-HT2 and 5-HT3).

Antidepressants and Suicide Warning

The Food and Drug Administration (FDA) has asked makers of 10 drugs to add or strengthen suicide-related warnings on their labels. The drugs of concern are Prozac, Paxil, Zoloft, Effexor, Celexa, Lexapro, Luvox, Remeron, and Wellbutrin. The FDA asked for explicit explanations of worrisome behavior changes to be placed in bold print under the prominent "warnings" section of those labels for such changes as agitation, anxiety, irritability, and recklessness. Physicians who prescribe any of these medications should monitor their patients closely for warning signs of suicide, especially when they first start the drug or change a dose.

> **Warning:**
>
> *Close observation of adult and pediatric patients for worsening depression or the emergence of suicidality when treated with Prozac (fluoxetine); Paxil (paroxetine); Zoloft (sertraline); Effexor (venlafoxine); Celexa (citalopram); Lexapro (escitalopram); Luvox (fluvoxamine); Remeron (mirtazapine); and Wellbutrin (bupropion).*

Selective Serotonin Reuptake Inhibitors (SSRIs)

Selective serotonin reuptake inhibitors are the result of research to find drugs that were as effective as tricyclic antidepressants but with fewer safety and tolerability problems. The SSRIs selectively inhibit serotonin reuptake and result in a potentiation of serotonergic neurotransmission. They are structurally diverse, with variations in their pharmacodynamic and pharmacokinetic profiles.

Actions

Specifically block reabsorption of serotonin. Inhibit neuronal reuptake of serotonin in the central nervous system (CNS), thus potentiating the activity of serotonin.

Uses

Depression, social anxiety disorder, obsessive compulsive disorder (OCD), and panic disorder (PD).

Contraindications

Hypersensitivity and concurrent Monoamine Oxidase inhibitor therapy (may result in serious potentially fatal reactions).

Adverse Reactions

Anxiety, dizziness, drowsiness, headache, insomnia, weakness, agitation, amnesia, confusion, constipation, diarrhea, dry mouth, nausea, sweating, tremor, ejaculatory disturbances, decreased libido, genital disorders, weight gain, weight loss, chills, and fever.

Dosage and Route

The dosage and route is determined by the physician. The dosage is individualized for each patient and regulated according to the effectiveness of the medication (see Table 19-2).

Implications for Patient Care

Observe the patient for any signs of hypersensitivity. Note the effectiveness of the drug. Are the symptoms improved? Observe for adverse reactions. Report any adverse reactions to the proper authority or to the physician. Monitor appetite and nutrition intake. Weigh weekly. Note weight gain or loss. Evaluate the patient for history of drug abuse and be aware of the possibility of misuse or abuse. **Be aware and ever alert to the possibility of suicide**.

 Patient Teaching

Inform patients that SSRIs may impair mental or physical abilities; therefore, they should not operate machinery or drive a motor vehicle. Advise patients to inform the physician if they are taking or plan to take any prescription or over-the-counter medication or alcohol. A female patient should advise the physician if she becomes pregnant, intends to become pregnant, or if she is breast-feeding an infant.

Instruct patients to take the medication as ordered. Inform patients to keep the medication out of the reach of children and to report any adverse reaction. Encourage patients to seek medical attention if symptoms do not improve. ◼

Serotonin-Norepinephrine Reuptake Inhibitor (SNRIs)

Serotonin-norepinephrine reuptake inhibitor such as venlafaxine (Effexor) are antidepressants that inhibit the reuptake of both serotonin and norepinephrine.

Effexor (venlafaxine HCl)

Effexor is a structurally novel antidepressant for oral administration. It is chemically unrelated to tricyclic, tetracyclic, or other available antidepressant agents.

Actions

It is believed that venlafaxine potentiates neurotransmitter activity of the central nervous system. It inhibits serotonin and norepinephrine reuptake and is a weak inhibitor of dopamine reuptake.

Uses

Indicated for the treatment of depression, generalized anxiety disorders (GAO), and social anxiety disorders (SAD) in adults.

TABLE 19-2 Selective Serotonin Reuptake Inhibitors

GENERIC NAME	TRADE NAME	ROUTE	USUAL DOSAGE	
fluoxetine	Prozac	Oral:	*Adults:*	Initially 20 mg/day in the morning. May be increased if needed after several weeks. Doses greater than 20 mg/day are given in 2 divided doses (morning and noon). Maximum dose is 80 mg/day.
			Geriatrics:	Initially 10 mg/day in the morning. May be increased, not to exceed 60 mg/day
fluvoxamine	Luvox	Oral:	*Adults:*	Initially 50 mg daily at bedtime. May increase by 50 mg every 4 to 7 days until desired effect is achieved. If daily dose is 100 mg or larger, give in 2 equally divided doses or give a larger dose at bedtime (not to exceed 300 mg/day).
			Children:	8 to 17 yrs: 25 mg at bedtime. May increase by 25 mg/day every 4 to 7 days (not to exceed 200 mg/day)
paroxetine	Paxil	Oral:	Depression:	
			Adults:	20 mg as a single dose in the morning. May be increased by 10 mg/day at weekly intervals (range 20 to 50 mg)
			Geriatrics:	Initially 10 mg/day. May be slowly increased (not to exceed 40 mg/day)
			Obsessive-compulsive disorder:	
			Adults:	Initially 20 mg/day. May increase by 10 mg/day every week up to 40 mg (range 40 to 60 mg/day)
			Panic disorder:	
			Adults:	Initially 10 mg/day. May increase by 10 mg/day every week up to 40 mg (not to exceed 60 mg/day)
sertraline	Zoloft	Oral:	Depression/obsessive-compulsive disorder:	
			Adults:	Initially 50 mg/day as a single dose in the morning or evening. After several weeks may be increased at weekly intervals up to 200 mg/day, depending on response
			Obsessive-compulsive disorder:	
			Children:	13 to 27 yrs: 50 mg once daily 6 to 12 yrs: 25 mg once daily
			Panic disorder:	
			Adults:	Initially 25 mg/day. May increase after 1 week to 50 mg/day

Contraindications

Hypersensitivity to venlafaxine.

Adverse Reactions

General weakness, sweating, nausea, constipation, anorexia, vomiting, sleepiness, dry mouth, dizziness, nervousness, anxiety, tremor, blurred vision, abnormal ejaculation or orgasm in men, and impotence.

Dosage and Route

Effexor is an oral antidepressant drug and the dosage is prescribed by the physician. The recommended starting dose is 75 mg/day. Depending on tolerability and the need for further clinical effect, the dose may be increased to 150 mg/day. When discontinuing Effexor after more than 1 week of therapy, it is generally recommended that the dose be tapered to minimize the risk of discontinuation symptoms. Patients who have received Effexor for 6 weeks or more should have their dose tapered gradually over a 2-week period.

Implications for Patient Care

Observe the patient for signs of hypersensitivity. Note the effectiveness of the drug. Are the symptoms improved? Observe for adverse reactions. Report any adverse reactions to the proper authority. Evaluate the patient for history of drug abuse and be aware of the possibility of misuse or abuse. Be aware and ever alert to the possibility of suicide.

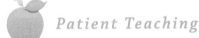

Patient Teaching

Inform the patient that Effexor may impair mental or physical abilities; therefore, one should not operate machinery or drive a motor vehicle. Advise patients to inform the physician if they are taking or plan to take any prescription or over-the-counter medication or alcohol. The patient should advise the physician if she becomes pregnant, intends to become pregnant, or is breast-feeding an infant. If the patient has high blood pressure, he or she should inform the physician, as Effexor can cause sustained increases in blood pressure. If the patient has liver or kidney disease, or a history of seizures, the physician should be informed before initiation of drug therapy.

Instruct the patient to take the medication as ordered. Inform the patient to keep the medication out of reach of children.

Inform the patient to report any adverse reactions to this medication, especially a rash or hives.

Encourage the patient to seek medical attention if symptoms do not improve. ■

FDA ALERT: Potentially Life-Threatening Serotonin Syndrome with Combined Use of SSRIs or SNRIs and Triptan Medications

There is the potential for life-threatening serotonin syndrome (a syndrome of changes in mental status, autonomic instability, neuromuscular abnormalities, and gastrointestinal symptoms) in patients taking 5-hydroxytryptamine receptor agonists (triptans) and selective serotonin reuptake inhibitors (SSRIs) or selective serotonin/norepinephrine reuptake inhibitors (SNRIs) concomitantly. This information is based on reports of serotonin syndrome occurring in patients treated with triptans and SSRIs/SNRIs, and the biological plausibility of such a reaction in people receiving two serotonergic medications. The FDA recommends that patients treated concomitantly with a triptan and an SSRI/SNRI be informed of the possibility of serotonin syndrome (which may be more likely to occur when starting or increasing the dose of an SSRI, SNRI, or triptan) and be carefully followed.

● Note

Triptans are a family of tryptamine-based drugs used as abortive medication in the treatment of migraine and cluster headaches. Examples include naratriptan (Amerge), almotriptan (Axert), sumatriptan (Imitrex), and rizatriptan (Maxalt). Tryptamine is a monoamine alkaloid found in plants, fungi, and animals. It is also the backbone for a group of compounds known collectively as tryptamines. This group includes many biologically active compounds, including neurotransmitters and hallucinogens. The most well-known tryptamines are serotonin, an important neurotransmitter, and melatonin, a hormone involved in regulating the sleep-wake cycle. ●

Health care providers should be alert to the highly variable signs and symptoms of serotonin syndrome. Common signs and symptoms of serotonin syndrome include restlessness, hallucinations, coma, loss of coordination, nausea, vomiting, diarrhea, fast heartbeat, fast changes in blood pressure, increased body temperature, and overactive reflexes.

If concomitant treatment with an SSRI or SNRI and triptan is clinically warranted, the patient should be carefully observed, particularly during treatment initiation and dose increases.

Tricyclic Antidepressants

Tricyclic antidepressants share a chemical configuration that is characterized by a three-ring or tricyclic structure. They are used in the treatment of depression.

Actions

The precise mechanism of action in humans is not known. These agents are believed to block norepinephrine and serotonin reuptake shortly after administration. Reuptake into nerve terminals is the primary mechanism for the termination of the action of norepinephrine and serotonin. They seem to elevate mood, increase physical activity and mental alertness, and improve appetite and sleep. In 60 to 70 percent of patients with endogenous depression, morbid preoccupation was reduced. Anticholinergic and alpha-adrenergic blocking activities are adverse actions to note.

Uses

Tricyclic antidepressants are used for the relief of symptoms of depression. Endogenous depression is more likely to be alleviated than other depressive states.

Contraindications

Hypersensitivity to tricyclic antidepressants.

Adverse Reactions

The most common adverse reactions of these agents are due to their blocking of parasympathetic nerve impulses (anticholinergic) and alpha-adrenergic blocking activities: flushing, diaphoresis, blurred vision, disturbance of accommodation, increased intraocular pressure, constipation, paralytic ileus, urinary retention, and dilatation of urinary tract.

Other adverse reactions that may occur are hypotension, particularly orthostatic hypotension; hypertension; tachycardia; palpitation; confusion; excitement; anxiety; insomnia; numbness, tingling and paresthesias of the extremities; ataxia; tremors; seizures; skin rash; nausea; vomiting; anorexia; diarrhea; dizziness; fatigue; headache; weight gain or loss; and drowsiness.

● **Note**

> **Cimetidine (Tagamet) may increase the bioavailability of certain tricyclic antidepressants. This drug interaction may produce severe anticholinergic adverse reactions, such as dizziness and orthostatic hypotension.** ●

Dosage and Route

The dosage and route are prescribed by the physician and individualized for each patient. See Table 19-3 for selected tricyclic antidepressants.

Implications for Patient Care

Observe the patient for any signs of hypersensitivity. Note the effectiveness of the drug. Are the symptoms improved? Observe for adverse reactions. Report any adverse reactions to the proper authority or to the physician.

TABLE 19-3 Selected Tricyclic Antidepressants

GENERIC NAME	TRADE NAME	ROUTE	USUAL DOSAGE		
desipramine HCl	Norpramin	Oral:	*Adults:*	100 to 200 mg daily	
			Adolescent and geriatrics:		
				25 to 100 mg daily	
imipramine HCl	Tofranil	Oral:	*Adults:*	Outpatients:	
				75 to 150 mg daily	
				Hospitalized patients:	
				100 to 300 mg daily	
			Adolescent and geriatrics:		
				30 to 40 mg daily; not to exceed 100 mg/day	
nortriptyline HCl	Pamelor	Oral:	*Adults:*	25 mg 3 to 4 times daily, up to 150 mg/day	
			Geriatrics:	30 to 50 mg/day in divided doses	
			Children:	12 yrs and older:	
				25 to 20 mg/day or 1 to 3 mg/kg/day in divided doses initially	
			Children:	6 to 12 yrs:	
				10 to 20 mg/day or 1 to 3 mg/kg/day in divided doses	
trimipramine maleate	Surmontil	Oral:	*Adults:*	Outpatients:	
				75 to 150 mg daily in divided doses	
				Hospitalized patients:	
				100 to 200 mg daily in divided doses	
			Adolescent and geriatrics:		
				50 to 100 mg/day	

Patient Teaching

Inform the patient that tricyclic antidepressants may impair mental or physical abilities or both; therefore, one should not operate machinery or drive a motor vehicle. Advise the patient not to arise suddenly. Teach the patient that alcohol and other central nervous system depressants have an additive effect and should not be used while taking these medications.

Instruct the patient to take the medications as ordered. Inform the patient to keep these medications out of the reach of children.

Inform the patient to report any adverse reactions to his or her physician. Encourage the patient to seek medical attention if symptoms do not improve. ■

Caution:

Tricyclic antidepressants should not be given together with monoamine oxidase inhibitors. When it is desired to replace a monoamine oxidase inhibitor with one of these agents, a minimum of 14 days should be allowed to elapse after the tricyclic antidepressant is discontinued.

The possibility of suicide in patients with depression remains until significant remission occurs. Potentially suicidal people should not have access to a large quantity of these agents.

Monoamine Oxidase Inhibitors

Monoamine oxidase inhibitors are antidepressants that inhibit the oxidase enzyme that breaks down monoamine transmitters (such as norepinephrine) in the body. They may be considered as the drugs of choice in such nonendogenous types of depression as agoraphobia and hysteroid dysphoria. They appear to be less effective than the tricyclic antidepressants in patients with endogenous depression, and their use generally requires strict dietary control.

Actions

Inhibit the monoamine oxidase enzyme that catalyzes the inactivation of catecholamines such as serotonin, norepinephrine, and dopamine, thereby increasing the brain concentrations of these substances. In theory, this increased concentration of monoamines in the brain stem is the basis for the antidepressant activity of Monoamine oxidase inhibitors. *In vivo* and *in vitro* studies demonstrated inhibition of amine-oxidase in the brain, heart, and liver.

Uses

May be used in agoraphobia, in hysteroid dysphoria, and in patients who have not responded to treatment with tricyclic antidepressants.

Contraindications

- In patients with known hypersensitivity to the drug.
- In patients with cerebrovascular defects or cardiovascular disorders.
- In the presence of pheochromocytoma.
- In combination with Monoamine oxidase inhibitors or with dibenzazepine-related entities, such as amoxapine.
- In combination with sympathomimetics.
- In combination with meperidine.
- In combination with cheese or other foods with a high tyramine content.
- In patients undergoing elective surgery.
- In patients with impaired renal or liver function.
- In combination with narcotics, alcohol, and hypotensive agents.
- with antiparkinsonism drugs.

Adverse Reactions

Orthostatic hypotension, drowsiness, dryness of the mouth, blurred vision, dysuria, constipation, restlessness, insomnia, weakness, nausea, diarrhea, abdominal pain, tachycardia, anorexia, edema, palpitation, chills, impotence, headache, dizziness, vertigo, tremors, muscle twitching, and photosensitivity are some of the adverse reactions.

Dosage and Route

The dosage and route are determined by the physician. The dosage is individualized for each patient and regulated according to the effectiveness of the medication. The patient has to be carefully monitored by the prescribing physician. See Table 19-4 for selected Monoamine oxidase inhibitors.

Implications for Patient Care

Observe the patient for any signs of hypersensitivity. Note the effectiveness of the drug. Observe for adverse reactions.

Warning:

Hypertensive crises may occur with the use of Monoamine oxidase inhibitors. These crises may be fatal.

TABLE 19-4 Monoamine Oxidase Inhibitors

GENERIC NAME	TRADE NAME	ROUTE	USUAL DOSAGE	
phenelzine sulfate	Nardil	Oral:	*Adults:*	Initial dose: 15 mg (one tablet) t.i.d. Early phase treatment: 60 mg/day or up to 90 mg/day Maintenance dose: 15 mg/day or every other day
tranylcypromine sulfate	Parnate	Oral:	*Adults:*	Starting dose: 20 mg/day 10 mg in A.M. and 10 mg in the afternoon Maintenance dose: 20 mg/day or 10 mg/day

Know the symptoms of marked elevation of blood pressure: occipital headache (which may radiate frontally), palpitation, neck stiffness or soreness, nausea or vomiting, sweating (sometimes with fever and sometimes with cold), and photophobia. Either tachycardia or bradycardia, chest pain, and dilated pupils may occur. Notify the physician immediately if these symptoms appear. The medication should be discontinued, and measures to lower the blood pressure should be initiated.

Patient Teaching

Instruct the patient to notify the physician immediately if headache, stiff neck, pounding heartbeat, or feelings of nausea or vomiting occur. Instruct the patient not to suddenly arise from a lying position. If the patient feels dizzy upon arising, instruct him or her to lie down until the dizziness disappears.

Inform the patient not to drink alcoholic or caffeine beverages or to take over-the-counter medications while using Monoamine oxidase inhibitors. Inform the patient to be sure to tell the physician about all other medications that he or she may be taking. If the patient is seeing more than one physician, then each physician should be informed of the patient's medication regimen. Advise the patient who is taking insulin or oral sulfonylureas to monitor blood glucose levels very carefully, as Monoamine oxidase inhibitors may have an additive hypoglycemic effect when taken with these drugs. The diabetic patient should discuss this information with his or her physician.

Be sure that the patient understands that large amounts of **tyramine** can lead to a hypertensive crisis. Provide the patient with a list of foods and beverages to *avoid*. You may use the following list. ■

When taking Monoamine oxidase inhibitors, the following foods and beverages should be *avoided*:

Cheese	Avocados	Chianti wine
Sour cream	Chocolate	Sherry
Pickled herring	Soy sauce	Beer
Liver	Fava beans	Protein foods that are aged
Canned figs	Yeast extracts	Chicken livers
Raisins	Meats prepared with	Pickles
Bananas	tenderizers	Yogurt

> ⚠ **Caution:**
>
> Effects of Monoamine Oxidase Inhibitors will continue for as long as 2 weeks after the Monoamine Oxidase Inhibitors is stopped. Foods and beverages containing tyramine must be avoided during this period.

ANTIMANIC AGENT(S)

Lithium is used for the treatment of the manic episode of bipolar disorder. *Bipolar disorder* is a major affective disorder that is characterized by episodes of mania and depression. It was previously called manic-depressive psychosis. Bipolar disorder is subdivided into three types: manic, depressed, and mixed. In the manic phase, there are excessive emotional displays such as excitement, euphoria, hyperactivity, boisterousness, impaired ability to concentrate, decreased need for sleep, exalted feelings, delusions of grandeur, and overproduction of ideas. In the depressive phase, there are marked apathy, underactivity, and feelings of profound sadness, loneliness, and guilt. In the mixed phase, elements of both mania and depression may be present.

Lithium

Actions

The specific biochemical mechanism of lithium action in mania is unknown. It counteracts mood changes without producing sedation. Studies have shown that lithium alters sodium transport in nerve and muscle cells and effects a shift toward intraneuronal metabolism of catecholamines.

Uses

Specific antimanic drug for prophylaxis and treatment of bipolar disorder (manic-depressive illness).

Warnings

Generally not given to patients with significant renal or cardiovascular disease, severe debilitation or dehydration, or sodium depletion, because the risk of lithium toxicity is high in such patients. Lithium may cause fetal harm when administered during pregnancy.

Adverse Reactions

Fine hand tremor, polyuria, and mild thirst may occur during initial therapy and may persist throughout the treatment. During the first few days of lithium administration, there may be transient and mild nausea and general discomfort.

Early signs of lithium intoxication are diarrhea, vomiting, drowsiness, muscular weakness, and lack of coordination. These signs may appear at serum lithium levels below 2.0 mEq/L. At higher levels, ataxia, giddiness, tinnitus, blurred vision, and polyuria may occur. Serum lithium levels above 3.0 mEq/L may cause a complex of signs and symptoms involving various organs and systems of the body. Refer to the *Physicians' Desk Reference* for further information.

Dosage and Route

The dosage is individualized according to the serum lithium level and the patient's clinical response. A threshold level of lithium in body tissues must be reached before it is effective. This may take three to five days of therapy. Lithium is available as the following:

    Eskalith—300-mg tablets and capsules; 450-mg controlled-release tablets

    Lithobid—300-mg slow-release tablets

Lithium carbonate—300-mg tablets and capsules

Lithium citrate syrup—8 mEq/5 ml (300 mg of lithium carbonate)

Implications for Patient Care

The patient should have a complete physical examination before the initiation of lithium therapy.

Close clinical observation and frequent monitoring of serum lithium levels are essential. Serum lithium levels should be determined two to three times weekly during the acute manic phase, then on a monthly basis during maintenance therapy. During the initial stage of therapy, the blood level should be maintained between 1 and 1.5 mEq/L of serum. During maintenance therapy, the blood level should be between 0.6 and 1.2 mEq/L of serum. Observe for adverse reactions. Report to the proper authority or to the physician.

 Patient Teaching

Patients and their family should be informed of the early symptoms of lithium intoxication or toxicity and instructed to discontinue the medication and contact the physician immediately.

Early Symptoms of Lithium Intoxication:
drowsiness, vomiting, muscle weakness, ataxia, dryness of the mouth, lethargy, abdominal pain, dizziness, slurred speech, diarrhea, tremor, and nystagmus

Inform patients that the metallic taste in the mouth may be temporary and will usually decrease with a lower dose of lithium. Teach the patients how to perform good oral hygiene. Advise patients to take the medication as prescribed and not to discontinue the medication unless symptoms of lithium intoxication occur.

To diminish nausea, lithium may be given with meals. Stress the importance of good nutrition, and emphasize that the patient should maintain a normal intake of sodium and fluids. Lithium may enhance sodium depletion, which could enhance lithium toxicity. Instruct patients to drink 10 to 12 8-ounce glasses of water daily to prevent possible toxicity. Patients should be advised to refrain from drinking caffeine liquids and alcoholic beverages. Instruct patients not to change the brand of the prescribed medication.

Advise female patients against becoming pregnant during the time they are taking lithium.

Advise patients to inform other health care providers of his or her lithium therapy.

Stress to the patients the importance of returning to their attending physician, as scheduled, for lithium blood analysis. ■

ANTIPSYCHOTIC AGENTS

Antipsychotic agents modify psychotic behavior and are called *neuroleptics*. Many antipsychotic agents are derivatives of phenothiazine (an organic compound used in the manufacture of certain antipsychotic drugs). Phenothiazines differ in their ability to produce sedation, **extrapyramidal** reactions, and anticholinergic effects. Thorazine, the first antipsychotic agent to be introduced in the early 1950s, is a phenothiazine derivative. It is available in a variety of forms and dosages such as tablets (10 mg, 25 mg, 50 mg, 100 mg, 200 mg), sustained-release (SR) capsules (30 mg, 75 mg, 150 mg, 200 mg, 300 mg), syrup (10 mg/5 mL), concentrate (30 mg/mL, 100 mg/mL), suppositories (25 mg, 100 mg), and injection (25 mg/mL).

Some antipsychotic agents are not phenothiazines, but resemble a phenothiazine in action. Others resemble tricyclic antidepressants, while some are miscellaneous compounds. Newer compounds antagonize dopamine and serotonin type 2 in the central nervous system, but they also have antihistaminic, anticholinergic, and alpha-antiadrenergic effects.

Neuroleptics

Actions

The precise mechanism of action is not known. They are believed to control the symptomatology of psychosis by reducing excessive dopamine activity, by blocking postsynaptic dopamine receptors in the cerebral cortex, basal ganglia, *limbic system*, brain stem, and hypothalamus.

Antipsychotic agents have varying degrees of antihistaminic, anticholinergic, and alpha-antiadrenergic activities. These activities account for a number of the adverse reactions associated with antipsychotic agents.

Uses

Antipsychotic agents are used in the treatment of acute and chronic schizophrenia, organic psychoses, the manic phase of bipolar affective disorder, and psychotic disorders.

Contraindications

Hypersensitivity to the specific antipsychotic agent. Most antipsychotic agents are contraindicated in those with hypersensitivity to the specific antipsychoticagent, in comatose patients, in patients receiving large doses of CNS depressants, and in patients with bone marrow depression, blood dyscrasia, or liver damage.

Adverse Reactions

Antipsychotic agents may cause a wide gamut of adverse reactions. Some that may occur are drowsiness, sedation, convulsive seizure, dryness of mouth, constipation, urinary retention, blurred vision, orthostatic hypotension, tachycardia, fainting, dizziness, dystonia, motor restlessness, nasal congestion, toxic psychosis, photosensitivity, jaundice, skin pigmentation, and ocular changes.

Other adverse reactions include *extrapyramidal symptoms* (EPS), symptoms that appear to be dose related and are the most frightening to the patient; *dystonia* difficult or bad muscle tone that may appear as spasm of the neck muscles, torticollis, rigidity of back muscles, carpopedal spasm, trismus, swallowing difficulty, oculogyric crisis, and protrusion of the tongue; *akathisia*, an inability to sit down, and a feeling of restlessness or urgent need of movement (pacing, fidgeting, and agitation are classic symptoms of akathisia; and *pseudo-parkinsonism*, a neuroleptic-induced reaction with symptoms that include masklike expression (facies), drooling, tremors, rigidity, bradykinesia, shuffling gait, postural abnormalities, and hypersalivation. These symptoms may occur within a few weeks to a few months after initiating therapy, and may be controlled by an anti-parkinsonism agent.

● *Note*

Levodopa *has not been found to be effective in the treatment of pseudo-parkinsonism.* ●

Warning:

Some antipsychotic agents have the following risks:

- Neuroleptic malignant syndrome *(NMS), a potentially fatal symptom complex, may occur. Clinical manifestations of NMS are hyperpyrexia, muscle rigidity, altered mental status, and evidence of autonomic instability (irregular pulse or blood pressure, tachycardia, diaphoresis, and cardiac dysrhythmia). Additional signs may include elevated phosphokinase, myoglobin-uria (rhabdomyolysis), and acute renal failure.*

- Hyperglycemia and diabetes mellitus *might occur in patients taking any of the following: Abilify (aripiprazole), Seroquel (quetiapine fumarate), clozapine, Risperdal (risperidone), or Zyprexa (olanzapine). Hyperglycemia, in some cases is associated with ketoacidosis, coma, or death, and has been reported in patients treated with atypical antipsychotic drugs.*

> ### Warning: *(continued)*
>
> - Cerebrovascular adverse events *(stroke, transient ischemic attack), including fatalities, were reported in elderly patients with dementia-related psychosis.*
> - Agranulocytosis, seizures, myocarditis, and other adverse cardiovascular and respiratory effects *were reported with clozapine.*
> - *Both conventional and atypical antipsychotics are associated with an increased risk of mortality in elderly patients treated for dementia-related psychosis. Antipsychotics are not indicated for the treatment of dementia-related psychosis.*
> - *According to a study published in the January 15, 2009, issue of the* New England Journal of Medicine, *patients aged 30 to 74 years who took atypical antipsychotic drugs such as risperidone (Risperdal), quetiapine (Seroquel), olanzapine (Zyprexa), and clozapine had a significantly higher risk of sudden death from cardiac arrhythmias and other cardiac causes than patients who did not take these medications.*

Tardive dyskinesias

These make up a syndrome characterized by rhythmical involuntary movement of the tongue, face, mouth, jaw, trunk, and extremities. These symptoms may appear in some patients on long-term therapy. They may also appear after drug therapy has been discontinued. Tardive (lateness) dyskinesia (difficult movement) may occur in patients of any age, but is more common in older women. There is no known effective treatment for this syndrome.

Dosage and Route

The dosage and route of administration are determined by the physician. The dosage is individualized for each patient and regulated according to the effectiveness of the medication. See Table 19-5 for selected antipsychotic agents.

TABLE 19-5   Selected Antipsychotic Agents

GENERIC NAME	TRADE NAME	ROUTE	USUAL DOSAGE	
aripiprazole	Abilify	Oral	*Adults:*	10 to 15 mg/day
			Adolescents:	2 mg/day
chlorpromazine HCl		Oral	*Adults:*	Excessive anxiety, tension and agitation: 10 mg t.i.d. or q.i.d. or 25 mg b.i.d. or t.i.d. More severe cases: 25 mg t.i.d.; daily dosage may be 200 to 800 mg
			Children:	Office patients, outpatients: $\frac{1}{4}$ mg/lb of body weight every 4 to 6 h, prn
clozapine		Oral	*Adults:*	Initially 25 mg 1 to 2 times daily. May be increased by 25 to 50 mg/day over a period of 2 weeks up to a target dose of 300 to 450 mg/day
fluphenazine HCl		Oral	*Adults:*	0.5 to 10 mg in divided doses

(continues)

TABLE 19-5 (*continued*)

GENERIC NAME	TRADE NAME	ROUTE	USUAL DOSAGE	
olanzapine	Zyprexa	Oral	*Adults:*	Initially 5 to 10 mg/day. May be increased at weekly intervals by 5 mg/day (not to exceed 15 mg/day)
perphenazine		Oral	Moderately disturbed nonhospitalized psychotic patients: 4 to 8 mg t.i.d. or 1 to 2 REPETABS b.i.d. (initially) Hospitalized psychotic patients: 8 to 16 mg b.i.d. to q.i.d. or 1 to 4 REPETABS b.i.d.; avoid dosage in excess of 64 mg daily	
promazine HCl	Sparine	Oral	*Adults:*	Psychotic disorders: 10 to 200 mg at 4 to 6 hour intervals; dose limit 1000 mg/day
			Children:	Over 12 years: 10 to 25 mg every 4 to 6 hours
quetiapine fumarate	Seroquel	Oral	*Adults:* *Schizophrenia:*	Initial dose of 25 mg twice a day, with increases in increments of 25 to 50 mg twice a day or three times a day on the second and third day, as tolerated, to a target dose range of 300 to 400 mg daily by the fourth day, given b.i.d. or t.i.d
			Bipolar Mania:	Initiated in twice daily doses totaling 100mg/da on Day 1, increased to 400 mg/day on Day 4 in increments of up to 100 mg/day required to maintain symptom remission
risperidone	Risperdal	Oral	*Adults:*	1 mg twice daily, increased by 3rd day to 3 mg twice daily
thioridazine HCl		Oral	*Adults:*	50 to 100 mg t.i.d. (starting dose); maximum to 800 mg a day Daily dosage range: 200 to 800 mg divided into 2 to 4 doses
			Children:	Ages 2 to 12 years: 0.5 to 3.0 mg/kg/day
Nonphenothiazines haloperidol	Haldol	Oral	*Adults:*	Moderate symptomatology: 0.5 to 2.0 mg b.i.d. or t.i.d. Severe symptomatology: 3.0 to 5.0 mg b.i.d. or t.i.d. Geriatric or debilitated: 0.5 to 2.0 mg b.i.d. or t.i.d. Chronic or resistant patients: 3.0 to 5.0 mg b.i.d. or t.i.d.
			Children:	3 to 12 years: Psychotic disorders: 0.05 mg/kg/day to 0.15 mg/kg/day

(*continues*)

TABLE 19-5 (*continued*)

GENERIC NAME	TRADE NAME	ROUTE	USUAL DOSAGE
loxapine		Oral	Initially 10 mg b.i.d. Severely disturbed: up to 50 mg/day Maintenance: 60 to 100 mg/day

molindone HCl	Moban	Oral	Initially 50 to 75 mg/day; increase to 100 mg/day in
			   3 to 4 days
			An increase to 225 mg/day may be required in patients with
			   severe symptomatology.
			Maintenance:
			Mild: 5 to 15 mg 3 to 4 times a day
			Moderate: 10 to 25 mg 3 to 4 times a day
			Severe: 225 mg/day

pimozide	Orap	Oral	Initially 1 to 2 mg a day in divided doses Maintenance: 0.2 mg/kg/day
thiothixene HCl	Navane	Oral	Initially (mild) 2 mg t.i.d. Severe: 5 mg b.i.d. Optimal dose: 20 to 30 mg daily

Implications for Patient Care

Patients who takes antipsychotic agents needs special care. It is essential that you understand the patients' diagnosis and their treatment regimen. Remember that drug therapy is only a part of the treatment plan. Patients need emotional, physical, and social support. It is important that their family be included in the planning and implementation of patient care.

Observe patients for signs of hypersensitivity and adverse reactions. Notify the proper authority or physician of any adverse reactions. Note the effectiveness of the medication. Are the symptoms improved?

Patient Teaching

Inform patients that antipsychotic agents may impair mental or physical abilities; therefore, one should not operate machinery or drive a motor vehicle while on these medications. Teach patients that alcohol and other central nervous system depressants have an additive effect and should not be used while on these medications.

Instruct patients to take the medications as ordered. If patients are unable to manage their own plan of treatment, inform the proper family member or other responsible person of any and all essential information.

Teach patients to report adverse reactions to their physician. Inform patients to avoid exposure toultraviolet rays (sunlight or artificial). Instruct patients not to suddenly arise from a lying position. Inform patients to be sure to tell the physician about all other medications that they may be taking. If a patient is seeing more than one physician, each physician should be informed of the patient's medication regimen.

Encourage patients to eat a balanced diet and to drink sufficient fluids. Keeping the mucous membranes moist will help relieve dryness of the mouth. If desired, patients may suck on ice chips or sugarless hard candy to help moisten the mouth. When a patients has constipation, the physician should order an appropriate stool softener, laxative, or both. ■

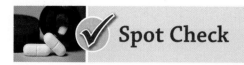 **Spot Check**

For each of the psychotropic agents given, list several aspects of patient teaching and several implications for patient care.

PSYCHOTROPIC AGENTS	PATIENT TEACHING	IMPLICATIONS FOR PATIENT CARE
benzodiazepines		
selective serotonin reuptake inhibitors		
tricyclic antidepressants		
lithium		

■ ■ REVIEW QUESTIONS

Directions. Select the best answer to each of the following multiple-choice questions, circling the letter of your choice.

1. The medical term that means pertaining to an emotion or mental state, or feeling, mood, or emotional response is known as _____.

   a. endogenous   c. limbic

   b. entrapyramidal   d. affective

2. Biochemical substances, epinephrine, norepinephrine, and dopamine are called _____.

   a. anticholinergics   c. metabolites

   b. catecholamines   d. adrenergics

3. Drugs that affect psychic function, behavior, or experience are called _____.

   a. psychotropic   c. adrenergic

   b. anticholinergic   d. antibiotic

4. _____ agents are chemical substances that relieve anxiety and muscle tension.

   a. Antidepressive

   b. Antipsychotic

   c. Antimanic

   d. Antianxiety

5. When a patient is taking benzodiazepines, it is your responsibility to teach the patient that _____.

   a. impairment of mental and/or physical abilities may occur

   b. alcohol and/or other CNS depressants have an additive effect

   c. physical dependence may occur

   d. all of these

6. Prozac (fluoxetine) is classified as a _____.

   a. selective serotonin reuptake inhibitor

   b. serotonin-norepinephrine reuptake inhibitor

   c. tricyclic antidepressant

   d. monoamine oxidase inhibitor

7. _____ agents are chemical substances that relieve the symptoms of depression.

   a. Antidepressive

   b. Antipsychotic

   c. Antimanic

   d. Antianxiety

8. The most common adverse reactions to tricyclic antidepressants are _____.

   a. flushing, diaphoresis, blurred vision, disturbance of accommodation

   b. increased intraocular pressure, constipation, paralytic ileus

   c. urinary retention and dilatation of urinary tract

   d. all of these

9. _____ _____ is a condition in which there is a decrease of systolic and diastolic blood pressure below normal due to a sudden change in body position.

   a. Orthostatic hypertension

   b. Orthostatic pneumonia

   c. Orthostatic hypotension

   d. none of these

10. Tricyclic antidepressants should not be given together with _____.

    a. protein foods that are aged

    b. cheese

    c. monoamine oxidase inhibitors

    d. caffeine

11. Wellbutrin (bupropion) is a monocyclic aminoketone used for the treatment of major depression, bipolar depression, chronic fatigue syndrome, cocaine addiction, nicotine addiction and _____.

    a. Parkinson's disease

    b. attention deficit/hyperactive disorder

    c. mild anxiety disorder

    d. alcoholism

12. Monoamine oxidase inhibitors may be used in _____.

    a. agoraphobia

    b. hysteroid dysphoria

    c. patients who have not responded to tricyclic antidepressants

    d. all of these

13. When a patient is taking MAO inhibitors, it is your responsibility to teach the patient _____.

    a. to notify the physician immediately if headache, stiff neck, pounding heartbeat, feelings of nausea, or vomiting occur

    b. not to arise suddenly from a lying position

    c. about foods and beverages to *avoid*

    d. all of these

14. Effects of monoamine oxidase inhibitors will continue for as long as 2 weeks after the MAOI is stopped. During this time period the patient should avoid foods that contain tyramine such as _____.

    a. cheese, sour cream, liver, canned figs, chicken livers

    b. raisins, bananas, avocados, chocolate, pickles, yogurt

    c. yeast extracts, Chianti wine, sherry, beer, protein foods that are aged

    d. all of these

15. _____ is used for the treatment of the manic episode of bipolar disorder.

    a. Nardil   b. Valium   c. Lithium   d. Elavil

16. The early signs of lithium intoxication are _____.

    a. diarrhea, vomiting, drowsiness, muscular weakness, and lack of coordination

    b. dryness of the mouth, lethargy, abdominal pain

    c. dizziness, slurred speech, tremor, and nystagmus

    d. all of these

17. During the initial stage of lithium therapy, the blood level should be maintained between _____.

    a. 2 to 3.0 mEq/L   c. 0.6 to 1.2 mEq/L

    b. 1 to 1.5 mEq/L   d. 1 to 3.5 mEq/L

18. When a patient is taking lithium, it is your responsibility to teach the patient _____.

    a. to recognize the early signs/symptoms of lithium intoxication

    b. how to perform good oral hygiene

    c. to refrain from drinking caffeine liquids and alcoholic beverages

    d. all of these

19. _____ _____ modify psychotic behavior and are called neuroleptics.

    a. Antidepressive agents   c. Antimanic agents

    b. Antipsychotic agents   d. Antianxiety agents

20. Adverse reactions to phenothiazines that appear to be dose-related and are most frightening to the patient are _____.

    a. dystonia, akathisia, and pseudo-parkinsonism

    b. dryness of the mouth, constipation, and tachycardia

    c. dizziness, nasal congestion, and blurred vision

    d. photosensitivity, jaundice, and skin pigmentation

21. _____ _____ is a syndrome characterized by rhythmical involuntary movement of the tongue, face, mouth, jaw, trunk, and extremities.

    a. Pseudo-parkinsonism   c. Toxic psychosis

    b. Tardive dyskinesias   d. none of these

22. When a patient is taking an antipsychotic agent, it is your responsibility to teach the patient _____.
    a. that impairment of mental and/or physical abilities may occur
    b. that alcohol and other CNS depressants have an additive effect
    c. to avoid exposure to ultraviolet rays
    d. all of these

Matching. Place the correct letter from Column II on the appropriate line of Column I:

Column I		*Column II*
23. ___B___ endogenous		A. a vasoconstrictor that affects sleep and sensory perception
24. ___C___ anticholinergic		B. produced or arising within a cell or organism
25. ___A___ serotonin		C. agent that blocks parasympathetic nerve impulses
		D. agent that stimulates parasympathetic nerve impulses

UNIT 20
Substance Abuse

OBJECTIVES

Upon completing this unit, you should be able to:

- Define the terms listed in the vocabulary.
- Describe problems that are associated with substance abuse.
- List the effects that alcohol has as a multisystem toxin and a central nervous system depressant.
- Be aware of some drugs that interact with alcohol.
- Complete the critical thinking questions and activities presented in this unit.
- Describe nicotine, club drugs, and inhalants as substances being abused.
- State the effects that amphetamines have upon the body.
- Describe methamphetamine and how it affects the body.
- Describe cocaine as a central nervous system stimulant and how it is used as an abused substance.
- State how barbiturates are abused, and explain their effects upon the body.
- Describe how narcotic analgesics are abused, and explain their effects upon the body.
- Describe marijuana as an abused substance.
- Describe how phencyclidine (PCP) is an abused substance, and its illegal use.
- State that lysergic acid diethylamide (LSD) is a hallucinogenic agent, and describe its effects upon the body.
- Describe prescription drug abuse and addiction.
- State the medical assistant's role in recognizing substance abuse and the action to take when substance abuse is suspected.
- List the warning signs of substance abuse in the workplace.
- Complete the Spot Check on interactions of selected drugs and alcohol.
- Answer the review questions correctly.

VOCABULARY

attention deficit/hyperactivity disorder (ADHD). A disease characterized by inappropriate inattention, impulsivity, and hyperactivity. It occurs in infancy, childhood, or both and may be known as hyperkinetic syndrome, hyperactivity, minimal brain damage, minimal brain dysfunction, and minimal cerebral dysfunction.

dependency (de-pend'en-cy). The psychic craving for a drug or a substance. It may or may not be accompanied by physiological dependency.

euphoria (u-for'e-a). A feeling of good health. It is a term that also means an exaggerated feeling of well-being; elation.

obesity (o-be'si-te). Excessive amount of fat on the body. *Exogenous* obesity is due to excessive intake of food.

tolerance (tol'er-ans). The progressive decrease in the effectiveness of a drug.

withdrawal (with-draw'al). The removal of a substance to which the individual has become addicted. Sudden withdrawal of certain substances can be very dangerous. This also refers to a set of physiological symptoms that occur when an individual is no longer taking a substance to which he or she has become addicted.

INTRODUCTION

Why do people use drugs? For hundreds of years, man has sought out substances that relieve pain, fight infection, as well as those that give pleasure. The modern Western culture in which we live places a reliance on such substances for everything from anxiety relief to a cure for some cancers.

This unit explores psychotropic (mood-altering) drugs and certain other substances our population has singled out for abuse. In this context, abuse can be defined as the misuse of a substance—legal or illegal—sufficient to cause the abuser mental, physical, emotional, or social harm. Abuse, in some instances, can lead to addiction or dependency. Addiction or dependency is the compulsive, continued use of a drug. Addiction can involve physical dependence, psychological dependence, or both.

It should be noted that not all drug abuse is related to illegal substances. Between 2 and 3 million Americans are addicted to prescription drugs, and hospital emergencies are as likely to involve legal drugs as they are illegal drugs.

Abused substances take many forms and are introduced into the body in a variety of ways. They can include substances like marijuana or tobacco; beverages containing alcohol; and pharmacological agents. They may be taken orally, smoked, inhaled, or injected.

Substance abuse can result in the development of drug tolerance, a condition wherein the person's body adjusts to the dosage of a particular drug, and larger amounts of the drug must be taken to achieve the desired effect. Physical dependency is often preceded or accompanied by tolerance. When a person with a physical dependency on a drug is forced to do without it, an illness results. Known as withdrawal, this condition may include flulike symptoms, nausea, shakes, sweats, tremors, and acute craving for the drug.

The abuse of alcohol, nicotine, certain drugs, and other chemical substances is a health and social problem that affects everyone. The cost of substance abuse runs into the billions of dollars, most of which goes to combat crime by drug users, to pay for property and personal injury resulting from accidents involving substance abuse, and for social and psychiatric services to victims of drug abuse. Increased taxation and higher insurance are pocketbook expenses that can be calculated in measurable terms. Not so easily measured is the absenteeism from school or work, the defective products produced by affected workers, and the waste of human potential epitomized by the addict.

How It Begins

One cannot become addicted to drugs without first starting to use them. Why people try drugs is open to debate, but research has shown that substance abuse occurs among people of all ages and socioeconomic levels. Environmental and social factors such as poverty, family dysfunction, and peer pressure are often cited as reasons for a person's willingness to try drugs, as is curiosity about the "feeling" derived from the experience.

Regardless of the reasons, people who try drugs risk addiction. True, not everyone who drinks becomes an alcoholic and not all substance abusers become drug addicts; however, far too many do. Addictive drugs, including nicotine and alcohol, are dangerous because most people believe that they are immune to addiction. Unfortunately, the body develops a tolerance for most abused substances. Increases in both dosage and frequency of use are needed to achieve the same degree of effect that was once possible with smaller or less frequent doses. Abuse with high doses of psychoactive substances leads to dependency. Physical dependency occurs when one or more of the body's physiologic functions become dependent on the presence of the abused drug. The body experiences withdrawal symptoms if the substance is not taken or ingested. Psychological dependency does not involve the body's physiologic functions; rather, it is a psychic craving for the effects produced by the abused substance.

◼️ Special Considerations: **OLDER ADULTS**

According to an article in the *Journal of the American Medical Association* (JAMA), doctors should prepare for an increase in the number of elderly people with alcoholism. A U.S. Census Bureau projection indicates that, by the year 2030, there will be more people over 65 years of age with alcoholism than people under 18 years of age.

Alcohol is a psychotropic drug that affects mood, judgment, behavior, concentration, and consciousness. It is a direct multisystem toxin and central nervous system depressant. Alcohol can cause drowsiness, incoordination, slurring of speech, sudden mood changes, aggression, belligerency, grandiosity, and uninhibited behavior. It can also cause stupor, coma, and death if taken excessively. Because of the increased susceptibility of older adults to the toxic effects of alcohol, a person can develop alcohol problems just by becoming older, and this may occur without necessarily increasing the amount of alcohol consumed. Manifestations of alcohol abuse in older adults are generally more subtle, atypical, and nonspecific than in younger people.

Alcohol interacts with at least half of the 100 most frequently used drugs on the market, and many of these drugs are used by older adults. Older people use more medications than any other age group. It is estimated that older adults use 30 percent of all prescribed medications and 40 percent of all over-the-counter medications.

Some Drugs That Interact with Alcohol

- *Antibiotics.* Chloramphenicol, furazolidone, griseofulvin, metronidazole, and some cephalosporins may interact with acute alcohol consumption and produce a disulfiram-like (Antabuse-like) reaction, which is a severe hypersensitivity to alcohol. Symptoms that may occur are flushing, chest pain, palpitations, tachycardia, hypotension, syncope (fainting), and arrhythmias.
- *Salicylates and aspirin.* Alcohol increases the tendency of salicylates to cause gastrointestinal bleeding. Aspirin increases alcohol absorption and results in elevated blood alcohol levels.
- *Acetaminophen* may increase susceptibility to acetaminophen-induced liver toxicity.
- *Tricyclic antidepressants.* Alcohol may accelerate the clearance of these antidepressants, and patients with depression who mix alcohol and these drugs may not achieve the appropriate blood levels of the antidepressant.
- *Sedatives and anxiolytics.* Alcohol enhances the sedative action and causes psychomotor impairment.
- *Monoamine oxidase inhibitors.* (MAOIs) may produce disulfiram-like (Antabuse-like) effects. Dark beers and red wines contain tyramine and may produce hypertensive episodes.
- *Opioids.* Respiratory depressant effects of both alcohol and opioids may be potentiated.
- *Anticoagulants.* Long-term drinkers metabolize warfarin more rapidly, and careful monitoring of anticoagulant therapy/blood studies is essential.
- *Cimetidine, ranitidine, and nizatidine.* These may increase blood alcohol levels by reducing alcohol metabolism in the stomach.
- *Oral hypoglycemic agents.* When ingested with alcohol, significant decreases in blood sugar levels may be produced.
- *Lithium* may reduce alcohol-induced intoxication as information processing in the brain is reduced.
- *Certain antihistamines.* Alcohol enhances sedative effect.
- *Certain cardiovascular drugs* may markedly increase alcohol's effects.

Special Considerations: **CHILDREN**

Alcohol abuse is the *number-one* drug problem of American children. Although most states have legal drinking ages of between 18 and 21 years of age, these laws have not prevented younger individuals from drinking. It is estimated that 3.3 million problem drinkers exist among the 14- to 17-year-olds, who make up 19 percent of the population.

The first drinking experience generally occurs at about 12 years of age, and the amount and frequency of drinking increases with age. Alcohol is a mind-altering drug that works as a depressant. The abusive effects of alcohol on a child's body systems can cause vomiting, diarrhea, ulcers, cirrhosis of the liver, pancreatitis, and brain damage.

Alcohol is also the drug most commonly abused by females of childbearing age. No "safe" level of alcohol intake during pregnancy is known. Three cans of beer per day, three glasses of wine or three mixed drinks per day, or repetitive binge drinking is known to increase the risk of alcohol-related infant defects. Maternal use of alcohol can cause spontaneous abortion and fetal alcohol syndrome (FAS), which includes growth retardation before and after birth, facial and cranial abnormalities, mental retardation, and developmental delay.

The U.S. Department of Education has designed a quiz for parents to help them learn about drug abuse and how it impacts families. To assist you in your learning about substance abuse, the quiz and its answers (in italic) are presented here:

1. What is the most commonly used drug in the United States?
   a. heroin
   b. cocaine
   c. *alcohol*
   d. marijuana
2. Name the three drugs most commonly used by children. *Alcohol, tobacco,* and *marijuana.*
3. Which drug is associated with the most teenage deaths? *Alcohol.*
4. Which of the following contains the most alcohol?
   a. a 12-ounce can of beer
   b. a cocktail
   c. a 12-ounce wine cooler
   d. a 5-ounce glass of wine
   e. *all contain equal amounts of alcohol (1.5 ounces)*
5. Crack is a particularly dangerous drug because it is _____.
   a. cheap
   b. readily available
   c. highly addictive
   d. *all of the above*
6. Fumes from which of the following can be inhaled to produce a high?
   a. spray paint
   b. model glue
   c. nail polish remover
   d. whipped cream canisters
   e. *all of the above*
7. People who have used alcohol and other drugs before their 20th birthday
   a. have no risk of becoming chemically dependent.
   b. are less likely to develop a drinking problem or use illicit drugs.
   c. *have an increased risk of becoming chemically dependent.*
      (Children who use alcohol before age 15 are very likely to have drug-related problems later in life.)
8. A speedball is a combination of which two drugs? *Cocaine and heroin.*
9. Anabolic steroids are dangerous because they result in
   a. development of female characteristics in males.
   b. development of male characteristics in females.
   c. stunted growth.
   d. damage to the liver and cardiovascular system.
   e. overly aggressive behavior.
   f. *all of the above*

10. How much alcohol can a pregnant woman safely consume?
    a. a 6-ounce glass of wine with dinner
    b. two 12-ounce cans of beer
    c. five 4-ounce shots of whiskey a month
    d. *none*
       (There have been no "safe" limits established.)

Critical Thinking QUESTIONS AND ACTIVITIES

Prepare a presentation on alcohol abuse among American children. Using the information in Special Considerations: Children, and any other reference that you need, ask yourself:

- What is the legal drinking age in the state where I live?
- How many problem drinkers exist among the 12- to 17-year-old age group?
- At what age do most children first try drinking?
- What are some of the abusive effects of alcohol on a child's body?
- What amount of beer, wine, or mixed drinks per day can increase the risk of alcohol-related infant defects?
- What quiz could I use to help others understand about drug abuse?

SOME SUBSTANCES BEING ABUSED

Many substances can be abused. Described in this section are nicotine, club drugs, inhalants, and selected groups of drugs.

Nicotine

According to the National Institute on Drug Abuse (NIDA), nicotine is one of the most heavily used addictive drugs in the United States. Cigarette smoking, since the beginning of the twentieth century, has been the method of choice for taking nicotine. Currently, 60 million Americans (ages 12 and older) are smokers. Like alcohol, tobacco products are legal for adults; yet according to NIDA, 4.1 million youths between the ages of 12 and 17 unlawfully obtain and use tobacco products.

Nicotine is highly addictive. It is both a stimulant and a sedative to the central nervous system and is absorbed readily from tobacco smoke in the lungs or as a consequence of chewing tobacco. Regular use of tobacco leads to nicotine accumulation in the body, thereby providing a continuous (24-hour) exposure to nicotine's effects on body systems.

It has been demonstrated that stress and anxiety affect nicotine tolerance and dependency. Corticosterone, a hormone released during stress, reduces the effects of nicotine; therefore, with stress, more nicotine must be consumed to achieve the same effect. This increases tolerance and leads to dependency. The use of tobacco products, aside from the addictive effects of nicotine, is accompanied by a host of health hazards. In addition to nicotine, cigarette smoke is primarily composed of a dozen or so gases (mainly carbon monoxide) and tar. The tar exposes the user to increased risk for lung cancer, emphysema, and bronchial disorders. The carbon monoxide increases the user's risk of cardiovascular diseases.

Those dependent on nicotine usually find it very difficult to quit because addiction to nicotine results in withdrawal symptoms. When deprived of cigarettes for as little as 24 hours, chronic smokers display increased anger, hostility, aggression, and loss of social cooperation. Approaches commonly employed by those attempting to break the cycle of nicotine dependency include (1) quitting "cold turkey," or abruptly stopping use of tobacco; (2) a gradual cessation program in which the smoker obtains decreasing amounts of nicotine from such sources as a transdermal patch or nicotine chewing gum; and (3) use of medications such as Zyban, which does not replace nicotine but helps to control nicotine craving and the associated urge to smoke.

Club Drugs and Inhalants

Beyond nicotine and alcohol is a plethora of legal and illegal substances sought out by many for their psychotropic effects. On the increase in popularity with young, beginning abusers are two distinct groups of substances, club drugs and inhalants. The term *club drug* categorizes a collection of dangerous substances used by teens and young adults at all-night dance events (raves), parties, dance clubs, and bars. According to the NIDA, uncertainties about the sources, chemicals, and possible contaminants used in the manufacture of many club drugs makes it extremely difficult to determine the toxicity and resulting medical consequences of these substances.

Commonly known by abbreviations and street names, the club drugs include MDMA (Ecstasy), GHB, Rohypnol, ketamine, methamphetamine, and LSD (see Table 20-1).

The NIDA warns that no club drug is benign. With some of these drugs, users risk long-term neurologic and cardiovascular damage, and because some club drugs are colorless, tasteless, and without odor, they are increasingly being used to intoxicate or sedate others, often preparatory to sexual assault (date rape) or pornographic photography.

Inhalants are breathable chemical vapors that produce psychoactive (mind-altering) effects. Most abused inhalants are legal substances commonly found in the home or workplace. Those most likely to abuse inhalants are young children in middle school experimenting with such substances and teens using nitrous oxide in combination with club drugs while attending "raves" or all-night dance parties. The popularity of inhalants tends to decrease among users as they grow older and move on to marijuana, LSD, and other illegal substances.

Nearly all inhalants produce effects similar to anesthetics by slowing down the body's functions. In sufficient concentrations, inhalants can cause intoxication lasting from a few minutes to several hours, depending on frequency of use. Serious, irreversible effects, including death, can result from the misuse of inhalants. Well documented are instances of brain damage and hearing loss associated with toluene (an ingredient found in paint sprays and some glues). Also well documented are peripheral neuropathies (limb spasms) associated with the hexane in glues, gasoline, or nitrous oxide from whipping cream containers or from small metal cylinders (see Table 20-2).

Nationally, estimates on inhalant deaths per year range from 100 to 1,000. Because researchers rely on surveys such as the NIDA's Monitoring the Future Survey (MTF), it is difficult to determine exactly how many youngsters use inhalants. However, when asked on the 1997 MTF if they had ever used inhalants, 21 percent of 8th graders, 18.3 percent of 10th graders, and 16.1 percent of 12th graders responded yes. In the same survey, almost 12 percent of 8th graders replied that their use had been within the past year.

GROUPS OF DRUGS

Amphetamines

Drugs of the amphetamine group are prescription medications designed for oral use in the treatment of exogenous obesity, narcolepsy, and attention deficit/hyperactivity disorder. *Amphetamine sulfate, dextroamphetamine sulfate* (Dexedrine), *methamphetamine sulfate* (Desoxyn), *methylphenidate HCl* (Ritalin), and *phenmetrazine HCl* have a high potential for abuse and are classed as Schedule II drugs under the Federal Controlled Substances Act. These drugs stimulate the central nervous system and cause increased alertness, elevation of mood, reduction of appetite, and a diminished sense of fatigue.

The misuse and abuse of amphetamines relate to the effects these drugs have upon the central nervous system. They have been taken to avoid sleep while studying or driving, and they have also been taken by athletes in an attempt to improve performance. Primarily, these drugs are abused by those seeking euphoric excitement, or by those who want to counter the effects of depressant drugs. Street names for amphetamines are *speed, crystal, bennies, wake-ups,* and *pep pills.*

Euphoria, excitement, anorexia, and insomnia are but a few of the possible effects of amphetamines. Those abusing these drugs may also experience dilated pupils, talkativeness, nervousness, agitation, dizziness, increased or decreased blood pressure, palpitations, tachycardia or bradycardia, pallor or flushing, dry mouth, abdominal pain, chills, fever, and fatigue.

If amphetamine use is abruptly stopped, heavy users exhibit withdrawal symptoms. These symptoms usually include fatigue, long but disturbed sleep, irritability, strong hunger, and deep depression that may lead to attempted suicide.

TABLE 20-1   Club Drugs

SUBSTANCES	STREET NAMES	PHYSIOLOGICAL EFFECTS	PSYCHOLOGICAL EFFECTS	ROUTE AND APPEARANCES
GHB (gamma hydroxy-butyrate)	Liquid Ecstasy, Scoop, Somatomax, Georgia Home Boy, Grievous Bodily Harm, G	Sedative, anabolic high dosage can slow heart rate and respiration to dangerous levels	Euphoric, intoxicant, anxiety relief	Oral: liquid, powder, tablet, or capsule
Ketamine (an injectable anesthetic that is primarily for veterinary use)	Special K, K, vitamin K, Cat Valiums	High dose: delirium, high blood pressure, impaired motor skills, respiratory distress	Weightless feeling, out-of-body or near-death sensation	Liquid or powder that is often snorted or smoked with tobacco or marijuana
LSD (lysergic acid diethylamide)	Acid, Boomers, Yellow Sunshine	Weakness, trembling, nausea, numbness, dilated pupils, loss of appetite, sweating	Hallucinogenic effect, hallucinogen persisting perception disorder (flashbacks)	Oral: tablets, capsules, liquid, or licked from absorbent paper
MDMA (methylenedioxymeth-amphetamine)	Ecstasy, XTC, Adam, Clarity, Lover's Speed, X	Stimulant, increased heart rate and blood pressure, involuntary teeth clenching, and muscle tension	Sense of alertness, psychedelic effect, hallucinogenic effect, increased stamina, anxiety, paranoia	Oral ingestion tablet or capsule
Methamphetamine	Speed, Ice, Chalk, Meth, Crystal, Crank Fire, Glass	Decreased appetite, physical activity, excited speech, cardiovascular damage	Short-term rush, flash, euphoria, agitation, aggression	Powder: oral ingestion or can be smoked, snorted, or injected
Rohypnol (flunitrazepam)	Rophies, Roofies, Roach, Rope, the "Date Rape" Drug, the Forget-Me Pill	Sedative-hypnotic, muscle relaxation, decreased blood pressure, dizziness	Anterograde amnesia (lack of recall for events while drugged)	Oral ingestion

Table 20-2 Inhalants Subject To Abuse

SUBSTANCES	PHYSIOLOGICAL EFFECTS	PSYCHOLOGICAL EFFECTS	HOW USED AND APPEARS
Medical anesthetic gases: nitrous oxide, chloroform, ether	General anesthetic used by medical professionals: restricts the pumping action of the heart, drops blood pressure, increases pulse rate	Laughing gas, mind-altering effect	Inhaled as vapor, often in large balloons
Volatile hydrocarbons, used as solvents in paint thinner, gasoline, nail polish remover, dry-cleaning fluids, glues, correction fluids, and as aerosol propellants for spray paint, fabric protectors, whipping cream, cooking oil, hair spray, air freshener, or in gases such as propane, butane, helium	Various effects: respiratory difficulty, heart palpitations, nerve cell damage, loss of sense of smell, irregular heartbeat, double vision, slows reaction time, loss of consciousness	Various effects: visual hallucinations and severe mood swings, dizziness, anxiety, poor memory, lack of concentration, confusion, intoxication, disorientation in time and space	Sniffing or snorting via the nose, *bagging* (inhaling fumes from a plastic bag), or *huffing* (stuffing an inhalant-soaked rag or sock into the mouth)
Volatile nitrates: amyl nitrate and products sold as room deodorizers, which use chemical variants of butyl nitrate	Vasodilation, face flushes, perspiration of head and neck, reduction in blood pressure, relaxation of involuntary muscles	Rushing sensation, light-headed or dizzy feeling, slowed perception of time	Yellowish-gold liquid in ampules

Methamphetamine

Methamphetamine is a powerfully addictive stimulant that dramatically affects the central nervous system and is a drug with high potential for widespread abuse. It is commonly known as *speed, meth,* and *chalk.* In its smoked form, it is often referred to as *ice, crystal, crank,* and *glass.* It is a white, odorless, bitter-tasting crystalline powder that easily dissolves in water or alcohol. The drug was developed early in this century from its parent drug, amphetamine, and was used originally in nasal decongestants and bronchial inhalers. Methamphetamine's chemical structure is similar to that of amphetamine, but it has more pronounced effects on the central nervous system. Like amphetamine, it causes increased activity, decreased appetite, and a general sense of well-being. The effects of methamphetamine can last 6 to 8 hours. After the initial "rush," there is typically a state of high agitation that can lead to violent behavior in some individuals.

Methamphetamine comes in many forms and can be smoked, snorted, orally ingested, or injected. The drug alters moods in different ways, depending on how it is taken. Immediately after smoking the drug or injecting it intravenously, users experiences an intense rush or "flash" that lasts only a few minutes and is described as extremely pleasurable. Snorting or oral ingestion produces euphoria—a high but not an intense rush. Snorting produces effects within 3 to 5 minutes, and oral ingestion produces effects within 15 to 20 minutes.

As with similar stimulants, methamphetamine most often is used in a "binge-and-crash" pattern. Because tolerance for methamphetamine occurs within minutes—meaning that the pleasurable effects disappear even before the drug concentration in the blood falls significantly—users try to maintain the high by bingeing on the drug.

As a powerful stimulant, methamphetamine, even in small doses, can increase wakefulness and physical activity and decrease appetite. A brief, intense sensation, or rush, is reported by those who smoke or inject methamphetamine. Oral ingestion or snorting produces a long-lasting high instead of a rush, which reportedly can continue for as long as half a day. Both the rush and the high are believed to result from the release of very high levels of the neurotransmitter dopamine into areas of the brain that regulate feelings of pleasure.

Methamphetamine has many effects on the brain and body. Short-term effects can include increased wakefulness, increased physical activity, decreased appetite, increased respiration, hyperthermia, irritability, tremors, convulsions, and aggressiveness. Hyperthermia and convulsions can result in death. Single doses of methamphetamine have also been shown to cause damage to nerve terminals in studies with animals. Long-term effects can include addiction, stroke, violent behavior, anxiety, confusion, paranoia, auditory hallucinations, mood disturbances, and delusions. Long-term use can also cause damage to dopamine neurons that persists long after the drug has been discontinued.

In addition to being addicted to methamphetamine, chronic methamphetamine abusers exhibit symptoms that can include violent behavior, anxiety, confusion, and insomnia. They also can display a number of psychotic features, including paranoia, auditory hallucinations, mood disturbances, and delusions (for example, the sensation of insects creeping on the skin, which is called formication). The paranoia can result in homicidal as well as suicidal thoughts.

With chronic use, tolerance for methamphetamine can develop. In an effort to intensify the desired effects, users may take higher doses of the drug, take it more frequently, or change their method of drug intake. In some cases, abusers forego food and sleep while indulging in a form of bingeing known as a "run," injecting as much as a gram of the drug every 2 to 3 hours over several days until the user runs out of the drug or is too disorganized to continue. Chronic abuse can lead to psychotic behavior, characterized by intense paranoia, visual and auditory hallucinations, and out-of-control rages that can be coupled with extremely violent behavior.

Although there are no physical manifestations of a withdrawal syndrome when methamphetamine use is stopped, there are several symptoms that occur when a chronic user stops taking the drug. These include depression, anxiety, fatigue, paranoia, aggression, and an intense craving for the drug.

Fetal exposure to methamphetamine also is a significant problem in the United States. At present, research indicates that methamphetamine abuse during pregnancy may result in prenatal complications, increased rates of premature delivery, and altered neonatal behavioral patterns, such as abnormal reflexes and extreme irritability. Methamphetamine abuse during pregnancy may be linked also to congenital deformities.

Methamphetamine is made illegally with relatively inexpensive over-the-counter ingredients. Pseudoephedrine is a key ingredient used to manufacture methamphetamine; the only difference is a single oxygen molecule. It is available for over-the-counter purchase in several forms of cold and cough remedies. Ten states have laws restricting sales of products containing pseudoephedrine. Oklahoma, the most strict state, requires the products to be kept behind the counter of pharmacies. Although the medicines can be bought by adults without a prescription, the customers must sign a registry and present a photo identification.

Cocaine

Like the amphetamines, cocaine is a central nervous system stimulant. This drug is extracted from the leaves of *Erythroxylon coca*, a plant that can be found in a number of South American countries. Cocaine hydrochloride (HCl), a fine, white, crystal-like powder, is the most available form of the drug and is used medically for surface anesthesia of the ear, nose, throat, rectum, and vagina. Cocaine has a high potential for abuse and is classified as a Schedule II drug under the Federal Controlled Substances Act.

As an abused substance, cocaine is usually sniffed or snorted into the nose, although some users inject it or smoke a form of the drug called *crack* or *freebase*. Cocaine is readily absorbed through mucous membranes, thus the reason for snorting it into the nasal passageway. Its effects begin within a few minutes, reach a peak within 15 to 20 minutes, and subside within an hour. These effects include dilated pupils, and increases in blood pressure, heart rate, breathing rate, and body temperature. The drug's high potential for abuse relates to its ability to cause feelings of euphoria, excitement, and a sense of well-being. In addition, other desirable effects are feeling more energetic or alert, and a reduction of appetite.

Crack or freebase cocaine is made by chemically converting cocaine HCl to a purified, altered form of the drug that is more suitable for smoking. This altered form of the drug resembles beige or brownish clumps of sugar, which, when smoked, produces an intense feeling of euphoria in less than 10 seconds. This instant "high" lasts only 5 to 25 minutes and is followed, almost immediately, by an equally intense depression. To avoid the depression, there is a strong need to smoke more of the drug. Crack can cause serious psychological dependency in as little as two weeks and, of those addicted to crack, experts predict nine out of ten will continue to abuse the drug despite efforts at rehabilitation.

Cocaine hydrochloride, although not as powerful as crack, is a very dangerous, dependency-producing drug. The feeling of well-being produced by cocaine can cause some of its users to center their lives around seeking and using this drug. Street names for cocaine are *blow, coke, flake, gold dust, nose candy, rock, snow*, and *white girl*. The street name for the combination of cocaine and heroin is *speedball*.

The adverse effects of cocaine use include perforated nasal septum, chills, fever, runny nose, ventricular fibrillation, cocaine psychosis, and death from respiratory and circulatory failure.

Barbiturates

The barbiturates are a group of drugs derived from barbituric acid. Although they may vary in onset of action, potency, and duration of effect, all are central nervous system depressants. Barbiturates are used medically as sedatives, to relieve anxiety, to treat insomnia, and in the control of epilepsy. Misuse of barbiturate drugs may grow out of poorly supervised prescription use of these agents. Patients may arbitrarily increase the dosage and frequency of use in response to self-perceived needs. Misuse of barbiturates can lead to their abuse because prolonged use results in tolerance and dependency.

Because of their potential for abuse, barbiturates are classified as Schedule II, III, and IV drugs under the Federal Controlled Substances Act. Those classified as Schedule II are *pentobarbital* and *secobarbital* (Seconal). Street names for barbiturates are *barbs, blues, downers, goofballs, yellow jacket* (pentobarbital), *red devil* (secobarbital), and *blue devil* (amobarbital). These drugs are generally taken orally in tablet or capsule form, but may be prepared as a solution for intravenous injection.

Relief from anxiety and sedation occurs when dosages of barbiturates are taken as prescribed. Higher doses may produce slurred speech, confusion, poor motor coordination, impaired judgment, and drowsiness. Very high doses can produce coma, respiratory arrest, circulatory collapse, and death.

Abrupt discontinuation of barbiturates can induce withdrawal symptoms that can be fatal. Such symptoms include apprehension, weakness, dizziness, tremors, nausea, vomiting, sweating, disturbed vision, insomnia, hypotension, headache, delirium, and convulsion.

Narcotic Analgesics (Opiates)

Opiates, sometimes referred to as narcotics, are a group of drugs derived from *opium*, some of which are used medically to relieve pain. Opiates have a high potential for abuse and can cause dependency if abused or when occasional use extends over a long period of time. Opium is a dark-brown substance obtained by air-drying the juice of unripe seed pods of Asian poppy plants. A number of other drugs, including *morphine, codeine*, and *heroin*, have been derived from opium. Other opiates, such as *meperidine* (Demerol) and *hydromorphone hydrochloride* (Dilaudid), are synthetic or semisynthetic drugs with morphine-like qualities.

The use of opium is prohibited in the United States. Heroin is a Schedule I drug under the Federal Controlled Substances Act because of its high abuse potential and the lack of any acceptable medical use. Other natural and synthetic opiates are listed as Schedule II drugs that have medical applications.

Heroin, sometimes called *junk* or *smack*, accounts for 90 percent of the opiate abuse in the United States, despite the fact that its sale or possession is illegal. Most street preparations are "cut" with other substances such as sugar or quinine and appear as a white or brownish powder. Because the effects of heroin (or morphine) are significantly diminished when taken orally, intravenous injection is the route of administration drug abusers prefer.

Patients beginning treatment with an opiate, and those misusing these drugs for the first time, often experience nausea, vomiting, itching, and restlessness. This initial unpleasantness precedes a feeling of relaxation, drowsiness, and euphoria. With continued use, the unpleasant effects of these drugs are diminished. Users develop a drug tolerance and larger dosages are required to produce the same effects. Drug dependence is easily established with opiate use. Finding and using the drug often become the primary focus in the lives of users. Because heroin use is very expensive, those addicted to this opiate often resort to criminal acts to pay for their habit.

The physical dangers associated with opiate abuse depend on the specific drug used, its source, the dose, and the route of administration. Most of the danger can be attributed to using too much of the drug, use of unsterile hypodermic needles, contamination of the drug itself, or combining the drug with other substances. Infections from contaminated solutions, syringes, and needles can cause liver disease, tetanus, serum hepatitis, and acquired immune deficiency syndrome (AIDS).

When the opiate-dependent person stops taking the drug, withdrawal symptoms become evident within four to six hours of the last dose. Symptoms include uneasiness, diarrhea, abdominal cramps, chills, sweating, nausea, runny nose, and tearing of the eyes. The intensity of withdrawal symptoms correlates with the dosage taken, the frequency of use, and the length of time that the user has been dependent on the drug. Withdrawal symptoms for most opiates grow stronger approximately 24 to 72 hours after they begin and subside within seven to ten days; however, symptoms such as sleeplessness and drug craving can last for months.

Marijuana

Two widely abused substances, marijuana and hashish, are obtained from the hemp plant *Cannabis sativa*. Both drugs owe their popularity to the same psychoactive component, *tetrahydrocannabinol*, better known as THC. The major differences in these two drugs are their appearance and the amount of THC each contains.

Marijuana is composed of the flowering tops and leaves of the plant. The seeds and stems of the plant may also be included when preparing marijuana for use by drug abusers. It may range in color from grayish-green to greenish-brown, and vary in texture from fine to coarse. The fine-textured marijuana resembles the spice oregano, whereas the coarse-textured drug looks like tea. The street names for marijuana are *Acapulco gold, grass, joint, Mary Jane, pot, reefer, roach, tea*, and *weed*.

Hashish is the dried resin extracted from the flowers, tops, and leaves of the female plant. This gummy extract, when dried, may range in color from light brown to black and in texture from soft to hard. Hashish also differs from marijuana in that an equal amount of hashish can contain five to ten times as much THC, thereby making it a much more potent drug.

Although it is possible to chew or swallow these substances, the most common method of use is by smoking. Marijuana is usually prepared for use as hand-rolled cigarettes, although it may be smoked in special pipes. Hashish is usually smoked in small pipes. Smoking these substances produces the euphoric effect of THC quicker than other methods of administration. The use of marijuana or hashish has been shown to produce moderate tolerance to the effects of THC; therefore, increased usage is required to produce similar effects.

The effects produced by marijuana and hashish are dose-related and can be influenced by such factors as the user's level of tolerance for the drug, the method of use, the concurrent use of other drugs such as alcohol, and the user's psychological state of mind. The use of moderate amounts of marijuana or hashish produces feelings of euphoria, relaxation, and drowsiness. The user may become less inhibited, talking and laughing more than usual. Coordination and judgment may be affected in much the same way as they are by alcohol. With larger doses, there is the tendency to misjudge the passage of time, and the user's perceptions of sound, color, and taste may be sharpened or distorted. In very large doses, the effects of cannabis may cause hallucinations. The effects of marijuana and hashish generally last for several hours. About 5 percent of regular users of these drugs will develop some degree of psychological dependence. Physical dependence and withdrawal symptoms are not usually associated with these drugs.

Aside from the euphoric effect that gives these drugs their high potential for abuse, they tend to increase heart rate, decrease pulmonary function, and increase appetite. Because of these effects, their use may aggravate an existing medical condition such as heart disease or hypertension. Although marijuana has been reported as beneficial in reducing nausea suffered by patients undergoing cancer chemotherapy, it remains classified as a Schedule I drug under the Federal Controlled Substances Act.

Phencyclidine

Phencyclidine (PCP) was originally developed for use as a surgical anesthetic; however, its unwanted and undesirable side effects caused its experimental use with humans to be discontinued. Today, the only legal use for phencyclidine is with animals through licensed veterinary clinics. Unfortunately, limiting this drug's use to veterinary medicine has not prevented its abuse by those acquainted with its psychoactive properties. PCP is readily available from illegal suppliers because it is easily made. The chemicals needed to manufacture this drug are readily available to illegal labs across the country that are interested in making a profit.

The street names for PCP are *angel dust, cosmos, jet, mist, peace pill, rocket fuel, superjoint, tranq,* and *whack.* Because it is cheaply manufactured, PCP is frequently used to "cut" more expensive drugs, thereby increasing the drug dealer's profits. It may be found as a powder, in tablet form, or as a capsule. In that, PCP is usually produced illegally; the size, shape, and color of the tablet or capsule may vary, making it possible to masquerade it as other popular street drugs.

For the same reasons that researchers discontinued medical use of PCP, many drug abusers have also labeled it as a bad drug. Its effects are often unpredictable and, because it is produced illegally, one cannot tell how much PCP is in a powder, tablet, or capsule. The most popular method for taking the drug is by sprinkling the powder on a marijuana cigarette and smoking the combination of drugs. Other methods include taking it orally in any of its available forms, or injecting a solution containing the drug.

Users of PCP often have difficulty describing its effects; however, most agree that it gives them a feeling that is different from other drugs. The psychoactive effects are described as hallucinogenic, sometimes pleasant, sometimes not, but usually associated with a world of fantasy. As the effects of the drug wear off, users report feeling depressed, irritated, and somewhat alienated from their surroundings. While under the influence of PCP, users may appear confused, expressionless, or intoxicated. Speech is often confused, vision distorted, and the user has difficulty thinking and remembering. Some users become violent and aggressive, whereas others withdraw and resist communicating with others. High doses of PCP can induce prolonged stupor or even coma for periods of a few days to several weeks. Long-term users of PCP are subject to recurring episodes of anxiety or depression, and regularly experience disturbances in memory, judgment, concentration, and perception, even after they have stopped taking the drug. Accidental death in which the victim fails to perceive danger is more likely to occur while under the influence of PCP than is death by chemical overdose. Users have been known to drown in shallow water, fall from buildings, and die of burns in circumstances that would have been avoided by less disoriented people.

Lysergic Acid Diethylamide

Lysergic acid diethylamide (LSD), or "acid" as it is sometimes called, is a hallucinogenic agent that has no accepted medical use. As such, LSD is classified as a Schedule I drug under the Federal Controlled Substances Act. The psychoactive effects of the drug are influenced by such factors as the environment in which it is being used, the user's personality, and the user's state of mind at the time the drug is taken. When LSD is taken in pleasant surroundings by a stable, unthreatened personality, the effect on the user can be pleasant and has been described as a "good trip." Alter any of these circumstances and this mood-related drug can provoke unpleasant hallucinations, a "bad trip."

LSD is usually taken orally, often by absorbing the drug in a sugar cube or other substance. Because it is an extremely potent drug, a dose as small as 25 mcg is capable of producing psychoactive effects in some users. Higher doses of LSD have been associated with such effects as alteration of perception wherein the user can "hear" colors, "taste" sounds, and see structural changes as they occur in objects. Those who use LSD may also experience mood changes that range from euphoria to deep depression.

Whether or not LSD produces lasting physical changes in those who take the drug is a subject that is under examination. There is some evidence that long-term use can cause chromosome damage and lead to subsequent birth defects. Incidents of serious adverse reactions to LSD have rarely been reported when the dosage taken was not excessive. There have been incidents where users suffered prolonged adverse psychological effects from LSD; however, the greatest danger presented by the drug appears to be from accidents and suicide attempts by those under its influence.

Spotlight

Prescription Drug Abuse and Addiction

Prescription drug abuse is defined as the intentional misuse of a medication outside of the normally accepted standards of its use. *Prescription drug misuse* is the taking of a medication in a manner other than that prescribed or for a different condition than that for which the medication is prescribed. An estimated 9 million people in the United States, aged 12 and older, use prescription drugs for nonmedical reasons.

There are three classes of prescription drugs that are most commonly abused:

- *Opioids* or narcotics, which are prescribed to treat pain. Examples: morphine, codeine, oxycodone (OxyContin), hydrocodone (Vicodin), hydromorphone (Dilaudid), and meperidine (Demerol).
- *CNS depressants*, which are used to treat anxiety and sleep disorders. Medications commonly prescribed for these purposes are:
    - Barbiturates, such as pentobarbital sodium.
    - Benzodiazepines, such as diazepam (Valium), chlordiazepoxide HCl (Librium), and alprazolam (Xanax) may be prescribed to treat anxiety, acute stress reactions, and panic attacks. The more sedating benzodiazepines, such as triazolam (Halcion) and estazolam may be prescribed for short-term treatment of sleep disorders.
- *Stimulants*, which are prescribed to treat narcolepsy, attention deficit/hyperactivity disorder, and obesity. Examples: dextroamphetamine (Dexedrine) and methylphenidate (Ritalin).

Prescription drug abuse affects many Americans, but some trends of concern can be seen among older adults, adolescents, and women. In addition, health care professionals may be at increased risk of prescription drug abuse because of ease of access, as well as their ability to self-prescribe drugs. In spite of this increased risk, recent surveys and research indicate that health care providers probably suffer from substance abuse, including alcohol and drugs, at a rate similar to rates in society as a whole, in the range of 8 to 12 percent.

Older adults use prescription medications approximately three times as frequently as the general population and have been found to have the poorest rates of compliance with directions for taking a medication. In addition, data suggest older adults may be prescribed inappropriately high doses of medications such as benzodiazepines and may be prescribed these medications for longer periods than are younger adults. Older people who take benzodiazepines are at increased risk for falls that cause hip and thigh fractures, as well as for vehicle accidents. In general, older people should be prescribed lower doses of medications, because the body's ability to metabolize many medications decreases with age.

Prescription drug abuse by teens and young adults is a growing problem in the United States. Many teens think these drugs are safe because they have legitimate uses, but taking them without a prescription to get high or "self-medicate" can be as dangerous and addictive as using street narcotics and other illicit drugs. Prescription medications, as all drugs, can cause dangerous interactions with other drugs or chemcials in the body.

A recent survey indicates that:

- One in five teens has abused a prescription (Rx) pain medication.
- One in five report abusing prescription stimulants and tranquilizers.
- One in ten has abused cough medication.
- More than 2.1 million teens abused prescription drugs in 2006.

Every day, 2,500 kids age 12 to 17 abuse a prescription painkiller for the first time, and more people are getting addicted to prescription drugs. Drug treatment admissions for prescription painkillers increased more than 300 percent from 1995 to 2005.

Parents are urged to safeguard all drugs in their homes, set clear rules, and talk to their teens about appropriate use of medications. Parents are advised to be good role models and also to properly conceal or dispose of old or unused medicines.

Though teen drug use is down overall nationwide, more teens abuse prescription drugs than any other illicit drug, except marijuana—more than cocaine, heroin, and methamphetamine combined.

Studies show that women are more likely than men to be prescribed an abusable prescription drug, particularly narcotics and antianxiety drugs. Overall, men and women have roughly similar rates of nonmedical use of prescription drugs. An exception is found among 12- to 17-year-olds. In this age group, young women are more likely than young men to use psychotherapeutic drugs nonmedically. Although most patients use medications as directed, abuse of and addiction to prescription drugs are public health problems for many Americans. Health care providers can play a role in preventing and detecting prescription drug abuse. About 70 percent of Americans, approximately 191 million people, visit a health care provider at least once every two years. Screening for any type of substance abuse can be incorporated into routine history taking with questions about what prescriptions and over-the-counter medicines the patient is taking and why.

The health care provider should be alert to the following situations that signal substance abuse:

- Any rapid increase in the amount of medication needed, which may indicate drug tolerance and a need for more of the drug.
- Frequent request for refills before the quantity prescribed should have been used.
- "Doctor shopping" by the patient. Moving from provider to provider in an effort to get multiple prescriptions for the drug they abuse.

Addiction to any drug, illicit or prescribed, is a brain disease and can be treated. No single type of treatment is appropriate for all individuals addicted to prescription drugs. Treatment must take into account the type of drug used and the needs of the individual.

RECOGNIZING SUBSTANCE ABUSE

As a member of a health care team, medical assistants are likely to encounter patients who are substance abusers. Aside from the usual disease conditions that might cause an individual to seek medical attention, those who abuse drugs are at greater risk of sustaining accidental injury or infection as a result of drug use. Additionally, there are patients who will attempt to simulate a disease condition that could result in a prescription for a dependency-producing drug.

Obvious signs of drug abuse are needle tracks on the arms or other parts of the patient's body. They may be observed when taking vital signs or doing other medical procedures. Less obvious indicators of possible drug abuse are jaundice, nasal ulceration, dilated or constricted pupils, slurred speech, confusion, impaired reflex action, neglected appearance, poor hygiene, and early withdrawal symptoms. When substance abuse is suspected, medical assistants should reflect a nonjudgmental attitude toward the patient and inform the physician at the earliest opportunity. All information obtained from patients, including evidence of drug abuse, is confidential. Those who provide health care are not allowed to disclose such information unless it becomes necessary to do so during a medical emergency.

SUBSTANCE ABUSE IN THE WORKPLACE

According to the National Institute on Drug Abuse, 10 to 23 percent of Americans abuse drugs and alcohol at work. Chemical dependency has an overwhelming impact on industry, with an annual cost of $140 billion as the result of absenteeism, waste, theft, lost productivity, and property damage.

Marijuana and cocaine are the most used illegal drugs, but alcohol and nicotine pose a far wider problem. It is estimated that 6 percent of all workers always have alcohol in their bloodstream. It is believed that one in three Americans use or have recently used drugs at work.

Warning Signs of Substance Abuse in the Workplace

- **Deteriorating Performance**

  Inconsistent work quality and low productivity

  Increased mistakes, poor concentration, carelessness

- **Poor Attendance or Absenteeism**

  Absenteeism and tardiness, particularly around weekends

  Increased physical complaints: vaguely defined illnesses

  Leaves early for lunch, long breaks, unexplained absences

- **Change in Attitude or Physical Appearance**

  Loss of pride in work: blames others for mistakes

  Avoids contact with coworkers and superiors

  Drastic change in appearance and hygiene

  Complaints from coworkers about covering up for him or her

- **Increasing Health and Safety Hazards**

  Increase in on-the-job accidents

  Carelessness in handling equipment

  Disregard for coworkers' safety

- **Emerging Domestic Problems**

  Complaints about family problems: talk of separation or divorce

  Recurring financial problems

ORGANIZATIONS AND HELP GROUPS

There are many organizations and help groups for substance abusers. They provide information via pamphlets and websites as well as referral assistance. The following list includes addresses, telephone numbers, and Internet website addresses for major substance abuse resource groups:

- Al-Anon/Alateen Family Group Headquarters, Inc.

  PO Box 862 Midtown Station

  New York, NY 10018-0862

  800-356-9996 (literature)

  800-344-2666 (meeting referral)

  http://www.al-anon.org

- Alcoholics Anonymous World Services, Inc
  475 Riverside Drive
  New York, NY 10115
  212-870-3400 (literature)
  212-647-1680 (meeting referral)
  http://www.alcoholics-anonymous.org
- American Council for Drug Education
  c/o Phoenix House
  164 West 74th Street
  New York, NY 10023
  800-488-DRUG
- Cocaine Anonymous World Services
  3740 Overland Avenue, Suite C
  Los Angeles, CA 90034
  http://www.ca.org
- Marijuana Anonymous World Services
  PO Box 2912
  Van Nuys, CA 91404
  800-766-6779
- Mothers Against Drunk Driving
  511 John Carpenter Freeway, Suite 700
  Irving, TX 75062
  800-GET-MADD
- Narcotics Anonymous World Services
  PO Box 9999
  Van Nyes, CA 91409
  818-773-9999
- National Clearinghouse for Alcohol and Drug Information
  800-729-6686
  http://www.health.org
- National Council on Alcoholism and Drug Dependency
  12 West 21st Street, 7th Floor
  New York, NY 10010
  800-NCA-CALL (will refer to local resources)
- National Institute on Drug Abuse
  800-662-HELP (treatment and referral hotline)
  888-644-6432 (Infofax in English/Spanish)
  http://www.nida.nih.gov
  http://www.drugabuse.gov

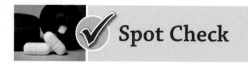

Spot Check

It is known that some drugs interact with alcohol. Give the interaction(s) of the following selected drug(s) when taken with alcohol:

DRUG(S)	INTERACTION(S)
antibiotics	
salicylates and aspirin	
acetaminophen	
anticoagulants	
cimetidine	
lithium	
certain antihistamines	

REVIEW QUESTIONS

Directions. Select the best answer to each of the following multiple-choice question, circling the letter of your choice.

1. _____ is the psychic craving for a drug, a substance.

   a. Euphoria   b. Tolerance   c. Dependency   d. Withdrawal

2. Amphetamines stimulate the central nervous system and cause _____.

   a. increased alertness, elevation of mood, and reduction of appetite

   b. decreased alertness, depression of mood, and stimulating of appetite

   c. increased sense of fatigue

   d. all of these

3. Street names for amphetamines are _____.

   a. speed, downers, and uppers

   b. speed, bennies, wake-ups, and pep pills

   c. speed, amphies, and pep pills

   d. speed, poppers, and pep pills

4. Sudden stoppage of amphetamines in a heavy user may cause the following withdrawal symptoms: _____.

   a. elation, loss of appetite, and restful sleep

   b. disturbed sleep, irritability, strong hunger, and deep depression

   c. disturbed sleep, elation, and anorexia

   d. all of these

5. Cocaine's high potential for abuse relates to its ability to cause _____.

   a. depression, excitement, and stimulation

   b. elation, stimulation, and irritability

   c. euphoria, excitement, and a sense of well-being

   d. none of these

6. _____ or _____ cocaine is made by chemically converting cocaine HCl to a purified, altered form of the drug that is more suitable for smoking.

   a. Crack or freebase   c. Smack or freebase

   b. Coke or freebase   d. all of these

7. The adverse effects of cocaine are _____.

   a. perforated nasal septum, chills, fever

   b. runny nose, ventricular fibrillation

   c. cocaine psychosis, and death from respiratory and circulatory failure

   d. all of these

8. Misuse of barbiturates can lead to their abuse because prolonged use results in _____.

   a. sedation and addiction   c. elation and addiction

   b. tolerance and dependency   d. none of these

9. Very high doses of barbiturates can produce _____.

   a. coma, respiratory arrest   c. death

   b. circulatory collapse   d. all of these

10. The following are all true statements about heroin except _____.

    a. it accounts for 90 percent of the opiate abuse in the United States

    b. it is a legal drug

    c. it is sometimes called junk or smack

    d. it is usually injected

11. The physical dangers associated with opiate abuse may include _____.

    a. the use of unsterile hypodermic needles, which could cause AIDS

    b. using too much of the drug

    c. contamination of the drug itself

    d. all of these

12. All of the following are true statements about marijuana except _____.

    a. it is usually smoked

    b. it causes feelings of euphoria, relaxation, and drowsiness

    c. its effects can be felt for several days

    d. regular users will develop some degree of psychological dependency

13. All of the following are true statements about PCP except _____.

    a. it is readily available from legal suppliers

    b. it is known as angel dust, cosmos, and peace pill

    c. its psychoactive effects are described as hallucinogenic

    d. some users become violent and aggressive

14. Lysergic acid diethylamide (LSD) is classified as a _____.

    a. Schedule I drug   c. Schedule III drug

    b. Schedule II drug   d. Schedule IV drug

15. Higher doses of LSD can cause the user to _____.

    a. "hear" colors

    b. "taste" sounds

    c. see structural changes as they occur in objects

    d. all of these

16. _____ are breathable chemicals that produce psychoactive vapors.

    a. Amphetamines   c. Opiates

    b. Barbiturates   d. Inhalants

17. All of the following are true statements about the abuse of butyl nitrite except _____.

    a. it is packaged in small bottles

    b. it is called "locker room" and "rush"

    c. it produces a "low" that lasts from a few seconds to several minutes

    d. it causes a decrease in blood pressure

18. The medical assistant should be aware of signs of possible substance abuse. These signs may include _____.

    a. needle tracks on the arms or other parts of the body

    b. jaundice, nasal ulceration, slurred speech

    c. dilated or constricted pupils, neglected appearance

    d. all of these

Matching. Place the correct letter from Column II on the appropriate line of Column I:

Column I	*Column II*

19. _____ euphoria

20. _____ tolerance

21. _____ dependency

22. _____ obesity

23. _____ amphetamines (street names)

24. _____ PCP (street names)

25. _____ withdrawal

A. removal of a substance

B. excessive amount of fat on the body

C. a feeling of good health

D. the progressive decrease in the effectiveness of a drug

E. angel dust, cosmos, and peace pill

F. speed, crystal, bennies, and pep pills

G. the psychic craving for a drug

H. the physical craving for a drug

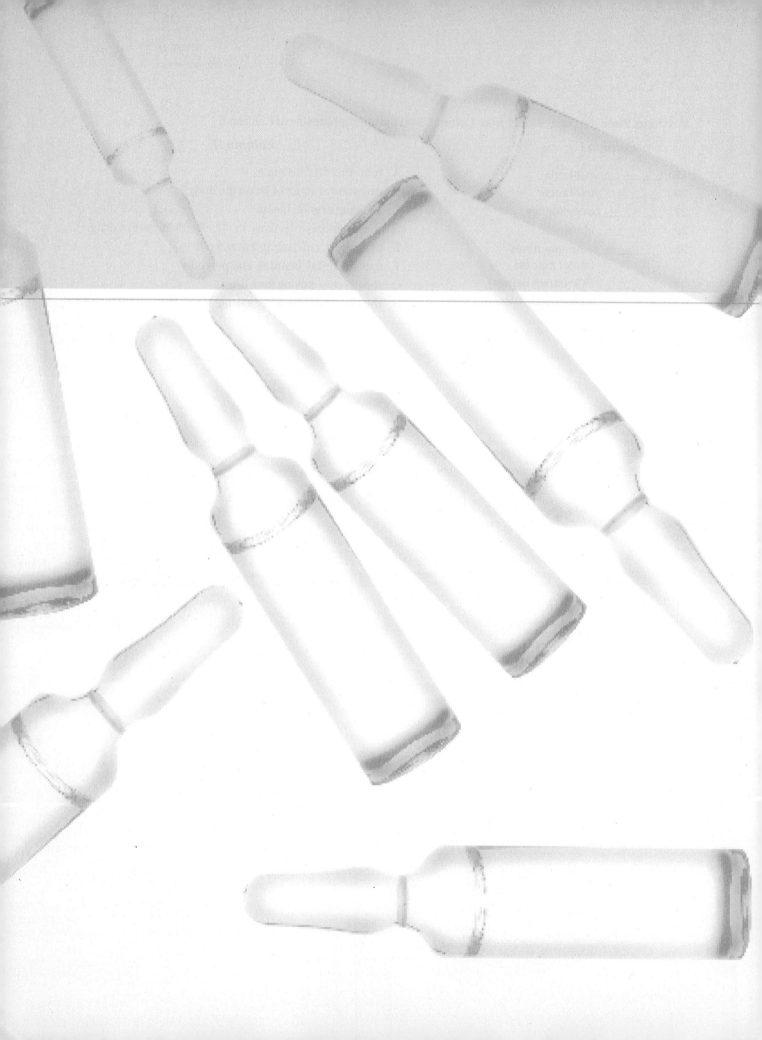

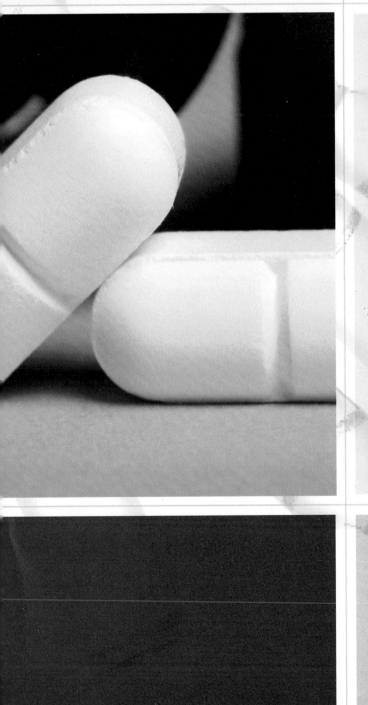

SECTION FOUR

Effects of Medications on Body Systems

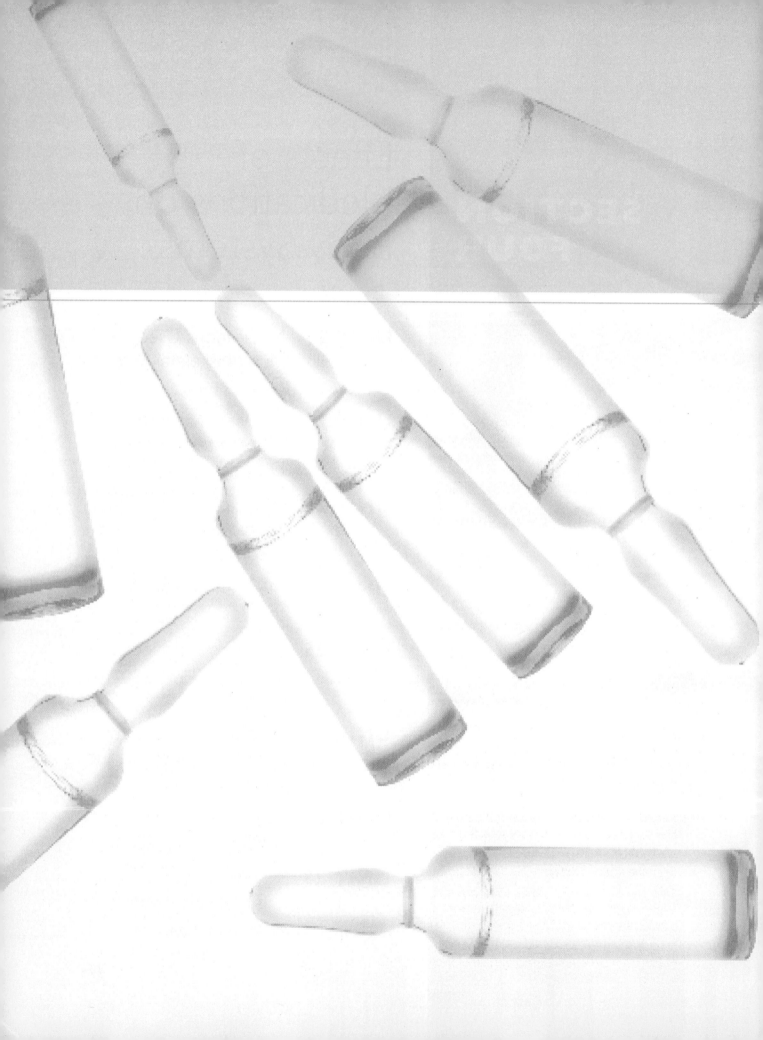

UNIT 21
Medications Used for Musculoskeletal System Disorders

OBJECTIVES

Upon completing this unit, you should be able to:

- Define the terms listed in the vocabulary.
- Describe the benefits and injuries associated with exercise.
- List the normal aging changes that can predispose older adults to falls.
- Explain why musculoskeletal injuries can be common in childhood.
- List ways that may be used to help prevent sports injuries during childhood.
- Complete the critical thinking questions and activities presented in this unit.
- State the actions, uses, contraindications, warnings, adverse reactions, dosage and route, implications for patient care, patient teaching, and special considerations for corticosteroids.
- State the usual anti-inflammatory dose, and adverse reactions of selected nonsteroidal anti-inflammatory agents.
- Describe disease-modifying antirheumatic drugs.
- Describe COX-2 inhibitors and give examples.
- Describe antitumor necrosis factor drugs.
- State the actions, uses, contraindications, adverse reactions, dosage and route, implications for patient care, and patient teaching for etanercept (Enbrel).
- State the actions, uses, contraindications, adverse reactions, dosage and route, implications for patient care, patient teaching, and special considerations for selected medications used to treat osteoporosis.
- Describe agents that are used to treat gout.
- State the actions, uses, types, usual dosage, adverse reactions, implications for patient care, patient teaching, and special considerations for selected skeletal-muscle relaxants.
- State the actions, uses, type, usual dosage, and adverse reactions of selected neuromuscular blocking agents.
- State the actions, uses, usual dosage, adverse reactions, implications for patient care, patient teaching, and special considerations for selected skeletal-muscle stimulants.
- Complete the Spot Check on selected nonsteroidal anti-inflammatory drugs.
- Answer the review questions correctly.

VOCABULARY

acetylcholine (as"e-til-ko'len). A neurotransmitter (ester of choline) that occurs in various tissues and organs of the body. It is thought to play an important role in the transmission of nerve impulses at synapses and myoneural junctions.

acetylcholinesterase (as"e-til-ko "lin-es'ter-as). An enzyme that inactivates the neurotransmitter acetylcholine. It catalyzes the breakdown of acetylcholine to acetic acid and choline. The enzyme is associated with neural structures and preferentially hydrolyzes acetylcholine.

anticholinesterase (an"ti-ko'lin-es' ter-as). A substance that inactivates the action of cholinesterase.

cyclooxygenase (si"klō-ŏk'sĭ-jĕn-ās). An enzyme involved in many aspects of normal cellular function and also in the inflammatory response.

(continues)

chrysotherapy (kris"o-ther'a-pe). The use of gold compounds as treatment; especially for rheumatoid arthritis.

corticosteroid (kor"ti-ko-ster'oyd). Any of a number of hormonal steroid substances (glucocorticoids, mineralocorticoids, and androgens) that are secreted by the adrenal cortex.

prostaglandins (pros'ta-gland-ins). A group of hormonelike unsaturated fatty acids that are present in many body tissues (brain, kidney, thymus, prostate gland, menstrual fluid, lung, seminal fluid, and pancreas). They are secreted in small amounts and effect changes in vasomotor tone, capillary permeability, smooth muscle tone, and autonomic and central nervous system.

receptor (re-sep'tor). A receiver; a cell component that combines with a drug or hormone to alter the function of the cell.

INTRODUCTION

The musculoskeletal system is made up of muscles, bones, ligaments, and tendons (see Figure 21-1). The skeleton consists of 206 interconnected bones that give the body its unique shape and provide support for its organs and tissues. There are more than 650 muscles in the body and those that attach to the skeleton are known as *skeletal muscles*. The maintenance of normal body posture and the production of movement in response to voluntary control are basic functions of these muscles.

Each skeletal muscle is activated by a motor nerve that has its origin at the spinal cord and terminates in fibers connected to muscle cells. The point at which a motor nerve fiber connects to a muscle cell is known as a *neuromuscular junction*. When an electrical impulse of sufficient strength passes from the spinal cord, over the motor nerve, to this junction, it causes the release of the cholinergic neurotransmitter acetylcholine. This substance passes across the neuromuscular junction and binds to specialized receptor sites on that part of the muscle opposite the nerve ending. The presence of acetylcholine sends electrical stimulation throughout the muscle, causing it to contract. This action is countered by the presence of acetylcholinesterase, an enzyme that destroys acetylcholine and readies muscle fibers for the next nerve impulse.

Because the musculoskeletal system is made up of living tissues and depends upon neuromuscular activity to function, this unit will cover medications for the relief of pain and inflammation, as well as drugs used to relax or stimulate skeletal muscles.

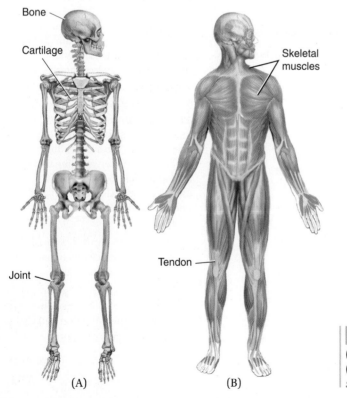

FIGURE 21-1

(A) Skeletal system: bones, cartilage, and joints;
(B) Muscular system: muscles and tendons.

Source: Delmar/Cengage Learning

Spotlight

Exercise—Benefits and Injuries

Each year, more and more evidence indicates that regular physical activity can help the human body maintain, repair, and improve itself. Regular aerobic and weight-bearing exercises, such as aerobic dance, brisk walking, weight lifting, and bicycling, improve heart and lung function and muscle tone. To maintain aerobic fitness, one needs to exercise three times a week for 20 to 30 minutes at the target heart rate.

Although exercise has many benefits, it also carries a number of risks due to the stresses placed on joints, muscles, tendons, and connective tissue. Injuries caused by sports and exercise are very common. Some of the most common types of injuries are bone bruises, bursitis, tendonitis, muscle cramps, sprains, stress fractures, strains, bone spurs, and pulled muscles.

In basketball, tennis, track, running, and brisk walking, the Achilles tendon is most commonly injured. This tendon can become inflamed or torn. In basketball and swimming, the tendons of the shoulder are commonly injured. In tennis, players are susceptible to tennis elbow, as are politicians who shake the hands of many people. Knee injuries account for many sports injuries, as well as presenting problems for many patients who engage in strenuous physical activity.

The best way to prevent injuries due to exercise and sports is to build muscle strength gradually. Muscles respond to increased use by becoming larger and stronger. Warm-up exercises are very important in conditioning the body and preparing it for exercise. Stretching exercises stimulate muscle circulation and help keep joints and tendons flexible.

The Aerobics and Fitness Association of America recommends the following guidelines for stretching before your workout:

1. A warm-up should include a balanced combination of static stretching and rhythmic limbering.
2. End a workout with static stretching.
3. Follow aerobic workouts with a sufficient cool-down period that includes hamstring and calf stretches.
4. After completing exercises for a specific muscle group, always stretch those muscles.

When there is a minor musculoskeletal injury, the first aid treatment is RICE (rest, ice, compression, and elevation). If the injury is severe, medical or surgical treatment should begin as soon as possible. Medical treatment may involve the use of anti-inflammatory drugs, analgesics, and skeletal-muscle relaxants.

It is wise to know one's body and to recognize any warning signs that could indicate injury. It is best to always seek advice from your physician before beginning any exercise program.

Some Benefits of Exercise

- It reduces the risk for heart disease.
- It may slow down the progression of osteoporosis.
- It reduces the levels of triglycerides, and raises the "good" cholesterol (high-density lipoproteins).
- Combined with a low-fat, low-calorie diet, it is effective in preventing obesity and in helping individuals maintain a proper body weight.
- It strengthens muscles and keeps joints, tendons, and ligaments more flexible.
- When older people improve their aerobic fitness, reaction times quicken. This may allow older person to stop a car 15 to 20 feet earlier than an older person who is not fit.

- Women who keep up aerobic exercise during pregnancy are less troubled by backaches, headaches, hot flashes, shortness of breath, and fatigue than sedentary mothers-to-be.
- According to a theoretical model developed by the RAND Corporation, every mile that you cover walking or running saves society an average of 24 cents in medical and other costs.

▪▪ Special Considerations: **OLDER ADULTS**

It has been estimated that approximately 50 percent of all accidental deaths in people over 65 years of age are a result of falls. Studies show that underlying medical problems and hazards in the environment cause about half of the falls; therefore, only half of the falls are truly accidental. As the body ages, certain normal changes can predispose older adults to falls.

Normal Aging Changes That Predispose Older Adults to Falls

- Poor vision.
- Bones lose strength, becoming more brittle. Such changes make the bones easier to break.
- Muscles, if not exercised, lose strength.
- Collagen and elastic fibers of tendons and ligaments degenerate, lose flexibility, and affect muscle activity. This can also cause a decrease in range of motion and make joints more painful.
- Decreased reaction time.
- Fall in blood pressure on sitting or standing.
- Decreased ability to judge exact height or depth of a surface.
- Medical problems such as osteoporosis, vertigo, mental confusion, heart valve, or rhythm abnormalities.
- Polypharmacy.

▪▪ Special Considerations: **CHILDREN**

Injury to the musculoskeletal system can be common in childhood. Approximately 200,000 children are admitted to hospitals each year with head injuries. Head injuries occur more frequently in males than in females and are prevalent during adolescence. Toddlers can also be prone to head injuries. The major complications of head injury are hemorrhage, swelling of the brain, compression of the brain stem, and infection.

School-age children are generally more prone to fractures because of bicycle accidents, falls on the playground, and sports injuries. Sports injuries are also common in adolescents. Concussion, injured ligaments, fractures, sprains, strains, muscle cramps, shin splints, and neck injury are some of the common sports injuries seen during adolescence. There are various ways to help prevent sports injuries. The following list offers some suggestions.

Prevention of Sports Injury

- Before and after sports activity, allow for adequate warm-up and cool-down periods.
- Year-round conditioning of the body, through a regular exercise program, is very important.
- Physical and mental ability should determine the choice of a sports activity.
- Sports activity should be supervised by a qualified adult.
- All participants should use safe and well-fitting athletic gear and equipment.
- All participants should follow safety rules and regulations of the sports activity.
- Proper nutrition and adequate fluids are necessary for children to perform at their best.

- Emergency services should be readily available in case of injury.
- Each child should have a physical examination before beginning any athletic activity.

■▪ Critical Thinking **QUESTIONS AND ACTIVITIES**

Regular physical activity can help the human body maintain, repair, and improve itself. Although exercise has many benefits, it also carries a number of risks due to stresses placed on joints, muscles, tendons, and connective tissue. Ask yourself:

- What are some of the common injuries due to exercise?
- What is the best way to prevent injuries due to exercise?
- What is the first aid treatment for a minor musculoskeletal injury?
- What is the medical treatment for a musculoskeletal injury?

ANTI-INFLAMMATORY DRUGS

Inflammation is a normal response to injury, infection, or irritation of living tissue. Redness, tenderness, pain, and swelling of the affected area are characteristics of the inflammatory process. Minor inflammations may occur as the result of a break in the skin or casual contact with a caustic substance. The more severe forms of inflammation are usually associated with rheumatic disorders such as arthritis.

Drugs that relieve the swelling, tenderness, redness, and pain of inflammation are known as anti-inflammatory agents. All but a few of these agents provide only symptomatic relief of pain and inflammation and do not treat its cause.

Steroidal anti-inflammatory agents are those that are chemically related to the naturally occurring hormone cortisone, which is secreted by the adrenal cortex. These agents are most often used in the treatment of local inflammatory disorders. Corticosteroids may be applied to the skin for topical treatment of dermatological conditions or injected into a joint, bursa, or skin lesion to reduce the effects of inflammation. The use of steroidal agents to treat systemic inflammatory disorders is limited by the array of serious side effects caused by these drugs.

Corticosteroids (Glucocorticoids)

Actions

Corticosteroids have potent anti-inflammatory effects in disorders of many organ systems. They also cause varied metabolic effects, and modify the body's immune responses to assorted stimuli.

Uses

Primary or secondary adrenocortical insufficiency, congenital adrenal hyperplasia, hypercalcemia associated with cancer, as adjunctive therapy in psoriatic arthritis, rheumatoid arthritis, ankylosing spondylitis, acute and subacute bursitis, acute nonspecific tenosynovitis, acute gouty arthritis, post-traumatic osteoarthritis, synovitis of osteoarthritis, epicondylitis, and in the treatment of certain collagen, dermatologic, ophthalmic, respiratory, hematologic, gastrointestinal, and neoplastic diseases, during allergic states, edematous states, and cerebral edema.

Contraindications

Contraindicated in patients with known hypersensitivity to any of the ingredients. They should not be used in patients with systemic fungal infections, idiopathic thrombocytopenia purpura, acute glomerulonephritis, amebiasis, or nonasthmatic bronchial disease, and by children under 2 years of age.

> ## Warning:
>
> 1. Corticosteroids may mask some signs of infection, and new infections may appear during their use.
> 2. Prolonged use may produce posterior subcapsular cataracts or glaucoma with possible damage of the optic nerves, and may enhance the establishment of secondary ocular infections due to fungi or viruses.
> 3. Use caution during pregnancy, lactation, active tuberculosis, and myocardial infarction.
> 4. Average and large doses of the drug(s) can cause elevation of blood pressure, salt and water retention, and increased excretion of potassium.
> 5. All corticosteroids increase calcium secretion.
> 6. Administration of live virus vaccines are contraindicated in patients receiving immunosuppressive doses of corticosteroids.
> 7. There are many precautions associated with corticosteroids. Please refer to a current drug reference book or visit www.Drugs@FDA.com.

Adverse Reactions

Sodium and fluid retention, congestive heart failure, potassium loss, hypokalemic alkalosis, hypertension, muscle weakness, steroid myopathy, loss of muscle mass, osteoporosis, peptic ulcer, pancreatitis, abdominal distention, poor wound healing, acne, ecchymosis, petechiae, depression, flushing, headache, mood changes, tachycardia, diarrhea, nausea, vertigo, convulsions, menstrual irregularities, development of cushingoid state, hirsutism, glaucoma, weight gain, increased appetite, malaise, hiccups.

Dosage and Route

The dosage and route of administration are determined by the physician and individualized for each patient (see Table 21-1).

Implications for Patient Care

Observe patients for evidence of fluid or electrolyte imbalance and any signs of adverse reactions. Monitor weight, intake and output ratio, vital signs, and serum electrolytes, and during long-term therapy, monitor blood sugar, urine glucose, and plasma cortisol levels. Protect patients from infection.

 Patient Teaching

Educate patients:

- to take the medication as prescribed.
- to be alert for signs of adverse reactions.
- to avoid the use of tobacco, alcohol, aspirin, caffeine, and over-the-counter medications unless they have the permission of the physician.
- to wear or carry a Medic Alert ID stating that they are on corticosteroid therapy.
- to avoid individuals who have respiratory infections and guard against other types of infection.
- to weigh themselves weekly and report gain of 5 pounds or more to the physician.
- to include in their diet foods high in potassium or low in sodium, and to take in an adequate amount of proteins, vitamins, and calcium. ▪

TABLE 21-1   Corticosteroids for Oral, Parenteral, and Local Injection

MEDICATION	ORAL DOSE	PARENTERAL DOSE	LOCAL INJECTION
methylprednisolone (Medrol)	4 to 48 mg/day	—	—
methylprednisolone acetate (Depo-Medrol)	—	IM: 40 to 120 mg every 1 to 4 weeks	4 to 80 mg, slow onset/ long duration
hydrocortisone (Cortef)	20 to 240 mg/day		

Special Considerations

- Prolonged corticosteroid therapy may result in a cushingoid state. Signs and symptoms include acne, moon face, hirsutism, buffalo hump, hypertension, protruding abdomen, girdle obesity, amenorrhea, glycosuria, purplish abdominal striae, edema, and thinning and atrophy of extremities.

- The effect of corticosteroids may be decreased by barbiturates, rifampin, ephedrine, or phenytoin.

- Corticosteroids may decrease the effect of anticoagulants, anticonvulsants, hypoglycemic agents, insulin, isoniazid, or neostigmine.

- Corticosteroids may increase digitalis toxicity as a result of increased potassium loss.

- The effect of corticosteroids may be increased by estrogens, salicylates, or indomethacin.

Nonsteroidal anti-inflammatory drugs (NSAIDs) are synthetic products that are unrelated to substances produced by the body (see Table 21-2). These agents are widely used in the treatment of inflammation, arthritis, and related disorders. Although the exact mechanism by which these agents act is not fully understood, their anti-inflammatory action is believed to result from inhibition of prostaglandins synthesis.

The most common adverse reactions associated with NSAIDs are nausea, vomiting, abdominal discomfort, diarrhea, constipation, gastric or duodenal ulcer formation, and gastrointestinal bleeding. Hematologic changes can occur, and other adverse reactions that may occur are jaundice, toxic hepatitis, visual disturbances, rash, dermatitis, and hypersensitivity reactions. Usually, these adverse reactions are associated with high doses and prolonged drug therapy.

Gastrointestinal disturbances may occur with the use of NSAIDs and can be severe and even fatal, especially in patients with a history of gastric or duodenal ulcers. For the diabetic patient, these agents can affect the blood glucose level; therefore, insulin dosage may require adjustment. For the patient taking warfarin, these drugs may potentiate the anticoagulant effect and increase the risk of bleeding. Based on research findings, it is

Warning:

Cardiovascular Risk

- NSAIDs may cause an increased risk of serious cardiovascular thrombotic events, myocardial infarction, and stroke, which can be fatal. This risk may increase wih duration of use. Patients with cardiovascular disease or risk factors for cardiovascular disease may be at greater risk.

- Motrin tablets are contraindicated for treatment of perioperative pain in the setting of coronary artery bypass graft (CABG) surgery.

Gastrointestinal Risk

- NSAIDs cause an increased risk of serious gastrointestinal adverse events including bleeding, ulceration, and perforation of the stomach or intestines, which can be fatal. These events can occur at any time during use and without warning symptoms. Elderly patients are at greater risk for serious gastrointestinal events.

TABLE 21-2 Nonsteroidal Anti-inflammatory Drugs

MEDICATION	USUAL ANTI-INFLAMMATORY DOSE	ADVERSE REACTIONS
acetylsalicylic acid (aspirin)	Oral: 3.6 to 5.4 g/day in divided doses	GI distress, tinnitus, rapid pulse, pulmonary edema
choline salicylate (Arthropan)	Oral: 1 to 2 tsp up to 4 times/day	See aspirin
diclofenac (Voltaren)	Oral: 50 mg 2 to 3 times daily	Dizziness, headache, GI bleeding, heartburn, abdominal pain, diarrhea, acute renal failure, rash, edema
diflunisal	Oral: 500 to 1000 mg/day in 2 divided doses	GI distress, dizziness, skin rash, headache, tinnitus
fenoprofen calcium (Nalfon)	Oral: 300 to 600 mg 3 to 4 times/day	GI distress, dizziness, headache, drowsiness, tinnitus
ibuprofen (Motrin)	Oral: 300 to 600 mg 3 to 4 times/day	GI distress, dizziness, headache, drowsiness, tinnitus
indomethacin (Indocin)	Oral, Rectal: 25 to 50 mg 2 to 3 times/day Sustained Release: 75 mg once/day	GI distress, headache, dizziness, drowsiness
ketoprofen	Oral: 150 to 300 mg, divided in 3 or 4 doses	Peptic ulcer, GI bleeding, nausea, malaise, diarrhea, anorexia, headache, dizziness, rash, tinnitus
meclofenamate sodium	Oral: 50 to 100 mg 3 to 4 times/day	GI distress
mefenamic acid (Ponstel)	Oral: 500 mg, then 250 mg every 6 hours for no more than 1 week	GI distress, skin rash
naproxen (Naprosyn)	Oral: 250 to 375 mg 2 times/day	GI distress, dizziness, headache, drowsiness, tinnitus
naproxen sodium (Aleve)	Oral: 275 to 550 mg twice daily (up to 1.65 g/day)	GI bleeding, anorexia, constipation, nausea, dizziness, drowsiness, headache, tinnitus, dyspnea, edema, palpitations, tachycardia, cystitis, renal failure, photosensitivity, rash, blood dyscrasias, anaphylaxis; may increase the risk of heart attack or stroke; should avoid taking the drug for more than 10 days
piroxicam (Feldene)	Oral: 20 mg/day as a single or divided dose	GI distress, dizziness, rash, rapid pulse
salsalate	Oral: 325 to 1000 mg 2 to 3 times/day	GI distress, tinnitus, rapid pulse, pulmonary edema
sulindac (Clinoril)	Oral: 150 to 200 mg 2 times/day	GI distress, dizziness, skin rash
tolmetin sodium (Tolectin)	Oral: 600 to 1800 mg/day in divided doses	GI distress, light-headedness, dizziness

recommended that patients taking warfarin should avoid NSAIDs. If given, these drugs should be introduced slowly and given in lower dosages whenever feasible. Prothrombin time should be monitored closely, especially during the first two weeks. When NSAIDs are stopped, there may be a loss of anticoagulant control. People who drink three or more alcoholic beverages daily and take Motrin should be warned of the risk of stomach bleeding.

Disease-Modifying Antirheumatic Drugs

Disease-modifying antirheumatic drugs (DMARDs) are also called slow-acting antirheumatic drugs (SAARDs) or second-line drugs. Although nonsteroidal anti-inflammatory drugs reduce pain and inflammation and improve stiffness and mobility in patients with rheumatoid arthritis, they do not slow the progression of joint damage. Disease-modifying antirheumatic drugs may influence the course of the disease progression; thereby, their introduction in early rheumatoid arthritis is recommended to limit irreversible joint damage. Examples of DMARDs are gold preparations (Aurolate, Ridaura, and Solganal), antimalarials (Plaquenil sulfate), penicillamine (Cuprimine), sulfasalazine (Azulfidine), leflunomide (Arava), and the immunosuppressants methotrexate (Rheumatrex), and azathioprine (Imuran). See Table 21-3.

Gold preparations are used in the long-term treatment of rheumatoid arthritis. These agents have been shown to be effective in reducing the progression of the disease, as well as relieving inflammation. The usefulness of gold therapy (**chrysotherapy**) is limited by the toxicity of these drugs. The adverse effects of gold compounds may occur shortly after administration, at any time during the course of therapy, or even after therapy has been discontinued.

The *antimalarial* drug *hydroxychloroquine sulfate* has been used as a second-line therapeutic agent for the treatment of rheumatoid arthritis. Treatment with this agent usually requires 6 to 12 months, and is complicated by its potential toxicity and the variability of beneficial effects produced. Ocular toxicity is the most serious complication and regular ophthalmologic examinations should accompany therapy with this drug.

Penicillamine, a chelating agent, has been shown to be effective in long-term treatment of rheumatoid arthritis. Its mechanism of action is not fully understood. Because penicillamine causes potentially serious adverse reactions, its use is recommended for those with long-standing progressive disease that has not responded to other agents.

Rheumatrex is a low-dose form of methotrexate approved for adult rheumatoid arthritis. It reduces inflammation, pain, swelling, and stiffness in adult rheumatoid arthritis. It is recommended for selected adults with severe, active, classical, or definite rheumatoid arthritis who have had insufficient response to other forms of treatment. The patient may see improvement within three to six weeks.

COX-2 Inhibitors

Recent advances in the understanding of the underlying causes of inflammation and pain have resulted in the development of a new class of drugs known as COX-2 inhibitors. The first drug of this class to be approved, Celebrex (celecoxib), is used for the treatment of osteoarthritis and rheumatoid arthritis, and a second drug, Mobic (meloxicam), is approved for the treatment of osteoarthritis.

Cyclooxygenase (COX) is an enzyme involved in many aspects of normal cellular function and also in the inflammatory response. Two forms, designated COX-1 and COX-2, have been identified. COX-2 is found in joints and other areas affected by inflammation. Inhibition of COX-2 reduces the production of compounds associated with inflammation and pain.

Celecoxib (Celebrex)

Actions

Believed to inhibit prostaglandin synthesis, primarily via inhibitory of cyclooxygenase-2 (COX-2).

Uses

For relief of the signs and symptoms of osteoarthritis, rheumatoid arthritis in adults, for the management of acute pain in adults, for the treatment of dysmenorrhea, and to reduce the number of adenomatous colorectal polyps in familial adenomatous polyposis (FAP).

Contraindications

Celebrex should not be given to patients with known hypersensitivity to celecoxib, and patients who have demonstrated allergic-type reactions to sulfonamides. It should not be given to patients who have experienced asthma,

TABLE 21-3 Disease-Modifying Antirheumatic Drugs

MEDICATION	USUAL ANTI-INFLAMMATORY DOSE	ADVERSE REACTIONS
auranofin (Ridaura)	Oral: 3 mg twice/day or 6 mg once/day	Loose stools or diarrhea, nausea, rash, pruritus, stomatitis, proteinuria
aurothioglucose (Solganal)	IM: 10 mg the 1st week, 25 mg the 2nd and 3rd week, then 50 mg thereafter until a total of 800 to 1000 mg has been given	Pruritus, "gold dermatitis," ulcerative stomatitis, hypersensitivity reactions, nephrotic syndrome with proteinuria, conjunctivitis
azathioprine (Imuran)	Oral: l mg/kg/day for 6 to 8 weeks; increase by 0.5 mg/kg/day every 4 weeks until response or up to 2.5 mg/kg/day, then decrease by 0.5 mg/kg/day every 4 to 8 weeks to minimal effective dose	Retinopathy, anorexia, nausea, vomiting, diarrhea, hepatotoxicity, alopecia, pulmonary edema, rash, anemia, leukopenia, chills, fever
gold sodium thiomalate (Myochrysine)	IM (Weekly): 1st injection 10 mg; 2nd injection 25 mg; then 25 to 50 mg weekly until a cumulative dose of 1000 mg has been given	Hypersensitivity reactions, nephrotic syndrome, stomatitis, dermatitis, colitis
hydroxychloroquine sulfate (Plaquenil Sulfate)	Oral: 200 to 600 mg daily	GI distress, visual disturbances, retinopathy, vertigo, tinnitus, nerve deafness, dermatologic reactions
leflunomide (Arava)	Oral: Loading dose of one 100-mg tablet per day for three days; daily maintenance dose is 20 mg, and doses higher than this are not recommended	Nephrotoxicity, diarrhea, alopecia, anorexia, abdominal pain, nausea, gastritis, hypertension, dizziness, rash
methotrexate (Rheumatrex)	Oral: 7.5 mg once weekly, or in divided doses of 2.5 mg at 12-hour intervals for three doses; not to exceed 20 mg/week	Nausea, mucositis, GI discomfort, rash, diarrhea, headache, hepatotoxicity, cirrhosis, bone marrow depression with anemia, leukopenia; potentially dangerous lung disease may occur, ulcerative stomatitis
penicillamine (Cuprimine)	Oral: initially 125 to 250 mg/day. Dosage increases of 125 to 250 mg/day at 1 to 3 month intervals, if necessary	Dermatologic reactions, GI distress, thrombocytopenia, cholestatic jaundice, membraneous glomerulopathy
sulfasalazine (Azulfidine)	Oral: 500 mg–1 g/day (as delayed-release tablet) for 1 week, then increase by 500 mg/day every week up to 2 g/day in 2 divided doses	Ataxia, confusion, dizziness, drowsiness, headache, mental depression, psychosis, restlessness

urticaria, or allergic-type reactions after taking aspirin or other NSAIDs. Severe, rarely fatal, anaphylactic-like reactions to NSAIDs have been reported in such patients. Celebrex should be used during pregnancy only if the potential benefit justifies the potential risk to the fetus.

Adverse Reactions

Abdominal pain, diarrhea, dyspepsia, flatulence, nausea, back pain, dizziness, headache, insomnia, pharyngitis, rash.

Dosage and Route

For osteoarthritis, the recommended oral dose is 100 to 200 mg per day administered as a single dose or as 100 mg twice per day. For rheumatoid arthritis, the recommended oral dose is 100 to 200 mg twice per day.

Implications for Patient Care

It is important that the patient understand that serious gastrointestinal toxicity such as bleeding, ulceration, and perforation of the stomach, small intestine or large intestine, can occur at any time, with or without warning symptoms, in patients treated with NSAIDs.

Patient Teaching

Educate patients:

- to promptly report signs or symptoms of gastrointestinal ulceration or bleeding, skin rash, unexplained weight gain, or edema to their physician.
- about the warning signs and symptoms of hepatotoxicity (nausea, fatigue, lethargy, pruritus, jaundice, right upper quadrant tenderness, and flulike symptoms). If these occur, patients should stop therapy and seek medical attention immediately.
- that one need not take the medicine with a meal. A high-fat meal will make the drug act more slowly.
- to not take with an antacid, as an antacid will actually make the drug less effective.
- to take the medicine for at least five days to get the full effect.
- that Celebrex seems to decrease the effect of angiotensin converting enzyme (ACE) inhibitors.
- that Celebrex also interferes with the action of diuretics.
- that Celebrex might increase lithium blood levels.
- that fluconazole increases blood levels of Celebrex.
- that if the pain is not reduced in a week or two, contact their physician. ■

> **Warning:**
>
> *Use of celecoxib (Celebrex) may be associated with an increased risk of adverse cardiovascular (CV) events, including cardiovascular death, acute myocardial infarction (MI), and stroke.*

Antitumor Necrosis Factor Drugs/Biological Response Modifiers

Antitumor necrosis factor drugs have evolved out of the biotechnology industry. Antitumor necrosis factor drugs seem to slow, if not halt altogether, the destruction of the joints by disrupting the activity of tumor necrosis factor (TNF), a substance involved in the body's immune response. An autoimmune response is a process by which the body's defense system malfunctions and begins to attack itself. This process appears to account for many types of arthritis including rheumatoid arthritis, lupus, myositis, and scleroderma. By blocking TNF, these agents act to preempt the autoimmune response. Examples include adalimumab (Humira), certolizumab pegol (Cimizia), infliximab (Remicade), and etanercept (Enbrel).

In 2008 the Food and Drug Administration ordered stronger warnings on four medications widely used to treat rheumatoid arthritis, Crohn's disease, juvenile arthritis, certain types of psoriasis, and other serious illnesses, stating that they can raise the risk of possible fatal fungal infections.

The drugs Enbrel, Remicade, Humira, and Cimzia work by suppressing the immune system to keep it from attacking the body. For patients with rheumatoid arthritis, the treatment provides relief from swollen and painful joints, but the drugs also lower the body's defenses to various kinds of infections. Of most concern are pulmonary and disseminated histoplasmosis, coccidioidomycosis, blastomycosis, tuberculosis, and other opportunistic infections that are not consistently recognized in patients taking TNF blockers. This has resulted in delays in appropriate treatment, sometimes resulting in death in patients taking TNF blockers. Health care professionals should be alert for signs and symptoms of possible systemic fungal infections, such as fever, malaise, weight loss, sweats, cough, shortness of breath, and/or other pulmonary infiltrates, or other serious systemic illness and initiate appropriate treatment immediately.

Etanercept (Enbrel)

Actions

This medicine binds specifically to tumor necrosis factor and blocks its interaction with cell surface TNF receptors. TNF is a naturally occurring cytokine that is involved in normal inflammatory and immune response.

Uses

Enbrel is indicated for reduction in signs and symptoms of moderately to severely active rheumatoid arthritis in patients who have had an inadequate response to one or more disease-modifying antirheumatic drugs. It can be used in combination with methotrexate in patients who do not respond adequately to methotrexate alone. It is indicated for reducing signs and symptoms of moderately to severe active polyarticular-course juvenile rheumatoid arthritis in patients who have had an inadequate response to one or more DMARDs. It is indicated for reducing signs and symptoms and inhibiting the progression of structural damage of active arthritis in patients with psoriatic arthritis. It is indicated for reducing signs and symptoms in patients with active ankylosing spondylitis. It is indicated for the treatment of adult patients (18 years or older) with chronic moderate to severe plaque psoriasis who are candidates for systemic therapy or phototherapy.

Contraindications

Enbrel should not be administered to patients with sepsis or with known hypersensitivity to Enbrel or any of its components.

Adverse Reactions

Reactions include erythema, itching, pain, or swelling at the injection site. Upper respiratory infections and sinusitis, headache, dizziness, asthenia, abdominal pain, rash, and dyspepsia.

Dosage and Route

The recommended dose of Enbrel for adult patients with rheumatoid arthritis is 25 mg given twice weekly as a subcutaneous injection.

Implications for Patient Care

Patients should be instructed in proper subcutaneous injection technique and how to measure and administer the correct dose of medication. The first injection should be performed under the supervision of a qualified health care professional.

Patient Teaching

Educate patients:

- to carefully read the Patient Information insert and to ask questions as necessary.
- that Enbrel can lower the ability of the immune system to fight infection, so one can be more prone to getting infections or make any infection that one has worse.

- that all medications have side effects and one should be aware of the possible serious side effects of Enbrel (serious infections, nervous system diseases, blood problems, heart problems, allergic reactions, and malignancies).

- that before starting on Enbrel, they should inform the physician about any active infection, history of infections, close contact with someone who has tuberculosis, symptoms of tuberculosis (dry cough, weight loss, fever, night sweats), nervous system disease, congestive heart failure, diabetes, or if one is scheduled major surgery or planned vaccination. ▪

Warning:

RISK OF INFECTIONS

Infections, including serious infections leading to hospitalization or death, have been observed in patients treated with Enbrel. Infections have included bacterial sepsis and tuberculosis. Patients should be educated about the symptoms of infection and closely monitored for signs and symptoms of infection during and after treatment with Enbrel. Patients who develop an infection should be evaluated for appropriate antimicrobial treatment and, in patients who develop a serious infection, Enbrel should be discontinued. Tuberculosis (frequently disseminated or extrapulmonary at clinical presentation) has been observed in patients receiving TNF-blocking agents, including Enbrel. Tuberculosis may be due to reactivation of latent tuberculosis infection or to new infection. Data from clinical trials and preclinical studies suggest that the risk of reactivation of latent tuberculosis infection is lower with Enbrel than with TNF-blocking monoclonal antibodies. Nonetheless, postmarketing cases of tuberculosis reactivation have been reported for TNF blockers, including Enbrel. Patients should be evaluated for tuberculosis risk factors and be tested for latent tuberculosis infection prior to initiating Enbrel and during treatment. Treatment of latent tuberculosis infection should be initiated prior to therapy with Enbrel. Treatment of latent tuberculosis in patients with a reactive tuberculin test reduces the risk of tuberculosis reactivation in patients receiving TNF blockers. Some patients who tested negative for latent tuberculosis prior to receiving Enbrel have developed active tuberculosis. Physicians should monitor patients receiving Enbrel for signs and symptoms of active tuberculosis, including patients who tested negative for latent tuberculosis infection.

AGENTS USED TO TREAT OSTEOPOROSIS

Osteoporosis is the loss of bone density and strength. It is a disease that leads to an increased risk of fracture. Osteoporosis is defined by the World Health Organization (WHO) in women as a bone mineral density, 2.5 standard deviations below peak bone mass (20-year-old healthy female average) as measured by DXA. Dual energy X-ray absorptiometry (DXA, formerly DEXA) is considered the gold standard for the diagnosis of osteoporosis. Osteoporosis is diagnosed when the bone mineral density is less than or equal to 2.5 standard deviations below that of a young adult reference population. This is translated as a T-score. WHO has established the following diagnostic guidelines:

- T-score of −1.0 or greater is "normal"
- T-score between −1.0 and −2.5 is "low bone mass" (or "osteopenia")
- T-score −2.5 or below is osteoporosis

Osteoporosis is most common in women after menopause, when it is called postmenopausal osteoporosis, but may also develop in men, and may occur in anyone in the presence of particular hormonal disorders and other chronic diseases or as a result of medications, specifically glucocorticoids, when the disease is called steroid- or glucocorticoid-induced osteoporosis (SIOP or GIOP).

Medications Used for Prevention and Treatment of Osteoporosis

Agents used to prevent or treat osteoporosis are known as antiresorptive medications and include bisphosphonates, calcitonin, estrogen, and estrogen agonists/antagonists. These drugs slow the bone loss that occurs in the breakdown part of the remodeling cycle. The goal of treatment with antiresorptive medications is to prevent bone loss and lower the risk of bone breakage.

Teriparatide (Forteo), a form of parathyroid hormone, is the first osteoporosis medication to increase the rate of bone formation in the bone remodeling cycle and is in a distinct category of osteoporosis medications called anabolic drugs. The goal of treatment with teriparatide is to build bone and lower the risk of bone breakage.

Antiresorptive Medications—Bisphosphonates

Actions

Bisphosponates inhibit osteoclast activity and reduce bone resorption and turnover. In postmenopausal women, they reduce the elevated rate of bone turnover, leading to, on average, a net gain in bone mass.

Uses

Indicated for the treatment and prevention of osteoporosis in postmenopausal women and for the treatment of osteoporosis in men. Also approved for the treatment of glucocorticoid-induced osteoporosis in men and women as a result of long-term use of steroid medications, such as prednisone and cortisone.

Contraindications

Contraindicated in patients with known hypersensitivity to any of the ingredients, uncorrected hypocalcemia, or the inability to stand or sit upright for at least 30 to 60 minutes.

Adverse Reactions

Side effects for all the bisphosphonates may include bone, joint, or muscle pain. Side effects of the oral tablets may include nausea, difficulty swallowing, heartburn, and irritation of the esophagus and gastric ulcer. Side effects that can occur shortly after receiving an IV bisphosphonate include flulike symptoms, fever, pain in muscles or joints, and headache. Inflammation of the eye (uveitis) is a rare side effect of all bisphosphonates.

There have been reports of osteonecrosis of the jaw (ONJ) with bisphosphonate medications.

> ⚠️ **Warning:**
>
> *The FDA informed health care professionals and patients of the possibility of severe and sometimes incapacitating bone, joint, and/or muscle (musculoskeletal) pain in patients taking bisphosphonates. Although severe musculoskeletal pain is included in the prescribing information for all bisphosphonates, the association between bisphosphonates and severe musculoskeletal pain may be overlooked by health care professionals, delaying diagnosis, prolonging pain and/or impairment, and necessitating the use of analgesics. The severe musculoskeletal pain may occur within days, months, or years after starting a bisphosphonate. Some patients have reported complete relief of symptoms after discontinuing the bisphosphonate, whereas others have reported slow or incomplete resolution. The risk factors for and incidence of severe musculoskeletal pain associated with bisphosphonates are unknown.*

Dosage and Route

The dosage and route of administration are determined by the physician and individualized for each patient (see Table 21-4).

TABLE 21-4   Medications Used to Prevent and/or Treat Osteoporosis

CLASS AND DRUG	BRAND NAME	FORM	FREQUENCY
Bisphosphonates			
Alendronate	Fosamax	Oral (tablet)	Daily/weekly
Alendronate	Fosamax Plus D™ (with 2,800 IU or 5,600 IU of Vitamin D₃)	Oral (tablet)	Weekly
Alendronate	Fosamax	Oral (liquid solution)	Weekly
Ibandronate	Boniva	Oral (tablet)	Monthly
Ibandronate	Boniva	Intravenous (IV)	Four times per year
Risedronate	Actonel	Oral (tablet)	Daily/weekly/twice monthly/monthly
Risedronate	Actonel with Calcium	Oral (tablet)	Weekly
Zoledronic Acid	Reclast	Intravenous (IV)	One time per year
Calcitonin			
Calcitonin	Fortical	Nasal spray	Daily
Calcitonin	Miacalcin	Nasal spray	Daily
Calcitonin	Miacalcin	Injection	Varies
Estrogen*			
Estrogen	Multiple Brands	Oral (tablet)	Daily
Estrogen	Multiple Brands	Transdermal (skin) patch	Twice weekly/weekly
Estrogen Agonists/ Antagonists *Also called Selective Estrogen Receptor Modulators (SERMs)*			
Raloxifene	Evista	Oral (tablet)	Daily
Parathyroid Hormone			
Teriparatide	Forteo	Injection	Daily

Implications for Patient Care

Patients taking the oral bisphosphonate tablets should stop taking the drug and contact their health care provider immediately when experiencing chest pain, new or worsening heartburn, or difficulty or painful swallowing. It is important that patients report these or other side effects to their health care provider.

Patient Teaching

Educate patients:

- To take the medication as prescribed.
- To be alert for signs of adverse reactions.
- To take the medication first thing in the morning at least 1 hour (60 minutes) before eating, drinking anything other than plain water, or taking any other oral medicine.
- To take the medication with 6 to 8 ounces of plain water. Do not take it with other drinks, such as mineral water, sparkling water, coffee, tea, dairy drinks, or juice.

- To swallow the medication whole. Do not chew or suck the tablet or keep it in the mouth to melt or dissolve.

- To wait at least 30 minutes to 1 hour (depending on the type of drug) before lying down. Patients may sit, stand, or do normal activities like read the newspaper or take a walk.

- Not to take other oral medicines including vitamins, calcium, or antacids at the same time as taking this medicine. Take vitamins, calcium, and antacids at a different time of the day.

- To drink a full glass of milk and call the local poison control center or emergency room right away if they've taken too much of this medicine. Patients should not make themselves vomit and should not lie down. ■

Special Considerations

- Bisphosphonates **are not** recommended for people with severe kidney disease or low blood calcium. People with certain problems of the esophagus may not be able to take the oral tablets.

- Patients should tell a health care provider (including a dentist) about all medicines they take, including prescription and nonprescription medicines, vitamins, and supplements.

Other Antiresorptive Medications

Calcitonin (Fortical and Miacalcin)

Calcitonin is approved for the treatment of osteoporosis in postmenopausal women who are at least five years beyond menopause. It is a naturally occurring hormone involved in calcium regulation and bone metabolism. Calcitonin slows bone loss and increases bone density in the spine. It reduces the risk of spine fractures but has not been shown to decrease the risk of non-spine fractures.

Calcitonin is available as an injection (dosage varies) or nasal spray (200 IU daily). An oral form of the drug is also being tested in clinical trials.

Estrogen Therapy (ET) and Hormone Therapy (HT)

Estrogen therapy (ET) and estrogen with progesterone hormone therapy (HT) are approved for the prevention of osteoporosis in postmenopausal women. ET and HT reduce bone loss, increase bone density in both the spine and hip, and reduce the risk of hip, spine, and other fractures in postmenopausal women. ET and HT are commonly available as a tablet or transdermal patch and in other forms. Estrogen and hormone medications come in a wide variety of doses.

Raloxifene (Evista)

Raloxifene is approved for the prevention and treatment of osteoporosis in postmenopausal women. Raloxifene is in a class of drugs called estrogen agonists/antagonists, also known as selective estrogen receptors modulators (SERMs), which have been developed to provide the beneficial effects of estrogens without their potential disadvantages. Raloxifene increases bone density and reduces the risk of spine fractures. There are no data showing that raloxifene reduces the risk of hip and other non-spine fractures.

Teriparatide – Parathyroid Hormone (PTH) (1-34) (Forteo)

Teriparatide, a type of parathyroid hormone, is approved for the treatment of osteoporosis in postmenopausal women and in men who are at high risk for a fracture. This medication rebuilds bone and significantly increases bone mineral density, especially in the spine.

Good candidates for teriparatide include those who have had an osteoporosis-related fracture and those with very low bone mineral density (T-scores lower than −3.0).

Teriparatide is self-administered as a daily injection from a preloaded pen containing a one-month supply of medication. It can be taken for a maximum of two years. At the end of two years, to retain the benefits of treatment with teriparatide, most experts recommend that patients start an antiresorptive medication.

AGENTS USED TO TREAT GOUT

Gout is a hereditary metabolic disease that is a form of acute arthritis. It is marked by inflammation of the joints and can affect any joint, but usually begins in the knee or foot. It is believed to be caused by excessive uric acid in the blood (hyperuricemia) and deposits of urates of sodium in and around joints.

Acute attacks of gout are extremely painful and may persist for several days to several weeks. Acute attacks should be treated as soon as possible and *colchicine*, a drug used for gout, may be administered either orally or intravenously. When given orally, an initial dose of 0.5 to 1.2 mg is administered. This dose may be given every 1 to 2 hours until pain is relieved or until nausea, vomiting, or diarrhea occur. The total dosage during a 24-hour period should not exceed 4 to 8 mg. When administered intravenously, an initial dose of 1 to 2 mg is usually given. This may be followed by doses of 0.5 mg every 6 hours until a satisfactory response is achieved. The total dosage during a 24-hour period should not exceed 4 mg. The major adverse reactions of colchicine are nausea, vomiting, and diarrhea. Other adverse reactions are gastrointestinal bleeding, neuritis, myopathy, alopecia, and bone marrow depression.

Once the acute attack of gout has been controlled, then drug therapy to control hyperuricemia can be initiated. The aim of treatment is to reduce the serum urate levels to below 6 mg/dL. Two types of drug therapy may be employed to reduce serum urate levels: uricosuric agents, such as *probenecid* (Benemid), which increase the urinary excretion of uric acid, and allopurinol (Zyloprim), which prevents the formation of uric acid in the body.

Sulfinpyrazone increases uric acid excretion by preventing the reabsorption of uric acid in the renal tubules. Because of this, urate stones may form in the kidneys, so patients are advised to drink 10 to 12 8-ounce glasses of water per day to ensure a urine output of more than 1 liter per day. Adverse reactions of sulfinpyrazone are nausea and vomiting.

Allopurinol, unlike the uricosuric agents, interferes with the conversion of purines to uric acid by inhibiting the enzyme xanthine oxidase. Two drugs, 6-mercaptopurine (Purinethol) and azathioprine (Imuran), are normally metabolized by the enzyme xanthine oxidase; their use must be avoided or dosage reduced when allopurinol is prescribed. The major adverse reactions of allopurinol are skin rashes and hepatotoxicity. Other adverse reactions are nausea, vomiting, abdominal pain, and hematologic changes.

SKELETAL MUSCLE RELAXANTS

Skeletal muscle relaxants, as shown in Table 21-5, are used to treat painful muscle spasms that may result from musculoskeletal strains, sprains, trauma, or disease. A muscle spasm is an involuntary contraction of one or more muscles and is usually accompanied by pain and the limitation of function.

Centrally acting muscle relaxants act by depressing the central nervous system and can be administered either orally or by injection. Individuals taking centrally acting muscle relaxants should be aware of the sedative effect produced by most of these drugs. Drowsiness, dizziness, and blurred vision may diminish the patient's ability to drive a vehicle, operate equipment, or climb stairs. The use of these agents in combination with other CNS depressants (alcohol, narcotic analgesics) may produce an additive effect; therefore, such use must be governed by caution.

Implications for Patient Care

Observe patients for signs of improvement and adverse reactions. Monitor blood studies (CBC, WBC, differential), liver function tests, and ECG in epileptic patients. Administer with meals to decrease GI distress.

TABLE 21-5   Skeletal Muscle Relaxants

MEDICATION	TYPE	USUAL DOSAGE	ADVERSE REACTIONS
baclofen (Lioresal)	Centrally acting agent	Oral: 5 mg 3 times/day; increased by 5 mg/dose every 3 days until optimum response is obtained, (maximum, 80 mg/day)	Hypotension, tinnitus, nasal congestion, blurred vision, nausea, dry mouth, dizziness, drowsiness, weakness
cyclobenzaprine HCl (Flexeril)	Centrally acting agent	Oral: 20 to 40 mg/day in 2 to 4 divided doses (maximum, 60 mg/day)	Edema of the face and tongue, pruritus, tachycardia, dry mouth, nausea, drowsiness, fatigue, blurred vision
dantrolene sodium (Dantrium)	Peripherally acting agent	Oral (Adult): initial 25 mg/day; increased to 25 mg 2 to 4 times/day, then, by increments, to 50 to 100 mg 4 times/day Oral (Child): 0.5 mg/kg twice/day; then, by increments of 0.5 mg to a maximum of 3 mg/kg 2 to 4 times/day	Drowsiness, muscle weakness, speech disturbances, tachycardia, diarrhea, nausea, anorexia, abdominal cramps, bloody or dark urine, burning with urination, blurred vision, pruritus, jaundice
diazepam (Valium)	Centrally acting agent	Oral (Adult): 2 to 10 mg 2 to 4 times daily IM (Adult): 2 to 10 mg as needed Oral (Child): 1 to 2.5 mg 3 to 4 times daily IM (Child): 1 to 2 mg as needed	Drowsiness, slurred speech, muscle weakness, vertigo, hypotension, tachycardia, urinary retention, nausea, xerostomia, blurred vision, hiccups, coughing, hepatic dysfunction, jaundice
metaxalone (Skelaxin)	Centrally acting agent	Oral (Adult, child over 12): 800 mg 3 to 4 times daily	Nausea, vomiting, gastrointestinal upset, drowsiness, headache, irritability, rash
methocarbamol (Robaxin)	Centrally acting agent	Oral (Adult): 1.5 g 4 times/day; then 1 to 1.5 g 4 times daily IM (Adult): 0.5 to 1 g at 8-hour intervals as necessary	Urticaria, pruritus, nasal congestion, rash, blurred vision, drowsiness, dizziness, headache, nausea
orphenadrine citrate (Norflex)	Centrally acting agent	Oral: 100 mg 2 times daily IM: 60 mg (may be repeated every 12 hours as needed)	Drowsiness, weakness, headache, dry mouth, nausea, urinary retention, blurred vision, dilated pupils

Patient Teaching

Educate patients:

- to take the medication as prescribed.
- that the drug should be tapered off over one to two weeks.
- that sudden discontinuance of the medication may cause insomnia, nausea, headache, spasticity, or tachycardia.
- not to use alcohol or other CNS depressants while on skeletal muscle relaxants.

- to avoid hazardous activities if drowsiness or dizziness occurs.
- not to use over-the-counter medications such as antihistamines, decongestants, and cough preparations unless prescribed by the physician. ■

Special Considerations

- Motor skill impairment, increased sedative effect, and respiratory depression may occur if taken with other CNS depressants (alcohol, narcotics, barbiturates, tricyclic antidepressants, antianxiety agents, and/or anticonvulsants).
- Cyclobenzaprine (Flexeril) may cause hyperpyrexia, excitation, and convulsions if taken with MAO inhibitors.
- May decrease the antihypertensive effect of guanethidine and clonidine (Catapres).
- May increase anticholinergic effects, including confusion and hallucinations, if taken with cholinergic blocking agents.

NEUROMUSCULAR BLOCKING AGENTS

Neuromuscular blocking agents are used to provide muscle relaxation and to reduce the need for deep general anesthesia in patients undergoing surgery. These drugs are also used to facilitate endotracheal intubation, to relieve laryngospasm, and to provide muscle relaxation in patients undergoing electroconvulsive therapy.

Neuromuscular blocking agents are of two types: competitive and depolarizing. The *competitive* drugs compete with the neurotransmitter acetylcholine for cholinergic receptor sites at the neuromuscular junction. These drugs act by occupying the receptor sites, thereby preventing the stimulation of muscle fibers by acetylcholine and causing paralysis of the affected muscle fibers. The *depolarizing* drugs are believed to mimic the action of acetylcholine in depolarizing muscle fibers but, because they are not readily destroyed by the enzyme cholinesterase, their prolonged action results in a persistent depolarization block and paralysis of muscle fibers.

SKELETAL MUSCLE STIMULANTS

Impaired neuromuscular transmission, thought to result from an autoimmune disorder, produces the condition known as *myasthenia gravis*. This disease, characterized by progressive weakness of skeletal muscles and their rapid fatiguing, is treated by the use of anticholinesterase muscle stimulants.

Skeletal muscle stimulant drugs, as shown in Table 21-6, act by inhibiting the action of acetylcholinesterase, the enzyme that halts the action of acetylcholine at the neuromuscular junction. By slowing the destruction of acetylcholine, these drugs foster accumulation of higher concentrations of this neurotransmitter and increase the number of interactions between acetylcholine and the available receptors on muscle fibers. The increase in the number of transmitter-receptor interactions improves muscle strength, but has no curative effect on the cause of the disease.

Implications for Patient Care

Observe patient for signs of improvement and adverse reactions. Monitor intake and output ratio and vital signs. Atropine sulfate must be available before administration of a skeletal muscle stimulant, because of the possibility of a cholinergic crisis (pronounced muscular weakness and respiratory paralysis caused by excessive acetylcholine). May be given with food to decrease GI distress, but better absorption takes place when given on an empty stomach. Discontinue drug if bradycardia, hypotension, bronchospasm, headache, dizziness, convulsions, or respiratory depression occur.

TABLE 21-6 Skeletal Muscle Relaxants

MEDICATION	TYPE	USUAL DOSAGE	ADVERSE REACTIONS
ambenonium chloride (Mytelase)	Cholinesterase inhibitor	Oral (Adult): 2.5 to 5 mg 3 to 4 times daily, increased every few days as needed Oral (Child): 0.3 mg/kg/day in 3–4 divided doses, then 1.5 mg/kg/day in 3 to 4 divided doses	Headache, incoordination, dizziness, fasciculations, respiratory depression, bradycardia, hypotension, nausea, diarrhea, blurred vision, urinary frequency
edrophonium chloride (Tensilon)	Cholinesterase inhibitor used in diagnosis of myasthenia gravis	IM (Adult): 10 mg IM (Child): 2 to 5 mg	Uncommon with usual doses; can cause weakness, muscle cramps, bradycardia, hypotension, nausea, diarrhea, respiratory paralysis
neostigmine bromide (Prostigmin Bromide)	Cholinesterase inhibitor	Oral: 15 to 30 mg 3 to 4 times/day, increased until maximum benefit is obtained (15 to 375 mg/day)	Fear, agitation, restlessness, nausea, epigastric discomfort, muscle cramps, fasciculations, pallor
neostigmine methylsulfate (Prostigmin Methylsulfate)	Cholinesterase inhibitor	IM, SC: 0.5 mg with subsequent dose based on individual response	See neostigmine bromide
pyridostigmine bromide (Mestinon)	Cholinesterase inhibitor	Oral: 60 to 600 mg/day in divided doses IM: 1/30 of oral dose	Acneiform rash, nausea, vomiting, diarrhea, miosis, bronchoconstriction, bradycardia, fasciculation

Patient Teaching

Educate patients:

- to take the medication as prescribed.
- to report any signs of cholinergic crisis to the physician without delay.
- that skeletal muscle stimulants are used to relieve symptoms and are not a cure for their disease. ■

Special Considerations

- These medications should not be given with other cholinergic agents.
- Because of the possibility of cholinergic crisis, emergency equipment and supplies should be available.
- Positive response to the medication includes increased muscle strength and hand grasp, improved gait, and absence of labored breathing.
- The effect of skeletal muscle stimulants may be decreased by aminoglycosides, anesthetics, or quinidine.
- Skeletal muscle stimulants may decrease the effects of gallamine, metocurine, pancuronium, and atropine.
- Skeletal muscle stimulants may increase the effects of succinylcholine (Anectine, Quelicin).

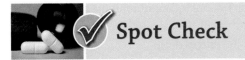 Spot Check

There are many nonsteroidal anti-inflammatory drugs that are used to treat the symptoms of inflammation. For each of the following drugs, give the usual anti-inflammatory dose and several adverse reactions:

DRUG(S)	USUAL ANTI-INFLAMMATORY DOSE	ADVERSE REACTIONS
acetylsalicylic acid (aspirin)		
ibuprofen (Motrin)		
naproxen (Naprosyn)		
piroxicam (Feldene)		

■ ■ REVIEW QUESTIONS

Directions. Select the best answer to each of the following multiple-choice questions, circle the letter of your choice:

1. _____ is a neurotransmitter that is thought to play an important role in the transmission of nerve impulses at synapses and myoneural junctions.
   a. Corticosteroid
   b. Prostaglandin
   c. Acetylcholine
   d. Acetylcholinesterase

2. _____ is an enzyme that destroys acetylcholine and readies muscle fibers for the next nerve impulse.
   a. Corticosteroid
   b. Prostaglandin
   c. Anticholinesterase
   d. Acetylcholinesterase

3. Drugs that relieve the swelling, tenderness, redness, and pain of inflammation are known as _____.
   a. analgesics
   b. anti-inflammatory agents
   c. antipyretics
   d. antibiotics

4. The Food and Drug Administration has indicated new labeling for Tylenol (acetaminophen) and Motrin (ibuprofen). For Motrin, the label warns of the risk of _____.

    a. stomach bleeding for those who drink three or more alcoholic beverages daily

    b. severe headache

    c. liver damage

    d. diarrhea

5. The Food and Drug Administration has indicated new labeling for Tylenol (acetaminophen) and Motrin (ibuprofen). For Tylenol, the label warns of the risk of _____.

    a. stomach bleeding for those who drink three or more alcoholic beverages daily

    b. severe headache

    c. liver damage

    d. diarrhea

6. The adverse reactions of aspirin include _____.

    a. GI distress   b. tinnitus   c. rapid pulse   d. all of these

7. The Food and Drug Administration has indicated new labeling for Tylenol (acetaminophen) and Motrin (ibuprofen). For Motrin, there is an additional warning about an allergy alert. It may cause _____.

    a. GI distress, rapid pulse

    b. hives, facial swelling, wheezing, and/or shock

    c. light-headedness, dizziness

    d. drowsiness, nausea

8. Disease-modifying antirheumatic drugs are recommended in early rheumatoid arthritis to _____.

    a. limit irreversible joint damage

    b. replace lost cartilage

    c. reduce pain and inflammation

    d. increase mobility of the joint

9. Antirheumatic agents that may be used in the treatment of rheumatoid arthritis include _____.

    a. gold preparations   c. pencillamine

    b. hydroxychloroquine sulfate   d. all of these

10. In patients treated with nonsteroidal anti-inflammatory drugs, it is important that the patients understand that serious gastrointestinal toxicity can occur at any time, with or without warning. Serious gastrointestinal toxicity includes _____.

    a. severe diarrhea

    b. impacted stool

    c. bleeding, ulceration, and perforation of the stomach, small intestine, or large intestine

    d. jaundice

11. Individuals taking centrally acting muscle relaxants should be advised that these agents may _____.

    a. cause drowsiness, dizziness, and blurred vision

    b. produce an additive effect when taken in combination with other CNS depressants

    c. impair their ability to drive a vehicle

    d. all of these

12. Antitumor necrosis factor drugs seem to do all of the following except _____.

    a. slow, if not halt the destruction of the joints

    b. act to preempt the autoimmune response

    c. replace lost cartilage

    d. have evolved out of the biotechnology industry

13. Serious infections and sepsis, including fatalities, have been reported with the antitumor necrosis factor drug _____.

   a. Enbrel (etanercept)

   b. Kineret (anakinra)

   c. Remicade (infliximab)

14. Drowsiness, dizziness, rash, erythemia, nausea, anorexia, jaundice, and liver damage are adverse reactions of _____.

   a. Valium   b. Robaxin   c. Paraflex   d. Norflex

15. Normal aging changes that predispose an older adult to falls include all of the following except _____.

   a. poor vision

   b. bone lose strength

   c. increased reaction time

   d. medical problems

16. Neuromuscular blocking agents may be used to _____.

   a. provide muscle stimulation   c. facilitate endotracheal intubation

   b. relieve laryngospasm   d. b and c

17. Headache, dizziness, and bradycardia are adverse reactions of _____.

   a. Tracrium   b. Mytelase   c. Mestinon   d. Prostigmin

18. All of the following are ways to help prevent sports injuries in children except _____.

   a. adequate warm-up and cool-down periods should be allowed

   b. the choice of a sports activity should not be determined by the child's physical and mental ability

   c. the child should have a regular exercise program

   d. proper nutrition and adequate fluids are necessary

19. Skeletal muscle stimulants act by _____.

   a. inhibiting the action of acetylcholinesterase

   b. inhibiting the action of cholinesterase

   c. inhibiting the action of prostaglandin

   d. none of these

20. Fear, agitation, restlessness, nausea, epigastric discomfort, muscle cramps, fasciculations, and pallor are adverse reactions of _____.

   a. Mytelase   c. Prostigmin bromide

   b. Tensilon   d. Mestinon

Matching. Place the correct letter from Column II on the appropriate line of Column I:

Column I	Column II
21. __C__ chrysotherapy	A. any number of hormonal steroid substances that are secreted by the adrenal cortex
22. __A__ corticosteroid	B. a group of hormonelike unsaturated fatty acids that are present in many body tissues
23. __B__ prostaglandins	C. the use of gold compounds as treatment, especially for rheumatoid arthritis
24. __E__ cyclooxygenase	D. a receiver; a cell component that combines with a drug or hormone to alter the function of the cell
25. __D__ receptor	E. an enzyme involved in normal cellular function and the inflammatory response
	F. an enzyme that inactivates the neurotransmitter acetylcholine

UNIT 22
Medications Used for Gastrointestinal System Disorders

OBJECTIVES

Upon completing this unit, you should be able to:

- Define the terms listed in the vocabulary.
- Describe the digestive process.
- State the treatment regimen for an ulcer associated with the *Helicobacter pylori* bacteria.
- List the changes that occur in gastrointestinal functioning of older adults.
- State the signs and symptoms of gastrointestinal disorders in children.
- Complete the critical thinking questions and activities presented in this unit.
- State the actions, uses, contraindications, adverse reactions, dosage and route, implications for patient care, patient teaching, and special considerations for selected antiulcer agents.
- State the usage, classifications, actions, usual dosage, onset of action, patient teaching, and special considerations for laxatives.
- State the usual dosage, adverse reactions, and special considerations for antidiarrheal agents.
- State the usual dosage and adverse reactions of selected anthelmintics.
- State the usual dosage and adverse reactions of selected antiprotozoal agents.
- State the usage, contraindications, and dosage of apomorphine HCl and ipecac syrup.
- Complete the Spot Check on selected drugs used to treat ulcers.
- Answer the review questions correctly.

VOCABULARY

amebiasis (am"e-bi'a-sis). Being infected with amebae. The disease is generally characterized by dysentery with diarrhea, weakness, prostration, nausea, vomiting, and abdominal pain.

chyme (kīm). A partially digested mass of food and digestive secretion found in the stomach and small intestines during digestion of food.

defecation (def-e-ka'shun). The process of emptying the bowel.

gastroesophageal reflux disease (gas'tro-e-sof"a-je-al re'flucks di'zez). A term for a range of symptoms that result from the exposure of the esophagus to gastric acid.

helminthiasis (hel-min-th'a-sis). A condition in which there is an intestinal infestation of parasitic worms.

histamine antagonist (his'ta-min an-tag'o-nist). An agent that inhibits the action of histamine at the histamine H_2 receptor site. The H_2 receptor site is located on the parietal cells of the stomach.

peptic ulcer (pep'tik ul'ser). An ulcer occurring in the lower end of the esophagus; along the lesser curvature of the stomach or in the duodenum.

INTRODUCTION

The gastrointestinal system enables the body to extract absorbable nutrients from food during the digestive process. During this process, food passes from the mouth, down the esophagus, to the stomach, where it is converted to a near-liquid mass by hydrochloric acid, various enzymes, and the churning motions of the stomach walls. This partially digested mass, known as chyme, leaves the acidic environment of the stomach through its lower orifice (pylorus) and passes into the first part of the small intestines (duodenum). Here, the acid chyme is made alkaline as it is mixed with bile, pancreatic juice, and intestinal secretions. As this near-liquid mass passes through the small intestines, the products of digestion are absorbed, pass into the blood and lymph, and are eventually carried throughout the body. The residue of digestion is passed into the ascending colon where reabsorption of water begins. The now semisolid waste passes from the ascending colon, through the transverse and descending colons, to the rectum. Here, it is stored until there is an opportunity for defecation (see Figure 22-1).

The digestive process involves a combination of mechanical and chemical processes coordinated by the autonomic nervous system. Typical complaints and disorders of the gastrointestinal system include dyspepsia (indigestion), pyrosis (heartburn), ulcers, nausea, vomiting, diarrhea, constipation, and infection. Many of these complaints may be the result of poor eating habits, stress, overindulgence, alcohol, caffeine, smoking, and nonsteroidal anti-inflammatory drugs (NSAIDs). However, research shows that most ulcers develop as a result of infection with bacteria called *Helicobacter pylori* (*H. pylori*). See Spotlight, Ulcers and *Helicobacter pylori* Bacteria.

Heartburn, a burning sensation in the substernal area, is caused by reflux of acid contents of the stomach into the lower esophagus (gastroesophageal reflux disease, GERD). GERD is an all-inclusive term for a range of symptoms that result from the exposure of the esophagus to gastric acid. Heartburn and regurgitation, a backward flowing of solids or fluids to the mouth from the stomach, are the most common symptoms, appearing as abdominal pain and burning sensations in the chest. GERD can evolve into erosive esophagitis (EE), a serious condition in which the gastric contents of the stomach pass upward and cause inflammation and tissue damage to the esophagus. If untreated,

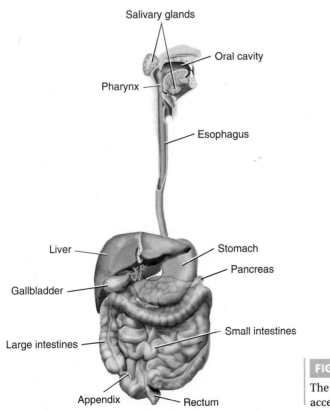

FIGURE 22-1

The gastrointestinal tract or alimentary canal and its accessory organs *Source: Delmar/Cengage Learning*

complications may occur, including hemorrhage, stricture, and Barrett's esophagus, inflammation with possible ulceration of the lower part of the esophagus, a condition associated with an increased risk of esophageal cancer.

Medications that are used to treat gastrointestinal system disorders or conditions described in this unit are antiulcer agents, laxatives, antidiarrheal agents, anthelmintics, antiprotozoal agents, antiemetics, and emetics.

Spotlight

Ulcers and *Helicobacter pylori* Bacteria

Approximately two-thirds of the world's population is infected with *Helicobacter pylori* (*H. pylori*). In the United States, *H. pylori* is more prevalent among older adults, African Americans, Hispanics, and lower socioeconomic groups. *Helicobacter pylori* is a spiral-shaped bacterium that is found in the gastric mucous layer or adherent to the epithelial lining of the stomach. *H. pylori* causes more than 90 percent of duodenal ulcers and up to 80 percent of gastric ulcers. Before 1982, when this bacterium was discovered, spicy food, acid, stress, and lifestyle were considered the major causes of ulcers. The majority of patients were given long-term medications, such as H_2 blockers, and more recently, proton pump inhibitors, without a chance for permanent cure. These medications relieve ulcer-related symptoms, heal gastric mucosal inflammation, and may heal the ulcer, but they do *not* treat the infection. When acid suppression is removed, the majority of ulcers, particularly those caused by *H. pylori*, recur. Because most ulcers are caused by *H. pylori*, appropriate antibiotic regimens can successfully eradicate the infection in most patients, with complete resolution of mucosal inflammation and a minimal chance for recurrence of ulcers.

Most people who are infected with *H. pylori never* suffer any symptoms related to the infection; however, *H. pylori* causes chronic active, chronic persistent, and atrophic gastritis in adults and children. Infection with *H. pylori* also causes duodenal and gastric ulcers. Infected people have a two- to sixfold increased risk of developing gastric cancer and mucosa-associated lymphoid tissue (MALT) lymphoma compared with their uninfected counterparts. The role of *H. pylori* in nonulcer dyspepsia remains unclear.

Approximately 25 million Americans suffer from **peptic ulcer** disease at some point in their lifetime. Each year there are 500,000 to 850,000 new cases of peptic ulcer disease and more than one million ulcer-related hospitalizations. The most common ulcer symptom is gnawing or burning pain in the epigastrium. This pain typically occurs when the stomach is empty, between meals and in the early morning hours, but it can also occur at other times. It may last from minutes to hours and may be relieved by eating or by taking antacids. Less common ulcer symptoms include nausea, vomiting, and loss of appetite. Bleeding can also occur; prolonged bleeding may cause anemia leading to weakness and fatigue. If bleeding is heavy, hematemesis, hematochezia, or melena may occur.

Several methods may be used to diagnose *H. pylori* infection. Serological tests that measure specific *H. pylori* IgG antibodies can determine if a person has been infected. The sensitivity and specificity of these assays range from 80 percent to 95 percent depending upon the assay used. Another diagnostic method is the breath test. In this test, the patient is given either 13C- or 14C-labeled urea to drink. *H. pylori* metabolizes the urea rapidly, and the labeled carbon is absorbed. This labeled carbon can then be measured as CO_2 in the patient's expired breath to determine whether *H. pylori* is present. The sensitivity and specificity of the breath test ranges from 94 percent to 98 percent. Upper esophagogastroduodenal endoscopy is considered the reference method of diagnosis. During endoscopy, biopsy specimens of the stomach and duodenum are obtained and the diagnosis of *H. pylori* can be made by several methods. One is the biopsy urease test, a colorimetric test based on the ability of *H. pylori* to produce urease; it provides rapid testing at the time of biopsy. Another method is the histologic identification of organisms, which is considered the gold standard of diagnostic tests. Culture of biopsy specimens for *H. pylori* requires an experienced laboratory and is necessary when antimicrobial susceptibility testing is desired.

Therapy for *H. pylori* infection consists of 10 days to 2 weeks of one or two effective antibiotics, such as amoxicillin, tetracycline (not to be used for children less than 12 years old), metronidazole, or clarithromycin, plus either ranitidine bismuth citrate, bismuth subsalicylate, or a proton pump inhibitor. Acid suppression by the H_2 blocker or proton pump inhibitor in conjunction with the antibiotics helps alleviate ulcer-related symptoms (abdominal pain, nausea), helps heal gastric mucosal inflammation, and may enhance efficacy of the antibiotics against *H. pylori* at the gastric mucosal surface. Currently, eight *H. pylori* treatment regimens are approved by the Food and Drug Administration (FDA); however, several other combinations have been used successfully. Antibiotic resistance and patient noncompliance are the two major reasons for treatment failure. Eradication rates of the eight FDA-approved regimens range from 61 percent to 94 percent, depending on the regimen used. Overall, triple therapy regimens have shown better eradication rates than dual therapy. Longer length of treatment (14 days versus 10 days) results in better eradication rates.

Special Considerations: **OLDER ADULTS**

With aging, certain changes occur in gastrointestinal functioning. The digestive system motion slows as muscle contractions become weaker. Glandular secretions decrease, causing a drier mouth and a lower volume of gastric juices. Atrophy of the mucosal lining may reduce the rate of nutrient absorption. Other changes that generally occur are the following:

- Teeth deteriorate.
- Taste buds decrease in functionality.
- Muscles associated with chewing weaken.
- Swallowing becomes more difficult.
- Peristalsis becomes slower.
- Gastric emptying becomes slower.
- Bile may become thicker; therefore, the emptying of the gallbladder may be slower.
- Liver size decreases.
- Blood flow through the liver is reduced.
- Liver enzyme activity is reduced.

The changes in the gastrointestinal system caused by aging generally increase the older person's risk for anorexia, bloating, indigestion, flatulence, diarrhea, and constipation. Constipation is one of the most frequent gastrointestinal complaints of older adults. Constipation may result from intestinal immotility, a diet low in bulk and roughage, lack of physical exercise, and an altered bacteria flora.

In addition to the changes cited, age-related and disease-related changes contribute to decreased ability of older adults to clear drugs through the liver and the renal system. Serum albumin concentration is lower, which tends to make available more free drug to tissues or to make available more drug to be eliminated from the body. A gradual decrease in blood flow to the internal organs in the abdomen reduces drug clearance through the liver or kidneys.

Older adults should be carefully evaluated before the initiation of any type of drug therapy. Reduced dosage and less frequent doses may be given to older adults to help avoid drug accumulation and adverse effects.

Special Considerations: **CHILDREN**

The gastrointestinal system of the child differs from that of the adult. The child who is not developing normally according to established growth parameters, such as height, weight, and head circumference, should be evaluated for gastrointestinal disorders. Signs and symptoms such as constipation, rectal bleeding, hematemesis, jaundice, nausea, and vomiting usually indicate GI disorders.

Children with nausea and vomiting will dehydrate more quickly than an adult. Fluid imbalances can quickly develop in infants and young children. It is important to accurately assess fluid intake and output and to seek medical attention if dehydration is suspected.

Signs of Dehydration

- Loss of body weight: mild dehydration up to 5 percent; moderate dehydration 5 percent to 10 percent; severe dehydration over 10 percent
- Irritable and lethargic
- Skin turgor—loss of elasticity
- Dry mucous membranes
- Eyeballs and fontanels—sunken
- Absent or decreased tearing and salivation
- Abnormal thirst
- Decreased urine output; specific gravity elevated
- Body temperature subnormal to elevated
- Rapid respirations
- Blood pressure normal to low
- Rapid pulse

▪▪ Critical Thinking QUESTIONS AND ACTIVITIES

There is now scientific proof showing that approximately 90 percent of duodenal ulcers and up to 80 percent of gastric ulcers are associated with *Helicobacter pylori* bacteria. Your patient is a 66-year-old male who has a history of dyspepsia, heartburn, nausea, vomiting, anorexia, and a "gnawing" pain in the epigastric region. His diagnosis is peptic ulcer disease. He states that he has taken Tagamet, Pepcid, Zantac, and numerous antacids, but none of these have seemed to cure his ulcer. Ask yourself:

- Could this patient have an ulcer caused by *H. pylori* bacteria?
- What does the *H. pylori* bacteria do to the lining of the stomach?
- Because the traditional medical treatment for an ulcer was not successful in this patient, what other treatment regimen could be prescribed?
- What are the reported problems associated with the drug regimen for ulcers caused by *H. pylori* bacteria?
- What are some of the side effects associated with the drug regimen that is used to treat ulcers caused by *H. pylori* bacteria?

ANTIULCER AGENTS

Antiulcer agents include antacids, histamine H_2 receptor antagonist, mucosal protective medications, and gastric acid pump inhibitors (proton-pump inhibitors, PPIs). Each of these classifications, along with selected drugs, is described in this unit.

ANTACIDS

Antacids are drugs that neutralize hydrochloric acid in the stomach. They are used to relieve acid indigestion, gas, and heartburn, and in the treatment of peptic ulcers. Ideally, an antacid should neutralize large amounts of acid with a small dose, should have a long-lasting effect, should not interfere with electrolyte balance, and should

TABLE 22-1   Nonsystemic Antacids

MEDICATION	USUAL DOSAGE	ADVERSE REACTIONS
aluminum phosphate (Phosphaljel)	Oral: 15 to 30 ml every 2 hours	Constipation
calcium carbonate, precipitated chalk (Tums)	Oral: 0.5 to 2 g 4 to 6 times daily, if necessary	Constipation, acid rebound, nausea, flatulence
dihydroxyaluminum sodium carbonate (Rolaids)	Oral: 1 to 2 tablets 4 or more times per day	Constipation, intestinal concentrations
magaldrate (Riopan)	Oral: 1 to 2 tablets, or 5 to 10 ml of suspension 4 times/day	Infrequent diarrhea or constipation
magnesium hydroxide (Milk of Magnesia)	Oral: 5 to 10 ml, or 1 to 2 tablets 1 to 3 hours after meals and at bedtime	Diarrhea, nausea, hypermagnesemia
magnesium oxide	Oral: 250 to 1500 mg with water or milk, 4 times/day after meals and at bedtime	Diarrhea, nausea, hypermagnesemia

not cause a secondary increase in gastric acidity. The majority of antacids are classified as nonsystemic agents because they remain largely in the gastrointestinal tract (see Table 22-1). These agents are useful for long-term treatment of ulcers and for occasional relief of gas, indigestion, and other complaints.

Sodium bicarbonate is a systemic antacid. It is readily absorbed and has a rapid onset and a short duration of action. For these and other reasons, this antacid is not indicated for use in long-term therapy.

Actions

Antacids act in a variety of ways. They may neutralize gastric acidity, cause hydrogen ion absorption, bind phosphates in the GI tract, buffer the acid, or reduce the surface tension of gas bubbles so that the gas may be more easily eliminated.

Uses

Relief of heartburn, acid indigestion, and gas, and in the symptomatic relief of hyperacidity associated with peptic ulcer, gastritis, peptic esophagitis, gastric hyperacidity, hiatal hernia, and postoperative gas pain.

Contraindications

Contraindicated in patients with hypersensitivity to any of the ingredients.

Adverse Reactions

Adverse reactions may vary with the type of preparation (see Table 22-1).

Dosage and Route

The dosage and route of administration are determined by the patient and the physician.

Implications for Patient Care

Patients should not take antacids for more than two weeks without the permission of the physician. Patients should not exceed the maximum dosage of any antacid or antacid mixture. Calcium carbonate and sodium bicarbonate may cause rebound hyperacidity. Patients with renal failure should not use large quantities of antacids containing magnesium. The magnesium cannot be excreted and may produce hypermagnesemia and toxicity.

Patient Teaching

Educate patients:

- *that aluminum-based and calcium carbonate antacids may cause constipation.*
- to increase their fluid intake to 2000 mL/day while taking an aluminum-based antacid to help relieve constipation, unless contraindicated.
- *that magnesium-based antacids may cause diarrhea.*
- to notify the physician if there is any difficulty with constipation or diarrhea.
- that liquid suspensions must be shaken well before taking.
- to store suspensions in a cool place.
- that chewable tablets should be chewed thoroughly before swallowing and then followed with 8 ounces of water. ■

Special Considerations

- Antacids should not be used in patients who are taking any form of tetracycline.
- Antacids should be used with caution in geriatric patients and those who have decreased GI motility, bowel obstruction, dehydration, renal disease, or sodium-restricted diets, or who are pregnant.
- Antacids may decrease absorption of cimetidine, iron, benzodiazepines, corticosteroids, anticholinergics, digitalis, and phenytoin (Dilantin).
- Levodopa absorption is increased by antacids.

Antacid Mixtures

Products that combine aluminum or calcium compounds with magnesium salts often prove more useful than the single-entity antacids listed in Table 22-1. These agents are commonly used in the treatment of peptic ulcers, acid indigestion, and heartburn. By combining the antacid properties of two single-entity agents, products have been created that provide the antacid action of both, yet tend to counter the adverse effects of each ingredient. For example, a product containing aluminum hydroxide (*a cause of constipation*) and magnesium hydroxide (*a cause of diarrhea*) will minimize these effects, while offering the sum of the antacid actions of both ingredients. Table 22-2 lists some common antacid mixtures.

HISTAMINE H$_2$-RECEPTOR ANTAGONIST

Histamine H$_2$-receptor antagonists inhibit both daytime and nocturnal basal gastric acid secretion and inhibit gastric acid stimulated by food, histamines, caffeine, insulin, and pentagastrin. There are four drugs of this type (cimetidine, ranitidine, famotidine, and nizatidine) that have been approved for the treatment of active duodenal ulcer, and for pathological hypersecretory conditions (Zollinger-Ellison syndrome). See Table 22-3.

Actions

Reduce gastric acid secretion by occupying H$_2$-receptor sites on parietal cells.

TABLE 22-2   Common Antacid Mixtures

MEDICATION	INGREDIENTS	USUAL DOSAGE	WARNINGS
Gaviscon	Aluminum hydroxide, magnesium carbonate (liquid), magnesium trisilicate (tablet)	Oral: 1 or 2 tablespoons, or 2 tablets (chewed), 1 hour after meals and at bedtime	Contraindicated in those with kidney disease, and those taking any form of tetracycline
Gelusil	Aluminum hydroxide, magnesium hydroxide, and simethicone	Oral: 2 or more teaspoons or tablets (chewed) after meals and at bedtime	See above
Maalox Plus	Aluminum hydroxide, magnesium hydroxide, and simethicone	Oral: 1 to 4 tablets chewed 4 times a day, 20 to 60 minutes after meals and at bedtime	See above
Mylanta	Aluminum hydroxide, magnesium hydroxide, and simethicone	Oral: 2 to 4 teaspoons or tablets (chewed), every 2 to 4 hours between meals and at bedtime	See above

TABLE 22-3   Histamine H_2-Receptor Antagonist

MEDICATION	USUAL DOSAGE	ADVERSE REACTIONS
cimetidine (Tagamet)	Active duodenal ulcer: 800 mg at bedtime Maintenance: 400 mg at bedtime Active gastric ulcer: 800 mg at bedtime or 300 mg 4 times a day with meals and at bedtime	Diarrhea, dizziness, somnolence, rash, headache, myalgia, arthralgia, facial edema, bradycardia, constipation, tiredness, confusion, jaundice, gynecomastia, impotence
famotidine (Pepcid)	Acute therapy: 1 (40-mg) tablet at bedtime Maintenance therapy: 1 (20-mg) tablet at bedtime	Headache, dizziness, diarrhea, constipation
nizatidine (Axid)	Active duodenal ulcer: 300 mg at bedtime Alternate dose: 150 mg b.i.d. Maintenance therapy: 150 mg at bedtime	Somnolence, sweating, urticaria, confusion, tachycardia, impotence, decreased libido
ranitidine (Zantac)	Active duodenal ulcer: 150 mg b.i.d. or 300 mg at bedtime Maintenance therapy: 150 mg at bedtime	Headache, malaise, dizziness, constipation, abdominal pain, diarrhea, insomnia, vertigo, arrhythmias, hepatitis, rash, blood dyscrasia, gynecomastia, impotence

Uses

Use for active duodenal ulcer and for pathological hypersecretory conditions (Zollinger-Ellison syndrome), short-term treatment of duodenal and gastric ulcers and maintenance therapy.

Contraindications

Contraindicated in patients with known hypersensitivity to any of the ingredients.

> ⚠ **Caution:**
>
> *Avoid use during pregnancy or breast-feeding, or for children under 16 years of age. Use caution in patients with hepatic disease or renal disease.*

Adverse Reactions

Histamine H_2-receptor antagonists are generally well tolerated. Adverse reactions vary with the specific drug and the length of use (see Table 22-3). Some adverse reactions that may occur are confusion, headache, depression, dizziness, anxiety, weakness, psychosis, tremors, convulsions, diarrhea, constipation, abdominal cramps, paralytic ileus, jaundice, rash, bradycardia, tachycardia, facial edema, malaise, insomnia, vertigo, gynecomastia, impotence, decreased libido, or blood dyscrasia.

Dosage and Route

Dosage and route of administration are determined by the physician and individualized for each patient (see Table 22-3).

Implications for Patient Care

Observe for signs of improvement and/or hypersensitivity. Monitor gastric pH (should be below 5), I&O ratio, BUN, CBC, liver function tests, creatinine, and prothrombin time.

Patient Teaching

Cimetidine and ranitidine: Educate patients:

- that gynecomastia and impotence may occur while using. Explain that both are reversible after discontinuation of the drug(s).
- that the medication may impair mental alertness; therefore, one should not operate machinery or drive a motor vehicle, until the response to the medication has been determined.

Famotidine: Educate patients:

- to report any signs of blood dyscrasia (bleeding, bruising, fatigue, and malaise) to the physician.
- that decreased libido may occur while using, but it is reversible after discontinuation of the drug.

Nizatidine: Educate patients:

- that false-positive tests for urobilinogen with Multistix may occur while taking this medication.
- that impotence and decreased libido may occur while using. Explain that both are reversible after discontinuation of the drug. ■

Special Considerations

- Patients with duodenal or gastric ulcers should avoid substances that may irritate the mucous membrane of the duodenum or stomach such as caffeine, nicotine, black pepper, alcohol, harsh spices, liquids and foods that are very hot or very cold, and over-the-counter medications, especially those that contain aspirin.
- The effect of the medication may be decreased with the use of antacids and ketoconazole (antifungal drug).

Maintenance of healing of erosive esophagitis: Adult oral dose: 20 mg daily

Pathological hypersecretory conditions: Adult oral dose: individualized for each patient. The recommended adult oral starting dose is 60 mg once a day. Doses should be adjusted to individual patient needs and should continue for as long as clinically indicated.

- *Aciphex* (rabeprazole sodium): Tablet, enteric-coated. Healing of erosive or ulcerative GERD: Adults: 20 mg once daily for 4 to 8 weeks. An additional 8 weeks of therapy may be considered for those who have not healed.

  Maintenance of healing of erosive or ulcerative GERD: Adults: 20 mg once daily

  Healing of duodenal ulcers: Adults: 20 mg once daily after the morning meal for up to 4 weeks

  Treatment of pathological hypersecretory conditions: Adults, initial: 60 mg once a day. Adjust dosage to individual patient needs (doses up to 100 mg/day bid have been used).

- *Prevacid* (lasoprazole): Delayed-release capsule, 15 mg once daily

- *Protonix* (pantoprazole sodium): Delayed-release tablet, 40 mg once daily. Swallow whole. Do not split, crush, or chew.

- *Nexium* (esomeprazole magnesium): "Little purple pill." Healing of erosive esophagitis: Adults: 20 mg or 40 mg once daily for 4 to 8 weeks.

  Maintenance of healing of erosive esophagitis: Adults: 20 mg once daily. Symptomatic gastroesophageal reflux disease: Adults: 20 mg once daily for 4 weeks.

  Risk reduction of NSAID-associated gastric ulcer: Adults: 20 mg or 40 mg once daily for up to 6 months.

  H. pylori eradication to reduce the risk of duodenal ulcer recurrence: Adults: Triple therapy: Nexium 40 mg once daily for 10 days; amoxicillin 1000 mg twice daily for 10 days, and clarithromycin 500 mg twice daily for 10 days.

Implications for Patient Care

It is important that patients understand not to chew or crush the tablets, or crush the tablets in food. This decreases how well the medication works.

Patient Teaching

Educate patients:

- to swallow the medication whole. Do not split, crush, or chew.
- to use the medication regularly as prescribed, at the same time each day to get the most benefit from it.
- to take the medication for the prescribed length of treatment even if the symptoms improve.
- to inform their physician if the condition persists or worsens.
- to inform their physician about *all* medications that are being taken before the initiation of drug therapy with a gastric acid pump inhibitor.
- to seek immediate medical attention if a serious allergic reaction occurs. Symptoms include rash, itching, swelling, dizziness, and trouble breathing. ■

LAXATIVES

Laxatives are commonly used to relieve constipation and to facilitate the passage of feces through the lower gastrointestinal tract. Normally, an active, healthy person who eats a balanced diet does not suffer from constipation. Occasionally, this condition results from travel, emotional stress, and other factors. More often, constipation results from decreased fluid intake, poor diet, lack of physical activity, eating constipating foods, and as a result of the action of certain drugs.

Several types of laxatives are in general use; see Tables 22-4 and 22-5. These agents have been grouped into the following classifications: *bulk-forming agents*, which absorb water, expand, and thereby stimulate peristaltic action; *lubricants*, which are various oils that soften the fecal mass and facilitate penetration of the fecal mass by intestinal fluids; *osmotic laxatives*, which help prevent the bowel from absorbing water so that the bulk volume increases; *saline laxatives*, which are salts that draw water into the intestinal lumen osmotically to mix with the stool and stimulate motility; *stool softeners*, which act as detergents, moistening and breaking up the feces; and *stimulant laxatives*, which act by irritating the intestinal mucosa or nerves in the intestinal wall (see Table 22-5).

TABLE 22-4 Various Types of Laxative Agents

MEDICATION	TYPE	USUAL DOSAGE	ONSET OF ACTION
bisacodyl (Dulcolax)	Stimulant	Oral (Adult): 10 to 15 mg Oral (Child): 5 to 10 mg Rectal: 10 mg if over 2 years of age; 5 mg if under 2 years old	Acts within 5 to 12 hours of oral administration; acts 15 to 60 minutes after rectal suppository insertion
docusate calcium (Surfak)	Stool softener	Oral (Adults): 50 to 200 mg/day Oral (Child 6 to 12 years): 40 to 120 mg, (Child 3 to 6 years): 20 to 60 mg, (Child under 3): 10 to 40 mg	Acts within 1 to 3 days after first administration
docusate sodium (Colace)	Stool softener	Oral: Same as docusate calcium	Same as docusate calcium
glycerin (Fleet Babylax)	Osmotic	Rectal (Adult and children 6 years and older): 2 to 3 g as a suppository or 5 to 15 ml as an enema	Acts within 15 to 30 min
lactulose (Cholac)	Osmotic	Oral (Adult): 15 to 30 mL/day; maximum dose up to 60 mL/day	Acts within 24 to 48 hours
lubiprostone (Amitiza)	Chloride Channel Activator	Oral (Adult): 24 mcg twice daily with food and water	Acts within 24 hours
magnesium hydroxide (milk of magnesia)	Saline	Oral (Adult): 15 to 30 mL Oral (Child 2 to 6 years): 5 to 15 mL Oral (Child under 2 years): 5 mL	Acts within 4 to 8 hours, depending upon dosage
methylcellulose (Cologel)	Bulk-forming	Oral (Adult): 5 to 20 mL 3 times/day Oral (Child): $\frac{1}{2}$ the adult dosage	Acts within 12 to 24 hours in most patients
mineral oil (liquid petrolatum)	Lubricant	Oral: 15 to 30 mL, usually in the evening	Acts within 6 to 12 hours
phenolphthalein (Ex-Lax)	Stimulant	Oral: 30 to 200 mg	Acts in 6 to 8 hours
polycarbophil (FiberCon)	Bulk-forming	Oral (Adult): 1 g 1 to 4 times daily or as needed (not to exceed 6 g/24 hr)	Acts within 12 to 24 hours
polyethylene glycol/electrolyte (GoLYTELY)	Osmotic	Oral (Adult): 30 to 60 mL single or divided dose or 10 to 20 mL as concentrate Oral (Children 6 to 12 years): 15 to 30 mL as single or divided dose Oral (Children 2 to 5 years): 5 to 15 mL as single or divided dose	Acts in 1 hour

(continues)

TABLE 22-4 (*continued*)

MEDICATION	TYPE	USUAL DOSAGE	ONSET OF ACTION
psyllium (Metamucil)	Bulk-forming	Oral (Adult): 1 to 2 rounded teaspoons, or 1 packet 1 to 3 times/day	Acts within 12 to 72 hours
		Oral (Child): 1 rounded teaspoon in $\frac{1}{2}$ glass/liquid 1 to 2 times/day	
senna, sennosides (Ex-Lax Gentle Nature Laxative Pills; Senokot)	Stimulant	Oral (Adult and children 12 years and older): senna: 0.5 to 2 g; sennosides: 12 to 50 mg 1 to 2 times daily	Acts within 6 to 12 hours
		Oral (Children 6 to 11 years): 50% of the adult dose	
		Oral, (Children 1 to 5 years): 33% of the adult dose	
		Rectal (Adult and children 12 years and older): 30 mg 1 to 2 times daily	Acts within $\frac{1}{2}$ to 2 hours

TABLE 22-5 Classification, Example, and Patient Teaching

CLASSIFICATION	EXAMPLE	PATIENT TEACHING
Bulk-forming	Metamucil	Do not take dry. Take with 8 ounces of water and follow with 8 ounces of water. If abdominal distention or unusual amount of flatulence occurs, notify your physician. Do not take within 1 hour of antacids, milk, or cimetidine. Report muscle cramps, pain, weakness, dizziness, or excessive thirst to your physician.
Chloride Channel Activator	Amitiza	The soft gelatin capsule should be taken twice daily with food and water to reduce potential symptoms of nausea. The capsule should be swallowed whole and should not be broken apart or chewed. Physicians and patients should periodically assess the need for continued therapy.
Stimulants	Dulcolax	Tablets should be swallowed. Do not crush or chew. Avoid milk or antacids within 1 hour of taking because the enteric coating may dissolve prematurely.
Saline	Milk of magnesia	Magnesium laxatives should not be taken by patients who have renal insufficiency. Only short-term use is recommended because of possibility of CNS or neuromuscular depression, or electrolyte imbalance. Medicine should be followed by 8 ounces of water. Chilling helps taste.
Lubricant	Mineral oil	Mineral oil may impair the absorption of fat-soluble vitamins (A, D, E, K). May increase effect of oral anticoagulants. Swallow carefully as access of oil into the pharynx, bronchi, and lung may produce a lipid pneumonia.
Osmotic	Cholac	Caution patient that this medication may cause belching, flatulence, or abdominal cramping. Patient should notify physician if this becomes bothersome or if diarrhea occurs.
Stool softener	Colace	May be taken alone or with 8 ounces of water. Store in cool environment, but do not freeze. Swallow tablets whole; do not chew. May be used safely by patients who should avoid straining.

Although relief of constipation is the leading reason for using a laxative, the agents are also used to prepare the bowel prior to surgery and before X-ray or proctoscopic examination of the lower GI tract. Laxatives are used after anthelmintic therapy to speed elimination of parasites, and as a means of reducing the strain of defecation in those with cardiovascular weaknesses.

Special Considerations

- Contraindicated in patients with hypersensitivity to any of the ingredients used in laxative preparations.

- Laxatives are contraindicated in patients with abdominal pain, nausea, vomiting, fecal impaction, intestinal obstruction, appendicitis, biliary tract obstructions, acute hepatitis, and/or in the third trimester of pregnancy.

- Side effects may include nausea, vomiting, diarrhea, anorexia, abdominal cramps, and electrolyte imbalance.

- It is claimed that approximately $400 million a year is spent on laxatives. Many patients abuse laxatives so you should evaluate each patient for signs of abuse. Laxative abuse causes the colon to become lazy and it stops responding to the defecation reflex, causing true constipation. If a patient is abusing laxatives, he or she should gradually reduce the dose or use a milder preparation, at the same time slowly increasing fiber and fluid intake until the defecation reflex returns to a normal state.

- Stimulant laxatives discolor alkaline urine red-pink and acid urine yellow-brown, and they may give a reddish color to feces.

- Administration of laxatives should be such that results will not interfere with a patient's daily activities.

ANTIDIARRHEAL AGENTS

Diarrhea is characterized by frequent defecation of loose, watery stools. It is not a disease; rather, it is a symptom that has been associated with numerous medical conditions. Diarrhea may be caused by infection, intoxication, allergy, malabsorption, inflammation, tumors of the GI tract, food poisoning, and certain medications.

Diarrhea may be described as *acute* when it has a sudden and severe onset, or *chronic* when it is of long-term duration. Acute diarrhea can cause water and salt depletion, resulting in dehydration and electrolyte imbalance.

Because diarrhea is a symptom of an underlying disorder, it is often more important to determine and treat its specific cause than it is to alleviate the diarrhea. When the specific cause of diarrhea can be diagnosed, therapy may involve the use of antiprotozoal agent, an antibacterial drug, or an adrenal corticosteroid. Should it become necessary, certain nonspecific antidiarrheal agents may be used to treat severe acute diarrhea when its cause is unknown. Table 22-6 lists some of these agents.

Special Considerations

- When diarrhea is severe or prolonged, the patient can become dehydrated and experience electrolyte imbalance. Monitor potassium, sodium, and chloride levels. Increase fluids if not contraindicated. Monitor bowel pattern.

- Patients using antidiarrheal agents should avoid over-the-counter products unless prescribed by their physician.

- Pepto-Bismol tablets should be chewed or allowed to dissolve in the mouth; do not swallow them. While taking this medicine, patients should avoid salicylates.

- Lomotil is contraindicated in patients with known hypersensitivity, severe liver disease, pseudomembranous enterocolitis, glaucoma, or electrolyte imbalance, and in children under 2 years of age. Use caution in patients with hepatic disease, renal disease, ulcerative colitis, and during pregnancy and lactation. Lomotil is a Schedule V controlled substance. This medication should not be used with MAO inhibitors because a hypertensive crisis may occur.

	TABLE 22-6	Nonspecific Antidiarrheal Agents

MEDICATION	USUAL ANTIDIARRHEAL DOSAGE	ADVERSE REACTIONS
bismuth subsalicylate (Pepto-Bismol)	Oral (Adult): 30 mL or 2 tablets, (maximum of 8 doses/day at 30 to 60-minute intervals) (Child 10 to 14 years): 20 mL as above (Child 6 to 10 years): 10 mL or 1 tablet (Child 3 to 6 years): 5 mL or $\frac{1}{2}$ tablet	Temporary darkening of stool and tongue
diphenoxylate HCl with atropine sulfate (Lomotil)	Oral (Adult): 5 mg 3 to 4 times/day as needed Oral (Child 2 to 12 years): 0.3 to 0.4 mg/kg/day of liquid in divided doses	Headache, sedation, dizziness, flushing, nausea, dry mouth, blurred vision
kaolin mixture with pectin (Kaopectate)	Oral (Adults): 4 to 8 tablespoons Oral (Children): Over 12 years: 4 tablespoons 6 to 12 years: 2 to 4 tablespoons 3 to 6 years: 1 to 2 tablespoons	Few adverse reactions. In the elderly and debilitated patients, constipation may occur.
loperamide HCl (Imodium)	Oral: 4 mg initially, then 2 mg after each unformed stool, maintenance dose: 4 to 8 mg/day	Drowsiness, abdominal discomfort or pain, nausea

- Imodium is contraindicated in patients with known hypersensitivity, severe ulcerative colitis, and pseudomembranous enterocolitis. Precautions are indicated in patients with liver disease, dehydration, bacterial disease, or during pregnancy and lactation, and in children under 2 years of age.

ANTHELMINTICS

Helminthiasis is a condition in which there is an intestinal infestation by parasitic worms. Infections of this type are a major cause of disease in many areas of the world and have been associated with unsanitary living conditions. Although most commonly found in the developing countries, worm infestations can occur in any society. The helminths that infest humans belong to two groups: *Nemathelminthes* (roundworms) and *Platyhelminthes* (flatworms). The roundworms, pinworms, hookworms, and other nemathelminthes of class *Nematoda* are the organisms responsible for the most common helminthic diseases worldwide and in the United States. The flatworms causing parasitic diseases are tapeworms and flukes. Most of these intestinal parasites can be eliminated by therapy with the appropriate anthelmintic (see Table 22-7).

ANTIPROTOZOAL AGENTS

Protozoa rival worms as the world's leading cause of disease and, although there has been great improvement in worldwide sanitation, developing countries continue to have a high incidence of parasitic disease. Travel and military service often expose Americans to such protozoal diseases as malaria, giardiasis, trichomoniasis, and amebiasis. Although not widespread in the United States, the organisms that cause this disease are becoming increasingly resistant to the drugs used in treating the disease. Antiprotozoal agents are listed in Table 22-8.

Trichomoniasis is primarily a disease of the vagina, although it can be present in the male urethra and the rectum of either sex. Infection by *Trichomonas vaginalis* is characterized by a thin, yellow, malodorous discharge and pruritus. Giardiasis is caused by the flagellate *Giardia lamblia*, which inhabits the small intestine. Many hosts are asymptomatic to the organism, which is increasingly found in the United States as a result of travel to and from other countries. Amebiasis is caused by *Entamoeba histolytica* and is transmitted by ingestion of mature cysts. Colonies develop in the intestinal tract, causing diarrhea and abdominal pain in many who are infected by the organism.

TABLE 22-7 Anthelmintics

MEDICATION	INFECTED BY	USUAL DOSAGE	ADVERSE REACTIONS
mebendazole	Roundworm, hookworm, whipworm, pinworm	Oral: 100 mg twice/day (morning and evening) for 3 consecutive days Oral: 100 mg as a single dose	Diarrhea, fever, dizziness, transient abdominal pain
niclosamide	Beef tapeworm, fish tapeworm Dwarf tapeworm	Oral (Adult): 4 tablets (2 g) as a single dose (Child): 2 to 3 tablets (dosage based on kg of body weight) Oral (Adult): 4 tablets/day for 7 days (Child): 2 to 3 tablets/day for 6 days (based on kg of body weight)	Drowsiness, dizziness, headache, irritability, skin rash, sweating, nausea, abdominal discomfort, edema of an arm, rectal bleeding, diarrhea
praziquantel (Biltricide)	Blood fluke Other flukes Tapeworms	Oral: 60 mg/kg in 3 divided doses at 4 to 6 hour intervals per day Oral: 75 mg/kg in 3 doses/same day Oral: 10 to 20 mg/kg as a single dose	Abdominal pain, nausea, anorexia, dizziness, headache, malaise, giddiness, pruritus, urticaria, fever
pyrantel pamoate (Antiminth)	Pinworm, roundworm	Oral: 11 mg/kg (5 mg/lb) in a single dose, (maxi-mum total dose 1 g)	Dizziness, drowsiness, headache, anorexia, nausea, abdominal distention, rash
thiabendazole (Mintezol)	Roundworm, pinworm, hookworm, threadworm	Oral (Patient less than 150 lb): 10 to 25 mg/kg in 2 doses per day; (Patient over 150 lb): 1.5 g in 2 doses per day	Hypotension, bradycardia, anorexia, nausea, vomiting, jaundice, cholestasis, liver damage, headache, blurred vision, malodor of urine

TABLE 22-8 Antiprotozoal Agents

MEDICATION	DISEASE	USUAL DOSAGE	ADVERSE REACTIONS
chloroquine HCl (Aralen HCl)	Malaria	IM (Adult): 160 to 200 mg of base repeated in 6 hours if necessary (maximum, 800 mg [base] in the first 24 hours) IM (Child): 5 mg base/kg repeated in 6 hours (maximum, 10 mg base/kg/24 hours)	Fatigue, irritability, psychoses, nightmares, heart block, hypotension, eczema, vomiting Abdominal cramps, visual disturbances
chloroquine phosphate (Aralen Phosphate)	Malaria Amebiasis (hepatic)	Oral (Adult): 600 mg of base, then 300 mg of base at 6, 24, and 48 hours Oral (Adult): 600 mg of base daily for 2 days, then 300 mg base/day for 2 to 3 wks	Same as above
furazolidone	Giardiasis	Oral (Adult): 100 mg 4 times daily (Child): 25 to 50 mg 4 times daily	Anorexia, nausea, vomiting, fever, hypotension, malaise

(continues)

TABLE 22-8 (*continued*)

MEDICATION	DISEASE	USUAL DOSAGE	ADVERSE REACTIONS
hydroxychloroquine sulfate (Plaquenil)	Malaria	Oral (Adult): 800 mg followed by 400 mg after 6 to 8 hours, then 400 mg on each of the next 2 days for a total of 2 g	GI distress, visual disturbances, retinopathy, vertigo, nerve deafness, tinnitus
iodoquinol (Yodoxin)	Amebiasis, Trichomoniasis	Oral (Adult): 650 mg 3 times/day for 20 days, to be taken after meals (Child): 30 to 40 mg/kg in 2 to 3 doses for 20 days, not to exceed 2 g per day	Headache, vertigo, muscle pain, paresthesias, blurred vision, optic atrophy, discoloration of hair and nails
metronidazole (Flagyl)	Amebiasis, Trichomoniasis, giardiasis	Oral (Trichomoniasis): 2 g in a single or divided dose (one day therapy) Oral (Amebiasis): (Adult): 500 to 750 mg 3 times/day for 5 to 10 days (Child): 35 to 50 mg/kg/day in 3 doses for 10 days	Rash, flushing, headache, vertigo, confusion, insomnia, depression, polyuria, cystitis, nausea, vomiting, anorexia, abdominal cramps, dry mouth, bitter taste, leukopenia
primaquine phosphate	Malaria	Oral: 15 mg of base daily for 14 days	Hemolytic anemia in patients with G6PD deficiency, nausea
pyrimethamine (Daraprim)	Malaria	Oral: 25 mg once weekly	Anorexia, vomiting, skin rash, folic acid deficiency

ANTIEMETICS

Antiemetics are agents that prevent or arrest vomiting. These drugs are the same as those listed in Unit 27, Table 27-10, for the treatment of vertigo, motion sickness, and the nausea associated with use of antineoplastic agents and radiation. For information on route, dosage, and adverse reactions of the various antiemetic agents, see Table 27-10.

EMETICS

Emetics are used to induce vomiting in people who have taken an overdose of oral drugs or who have ingested certain poisons. An emetic agent should not be given to a patient who is unconscious, in shock, or in a semicomatose state. Emetics are also contraindicated in individuals who have ingested strongly caustic substances, such as lye or acid, because their use could result in additional injury to the patient's esophagus.

Apomorphine hydrochloride acts on the chemoreceptor trigger zone of the medulla and causes vomiting in adults in 2 to 10 minutes. This emetic is more effective when the stomach is full; therefore, 200 to 300 ml of water should be given prior to its injection. The usual adult dose is 5 mg by the subcutaneous route. Apomorphine HCl is available as a hypodermic tablet, which must be dissolved to facilitate injection. The drug is not stable and should be protected from light during storage. Apomorphine HCl should not be used if the solution is green or brown in color.

Ipecac syrup is available without a prescription from local pharmacies in amounts up to 30 mL. Some physicians advise parents of young children to keep a small amount of this emetic on hand for use in an emergency. Ipecac syrup causes less CNS depression than apomorphine HCl, especially in young patients. It acts directly on the chemoreceptor trigger zone of the medulla and reflexly on the gastric mucosa to cause vomiting. The usual dose for adults is 20 mL followed by one or two full glasses of water. For children between 1 and 12 years of age, the usual dose is 15 mL (one tablespoonful) followed by one to one and a half full glasses of water. The usual dose for infants 9 to 12 months of age is two teaspoonsful followed by one half to one full glass of water. Ipecac syrup will usually cause vomiting within 20 minutes of administration and the dosage can be repeated should vomiting not occur within this time. Activated charcoal may be used *after* vomiting has subsided to absorb the remaining poison.

 Spot Check

There are several medications that may be used to treat ulcers. For each of the selected drugs listed, give the usual dosage and several adverse reactions:

DRUG	USUAL DOSAGE	ADVERSE REACTIONS
Tagamet (cimetidine)		
Pepcid (famotidine)		
Axid (nizatidine)		
Zantac (ranitidine)		
Carafate (sucralfate)		
Cytotec (misoprostol)		

■ ■ REVIEW QUESTIONS

Directions. Select the best answer to each of the following multiple-choice questions, circling the letter of your choice:

1. During the digestive process, a partially digested mass, known as _____, leaves the stomach and passes into the small intestines.
   a. bolus
   b. chyme
   c. bile
   d. chole

2. Typical complaints and disorders of the gastrointestinal system include _____.
   a. dyspepsia, dysphagia, and pyrosis
   b. dyspepsia, pyrosis, and nausea
   c. dyspepsia, dysphonia, pyrosis
   d. dyspepsia, dysphasia, pyrosis

3. _____ are drugs that neutralize hydrochloric acid in the stomach.
   a. Antispasmodics
   b. Antagonists
   c. Antacids
   d. Agonists

4. Magnesium-based antacids may cause diarrhea.
   a. True
   b. False

5. Antacid mixtures are commonly used in the treatment of _____.
   a. peptic ulcers
   b. acid indigestion
   c. heartburn
   d. all of these

6. Products that contain magnesium hydroxide frequently cause _____.
   a. constipation
   b. diarrhea
   c. belching
   d. vomiting

7. Tagamet and Zantac are _____.
   a. histamine agonists
   b. histamine antagonists
   c. antispasmodics
   d. antacids

8. _____ mixes with gastric acid to form a pastelike coating that prevents further damage by ulcerogenic secretions.
   a. Tagamet
   b. Zantac
   c. Carafate
   d. cimetidine

9. Sucralfate (Carafate) is a/an _____ agent that is used to prevent further damage by ulcers.
   a. antacid
   b. cytoprotective
   c. proton pump inhibitor
   d. histamine H$_2$-receptor

10. When taking misoprostol (Cytotec), one should avoid _____.
    a. aluminum-containing antacids
    b. grapefruit
    c. magnesium-containing antacids
    d. simethicone

11. When taking pantoprazole (Protonix), the delayed-release tablet should be swallowed whole. This drug is a/an _____.
    a. mucosal protective medication
    b. gastric acid pump inhibitor
    c. antacid
    d. histamine H$_2$-receptor antagonist

12. Polycarbophil (FiberCon) is a/an _____ laxative.
    a. osmotic
    b. saline
    c. bulk-forming
    d. stimulant

13. _____ are various oils that soften the fecal mass and facilitate its passage through the colon.

    a. Stimulants   c. Stool softeners

    b. Bulk-forming agents   d. Lubricants

14. Docusate sodium (Colace) is a _____.

    a. stimulant laxative   c. bulk-forming laxative

    b. saline laxative   d. stool softener

15. _____ is characterized by frequent defecation of loose, watery stools.

    a. Constipation   b. Diarrhea   c. Dehydration   d. all of these

16. Temporary darkening of the stool and tongue is an adverse reaction of _____.

    a. Pepto-Bismol   b. Lomotil   c. Imodium   d. Laudanum

17. A condition in which there is an intestinal infestation by parasitic worms is known as _____.

    a. giardiasis   b. amebiasis   c. helminthiasis   d. trichomoniasis

18. Diarrhea, fever, dizziness, and transient abdominal pain are adverse reactions of _____.

    a. Niclocide   b. Mintezol   c. Vermox   d. Vansil

19. The following are all protozoal diseases except _____.

    a. malaria   b. giardiasis   c. amebiasis   d. monilia

20. _____ are agents that prevent or arrest vomiting.

    a. Emetics   b. Antacids   c. Antiemetics   d. Antidiarrheals

21. Apomorphine HCl and ipecac syrup are _____.

    a. antiemetics   b. emetics   c. antispasmodics   d. antacids

Matching. Place the correct letter from Column II on the appropriate line of Column I:

Column I		*Column II*
22. ___C___ amebiasis		A. an intestinal infestation of parasitic worms
23. ___D___ defecation		B. a partially digested mass of food
24. ___B___ chyme		C. being infected with amebae
25. ___A___ helminthiasis		D. the process of emptying the bowel
		E. being infected with helminths

UNIT 23
Medications Used for Cardiovascular System Disorders

OBJECTIVES

Upon completing this unit, you should be able to:

- Define the terms listed in the vocabulary.
- State the function of the cardiovascular system.
- List the warning signs of a heart attack.
- List the established risk factors for heart disease.
- Explain why age is directly related to the development of heart disease.
- Explain why age complicates the treatment regimen for older adults.
- Describe two causes of congenital heart disease.
- Complete the critical thinking questions and activities presented in this unit.
- Describe three ways that drugs may affect heart action.
- Explain the action of digitalis products.
- State the usual initial or digitalizing dose, the usual maintenance dose, and adverse reactions of selected digitalis products.
- State the actions, uses, contraindications, warnings, adverse reactions, dosage and route, implications for patient care, patient teaching, and special considerations for digitalis preparations, antihypertensive agents, anticoagulants, antiplatelet drugs, hematinic agents, agents used in treating megaloblastic anemia, and antihyperlipidemic agents.
- Describe hemostatic agents and their uses.
- Complete the Spot Check on selected drugs that are used to treat cardiovascular system disorders.
- Answer the review questions correctly.

VOCABULARY

angiotensin (an"je-o-ten'sin). A vasopressor substance that is formed in the body by interaction of renin and angio tensinogen.

atherosclerosis (ăth"ĕr-ō"sklē-rō"sĭs). The building up of fatty plaques and hardening of the arteries.

glycoside (gli"ko'sid). A substance that is derived from plants, and upon hydrolysis yields a sugar plus additional products.

hypokalemia (hi"pō-kǎ-lĕ'mē-a). A deficient amount of potassium in the blood. This condition can cause muscle weakness, thirst, dizziness, mental confusion, paralysis, tetany, and postural hypotension.

mast cells. Connective tissue cells that contain heparin and histamine.

megaloblastic anemia (meg"a-lo-blast'ik a-ne'me-a). An anemia in which megaloblasts (large-size nucleated abnormal red blood cells) are found in the blood. Also known as pernicious anemia.

plasminogen (plaz-min'o-jen). A protein that is found in many body tissues and fluids. It is important in the prevention of fibrin clot formation.

INTRODUCTION

The heart and a complex network of arteries, veins, and capillaries make up the cardiovascular system. The arteries take blood away from the heart to the various organs of the body. Blood, leaving the left side of the heart, enters the aorta and is carried by even smaller arteries to all parts of the body. Within the tissues, arterioles empty into microscopic vessels known as *capillaries*. The thin, porous walls of these vessels are easily penetrated by molecules of sugars, salts, gases, and other substances needed by surrounding cells. In this network of capillaries, the primary function of the circulatory system is carried out. That function is to bring oxygen and needed nutrients to the cells adjacent to the capillary, and to pick up carbon dioxide and metabolic waste that need to be removed from the body.

As blood passes through the capillaries, it enters into venules. These veins link up with larger and larger veins and ultimately carry the blood back to the heart. Venous blood enters the right side of the heart and is pumped out again into the pulmonary artery, which takes it to the lungs. Once in the lungs, the waste carbon dioxide in the venous blood is removed and a new supply of oxygen is absorbed. The blood is now ready to circulate back through the left side of the heart and the arteries to supply the needs of the body once again. See Figure 23-1 for a drawing of the cardiovascular system.

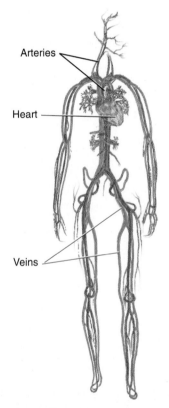

Arteries

Heart

Veins

FIGURE 23-1

Cardiovascular system: Heart, arteries, veins, capillaries, and blood
Source: Delmar/Cengage Learning

Spotlight

Heart Disease

In the United States, one out of four adults is at risk for heart disease. Coronary heart disease (CHD) is the leading cause of death for men and women (see Figure 23-2). According to the American Heart Association, someone in the United States suffers from a CHD-related event about every 29 seconds, and someone dies from such an event about every minute. The lifetime risk of having coronary heart disease after age 40 is 49 percent for men and 32 percent for women. As women get older, the risk increases almost to that of men.

One in 10 American women 45 to 64 years of age has some form of heart disease, and this increases to one in four women over 65. Heart disease kills far more women than breast cancer does. The common misconception that heart disease is a man's disease may cause women to be misinformed about heart disease, the risk factors associated with developing heart disease, and lifestyle changes.

Researchers have found that refined carbohydrates may be as bad for the heart as saturated fats. The Boston School of Public Health analyzed the eating habits of 75,000 women over 10 years to track the effects of foods with a high glycemic load, the starchy carbohydrates (white bread, white rice, white potatoes, and low-fiber cereal), that send blood sugar soaring. Why such starches make trouble for the heart is not fully understood. Evidence does suggest that easily digested foods that dump torrents of sugar into the bloodstream may reduce levels of good cholesterol, raise triglyceride levels, and interfere with the body's ability to use insulin. Research shows that foods with a low glycemic load such as whole grain breads and cereals, fruits, vegetables, and legumes may, if anything, help to keep the heart healthy and the arteries clear.

The primary cause of coronary heart disease is **atherosclerosis** or the building up of fatty plaques and hardening of the arteries. It has been discovered that the real danger of this condition comes when the plaque fractures or cracks, causing clotting material to be released and a blood clot to form inside the vessel. The clot can go on to partially block the vessel and create chest pain, or completely block the artery causing a myocardial infarction (heart attack).

It is estimated that 1.5 million Americans will have a heart attack this year. About 600,000 will die and, of this number, 350,000 will die before they reach medical help. It is said that the average heart attack victim waits three hours after symptoms occur to seek help. Many times they try to ignore the symptoms or say, "It's just indigestion."

Cross sections through a coronary artery
undergoing progressive atherosclerosis
and arteriosclerosis

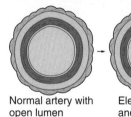

— Small
   atheroma

Normal artery with
open lumen

Elevated cholesterol
and blood fats

— Enlarging
   atheroma

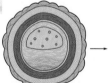

Moderate athero-
sclerotic narrowing
of lumen

Moderate
myocardial ischemia
↓
Angina pectoris

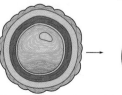

Occlusion of
left coronary
artery
Myocardial infarction
("heart attack") on left
side of the heart

Complete/almost complete
occlusion, with hardening
due to calcium deposition

Severe acute
myocardial ischemia
and infarction

FIGURE 23-2

The natural history of coronary heart disease *Source: Delmar/Cengage Learning*

A recent study notes that inflammation is a powerful trigger for a heart attack. Those who have high levels of inflammation are more likely to die from heart attacks and strokes. A C-reactive protein (CRP) test can be performed to indicate the presence of bacterial infections, but not viral infections in the body. CRP appears in the blood 6 to 10 hours after an acute inflammatory process or tissue destruction (necrosis), or both, and it peaks within 48 to 72 hours. It is not normally present in the adult or child; a 1:2 titer indicates a positive result.

Abundant evidence exists that low-density lipoprotein (LDL) particle size is an important determinant of coronary heart disease risk. Several studies have shown that individuals with predominantly small, dense LDL particles (subclass pattern B) are at increased risk for CHD even when levels of LDL are not elevated. To determine the lipoprotein profile, a physician will order a special test such as the NMR (nuclear magnetic resonance) LipoProfile.

The American Heart Association lists the following as warning signs of heart attack:

- Pressure, fullness, squeezing pain in the center of the chest that lasts two minutes or longer
- Pain that spreads to the shoulders, neck, or arms
- Dizziness, fainting, sweating, nausea, or shortness of breath

Chest pain can be caused by a variety of conditions, including angina, myocardial infarction, stress, anxiety, and gastrointestinal disorders. It is essential that the physician determine the cause of the pain and treat it appropriately.

The Two Primary Causes of Chest Pain

	ANGINA PECTORIS	MYOCARDIAL INFARCTION
Cause(s):	Decreased blood flow through the coronary arteries that causes less oxygen to reach the myocardium.	Occlusion of a coronary artery. Area becomes necrotic (infarct). May be caused by an embolus, vasoconstriction of the arteries, or sudden atherosclerotic changes in the vessels.
Predisposing Factors:	<ul><li>atherosclerosis</li><li>hypertension</li><li>diabetes mellitus</li><li>syphilis</li><li>rheumatic heart disease</li></ul>	<ul><li>atherosclerosis</li><li>hypertension</li><li>diabetes mellitus</li><li>obesity</li><li>family history</li><li>smoking</li><li>blood cholesterol level: 200 to 239 borderline high 240 high LDL 130 to 159 borderline/160 high risk</li></ul>
Symptoms:	Sudden, agonizing pain in the substernal region, may radiate to left shoulder and arm, up to jaw; skin cold and clammy; pulse normal; B/P little or no change; anxious, apprehensive	Severe, crushing pain in the substernal region and upper abdomen, radiates to shoulders, arms, jaw; skin cold and clammy; pulse rapid, weak, irregular; nausea and possible vomiting; B/P drops; extremely apprehensive

Established Risk Factors

- Male age 55 or older
- Female age 65 or older
- Female under age 65 with premature menopause
- Smoker
- Hypertension
- Diabetes mellitus

- Hyperlipidemia
- Family history of early heart disease (parent or sibling; male less than 55, female less than 65)
- Obesity

■ Special Considerations: **OLDER ADULTS**

More than 2.7 million people over 60 years of age live with heart disease. Four out of five people who die of heart attacks are 65 years of age or older. With maturity, the body begins the inevitable process of aging, and the body's ability to restore and repair itself decreases. The heart must work harder to pump against the hardening of the arteries and an increasing systolic blood pressure that is common as one ages. Reduced blood flow, elevated blood lipids (fats), and defective endothelial repair common in aging accelerates the course of cardiovascular disease (see Figure 23-3).

Age is directly related to the development of heart disease, and age complicates the treatment regimen for older adults because of the normal physiologic changes that occur with aging, the presence of chronic diseases such as arthritis, diabetes, COPD, and others in addition to heart disease, the taking of multiple drugs (polypharmacy), and the possibility of nutritional deficiencies or substance abuse. The functional, cognitive, and sensory capacities of older adults should be carefully evaluated before and during drug therapy. Some other factors that can affect the actions, absorption, metabolism, and excretion of cardiovascular drugs are:

- Slowed intestinal motility. With aging, blood flow to the entire digestive system decreases, thereby slowing drug entry into the general circulation. This delay in absorption may weaken a drug's potency and extend the duration of action.
- Decrease in lean body mass and total body water makes it necessary for smaller dosages of some medications to maintain therapeutic levels without causing toxicity.

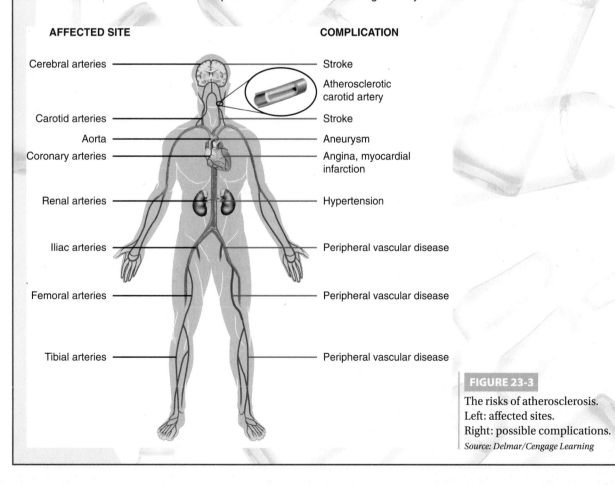

AFFECTED SITE

- Cerebral arteries
- Carotid arteries
- Aorta
- Coronary arteries
- Renal arteries
- Iliac arteries
- Femoral arteries
- Tibial arteries

COMPLICATION

- Stroke
- Atherosclerotic carotid artery
- Stroke
- Aneurysm
- Angina, myocardial infarction
- Hypertension
- Peripheral vascular disease
- Peripheral vascular disease
- Peripheral vascular disease

FIGURE 23-3

The risks of atherosclerosis.
Left: affected sites.
Right: possible complications.
Source: Delmar/Cengage Learning

- Low serum albumin levels in older adults may allow too much free circulation of drugs that bind with albumin, such as digoxin. The increased risk of adverse effects and toxicity may occur because the drug's plasma concentration is too high.
- Age- or disease-related cardiovascular changes can slow drug distribution to tissues and prolong the time until onset and duration of action.
- The efficiency of the kidneys and liver can decline with age, decreasing their ability to excrete drugs, which may necessitate drug dosage reductions.

Special Considerations: CHILDREN

Pulse, respiration, blood pressure, and hematologic values vary with the age of the child. In the newborn, the pulse may vary from 110 to 160 beats per minute, respirations 35 to 50 per minute, and blood pressure 52/26 to 80/46. The newborn's circulation begins to function shortly after birth and if proper adaptations do not take place, congenital heart disease may occur. Annually, approximately 25,000 babies in the United States are born with congenital heart defects.

The development of the fetal heart is usually completed during the first 2 months of intrauterine life. It is completely formed and functioning by 10 weeks, and most congenital heart defects develop before the tenth week of pregnancy. Pediatric cardiologists have recognized more than 50 congenital heart defects. If the left side of the heart is not completely separated from the right side, various septal defects develop. If the four chambers of the heart do not occur normally, complex anomalies form such as tetralogy of Fallot, a congenital heart defect involving pulmonary stenosis, ventricular septal defect, dextroposition of the aorta, and hypertrophy of the right ventricle.

The causes of congenital heart disease may be classified as exogenous or endogenous. Viruses and alcohol are the most common causes of exogenous congenital heart disease, and chromosomal abnormalities are among the most important endogenous causes.

- **Viruses:** During the first 3 months of pregnancy, the rubella (German measles) virus is associated with a high incidence of congenital heart disease in infants. It is believed that the virus enters the fetal circulation and damages the developing heart.
  Prevention: Rubella can be prevented by immunization.
- **Alcohol:** Alcohol affects the fetal heart directly and interferes with its development. Fetal alcohol syndrome is often associated with heart defects.
  Prevention: There is no "safe" level of alcohol consumption for a pregnant female. All alcohol should be avoided during pregnancy.

Critical Thinking QUESTIONS AND ACTIVITIES

Your patient is a 72-year-old male who has been admitted with angina pectoris and hypertension. He complains of having experienced a sudden, agonizing pain in his chest that radiated to his left shoulder, his skin is cold and clammy, and he appears anxious. His physician has ordered blood studies, a chest X-ray, and an electrocardiogram stat. He has asked that the patient continue his sublingual nitroglycerin PRN and atenolol (Tenormin) 50 mg once daily. Using the information in Special Considerations: Older Adults and any other reference that you need, ask yourself:

- What are some of the factors that cause angina pectoris and hypertension in older adults?
- What are some factors that may complicate the treatment regimen for older adults?
- What are some other factors that can affect the actions, absorption, metabolism, and excretion of cardiovascular drugs?
- What type of cardiovascular drug is nitroglycerin?
- What should I teach the patient about this medication?
- What type of cardiovascular drug is atenolol (Tenormin)?
- What should I teach the patient about the medication?

HOW DRUGS AFFECT THE HEART

The agents discussed in this unit may affect heart action in one or more of the following ways:

1. Exert a positive or negative *inotropic effect* by increasing or decreasing the force of myocardial contraction.
2. Exert a positive or negative *chronotropic effect* by increasing or decreasing heart rate.
3. Exert a positive or negative *dromotropic effect* by increasing or decreasing the conduction of electrical impulses through the heart muscle.

Digitalis

In the treatment of congestive heart failure, therapy usually includes the use of a digitalis drug together with a diuretic, a low-sodium diet, and a reduction of physical activities. This combination of drugs, diet, and change in lifestyle is designed to increase cardiac output while reducing pulmonary congestion and the lower-body edema that is characteristic of this disorder.

Digitalis is obtained by crushing the dried leaves of the plant *Digitalis purpurea* or purple foxglove into a powder. A similar drug, digoxin, is obtained from the leaves of *Digitalis lanatas*. The primary use for these and other digitalis compounds is the treatment of various types of heart failures and, together, they belong to a chemical classification known as *cardiac glycosides*. These drugs exert a positive inotropic effect on the heart. They strengthen the heart muscle (myocardium), increase the force of systolic contraction, slow the heart, and improve the muscle tone of the myocardium. As a result of these effects on the heart, there is a decrease in venous pressure as the heart takes in larger amounts of venous blood. Improving the effectiveness of the heart's pumping action reduces the size of the heart and increases the flow of blood to the kidneys, thereby causing a diuretic effect and the removal of some excess fluid from the body. Additional fluids are removed through the use of diuretic drugs. See Unit 25 for a discussion of diuretic agents.

The pharmacologic actions of all digitalis compounds are similar, but these products differ in their potency, onset of action, and the rate at which they are absorbed. Digitalis drugs may be given parenterally, although the oral route is generally preferred.

When first started, an *initial* or *digitalizing* dose is often given to bring the serum level of the drug up to the desired level. The effect of the initial dose is then sustained by smaller daily *maintenance doses*. When a digitalizing dose is not given, the administration of maintenance doses over a period of about seven days will usually result in sufficient accumulation of the drug to produce the desired serum level. The amount of the initial and maintenance doses may vary, depending upon the size of the patient and whether or not there is normal renal or hepatic function. Frequently, maintenance doses of digitalis drugs must be taken throughout the remainder of a patient's lifetime.

Digitalis intoxication can occur when there is excess accumulation of the drug in the body. This can occur when the initial or digitalizing dose is administered too rapidly, or from maintenance doses that are larger than necessary. The difference between therapeutic and toxic doses of digitalis is generally not great. Signs of digitalis intoxication have been reported in up to 20 percent of hospitalized patients receiving the drug; therefore, those who administer this medication should observe the patient for possible toxic reactions.

Digitalis Preparations

Actions

Digitalis drugs strengthen the heart muscle, increase the force and velocity of myocardial systolic contraction (positive inotropic effect), slow the heart rate (negative chronotropic effect), and decrease conduction velocity through the atrioventricular (AV) node.

Uses

Congestive heart failure, atrial fibrillation, atrial flutter, paroxysmal atrial tachycardia.

Contraindications

Contraindicated in patients with known hypersensitivity to any of the ingredients and in ventricular fibrillation.

Caution:

1. *Anorexia, nausea, vomiting, and arrhythmias may be indications of digitalis intoxication.*
2. *Use caution in patients with renal disease, severe respiratory disease, acute myocardial infarction, AV block, or hypothyroidism. Also use caution in geriatric patient and during pregnancy/lactation.*

Adverse Reactions

Reactions can include unifocal or multiform ventricular premature contractions, ventricular tachycardia, atrioventricular dissociation, atrial tachycardia, excessive slowing of the pulse (clinical signs of digitalis overdose), complete heart block, anorexia, nausea, vomiting, diarrhea, blurred vision, headache, weakness, dizziness, apathy, psychosis, gynecomastia, maculopapular rash, drowsiness, confusion, or depression.

Dosage and Route

The dosage and route of administration are determined by the physician and are individualized for each patient.

Implications for Patient Care

Assess the apical pulse for one minute before administering digitalis drugs. Withhold the medication if the pulse is below 60 or the minimum specified by the prescribing physician. Monitor intake and output ratio, daily weight, liver function studies, serum electrolytes, creatinine, and drug levels. Be alert for signs of digitalis toxicity and hypokalemia. Evaluate the therapeutic response of medication (decreased edema, weight loss, increased urine output, improved heart rate, and rhythm).

Signs and Symptoms of Digitalis Toxicity

The most common early symptoms of digitalis toxicity are anorexia, nausea, vomiting, and arrhythmias. Other signs and symptoms according to body system are the following:

Gastrointestinal: anorexia, nausea, vomiting, diarrhea, abdominal pain.

Nervous system: headache, restlessness, irritability, drowsiness, depression, confusion, disorientation, insomnia, psychosis, convulsions, coma, blurred or yellow vision.

Cardiovascular: bradycardia, tachycardia, atrial tachycardia with varying AV block, ventricular bigeminy, ventricular tachycardia, second-degree AV block, complete AV block.

Musculoskeletal: severe weakness.

Patient Teaching

Educate patients:

- about possible adverse reactions and the signs and symptoms of digitalis toxicity.
- to notify their physician without delay if toxic symptoms appear.
- about the importance of taking the medication as prescribed.

- not to stop taking the drug unless the physician so orders.

- to avoid over-the-counter medications unless ordered by the physician.

- to include foods high in potassium (unless the patient is taking a potassium-sparing diuretic) and low in sodium in their diet.

- and their family how to take a pulse and how to recognize changes in rate, volume, and rhythm.

- to weigh themselves weekly and report weight gain of 5 pounds or more to the physician.

- to wear or carry a Medic Alert ID stating that they are on digitalis. ∎

Special Considerations

- Potassium-depleting corticosteroids and diuretics may be major contributing factors to digitalis toxicity.

- Rapid intravenous administration of calcium may produce serious arrhythmias in patients receiving digitalis.

- Quinidine, verapamil, and amiodarone cause a rise in serum digoxin concentration, with the implication that digitalis intoxication may result.

- Antacids, kaolin-pectin, sulfasalazine, neomycin, cholestyramine, and certain anticancer drugs may interfere with intestinal digoxin absorption, resulting in unexpectedly low serum concentration.

- The additive effects of beta-adrenergic blockers or calcium channel blockers and digitalis can result in complete heart block.

- There are numerous precautions and drug interactions associated with digitalis drugs. Please refer to a current drug reference source for more information.

Antiarrhythmic Agents

The heartbeat is controlled by neuromuscular tissue within the heart. The sinoatrial node (SA), located in the upper wall of the right atrium, is considered to be the source of the heartbeat and is referred to as the *pacemaker* of the heart.

Normally, impulses from the sinoatrial node cause contraction of both left and right atria. The impulse also stimulates the atrioventricular node (AV) below the endocardium of the right atrium, which, in turn, transmits the impulse to the atrioventricular bundle (bundle of His) and causes contraction of the left and right ventricles.

Disorders of the SA node that interfere with impulse formation or disorders with the conduction system (AV node, bundle of His) result in a variety of cardiac arrhythmias. The term *arrhythmia* means irregularity or loss of rhythm and is commonly used to describe an irregular heartbeat. Some cardiac arrhythmias do not require treatment, whereas others may result in death if not treated by drug therapy or the use of an artificial pacemaker.

Antiarrhythmic drugs are used to control many cardiac arrhythmias. Some of the drugs used to treat this condition are found in Table 23–1.

Vasopressors and Vasodilators

There are many uses for drugs that act to either constrict or dilate the walls of blood vessels. Based simply upon their primary action, these medications can be classified as vasopressors and vasodilators.

Vasopressors are drugs that cause contraction of the muscles associated with capillaries and arteries, thereby narrowing the space through which the blood circulates. This narrowing increases the resistance to blood flow and results in an elevation of blood pressure. Drugs classified as vasopressors are useful in the treatment of patients suffering from shock (see Table 23–2).

Vasodilators are medications that cause the relaxation of blood vessels. This action dilates the vessels, thereby increasing their ability to carry blood. This eases resistance to blood flow and lowers blood pressure. Vasodilators may be classified as coronary or peripheral vasodilators.

Coronary vasodilators are used primarily for the treatment of *angina pectoris*, a condition caused by an insufficient supply of blood to the heart. The treatment of this condition usually involves the nitrate group of drugs. Nitrate tablets are rapidly absorbed through the mucous membrane of the mouth or stomach (see Table 23-3).

TABLE 23-1　Antiarrhythmic Drugs

MEDICATIONS	USUAL DOSAGE	ADVERSE REACTIONS
disopyramide (Norpace)	Oral: 600 mg/day in divided doses (150 mg every 6 hours) Less than 110 pounds (50 kg): 100 mg every 6 hours	Hypotension, nausea, congestive heart failure, urinary retention, headache
(Norpace CR)	Oral: 600 mg/day in divided doses (300 mg every 12 hours) Less than 110 pounds (50 kg): 200 mg every 12 hours	Dry mouth, malaise, constipation, blurred vision, dry nose, eyes, and throat
flecainide acetate (Tambocor)	Oral: 100 mg every 12 hours with increases of 50 mg b.i.d. every 4 days until efficacy is achieved	Chest discomfort and tinnitus, leg cramps, blurred vision, ataxia, dry mouth, nasal congestion, nausea
lidocaine HCl (Xylocaine HCl)	IM: 2 mg/lb (4.3 mg/kg) of 10% solution as needed	Light-headedness, visual disturbances, tinnitus, muscle twitches
propranolol HCl (Inderal)	Oral: 10 to 30 mg 3 to 4 times daily before meals and at bedtime	Light-headedness, mental depression and insomnia, nausea, vomiting, visual disturbances. Most adverse reactions are mild and transient.
quinidine sulfate (Extentabs)	Oral: 200 to 300 mg 3 to 4 times daily	Tinnitus, visual disturbances, nausea, vomiting, headache, vertigo. Hypersensitivity to the drug may cause angioedema, acute asthmatic episode, and sometimes vascular collapse.

TABLE 23-2　A Vasopressor

MEDICATIONS	USUAL DOSAGE	ADVERSE REACTIONS
phenylephrine HCl (Neo-Synephrine 1% Injection)	IM, SC: 2 to 5 mg	Headache, reflex bradycardia, excitability, restlessness

TABLE 23-3　Coronary Vasodilators

MEDICATIONS	USUAL DOSAGE	ADVERSE REACTIONS
isosorbide dinitrate (Isordil)	Sublingual: 2.5 to 5 mg every 3 hours Chewable: 5 mg initially every 2 to 3 hours Oral: 5 to 20 mg 4 times daily Oral (sustained-release): 40 mg every 6 to 12 hours	Headache, hypotension, cutaneous vasodilation with flushing, transient episodes of dizziness
nitroglycerin (Nitrolingual Spray) (Nitrostat) (Nitro Dur Transderm)	Topical: Spread in a thin layer over a 2- to 6-inch area every 3 to 4 hours when needed Sublingual: 0.15 to 0.6 mg under tongue as needed for acute angina Oral (sustained-release): 2.5 mg 3 to 4 times daily Transdermal: 2.5 to 20 mg released over a 24-hour period Lingual aerosol: 1 to 2 metered doses onto or under the tongue Transmucosal: 1 mg placed on the oral mucosa between cheek and gum	Headache, hypotension, cutaneous vasodilation with flushing, and occasional drug rash or exfoliative dermatitis

(*continues*)

TABLE 23-3 (continued)

MEDICATIONS	USUAL DOSAGE	ADVERSE REACTIONS
pentaerythritol tetranitrate	Oral (sustained-release): 10 to 40 mg 4 times a day	Rash, headache, mild gastrointestinal distress, cutaneous vasodilation with flushing, transient episodes of dizziness

TABLE 23-4 Peripheral Vasodilators

MEDICATIONS	USUAL DOSAGE	ADVERSE REACTIONS
cyclandelate (Cyclospasmol)	Oral: Initial dose, 1200 to 1600 mg per day in divided doses before meals and at bedtime; with clinical response, reduce dose by 200 mg decrements until maintenance dose (400 to 800 mg/day) is reached	Gastrointestinal distress, mild flush, headache, feeling of weakness, or tachycardia
isoxsuprine HCl (Vasodilan)	Oral: 10 to 20 mg 3 to 4 times daily IM: 5 to 10 mg 2 to 3 times daily	Occasional hypotension, tachycardia, nausea, dizziness, chest pain, rash
nylidrin HCl (Arlidin)	Oral: 3 to 12 mg 3 to 4 times daily	Trembling, nervousness, weakness, dizziness, nausea and vomiting
papaverine HCl	Oral (sustained-release): 150 mg every 8 to 12 hours	Nausea, abdominal distress, anorexia, constipation, headache, drowsiness, sweating

Peripheral vasodilators are used in the treatment of peripheral vascular disease (PVD), although many are classified by the Food and Drug Administration as only "possibly effective." They are used for the relief of symptoms of cerebral and peripheral vascular insufficiency (see Table 23-4).

Antihypertensive Agents

Hypertension affects approximately 50 million individuals in the United States and approximately 1 billion worldwide. In hypertension, also known as high blood pressure, blood is forced through the heart and vessels throughout the body with a greater force than is necessary. Over time, hypertension damages the heart and blood vessels. When left untreated, those with hypertension are at risk for stroke and progressive deterioration of cardiac and renal function.

Normal blood pressure for adults age 18 and over is a systolic blood pressure reading less than 120 mm Hg and a diastolic less than 80 mm Hg. Prehypertension is a new classification that impacts approximately 45 million American adults and is defined as a systolic of 120 mm Hg to 139 mm Hg and a diastolic of 80 mm Hg to 89 mm Hg. Individuals at the upper end of the prehypertension blood pressure range are twice as likely to progress to hypertension. Hypertension is defined as a systolic pressure of 140 mm Hg or higher or a diastolic of 90 mm Hg or higher.

The National Heart, Lung, and Blood Institute (NHLBI) classifies blood pressure into categories and provides guidelines for the prevention and treatment of hypertension.

The classification of hypertension is as follows:

	Systolic (mm Hg)	Diastolic (mm Hg)
Normal	<120	<80
Prehypertension	120–139	80–89
Stage 1	140–159	90–99
Stage 2	>160	>100

The overall goal in treating hypertension is to prevent other health-related complications and death from hypertension. The relationship between blood pressure and risk of cardiovascular disease events is continuous, consistent, and independent of other risk factors. The higher the blood pressure, the greater is the chance of heart attack, heart failure, stroke, and kidney disease.

In initiating drug therapy for the treatment of hypertension, several factors are considered: the degree of blood pressure elevation, the presence of target organ damage, and the presence of clinical cardiovascular disease or other risk factors, such as smoking, diabetes, and obesity.

There are various classes of drugs used in the treatment of hypertension, including diuretics, beta-blockers, angiotensin-converting enzymes (ACE) inhibitors, **angiotensin** antagonists, calcium channel blockers (CCBs), alpha-blockers, alpha-beta-blockers, nervous system inhibitors, and vasodilators.

- *Diuretics* decrease reabsorption of sodium chloride by the kidneys, thereby increasing the amount of salt and water excreted in the urine. They are sometimes called "water pills."
- *Beta-blockers* reduce nerve impulses to the heart and blood vessels. This makes the heart beat slower and with less force. Blood pressure drops and the heart works less hard.
- *Angiotensin-converting enzyme inhibitors* prevent the formation of a hormone called angiotensin II, which normally causes blood vessels to narrow. The ACE inhibitors cause the vessels to relax and blood pressure goes down.
- *Angiotensin antagonists* shield blood vessels from angiotensin II. As a result, the vessels become wider and blood pressure goes down.
- *Calcium channel blockers* block the flow of calcium ions into myocardial muscle cells and myocardial pacemaker cells. This causes the blood vessels to relax and pressure goes down.
- *Alpha-blockers* reduce nerve impulses to blood vessels, thus allowing blood to pass more easily and causing the blood pressure to go down.
- *Nervous system inhibitors* relax blood vessels by controlling nerve impulses. This causes the blood vessels to become wider and the blood pressure to go down.
- *Vasodilators* act on arteries, veins, or both to reduce blood pressure. They relax smooth muscle, thereby reducing blood pressure.

It is recommended that diuretics be used as initial therapy for most patients with hypertension, either alone or in combination with one of the other classes. Patients with Stage 1 hypertension are generally started on a diuretic, but other classes of medication can also be considered. Patients diagnosed with Stage 2 hypertension typically need a two-drug combination consisting of a diuretic along with one of the other drugs from the antihypertensive class (see Table 23-5).

Implications for Patient Care

Assess blood pressure for therapeutic response to the prescribed medication. Monitor blood studies (neutrophils, decreased platelets, potassium, and sodium levels) and renal studies (protein, BUN, creatinine—increased levels may indicate nephrotic syndrome). Be aware of possible adverse reactions to the prescribed medication.

Patient Teaching

Educate patients:

- to take the medication as prescribed.
- that they may have to take high blood pressure medicine for the rest of their lives.
- that the medication does not cure hypertension, but helps to control it, and that they must continue to take the medication even if they feel better.
- to be aware of possible adverse reactions.

TABLE 23-5 Selected Antihypertensive Agents

CLASS	GENERIC NAME (TRADE NAME)	USUAL DOSAGE RANGE
Thiazide diuretics	chlorothiazide (Diuril)	125 to 500 mg/day
	chlorthalidone (generic)	12.5 to 25 mg/day
	hydrochlorothiazide (Microzide)	12.5 to 50 mg/day
	indapamide	1.25 to 2.5 mg/day
	metolazone	0.5 to 1.0 mg/day
	polythiazide	2 to 4 mg/day
Loop diuretics	bumetanide (Bumex)	0.5 to 2 mg/day
	furosemide (Lasix)	20 to 80 mg/day
	torsemide (Demadex)	2.5 to 10 mg/day
Potassium-sparing diuretics	amiloride	5 to 10 mg/day
	triamterene (Dyrenium)	50 to 100 mg/day
Aldosterone receptor blockers	eplerenone (Inspra)	50 to 100 mg/day
	spironolactone (Aldactone)	25 to 50 mg/day
Beta-blockers	atenolol (Tenormin)	25–100 mg/day
	betaxolol (Kerlone)	5–20 mg/day
	bisoprolol (Zebeta)	2.5–10 mg/day
	metoprolol (Lopressor)	50–100 mg/day
	nadolol (Corgard)	40–120 mg/day
	propranolol (Inderal)	40–160 mg/day
Beta-blockers with intrinsic sympathomimetic activity	acebutolol (Sectral)	200 to 800 mg/day
	penbutolol (Levatol)	10 to 40 mg/day
	pindolol (generic)	10 to 40 mg/day
Combined alpha- and beta-blockers	carvedilol (Coreg)	12.5 to 50 mg/day
	labetalol (Trandate)	200 to 800 mg/day
ACE inhibitors	benazepril (Lotensin)	10 to 40 mg/day
	captopril (Capoten)	25 to 100 mg/day
	enalapril (Vasotec)	2.5 to 40 mg/day
	fosinopril (Monopril)	10 to 40 mg/day
	lisinopril (Prinivil, Zestril)	10 to 40 mg/day
	moexipril (Univasc)	7.5 to 30 mg/day
	perindopril (Aceon)	4 to 8 mg/day
	quinapril (Accupril)	10 to 40 mg/day
	ramipril (Altace)	2.5 to 20 mg/day
	trandolapril (Mavik)	1 to 4 mg/day
Angiotensin II antagonists	candesartan (Atacand)	8 to 32 mg/day
	eprosartan (Teveten)	400 to 800 mg/day
	irbesartan (Avapro)	150 to 300 mg/day
	losartan (Cozaar)	25 to 100 mg/day
	olmesartan (Benicar)	20 to 40 mg/day
	telmisartan (Micardis)	20 to 80 mg/day
	valsartan (Diovan)	80 to 320 mg/day
Calcium channel blockers non-dihydropyridines	diltiazem extended release (Cardizem CD, Dilacor XR, Tiazac)	180 to 420 mg/day
	diltiazem extended release (Cardizem LA)	120 to 540 mg/day
	verapamil immediate release (Calan, Isoptin)	80 to 320 mg/day
	verapamil long-acting (Calan SR, Isoptin SR)	120 to 360 mg/day
	verapamil (Coer Covera HS, Verelan PM)	120 to 360 mg/day

(continues)

TABLE 23-5 *(continued)*

CLASS	GENERIC NAME (TRADE NAME)	USUAL DOSAGE RANGE
Calcium channel blockers dihydropyridines	amlodipine (Norvasc)	2.5 to 10 mg/day
	felodipine (Plendil)	2.5 to 20 mg/day
	isradipine (Dynacirc CR)	2.5 to 10 mg/day
	nicardipine sustained release (Cardene SR)	60 to 120 mg/day
	nifedipine long-acting (Adalat CC, Procardia XL)	30 to 60 mg/day
	nisoldipine (Sular)	10 to 40 mg/day
Alpha1-blockers	doxazosin (Cardura)	1 to 16 mg/day
	prazosin (Minipress)	2 to 20 mg/day
	terazosin (Hytrin)	1 to 20 mg/day
Central alpha2-agonists and other centrally acting drugs	clonidine (Catapres)	0.1 to 0.8 mg/day
	clonidine patch (Catapres-TTS)	0.1 to 0.3 mg/day
	guanfacine	0.5 to 2 mg/day
	reserpine	0.05 to 0.25 mg/day

- to avoid alcohol, over-the-counter drugs (especially cough, cold, and allergy medicines).
- not to operate hazardous machinery or drive a motor vehicle if dizziness occurs.
- about the factors that tend to increase blood pressure: obesity, smoking, consumption of alcohol, stress, lack of exercise, and excessive intake of sodium.
- in ways to reduce the factors that may be contributing to hypertension.
- who is taking diuretics that may deplete potassium to eat foods rich in potassium. (See Unit 25 for more information on diuretics.) ■

DRUGS THAT AFFECT THE BLOOD

A number of medications have been developed that affect the clotting of blood. Simply put, these drugs either assist in the clotting process or work to inhibit the formation of a clot. The formation of a blood clot within a blood vessel is a life-threatening event; therefore, agents that interfere with the clotting process are important. These drugs are the anticoagulants and the thrombolytic agents.

Anticoagulants are used therapeutically after a *thrombus* or blood clot has formed. They do not alter the size of an existing thrombus; however, they do act to prevent further growth and reduce the possibility of embolization. If a thrombus is detached from the point at which it formed, it becomes an *embolus* moving within the vascular system. An embolus that occludes (blocks) the flow of blood can cause serious damage to an organ, as in the case of a coronary embolism.

Thrombolytic agents will dissolve existing fresh thrombi and emboli. These drugs diffuse into the clot and activate plasminogen that is trapped therein. **Plasminogen** is a protein that is important in the prevention of fibrin clot formation. After a thrombolytic agent has been employed, anticoagulants are used to prevent recurrence of a blood clot.

Heparin

Heparin is a potent anticoagulant that has been used for that purpose for many years. It is produced by **mast cells** found in the liver, lungs, and other parts of the body. Clinically, heparin is used during open heart surgery, during renal hemodialysis, and in the treatment of deep venous thrombosis or pulmonary infarction. Subcutaneous administration of low doses of heparin has been shown to diminish postoperative pulmonary embolism in older adults. The administration of heparin is by either *subcutaneous* or *intravenous* injection.

Actions

Prevents conversion of fibrinogen to fibrin.

Uses

Use in anticoagulant therapy in prophylaxis and treatment of venous thrombosis and its extension. Use also for prevention of postoperative deep venous thrombosis and pulmonary embolism, prevention of clotting in arterial and heart surgery, prophylaxis and treatment of peripheral arterial embolism, atrial fibrillation with embolization, disseminated intravascular clotting syndrome, as an anticoagulant in blood transfusions, extracorporeal circulation, and dialysis procedures, and in blood samples for laboratory purposes.

Contraindications

Contraindicated in patients with known hypersensitivity to any of its ingredients and in patients with severe thrombocytopenia and uncontrollable active bleeding.

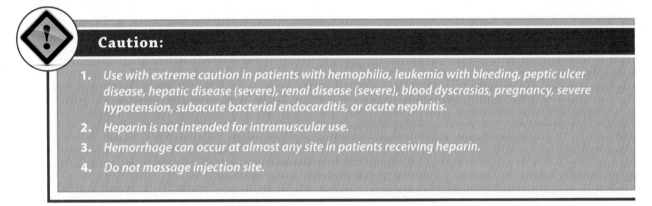

Caution:

1.   Use with extreme caution in patients with hemophilia, leukemia with bleeding, peptic ulcer disease, hepatic disease (severe), renal disease (severe), blood dyscrasias, pregnancy, severe hypotension, subacute bacterial endocarditis, or acute nephritis.
2.   Heparin is not intended for intramuscular use.
3.   Hemorrhage can occur at almost any site in patients receiving heparin.
4.   Do not massage injection site.

Adverse Reactions

Reactions include hemorrhage; local irritation, erythema, mild pain, hematoma, or ulceration may follow deep subcutaneous injection. Hypersensitivity reaction may include chills, fever, and urticaria. Other adverse reactions are asthma, rhinitis, lacrimation, headache, nausea, vomiting, and anaphylactoid reactions, including shock.

Dosage and Route

The dosage and route of administration (IV or subcutaneous) are determined by the physician and are individualized for each patient.

Implications for Patient Care

Parenteral drug products should be inspected visually for particulate matter and discoloration prior to administration. Slight discoloration does not alter potency. *Never administer by intramuscular injection.* The dosage of heparin should be adjusted according to the patient's coagulation test results; these should be monitored very carefully. Be aware of signs of bleeding: petechiae, ecchymosis, black tarry stools, bleeding gums, and hematuria. Be alert for signs of adverse reactions.

Patient Teaching

Educate patients:

- about the purpose of the medication.
- about adverse reactions. ■

Special Considerations

Heparin sodium is not effective by oral administration and should be given by intermittent intravenous injection, intravenous infusion, or deep subcutaneous injection.

Oral Anticoagulants

Anticoagulants that are administered *orally* do not produce an immediate effect. Their action is usually evident within 12 to 24 hours of administration. As with other anticoagulants, the use of these drugs may produce a cumulative effect; therefore, dosages must be individualized and based upon the patient's clotting time, using a blood coagulation test (see Table 23-6).

Warfarin Sodium (Coumadin)

Actions

Coumadin and other coumarin anticoagulants act by inhibiting the synthesis of vitamin–K dependent coagulation factors.

Uses

Indicated for the prophylaxis or treatment of venous thrombosis and its extension, pulmonary embolism, atrial fibrillation with embolization, and as an adjunct in the prophylaxis of systemic embolism after myocardial infarction.

Contraindications

Contraindicated in patients with known hypersensitivity to any of its ingredients and in patients where the hazard of hemorrhage might be greater than the potential clinical benefits of anticoagulation such as pregnancy, hemorrhagic tendencies or blood dyscrasias, recent or contemplated surgery, bleeding tendencies associated with active ulceration or overt bleeding, threatened abortion, and in unsupervised senility, alcoholism, or psychosis.

Caution:

1. Hemorrhage can occur at almost any site in patients on anticoagulant therapy.
2. Anticoagulant therapy with Coumadin may enhance the release of atheromatous plaque emboli.
3. Use caution during lactation, severe to moderate hepatic or renal insufficiency, trauma that may result in internal bleeding, surgery or trauma resulting in large exposed raw surfaces, and in patients with indwelling catheters, severe to moderate hypertension, known or suspected deficiency in protein C, polycythemia vera, vasculitis, severe diabetes, and severe allergic and anaphylactic disorders.

Precautions:

1. A patient receiving Coumadin must have periodic and carefully monitored prothrombin time or other suitable coagulation tests.
2. There are numerous factors that can affect anticoagulant response. Please refer to a current drug reference book or visit www.Drugs@FDA.gov for additional information.

Adverse Reactions

Reactions can include hemorrhage or necrosis of the skin and other tissue. Other adverse reactions are alopecia, urticaria, dermatitis, fever, nausea, diarrhea, abdominal cramping, systemic cholesterol microembolization, a syndrome called "purple toe," cholestatic hepatic injury, and hypersensitivity reactions.

TABLE 23-6	Anticoagulants	
MEDICATIONS	**USUAL DOSAGE**	**ADVERSE REACTIONS**
enoxaparin (Lovenox)	SC (Adult): Prophylaxis before knee or hip surgery: 30 mg twice daily starting within 24 hours post-op and continued for 7 to 10 days or until ambulatory (up to 14 days) Prophylaxis before abdominal surgery: 40 mg twice daily starting within 24 hours post-op and continued for 7 to 10 days or until ambulatory (up to 14 days) Systemic anticoagulants: 1 mg/kg every 12 hours	Hemorrhage, anemia, thrombocytopenia, dizziness, headache, nausea, vomiting, pruritus, rash, urticaria, fever
warfarin sodium (Coumadin)	Oral (Adult): 40 to 60 mg the first day, followed by 2 to 10 mg daily	Hemorrhage, alopecia, dermatitis, urticaria

Dosage and Route

The dosage and route of administration are determined by the physician and individualized for each patient (see Table 23-6).

Implications for Patient Care

Assess prothrombin time and therapeutic response to medication. Monitor blood pressure, blood studies (hematocrit, platelet count), and stools and urine for blood. Be aware of signs of bleeding. Be alert for signs of adverse reactions.

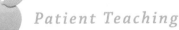 *Patient Teaching*

Educate patients:

- about the purpose of the medication.
- about adverse reactions.
- to take the medication as prescribed and to have periodic (monitored) prothrombin time evaluations.
- to avoid alcohol, salicylates (aspirin), large amounts of green vegetables, or drastic changes in dietary habits, which may affect Coumadin therapy.
- that Coumadin may cause a red-orange discoloration of alkaline urine. ■

Special Considerations

Patients should notify the physician if any illness, such as diarrhea, infection, or fever, develops or of any unusual symptoms, such as pain, swelling, prolonged bleeding from cuts, increased menstrual bleeding, nosebleeds, bleeding of gums from brushing of teeth, unusual bleeding or bruising, red or dark-brown urine, or red or tarry stools.

Antiplatelet Drugs

Antiplatelet drugs help reduce the occurrence of and death from vascular events such as heart attacks and strokes. Aspirin is considered to be the reference standard antiplatelet drug and is recommended by the American Heart Association for use in patients with a wide range of cardiovascular diseases.

Plavix (clopidogrel) is another antiplatelet drug that is approved by the Food and Drug Administration for many of the same indications as aspirin. Plavix may provide valuable therapeutic benefit over aspirin in patients with peripheral arterial disease and patients who have suffered stroke or myocardial infraction for whom aspirin fails to achieve a therapeutic benefit. The recommended dosage of Plavix is 75 mg (tablet) once daily. Other antiplatelet agents include dipyridamole (Persantine) and ticlodipine (Ticlid).

Caution:

New data shows that when clopidogrel (Plavix) and omeprazole (Prilosec/Prilosec OTC) are taken together, the effectiveness of clopidogrel is reduced. Patients at risk for heart attacks or strokes who use clopidogrel to prevent blood clots will not get the full effect of this medicine if they are also taking omeprazole. Separating the dose of clopidogrel and omeprazole in time will not reduce this drug interaction.

Aspirin may be recommended by physicians to reduce the risk of a second heart attack, to reduce the risk of having a heart attack, or to reduce the risk of a stroke. Aspirin has been shown to inhibit an essential enzyme that cells use to manufacture prostaglandin, a hormonelike substance that takes an active role in many cellular activities. By inhibiting prostaglandin production, it also inhibits platelet clumping, the first stage of the blood-clotting process.

Aspirin helps keep platelets from sticking together to form clots. With this clotting activity reduced, the blood flows more freely and oxygen is more easily supplied to the heart, brain, and other organs. Clots are less likely to form, thus reducing the possibility of a clot forming and breaking away and lodging in the heart or brain.

It is generally recommended that an individual take aspirin (81 mg, 162 mg, or 325 mg) per day to prevent thromboembolic disorders.

Contraindications

This medicine should not be used in patients with hypersensitivity, gastrointestinal bleeding, bleeding disorders, children under 3 years of age, children with flulike symptoms, pregnancy, lactation, vitamin K deficiency, and peptic ulcer.

Precautions

Use caution in patients with anemias, hepatic or renal disease, and Hodgkin's disease.

Adverse Reactions

Reactions can include thrombocytopenia, agranulocytosis, leukopenia, neutropenia, hemolytic anemia, increased prothrombin time, drowsiness, dizziness, confusion, convulsions, headache, flushing, hallucinations, coma, nausea, vomiting, GI bleeding, heartburn, anorexia, rash, urticaria, bruising, ototoxicity, tinnitus, hearing loss, rapid pulse, hyperpnea, hypoglycemia, hypokalemia, hepatotoxicity, renal dysfunction, visual changes, and edema.

Implications for Patient Care

Assess liver, renal, and blood studies. Monitor prothrombin time and intake and output ratio. Decreased output may indicate renal failure (long-term therapy). Be aware of adverse reactions, especially hepatotoxicity (dark urine, clay-colored stool, jaundice, itching, abdominal pain, fever, diarrhea), allergic reactions (rash, urticaria), renal dysfunction (decreased urine output), ototoxicity (tinnitus, loss of hearing), visual changes (blurring, halos, corneal or retinal damage), or edema in feet, ankles, or legs.

Patient Teaching

Educate patients:

- to take the medication as prescribed.
- about adverse reactions.
- to visit their physician on a regular basis.
- to have liver, renal, and blood studies performed.
- not to take over-the-counter medications unless prescribed by their physician.
- to avoid alcohol, caffeine, and nicotine. ■

Special Considerations

- Patients taking anticoagulant drugs should not take aspirin unless prescribed by their physician. Prothrombin time should be performed on a regular basis and monitored carefully.
- Antacids, steroids, and urinary alkalizers may decrease the effectiveness of the drug.
- Anticoagulants, insulin, and methotrexate may increase the effectiveness of the drug.

Thrombolytic Agents

Approximately 80 percent of all acute myocardial infarctions (MIs) caused by a thrombus that occludes a coronary artery. Unless contraindicated, thrombolytic therapy is the treatment of choice for an MI patient who reaches the hospital within six hours of the onset of chest pain. In some hospitals, the time period for administering thrombolytic agents has been extended to 12 and 24 hours.

Thrombolytic agents act to dissolve an existing thrombus when administered soon after its occurrence. These agents dissolve the clot, reopen the artery, restore blood flow to the heart, and prevent further damage to the myocardium.

Thrombolytic agents that have been approved for treating acute myocardial infarction are streptokinase (Kabikinase, Streptase); anistreplase—which is also called APSAC; alteplase (Activase); urokinase, which is currently used to dissolve obstructive thrombi in the peripheral circulation and acute pulmonary emboli; and a single-chain urokinase plasminogen activator, which converts to urokinase at the site of the clot.

Contraindications

Avoid use with hypersensitivity, active internal bleeding, recent (within 2 months) cerebrovascular accident, intracranial or intraspinal surgery, intracranial neoplasm, or severe uncontrolled hypertension.

Caution:

1. *Bleeding is the most common complication encountered during thrombolytic therapy. Internal bleeding may involve the gastrointestinal tract, genitourinary tract, retroperitoneal or intracranial sites. Superficial or surface bleeding may occur at invaded or disturbed sites (venous cutdown, arterial puncture, sites of recent surgical intervention). Intramuscular injections and nonessential handling of the patient should be avoided during treatment.*

2. *Should serious bleeding (not controlled by local pressure) occur, treatment with a thrombolytic agent should be stopped immediately.*

3. *Each patient being considered for therapy must be carefully evaluated and anticipated benefits weighed against potential risks associated with thrombolytic therapy.*

Adverse Reactions

Bleeding, allergic reactions, anaphylactic and anaphylactoid reactions, and fever are some reactions.

Hemostatic Agents

*Hemostat*ic agents may be administered systemically to overcome specific coagulation defects, or applied topically to control surface bleeding. Certain of these drugs are used in the treatment of hemophilia (ProPlex) and for hypofibrinogenemia (Amicar, vitamin K). Other products, known as *locally absorbable* hemostatics, are applied topically to control capillary oozing and surface bleeding. Examples of these are gelatin sponge (Gelfoam), oxidized cellulose (Surgicel), microfibrillar collagen (Avitene), and thrombin.

Hematinic Agents: Irons

Oral hematinic agents that are used to treat iron deficiency anemia are ferrous fumarate, ferrous gluconate, and ferrous sulfate. These iron preparations are available in various trade name products such as Femiron, Feostat, Ircon, and Palmrion (ferrous fumarate); Fergon, Ferralet, and Simiron (ferrous gluconate); and Feosol, Fer-in-Sol, Ferolix, Irospan, and Slow-Fe (ferrous sulfate). See Table 23-7.

Actions

Hematinic agents provide the body with iron that is needed for red blood cell development, energy, and oxygen transport.

Uses

Use for iron deficiency and iron-deficiency anemia.

Contraindications

This medicine is contraindicated in patients with known hypersensitivity and in patients with ulcerative colitis, regional enteritis, hemosiderosis, hemochromatosis, peptic ulcer disease, hemolytic anemia, and cirrhosis.

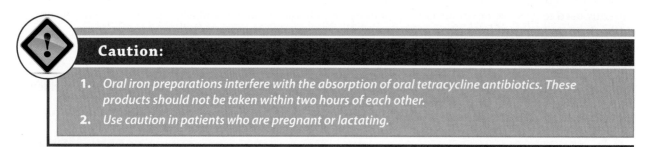

Caution:

1. *Oral iron preparations interfere with the absorption of oral tetracycline antibiotics. These products should not be taken within two hours of each other.*
2. *Use caution in patients who are pregnant or lactating.*

Adverse Reactions

Reactions include nausea, constipation, epigastric pain, vomiting, diarrhea, and tarry stools.

TABLE 23-7   Hematinic Agents: Iron Preparations

MEDICATION	USUAL DOSAGE
ferrous fumarate	Oral (Adult): 200 mg t.i.d.–q.i.d.
ferrous gluconate	Oral (Adult): 200 to 600 mg t.i.d.
ferrous sulfate	Oral (Adult): 0.750 to 1.5 g/day in divided doses t.i.d.

Dosage and Route

The dosage and route of administration are determined by the physician and are individualized for each patient (see Table 23-7).

Implications for Patient Care

Assess hematocrit, hemoglobin, reticulocyte, and bilirubin determinations before initiation of therapy and monthly during treatment. Liquid preparation should be diluted and given through a plastic straw to avoid discoloration of tooth enamel. Store medication in a tight, light-resistant container. Monitor patient for signs of toxicity: nausea, vomiting, diarrhea (green then tarry stools), hematemesis, pallor, cyanosis, shock, or coma. Assess patient's nutritional needs. Evaluate therapeutic response.

Patient Teaching

Educate patients:

- about the purpose of the medication.
- about adverse reactions.
- to take the medication as prescribed.
- to have monthly blood studies evaluated by their physician.
- to take the medication between meals for best absorption and not to take with milk or antacids.
- to take liquid iron preparations through a plastic straw.
- that iron may cause dark-green or black stools.
- about the proper method of storage for the medication.
- to include iron-rich foods in their diet. (Foods rich in iron are liver, beef, veal, lamb, pork, turkey, chicken, oysters, eggs, peanut butter, soybeans, dried apricots, peaches, prunes, dates, figs, raisins, molasses, dried beans, enriched breads and cereals, and dark-green leafy vegetables.)
- that tablets should not be crushed.
- to contact a physician or poison control center immediately in case of accidental overdose.
- not to substitute one iron preparation for another. ▪

Iron Dextran (Imferon)

Iron dextran (Imferon) is a parenteral preparation that is available for IM or IV administration. It is administered only after test dose of 0.5 mL by preferred route and if well tolerated, the remaining portion of the dose is administered after a one-hour wait. The Z-track method of intramuscular injection is used and a 19- to 20-gauge, 2- to– 3-inch needle is used for the average adult patient. For patients who are larger than average, a longer needle is used to ensure that the drug is deep in muscle tissue, as the drug may be irritating to subcutaneous tissue and cause discoloration. IV injection is administered only by physicians.

Contraindications

Avoid use with hypersensitivity, all anemias excluding iron deficiency anemia, and hepatic disease.

Adverse Reactions

Reactions include headache, paresthesia, dizziness, shivering, weakness, seizures, nausea, vomiting, abdominal pain, rash, pruritus, urticaria, fever, sweating, chills, brown skin discoloration at injection site, necrosis, sterile abscess, phlebitis, chest pain, shock, hypotension, tachycardia, dyspnea, leukocytosis, and anaphylaxis.

Implications for Patient Care

Assess patient for signs of adverse reactions. Monitor cardiac status: chest pain, hypotension, and tachycardia. Monitor for hypersensitivity reaction: rash, pruritus, fever, chills, and anaphylaxis. Store medication at room temperature in a cool environment. Patient should remain in the recumbent position for 30 minutes after an injection of Imferon.

AGENTS USED IN TREATING MEGALOBLASTIC ANEMIAS

Megaloblastic anemias result from decreased erythrocyte formation and the immaturity, fragility, and early destruction of these cells. There is a defective DNA synthesis, usually from vitamin B_{12} or folic acid deficiency. Agents used to treat megaloblastic anemias include folic acid (Folvite) and vitamin B_{12}.

Folic Acid (Vitamin B_9)

Actions

It increases red blood cell, white blood cell, and platelet formation in megaloblastic anemias.

Uses

Folic acid is used for megaloblastic or macrocytic anemia caused by folic acid deficiency, as well as liver disease, alcoholism, hemolysis, and intestinal obstruction. Use caution during pregnancy.

Contraindications

Folic acid is contraindicated in patients with hypersensitivity, anemias other than megaloblastic or macrocytic anemia, and vitamin B_{12} deficiency.

Adverse Reactions

Bronchospasm.

Dosage and Route

Megaloblastic or macrocytic anemia: Oral, IM, SC (adult and child over 4 years of age) 1 mg every day times 4 to 5 days.

Implications for Patient Care

Assess folate blood levels. Store medication in a light-resistant container. Evaluate therapeutic response and nutritional status of patient.

Patient Teaching

Educate patients:

- about sources of folic acid (meat, eggs, green leafy vegetables).
- about the therapeutic response.
- how to properly store the medication. ■

Cyanocobalamin (Vitamin B$_{12}$)

Actions

Replaces vitamin B$_{12}$ that the body would normally absorb from the diet.

Uses

It is used for vitamin B$_{12}$ deficiency, pernicious anemia, and vitamin B$_{12}$ malabsorption syndrome.

Contraindications

Do not use in patients with hypersensitivity or optic nerve atrophy. Use caution during pregnancy and lactation.

Adverse Reactions

Flushing, optic nerve atrophy, diarrhea, congestive heart failure, peripheral vascular thrombosis, pulmonary edema, itching, rash, and hypokalemia are possible reactions.

Dosage and Route

Pernicious anemia: IM (adult) 100 to 1000 micrograms every day times 2 weeks, then 100–1000 micrograms every month.

Implications for Patient Care

Assess gastrointestinal function, potassium blood level, and complete blood count. Be aware of signs of adverse reactions. Evaluate therapeutic response and nutritional status of patient.

Patient Teaching

Educate patients:

- about the importance of taking the medication exactly as prescribed by their physician.
- that treatment is for life when one has pernicious anemia.
- about foods rich in vitamin B$_{12}$. ■

Epoetin Alfa (Epogen)

Epogen is an erythropoiesis-stimulating agent (ESA) that stimulates red blood cell production (erythropoeisis). ESAs, structurally and biologically, are similar to naturally occurring protein erythropoietin.

Actions

It stimulates the production of red blood cells.

Uses

Used for anemia associated with chronic renal failure or in AIDS patients.

Contraindications

Do not use in patients with uncontrolled hypertension, known hypersensitivity to mammalian cell-derived products and known hypersensitivity to albumin (human).

Warnings:

INCREASED MORTALITY, SERIOUS CARDIOVASCULAR and THROMBOEMBOLIC EVENTS, and TUMOR PROGRESSION

Renal failure: Patients experienced greater risks for death and serious cardiovascular events when administered erythropoiesis-stimulating agents (ESAs) to target higher versus lower hemoglobin levels (13.5 versus 11.3 g/dL; 14 versus 10 g/dL) in two clinical studies. Individualize dosing to achieve and maintain hemoglobin levels within the range of 10 to 12 g/dL.

Cancer:

- *ESAs shortened overall survival and/or time-to-tumor progression in clinical studies in patients with breast, non-small cell lung, head and neck, lymphoid, and cervical cancers when dosed to target a hemoglobin of ≥ 12 g/dL*
- *The risks of shortened survival and tumor progression have not been excluded when ESAs are dosed to target a hemoglobin of < 12 g/dL.*
- *To minimize these risks, as well as the risk of serious cardio- and thrombovascular events, use the lowest dose needed to avoid red blood cell transfusions.*
- *Use only for treatment of anemia due to concomitant myelosuppressive chemotherapy.*
- *Discontinue following the completion of a chemotherapy course.*

Perisurgery: EPOGEN increased the rate of deep venous thromboses in patients not receiving prophylactic anticoagulation. Consider deep venous thrombosis prophylaxis.

Adverse Reactions

Reactions include hypertension, headache, arthralgia, nausea, edema, fatigue, diarrhea, vomiting, chest pain, skin reactions, asthenia, dizziness, clotted vascular access, seizure, and myocardial infarction.

Dosage and Route

Starting dose: 50 to 100 U/kg three times weekly IV for dialysis patients; IV or SC for nondialysis patients. Reduce dose when (1) target range is reached, or (2) hematocrit increases above four points in any two-week period. Increase dose if hematocrit does not increase by five to six points after eight weeks of therapy, and hematocrit is below target range.

Implications for Patient Care

Carefully monitor blood pressure for signs of hypertension. Assess hematocrit for therapeutic range. Do not shake the container, as shaking may denature the glycoprotein, rendering it biologically inactive. Inspect parenteral drug product for particulate matter and discoloration. Do not use vial if either or both are apparent. Use aseptic technique. Use only one dose per vial; do not reenter vial. Discard unused portions. Do not administer in conjunction with other drug solutions.

Patient Teaching

Educate patients:

- that this drug may cause seizures within the first 90 days of treatment.
- not to drive, operate hazardous equipment, or engage in dangerous activites until effect of drug is noted.

- that even though the medication may make the patient feel much better, it is important to continue all other treatments as prescribed by the physician.
- to report any side effects to the physician. ▨

ANTIHYPERLIPIDEMIC AGENTS

Antihyperlipidemic agents are used to lower abnormally high blood levels of fatty substances (lipids) when other treatment regimens fail. Lipids may accumulate in the walls of blood vessels as atherosclerotic plaques, and this accumulation can contribute to hypertension, increase the risk of coronary artery disease, and decrease the flow of oxygenated blood to the heart and other body organs.

Lipids include sterols (cholesterol and cholesterol esters), free fatty acids (FFA), triglycerides (glycerol esters of FFA), and phospholipids (phosphoric acid esters of lipid substances). Lipids may be exogenous (derived from foods and oils that are high in saturated fat) and endogenous (produced by the liver from the end products of lipid and carbohydrate metabolism).

Saturated fats (usually solid at room temperature) raise low-density liproprotein cholesterol, the fatty substance that can accumulate in the walls of blood vessels. Foods high in saturated fats include butter, cheese, chocolate, coconut oil, egg yolk, lard, meats, palm oil, whole milk, shellfish, and sardines. Other types of lipoprotein include very low-density lipoprotein (VLDL) and high-density lipoprotein (HDL). High-density lipoproteins are "H"ighly "D"esirable and are known as the "good type of cholesterol." Elevations in total cholesterol and low-density lipoprotein are associated with the development of coronary heart disease (see Table 23–8).

Antihyperlipidemic agents are not usually the first treatment of choice for lowering lipids in the blood. Diet, weight and stress management, exercise, and proper treatment of other conditions such as hypertension and diabetes are tried before the physician prescribes an antilipidemic agent.

Various medications can lower blood cholesterol levels. They may be prescribed individually or in combination with other drugs. Some of the common types of cholesterol-lowering drugs include statins, resins (cholestryamine, colestipol, and coleseveiam) and nicotinic acid (niacin), gemfibrozil, and clofibrate (see Table 23–9).

Statins are very effective for lowering LDL ("bad") cholesterol levels and have few immediate short-term side effects. They interrupt the formation of cholesterol from the circulating blood. *Resins* are also called bile acid-binding drugs. They work in the intestines by promoting increased disposal of cholesterol. *Nicotinic acid* (niacin) works in the liver by affecting the production of blood fats. It is used to lower triglycerides and LDL cholesterol, and raise HDL ("good") cholesterol. It is accessible to patients as over-the-counter preparations and as "dietary supplements." The Food and Drug Administration (FDA) regulates OTC niacin, so the content is assured. The FDA does not regulate "dietary supplements" that may contain widely variable amounts of niacin. Dietary supplement niacin must not be used as a substitute for prescription niacin. *Gemfibrozil* (Lopid) lowers blood fats and raises HDL cholesterol levels.

Implications for Patient Care

Assess cholesterol blood level, liver function studies, and renal function studies in patients with compromised renal system. A slit lamp examination of the eye should be performed one month after treatment begins and then annually (lens opacities may occur). Evaluate the therapeutic response to medication. Administer medication as prescribed.

TABLE 23-8 Cholesterol Values and Associated Risk Level

TOTAL CHOLESTEROL	LDL	RISK LEVEL
<200 mg/dL	<100 mg/dL	Desirable
200–239 mg/dL	130–159 mg/dL	Borderline high
240 mg/dL	160–189 mg/dL	High
>241 mg/dL	>190 mg/dL	Very high

TABLE 23-9   Selected Antihyperlipidemic Agents

MEDICATIONS	USUAL DOSAGE	ADVERSE REACTIONS
atorvastatin calcium (Lipitor)	10 mg orally once daily	Constipation, flatulence, dyspepsia, and abdominal pain
coleseveiam (Welchol)	6 tablets once a day or 3 tablets twice a day with meals and a liquid. Also available as an oral suspension. Use 1 packet daily as directed.	Gas, constipation, infection, upset stomach, headache
colestipol (Colestid)	15 to 30 g/day in 2 to 4 divided doses	Constipation, abdominal pain, nausea, fecal impaction, vomiting, hemorrhoids, flatulence, peptic ulcer, steatorrhea
fluvastatin sodium	20 mg orally once daily at bedtime	Rash, back pain, coughing, dyspepsia, diarrhea, abdominal pain, nausea, constipation, flatulence, dizziness, headache
gemfibrozil (Lopid)	600 mg b.i.d. orally 30 minutes before morning and evening meal	Nausea, flatulence, diarrhea, epigastric pain, abdominal pain
lovastatin (Mevacor)	20 to 80 mg daily, orally	Muscle pain and inflammation, increase liver function studies, rhabdomyolysis, acute muscle deterioration, headache, skin rash, pruritus, nausea, diarrhea, constipation, gas
niacin	300 to 600 mg daily, orally	Flushing, skin rash, pruritus, GI upset, exacerbation of peptic ulcer, hyperglycemia, hyperuricemia
pravastatin (Pravachol)	10 or 20 mg once daily at bedtime	Gas, stomach pain or cramps, diarrhea, constipation, heartburn, headache, blurred vision, dizziness, rash or itching, muscle pain
probucol (Lorelco)	500 mg b.i.d., orally	Nausea, diarrhea, prolonged QT interval on ECG, increased risk of ventricular tachycardia and fibrillation, insomnia, headache
simvastatin (Zocor)	5 to 10 mg orally once a day in the evening range 5 to 40 mg/day single dose in the evening	Muscle cramps, myalgia, tremor, dizziness, headache, vertigo, memory loss, anorexia, vomiting, constipation, diarrhea, alopecia, pruritus, gynecomastia, loss of libido, blurred vision

Patient Teaching

Educate patients:

- to take the medication as prescribed.
- about adverse reactions.
- to report any adverse reactions to their physician.
- to continue to see their physician on a regular basis for cholesterol and liver function tests.
- about diet, exercise, lifestyle changes, and stress management.
- to avoid eating or drinking grapefruit products while taking a statin drug such as Lipitor, Lescol, Mevacor, Pravachol, or Zocor. ■

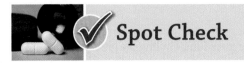

Spot Check

There are many medications that may be used to treat circulatory system disorders. For each of the selected drugs and/or drug classifications, list several aspects of patient teaching and several implications for patient care:

DRUG(S)	PATIENT TEACHING	IMPLICATION FOR PATIENT CARE
digitalis		
antiarrhythmics		
vasopressors		
nitrates		
antihypertensives		
anticoagulants		
antihyperlipidemic		

REVIEW QUESTIONS

Directions. Select the best answer to each of the following multiple-choice questions, circling the letter of your choice:

1. A protein that is found in many body tissues and fluids, and is important in the prevention of fibrin clot formation is _____.

    a. glycoside
    b. angiotensin
    c. plasminogen
    d. a mast cell

2. The primary function of the circulatory system is carried out in the _____.

    a. arteries   b. veins   c. aorta   d. capillaries

3. Inotropic effect means _____.

    a. increasing or decreasing heart rate
    b. increasing or decreasing the force of myocardial contraction
    c. increasing or decreasing the conduction of electrical impulses
    d. all of these

4. Cardiac glycosides (digitalis drugs) _____.

    a. strengthen the myocardium
    b. increase the force of the systolic contraction
    c. slow the heart and improve muscle tone
    d. all of these

5. Prehypertension is a new classification that impacts approximately 45 million Americans. It is defined as a systolic of _____ mm Hg and a diastolic of 80 mm Hg to 89 mm Hg.

    a. 140 to 146
    b. 146 to 150
    c. 120 to 139
    d. 112 to 118

6. Adverse reactions to procainamide HCl are _____.

    a. anorexia, nausea, vomiting, and bitter taste
    b. orthostatic hypotension, diarrhea, and muscle weakness
    c. angioedema, depression, and malaise
    d. constipation, blurred vision, and hypotension

7. Vasopressors are drugs _____.

    a. that cause dilation of the muscles associated with capillaries and arteries
    b. that cause contraction of the muscles associated with capillaries and arteries
    c. that are useful in the treatment of patients suffering from shock
    d. b and c

8. Coronary vasodilators are used primarily for the treatment of _____.

    a. congestive heart failure
    b. angina pectoris
    c. hypertension
    d. peripheral vascular disease

9. There are various classes of drugs used in the treatment of hypertension. The classification _____ reduces nerve impulses to the heart and blood vessels.

    a. diuretics
    b. calcium channel blockers
    c. beta-blockers
    d. angiotensin-converting enzymes

10. Drugs used in the treatment of hypertension may be categorized as _____.

   a. diuretics
   c. angiotensin antagonists
   b. vasodilators
   d. all of these

11. Heparin is a potent _____.

   a. anticoagulant
   c. antihypertensive agent
   b. antiarrhythmic
   d. vasopressor

12. Agents used in the treatment of megaloblastic anemias include _____.

   a. folic acid   b. folate sodium   c. vitamin B_{12} d. all of these

13. In the treatment of congestive heart failure, therapy usually includes _____.

   a. a low-sodium diet
   c. a digitalis drug
   b. a reduction of physical activities
   d. all of these

14. The pharmacologic actions of all digitalis compounds are similar, but these products differ in their _____.

   a. potency
   c. the rate of absorption
   b. onset of action
   d. all of these

15. It is generally recommended that an individual take aspirin, _____ mg per day to prevent thromboembolic disorders.

   a. 80, 160, or 320
   c. 84, 164, or 324
   b. 81, 162, or 325
   d. 82, 163, or 326

16. The term _____C_____ means irregularity or loss of rhythm.

   a. bradycardia
   c. arrhythmia
   b. tachycardia
   d. anrhythmia

17. The treatment of angina pectoris usually involves the _____ group of drugs.

   a. nitrate
   c. thrombolytic
   b. anticoagulant
   d. hemostatic

18. _____ can be defined as a condition wherein the patient has a higher arterial blood pressure than that judged to be normal.

   a. Hypotension
   c. Pulse pressure
   b. Hypertension
   d. Venous pressure

Matching. Place the correct letter from Column II on the appropriate line of Column I:

Column I		Column II
19.	__D__ atherosclerosis	A. a protein that is found in many body tissues and fluids. It is important in the prevention of fibrin clot formation
20.	__E__ angiotensin	
21.	__B__ hypokalemia	B. a deficient amount of potassium in the blood
22.	__F__ glycoside	C. an anemia in which megaloblasts are found in the blood
23.	__G__ hyperlipidemia	D. the building up of fatty plaques and hardening of the arteries
24.	__C__ megaloblastic anemia	
25.	__A__ plasminogen	E. a vasopressor substance that is formed in the body by interaction of renin and angiotensinogen
		F. a substance that is derived from plants, and upon hydrolysis yields a sugar plus additional products
		G. abnormally elevated concentration of lipids in the blood
		H. an increased amount of fibrinogen in the blood

UNIT 24
Medications That Affect the Respiratory System

OBJECTIVES

Upon completing this unit, you should be able to:

- Define the terms listed in the vocabulary.
- Describe respiration.
- Describe the causes of respiratory conditions and/or diseases.
- Describe the various drug classifications that are used for respiratory system conditions and diseases.
- Identify selected drugs according to each described classification.
- Understand the actions, uses, contraindications, warnings, adverse reactions, dosage and route, implications for patient care, patient teaching, and special considerations for selected drugs that affect the respiratory system.
- Describe tuberculosis, listing the symptoms, diagnosis, and treatment regimen.
- Explain why there may be an increased risk of developing tuberculosis in older adults.
- Explain why a child may be at greater risk of contracting tuberculosis.
- Complete the critical thinking questions and activities presented in this unit.
- Complete the Spot Check on recommended children's dosages for selected antituberculosis drugs.
- Answer the review questions correctly.

VOCABULARY

allergic rhinitis (a-ler′jik ri-ni′tis). Inflammation of the nasal mucosa that is due to the sensitivity of the nasal mucosa to an allergen. Also known as hay fever.

common cold. A general term for *coryza*. An inflammation of the respiratory mucous membranes caused by a rhinovirus.

histamine (his′ta-min). A substance that is normally present in the body. When released from injured cells, it causes increased mucous secretions, dilation of capillaries, constriction of bronchial smooth muscle, and increased gastric secretions.

pruritus (proo-ri′tus). Severe itching.

rhinorrhea (ri″no-re′a). Flow of thin watery discharge from the nose.

rhinovirus (ri′no-vi′rus). One of a subgroup of viruses that cause the common cold in humans.

urticaria (ur-ti-ka′re-a). A vascular reaction of the skin that is characterized by wheals and severe itching. Also known as hives.

INTRODUCTION

The principal organs of the respiratory system are the nose, pharynx, larynx, trachea, bronchi, and lungs. These structures provide for the passage of respiratory gases to and from the lungs during the act of breathing. The lungs do not contain muscle tissue; therefore, they are dependent upon the movement of surrounding structures (the rib cage and the diaphragm) to function. The contraction of the intercostal (rib) muscles and the diaphragm expands the volume of the thoracic cavity and causes the intake (inspiration) of air into the lungs. The relaxation of these muscles decreases the volume of the cavity and forces air out of the lungs (expiration). The rhythmic contraction and relaxation of rib and diaphragm muscles involved in breathing are controlled by nerve impulses from the respiratory center of the brain.

The act of breathing brings oxygen-rich air into the lungs, where a very important exchange of gases occurs. Air that enters the lungs travels through a multibranched network of smaller and smaller bronchial tubes until it reaches clusters of tiny, thin-walled air sacs called *alveoli*. There are about 300 million alveoli, each in close contact with equally thin-walled capillaries filled with pulmonary blood. This close contact between air- and oxygen-poor blood allows an exchange of gases to take place. Carbon dioxide, carried from tissue cells by pulmonary blood, is released into the air to be exhaled. As this gas is given up, oxygen molecules diffuse from the air into the blood and are carried to body cells that use oxygen in metabolizing foods (see Figure 24-1).

Respiratory conditions and diseases may be caused by allergies, pathogenic microorganisms such as bacteria and viruses, fungi, and environmental and hereditary factors. The common cold (coryza) is the most frequent infection in all age groups in the United States. It is caused by the rhinovirus, one of a species of picornaviruses. There are more than 200 rhinoviruses that can infect the nose and throat and cause the common cold. Rhinoviruses affect the average adult two to three times a year and children an average of twelve times a year. There is no cure for the common cold, and it generally runs its course with or without treatment. It is estimated that there are 71 million colds a year in the United States.

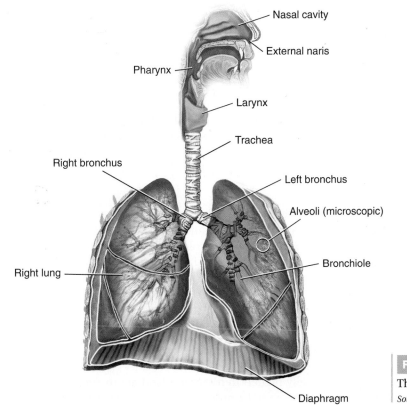

FIGURE 24-1

The organs of the respiratory system

Source: Delmar/Cengage Learning

Some researchers feel that the cold virus is spread by direct contact with an infected person or the things he or she has contaminated. Other researchers say the viruses float through the air, taking root in nasal mucosa of unsuspecting passersby. Regardless of the method by which the virus is spread, the common symptoms—sniffling, sneezing, hacking cough, and malaise—are experienced by many during a year. Antihistamines, decongestants, antitussives, analgesics, and antipyretics are some of the medications that may be used to treat symptoms of the common cold. *In children, aspirin should not be used as an antipyretic because of the risk of Reye's syndrome.*

Pathogenic organisms are the cause of many respiratory diseases, such as sinusitis, laryngitis, pharyngitis, pleuritis, bronchitis, pneumonia, tuberculosis, pneumocystis pneumonia, and bronchomycosis. Antimicrobials— antibiotics and antifungals—are the drugs of choice for the treatment of respiratory diseases caused by pathogenic microorganisms.

Pertussis (whooping cough) is a very contagious disease caused by a type of bacteria called *Bordetella pertussis.* It is a serious infection that spreads easily from person to person. Pertussis is on the rise in the United States and affects adults as well as children. The infection causes coughing spells so severe that it can be hard to breathe, eat, or sleep. It can lead to cracked ribs, pneumonia, or hospitalization.

The disease starts like the common cold, with runny nose or congestion, sneezing, and mild cough or fever, but after one to two weeks, severe coughing begins. Children with the disease cough violently and rapidly, over and over, until the air is gone from their lungs and they are forced to inhale with a loud "whooping" sound. Adults rarely have the classic "whoop."

People with pertussis usually spread the disease by coughing or sneezing while in close contact with others, who then breathe in the pertussis bacteria. Many infants who get pertussis are infected by older siblings or parents who might not even know they have the disease. Whooping cough is most contagious before the coughing starts, so the most effective way to prevent it is through immunization. In the United States, the recommended pertussis vaccine for children is called DTaP; for adolescents 11 to 18 and adults 19 to 64 years of age, the vaccine is called Tdap. See Unit 16 for more information on immunizations.

Environmental factors such as smoke, chemicals, metals, and gases may cause certain respiratory diseases such as pneumoconiosis and emphysema (chronic obstructive pulmonary disease, COPD). Bronchodilators and mucolytics are the drugs of choice for the treatment of respiratory diseases that may be caused by environmental factors.

Antihistamines, decongestants, antitussives, expectorants, mucolytics, bronchodilators, glucocorticoids, leukotriene receptor antagonists (blockers), cromolyn sodium, and drugs used to treat tuberculosis are described in this unit.

● *Note*
_____

Many of the medications described in this unit may be given in combination with each other. This is especially true with antihistamines, decongestants, and antitussive agents. When this occurs, one should be aware of the combined effects of the drugs, the possible adverse reactions, contraindications, warnings, and special considerations for each. ●

The FDA has issued a public health advisory that states it strongly recommends that over-the-counter (OTC) cough and cold products should not be used for infants and children under 2 years of age because serious and potentially life-threatening side effects could occur. Also, multisymptom cold medicines may include a decongestant, cough suppressant, pain or fever reliever, and/or antihistamine and should not be given to a child under 2 years of age. One must be aware that if a multisymptom medicine is used and an additional acetaminophen (Tylenol) product is given, then an overdose may occur.

ANTIHISTAMINES

Antihistamines are chemical agents that are structurally related to histamine and act to counter its effects by blocking histamine 1 (H₁) receptors. They do not interfere with the production and release of histamine.

Actions

Antihistamines appear to compete with histamine for cell receptor sites on effector cells. Histamine-related allergic reactions and tissue injury are blocked or diminished in intensity.

Uses

The primary use for antihistamine agents is the treatment of allergy symptoms that have resulted from the release of histamine. They are effective in the treatment of perennial and seasonal allergic rhinitis, contact dermatitis, urticaria, pruritus, for amelioration of allergic reactions to substances such as blood, plasma, insect stings, plant poisons, and as an adjunctive therapy during anaphylactic shock. Some antihistamines are used for the prevention and control of motion sickness and others are used in combination cold remedies to decrease mucus secretion and at bedtime for sedation.

Contraindications

Antihistamines are contraindicated in patients who are known to be hypersensitive to any of the ingredients. They should not be used in newborn or premature infants and during breast-feeding.

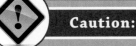

Caution:

Antihistamines should be used with considerable caution in patients with narrow-angle glaucoma, stenosing peptic ulcer, liver function problems, pyloroduodenal obstruction, symptomatic prostatic hyperplasia, or bladder-neck obstruction.

Adverse Reactions

The most frequent adverse reactions to antihistamines are sedation, sleepiness, dizziness, disturbed coordination, epigastric distress, and thickening of bronchial secretions. Other adverse reactions are dryness of mouth, nose, and throat, as well as hypotension, headache, palpitations, nervousness, tremor, irritability, vertigo, tinnitus, anorexia, nausea, vomiting, diarrhea, constipation, wheezing, and nasal stuffiness.

Dosage and Route

The dosage and route of administration are determined by the manufacturer, but a physician should be consulted when needed. See Table 24-1 for selected antihistamines.

Implications for Patient Care

You should know that many antihistamines have an atropine-like action and, therefore, should be used with caution in patients with a history of bronchial asthma, increased intraocular pressure, hyperthyroidism, cardiovascular disease, or hypertension.

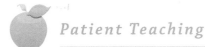

Patient Teaching

Educate patients that:

- antihistamines may impair mental alertness; therefore, they should not operate machinery or drive a motor vehicle until their response to the medication has been determined.
- alcohol or other sedative drugs may enhance the drowsiness caused by antihistamines.

TABLE 24-1 Antihistamines

MEDICATION	USUAL DOSAGE	ADVERSE REACTIONS
azatadine maleate	Oral (Adult): 1 to 2 mg twice daily	Drowsiness, dizziness, epigastric distress, thickening of bronchial secretions
azelastine (Astelin)	Nasal spray (Adult and children 12 years old and over): two sprays in each nostril twice daily	Drowsiness, headache, itching or burning of the nasal mucosa, bitter or metallic taste in the mouth
cetirizine (Zyrtec)	Oral (Adult): 5 to 10 mg once daily Oral (Child 6 to 11): 5 mg once daily	Dizziness, fatigue, pharyngitis, dry mouth
chlorpheniramine maleate (Chlor-Trimeton)	Oral (Adult): 6 to 16 mg/daily or 8 to 36 mg/daily (time-release form) IM, SC (Adult): 5 to 20 mg Oral (Child 6 to 11): 3 to 8 mg/day	Drowsiness, excitability in children
clemastine fumarate (Tavist, Tavist–1)	Dosage should be individualized according to the needs and response of the patient. Refer to a drug reference book	Drowsiness, urticaria, drug rash, anaphylactic shock, photosensitivity, chills, dryness of the mouth, nose, and throat
diphenhydramine HCl (Benadryl)	Oral (Adult): 25 to 50 mg 3 to 4 times daily Deep IM (Adult): 10 to 100 mg 3 to 4 times daily Oral (Child over 20 lb): 12.5 to 25 mg 3 to 4 times daily Deep IM (Child): 5 mg/kg/day in 4 divided doses	Drowsiness, dizziness, epigastric distress, thickening of bronchial secretions
fexofenadine (Allegra)	Oral (Adult): 60 mg twice daily Oral (Child 12 and older): 60 mg twice daily	Drowsiness, fatigue, dyspepsia, dysmenorrhea
ketotifen fumarate (Zaditor)	Ophthalmic (Adults and children over 3 years old): 1 drop in the affected eye(s) twice a day, every 8 to 12 hours	Headache, conjunctival infection, rhinitis, burning or stinging, eye pain, photophobia, rash
loratadine (Claritin)	Oral (Adult and children over 14 years old): 10 mg every 24 hours	Headache, drowsiness, fatigue, dry mouth

- antihistamines should not be taken if monoamine oxidase inhibitor(s) or anticoagulants are part of the patient's drug regimen.
- antihistamines may cause the respiratory tract to dry and mucus to thicken; therefore, when taking antihistamines, patients should drink plenty of fluids to thin secretions and keep tissue moist. ■

Special Considerations

- The action of oral anticoagulants may be diminished by antihistamines.
- Antihistamines have additive effects with alcohol and other CNS depressants (for example, tranquilizers, sedatives, hypnotics).
- Antihistamines are most likely to cause dizziness, sedation, and hypotension in patients over 60 years of age.
- Antihistamines should only be taken when needed. One may develop tolerance to a certain antihistamines.

DECONGESTANTS

Congestion of the nasal mucosa may occur as a result of infection, allergy, inflammation, or emotional upset. Decongestants are commonly used for symptomatic relief of nasal congestion.

Actions

Decongestants act by stimulating alpha-adrenergic receptors of vascular smooth muscle. As a result, dilated arterioles in the nasal mucosa are constricted. This reduces blood flow to the affected area, slows the formation of mucus, improves drainage, and opens obstructed nasal passages.

Uses

For the temporary relief of nasal congestion associated with the common cold, hay fever and other upper respiratory allergies, and sinusitis.

Contraindications

Decongestants are contraindicated in patients who are allergic to adrenergic agents or have narrow-angle glaucoma, and patients who are taking MAO inhibitors or tricyclic antidepressants.

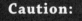

Caution:

1. If recommended dosage is exceeded, nervousness, dizziness, sleeplessness, rapid pulse, or high blood pressure may occur.
2. Medication should not be taken for more than seven days. If symptoms do not improve or fever occurs, patient should see a physician.
3. Patients with heart disease, hypertension, thyroid disease, glaucoma, diabetes, or prostatic hyperplasia should not take decongestants without the permission of their physician.
4. Patients who are pregnant or nursing babies should not take decongestants without the permission of their physician.

Adverse Reactions

Reactions include rebound nasal congestion, dryness and stinging of the mucosa, sneezing, light-headedness, headache, anxiety, palpitations, drowsiness, nausea, vomiting, and anorexia.

Dosage and Route

The dosage and route of administration are determined by the manufacturer, but a physician should be consulted when needed. See Table 24-2 for selected decongestants.

Implications for Patient Care

Because most decongestants are taken as over-the-counter medications, the implications for patient care mainly involve teaching the patient about the medication.

TABLE 24-2 Decongestants

MEDICATIONS	USUAL DOSAGE	ADVERSE REACTIONS
oxymetazoline HCl (Afrin)	Topical (Adults and children over 6 years): 2 to 3 drops or sprays of 0.5% solution in each nostril twice daily Topical (Children 2 to 5 years): 2 to 3 drops of 0.025% solution in each nostril twice daily	Mild adverse effects include dryness and stinging of the mucosa, sneezing, light-headedness, and headache
phenylephrine HCl (Coricidin) (Neo-Synephrine HCl)	Topical (Adults and older children): several drops of a 0.25 to 1.0% solution in each nostril as needed Topical (Infants): 0.125% solution used as above	Drowsiness, excitability in children, rebound nasal congestion, anxiety
pseudoephedrine HCl (Sudafed)	Oral (Adult): 60 mg 3 to 4 times daily Oral (Child): 4 mg/kg daily in four divided doses	Drowsiness, rebound nasal congestion, anxiety, headache, palpitation
xylometazoline HCl (Sinutab Long-Lasting Sinus Spray)	Topical (Adult): 2 to 3 drops of 0.1% solution or 1 to 2 inhalations of the 0.1% spray in each nostril every 8 to 10 hours Topical (Child): 2 to 3 drops of 0.05% solution in each nostril every 8 to 10 hours Topical (Infant): 1 drop of 0.05% solution in each nostril every 6 hours if necessary	Mild adverse effects include local stinging, sneezing, dryness of the nose, headache, drowsiness, palpitations; chronic swelling of the nasal mucosa possible with prolonged or excessive use

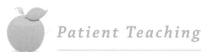 *Patient Teaching*

Educate patients that:

- long-term use of nasal sprays or solutions increases the risk of sensitization, which often causes a rebound effect or an increase in symptoms.
- decongestants should not be taken if antihypertensive agents, MAO inhibitors, or tricyclic antidepressants are part of the medication regimen. ■

Special Considerations

- Topical decongestants must be administered correctly to avoid systemic absorption.
- Physician should be notified if irregular heartbeat, insomnia, dizziness, or tremors occur.
- Environmental humidification may decrease drying of the mucosa.

ANTITUSSIVES

Cough is a physiologic reflex. It is a protective action that clears the respiratory tract of secretions and foreign substances. Coughing helps to maintain an open airway in individuals with asthma, chronic obstructive pulmonary disease, and cystic fibrosis. In other individuals, coughing may be associated with smoking, viral upper respiratory infections, allergy, and numerous other causes. Often, cough can be alleviated by treating the underlying cause. Although antitussives have no effect on the underlying condition, they ease respiratory discomfort, facilitate sleep, and reduce irritation.

Actions

Nonnarcotic antitussive agents anesthetize the stretch receptors located in the respiratory passages, lungs, and pleura by dampening their activity and thereby reducing the cough reflex at its source. Narcotic antitussive agents depress the cough center that is located in the medulla, thereby raising its threshold for incoming cough impulse.

Uses

Antitussives are used for symptomatic relief of cough.

Contraindications

Antitussive agents are contraindicated in individuals who are hypersensitive to any of the ingredients. They should not be used by newborn or premature infants, pregnant women, and during breast-feeding.

Adverse Reactions

Nonnarcotic antitussive agents may produce sedation, headache, mild dizziness, pruritus, nasal congestion, constipation, nausea, and GI upset. Narcotic antitussive agents may produce nausea, vomiting, constipation, light-headedness, and drowsiness.

Dosage and Route

The dosage and route of administration are determined by the manufacturer, but a physician should be consulted when needed. See Table 24-3 for selected antitussives.

Implications for Patient Care.

Because most nonnarcotic antitussives are taken as over-the-counter medications, the implications for patient care mainly involve teaching the patient about the medication. For narcotic antitussives, you should monitor the patient for signs of improvement, adverse reactions, dependency, and tolerance.

 Patient Teaching

Educate patients that:

- narcotic antitussive agents may be habit-forming and that they may cause drowsiness.
- the medication may impair mental alertness; therefore, patients should not operate machinery or drive a motor vehicle until their response to the medication has been determined.

TABLE 24-3   Antitussives

MEDICATION	USUAL DOSAGE	ADVERSE REACTIONS
benzonatate (Tessalon)	Oral (Adults and children over 10): 100 mg 3 to 6 times daily Oral (Children under 10 years): 8 mg/kg/day in 3 to 6 divided doses	Mild adverse effects, including constipation, rash, drowsiness, nasal congestion, headache, and hypersensitivity reactions
codeine codeine phosphate codeine sulfate	Oral (Adults): 10 to 20 mg every 4 to 6 hours (maximum 120 mg/24 hrs) Oral (Children 6 to 12): 5 to 10 mg every 4 to 6 hours (maximum of 60 mg/day) Oral (Children 2 to 6): 2.5 to 5 mg every 4 to 6 hours (maximum of 30 mg/day)	Respiratory and circulatory depression with overdose (particularly with children), nausea, vomiting, constipation, light-headedness, drowsiness

- medication should not be chewed or allowed to dissolve in the mouth because it could anesthetize the throat and lead to choking.
- liquid medication should not be taken with or followed by water, as this could diminish its effect. ▨

EXPECTORANTS AND MUCOLYTICS

Among the drugs used to treat a cough are expectorants and mucolytics. An expectorant is an agent that stimulates and decreases the *thickness* of respiratory tract secretions. Mucolytics are drugs that reduce the *viscosity* of respiratory tract fluids. The actions of these medications are theoretically useful in treating coughs, because such actions should facilitate removal of irritants and phlegm. Despite studies that show some agents to be effective, conclusive evidence of the effectiveness of these medications is yet to be reported.

Expectorants

Actions

Expectorants enhance the output of lower respiratory tract fluids and help make them less viscid. This promotes and facilitates the removal of mucus.

Uses

Use an expectorant to help loosen phlegm (mucus) and thin bronchial secretions to make cough more productive.

Contraindications

Expectorants are contraindicated in patients who are hypersensitive to any of the ingredients and those with persistent cough.

Adverse Reactions

Reactions include drowsiness, nausea, vomiting, and anorexia.

Dosage and Route

The dosage and route of administration are determined by the physician. See Table 24-4 for selected expectorants.

Implications for Patient Care

You should monitor the patient for signs of improvement and adverse reactions.

Patient Teaching

Educate patients:

- on how to cough to facilitate the removal of phlegm and the proper disposal of the coughed-up secretions. (Patients should be in the upright position, take several slow, deep breaths, place a tissue over their mouth, and then cough. The color, amount, and character of the sputum should be noted. The tissue should be placed in a proper container.)
- to drink plenty of fluids to help keep mucous membranes moist and loosen secretions. ▨

TABLE 24-4 Expectorants and Mucolytics

MEDICATION	USUAL DOSAGE	ADVERSE REACTIONS
EXPECTORANTS		
guaifenesin (Robitussin)	Oral (Adults): 100 to 400 mg every 4 hours (maximum, 2400 mg/day) Oral (Children 6 to 12): 100 to 200 mg as above (maximum, 1200 mg/day) Oral (Children 2 to 6): 50 to 100 mg as above (maximum, 600 mg/day)	Drowsiness, nausea, vomiting, anorexia
saturated solution of potassium iodide	Oral (Adults): 0.3 to 0.6 mL diluted in 1 glassful of water, fruit juice, or milk 3 to 4 times daily	Skin rash, swelling or tenderness of salivary glands
terpin hydrate and codeine elixir	Oral (terpin hydrate and codeine elixir): 5 mL 3 to 4 times a day	Gastrointestinal upset
MUCOLYTICS		
acetylcysteine (Mucomyst)	Nebulization-face mask, mouth piece, tracheostomy: 3 to 5 mL of 20% solution, or 6 to 10 mL of 10% solution 3 to 4 times/day	Stomatitis, nausea, vomiting, fever, rhinorrhea, drowsiness, clamminess, chest tightness, bronchoconstriction

Special Considerations

- Patients should notify the physician if cough does not improve or if they develop a fever, rash, or persistent headache.
- Environmental humidification may decrease drying of the mucosa and help loosen secretions.
- Saturated solution of potassium iodide (SSKI) should be diluted in water or fruit juice before administering.

Mucolytics

Actions

Mucolytics (Mucomyst) break chemical bonds (disulfide linkage) in mucus, thereby lowering the viscosity.

Uses

Use as an adjuvant therapy for patients who have abnormal, viscid, or thickened mucous secretions in such conditions as chronic obstructive pulmonary disease(s), cystic fibrosis, and pneumonia.

Contraindications

Mucolytics are contraindicated in patients who are hypersensitive to any of Mucomyst's ingredients.

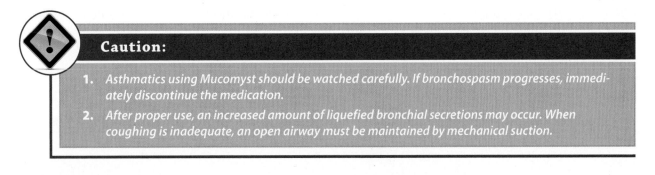

Caution:

1. *Asthmatics using Mucomyst should be watched carefully. If bronchospasm progresses, immediately discontinue the medication.*
2. *After proper use, an increased amount of liquefied bronchial secretions may occur. When coughing is inadequate, an open airway must be maintained by mechanical suction.*

Adverse Reactions

Most patients tolerate Mucomyst very well. Adverse reactions that may occur are stomatitis, nausea, vomiting, fever, rhinorrhea, drowsiness, clamminess, chest tightness, and bronchospasm.

Dosage and Route

The dosage and route of administration are determined by the physician. See Table 24-4 for Mucomyst.

Implications for Patient Care

You should know that this medication should not be mixed with antibiotics, iron, copper, or rubber products.

Patient Teaching

Educate patients:

- about good oral hygienic practices.
- that the unpleasant odor experienced with use of Mucomyst will decrease after repeated use, and that discoloration of solution after the bottle is opened does not impair the effectiveness of the medication.
- medication should be stored in a refrigerator and used within 96 hours of opening.
- medication should be given one-half to one hour before meals for better absorption and to decrease nausea. ■

Special Consideration

Mucolytics may be used as an antidote for acetaminophen overdose.

BRONCHODILATORS

Bronchodilators are used to improve pulmonary airflow in patients with chronic obstructive pulmonary disease and asthma. They may be classified as sympathomimetics (beta-adrenergic agents), as shown in Table 24-5, xanthines (phosphodiesterase inhibitors), as shown in Table 24-6, leukotriene receptor antagonists (blockers), and anticholinergic agents.

Actions

Sympathomimetics act on beta-2 adrenoreceptors to relax smooth muscle cells of the bronchi. They also produce a vasoconstriction response throughout the body by stimulating alpha receptors. This response reduces edema in the bronchial mucosa. Some sympathomimetics also stimulate beta-1 receptors and this results in an increased heart rate and its force of contraction. Xanthine bronchodilators relax smooth muscle of the bronchial airways and pulmonary blood vessels by blocking phosphodiesterase, which increases adenosine monophosphate (AMP). By preventing the breakdown of cyclic AMP, smooth muscles relax and bronchodilation occurs, thus relieving dyspnea. They may also produce cardiac stimulation, coronary vasodilation, stimulation of skeletal muscles, cerebral stimulation, and diuresis.

Uses

Bronchodilators are used in the prevention and relief of bronchospasm in patients with asthma, bronchitis, and emphysema.

TABLE 24-5 Sympathomimetic Bronchodilators

MEDICATION	USUAL DOSAGE	ADVERSE REACTIONS
epinephrine epinephrine HCl	IM, SC (Adults): 0.2 to 0.5 mL of 1 : 1,000 solution every 2 hours as necessary IM, SC (Children): 0.01 mg/kg every 4 hours as needed (maximum of 0.5 mg/day)	Anxiety, headache, palpitations, tremor, tachycardia
ephedrine sulfate	Oral, SC (Adults): 25 to 50 mg every 3 to 4 hours as needed. (Children 2 to 6 years): 0.3 to 0.5 mg/kg every 4 to 6 hours (Children 6 to 12 years): 6.25 to 12.5 mg every 3 to 4 hours as needed	Tremors, anxiety, insomnia, headache, confusion, anorexia, nausea, dyspnea
isoproterenol HCl (Isuprel)	Inhalation: 1 to 2 deep inhalations from nebulizing unit; dose may be repeated up to 5 times daily	Tachycardia, palpitations, headache, nervousness
metaproterenol sulfate (Alupent)	Inhalation (Adults and children 12 and older): Usual single dose is 2 to 3 inhalations, every 3 to 4 hours. Total dosage should not exceed 12 inhalations	Tachycardia, hypertension, palpitations, nervousness, tremor, nausea, vomiting

TABLE 24-6 Xanthine Bronchodilators

MEDICATION	USUAL DOSAGE	ADVERSE REACTIONS
aminophylline	Oral (Adults): 500 mg, then, 250 to 500 mg every 6 to 8 hours. (Children): 7.5 mg/kg, then 3 to 6 mg/kg every 6 to 8 hours Rectal (Adults): 250 to 500 mg every 6 to 8 hours IM (Adults): 500 mg as necessary	Anxiety, restlessness, insomnia, headache, palpitations, nausea, vomiting, anorexia, increase in blood pressure
dyphylline (Lufyllin)	Oral (Adults): Up to 15 mg/kg every 6 hours IM (Adults): 250 to 500 mg (1 to 2 mL) every 2 to 6 hours (maximum of 15 mg/kg every 6 hours)	Headache, nausea, palpitations
theophylline (Elixophyllin)	Oral (Adults and children): 6 mg/kg initially, followed by 3 to 4 mg/kg every 4 to 6 hours	Nausea, vomitting, headache, dizziness, nervousness, epigastric pain
theophylline (Theo-24)	Oral (Adults): Initially 400 mg as single daily dose. Maximum without serum monitoring: 13 mg/kg/day, up to 900 mg/day. (Children): 30 to 35 kg: Initially 300 mg once daily	Cardiac arrhythmias, nausea, headaches, diuresis, rash

Contraindications

Bronchodilators are contraindicated in patients who are hypersensitive to any of the ingredients.

Caution:

1. *The potential for paradoxical bronchospasm should be kept in mind, and if it occurs, discontinue the medication immediately.*
2. *Metered-dose aerosol units are under pressure. Do not puncture, use, or store near heat or flame.*

Adverse Reactions

Palpitations, increase in blood pressure, tremors, nausea, vomiting, dizziness, heartburn, nervousness, urticaria, and headache are possible reactions.

Dosage and Route

The dosage and route of administration are determined by the physician. See Table 24-5 for selected sympathomimetic bronchodilators, Table 24-6 for selected xanthine bronchodilators, and Table 24-7 for glucocorticoids.

Implications for Patient Care

You should be aware that many sympathomimetic bronchodilators may also stimulate beta-1 receptors located in the heart. They may be dangerous to use in patients who have heart disease. Monitor all patients for changes in cardiac function and blood pressure. With xanthine bronchodilators, monitor the patient for disruption of cardiac function, insomnia, and hyperexcitability. Be aware of increased potential for convulsive activity. The serum levels of the medication should be checked on a regular basis. Therapeutic range should be 10 to 20 mcg/mL.

Patient Teaching

Sympathomimetic Bronchodilators. Educate patients:

- to take the medication as prescribed and not to exceed the dosage.
- to notify the physician immediately if symptoms do not improve, if they experiences bronchial irritation, dizziness, chest pain, or insomnia.
- not to take any other medication unless it is prescribed by the physician.
- to drink plenty of fluids, especially water, to help moisten mucous membranes and reduce the thickness of mucus.
- that the medication should be protected from light, and if the color of the solution changes, it should be discarded.

Xanthine Bronchodilators. Educate patients:

- that oral xanthine bronchodilators may be taken with food to avoid GI upset, but the medicine should not be crushed or chewed.
- that cola drinks, coffee, tea, and chocolate contain xanthine and they should not be consumed while on medication. ■

TABLE 24-7 Glucocorticoids

MEDICATION	USUAL DOSAGE	ADVERSE REACTIONS
flunisolide (Aerobid)	Inhalation (Adults): 2 inhalations twice daily, morning and evening. Maximum 8 inhalations/day. (Children 6 to 15): 2 inhalations twice daily	Diarrhea, nausea, sore throat, headache, URI, dizziness
triamcinolone acetonide (Azmacort)	Inhalation (Adults): 2 inhalations 3 to 4 times daily. Maximum 16 inhalations daily (Children 6 to 12): 1 to 2 inhalations 3 to 4 times daily. Maximum 12 inhalations daily	Hoarseness, dry mouth and throat, wheezing, cough, oral fungal infections

Special Considerations

- Sympathomimetic bronchodilators should not be used with MAO inhibitors because sympathomimetic activity could be increased and hypertensive crisis might occur.
- Patients using antihistamines, tricyclic antidepressants, and thyroid hormone may experience greater sympathomimetic activity with the use of a sympathomimetic bronchodilator.
- Xanthine bronchodilators may enhance CNS stimulation of ephedrine, sympathomimetics, and amphetamines.
- Certain antibiotics (erythromycin, lincomycin, and clindamycin) may increase blood levels of xanthines.
- Xanthines may interact with beta-blocking agents, digitalis, anticoagulants, lithium, and furosemide.

LEUKOTRIENE RECEPTOR ANTAGONISTS (BLOCKERS)

Leukotriene receptor antagonists (blockers) are used for the treatment and management of asthma. These agents block cysteinyl leukotrienes and leukotriene receptor occupation, that have been correlated with the pathophysiology of asthma, including airway edema, smooth muscle contraction, and altered cellular activity associated with the inflammatory process, which contribute to the signs and symptoms of asthma.

Medications included in this classification are Accolate (zafirlukast) and Singulair (montelukast sodium). Accolate is used as a long-term control agent in the management of asthma. The dosage of Accolate for adults and children 12 years and older is a 20-mg tablet twice daily. Accolate is also now available in a 10-mg, nonflavored mini-tablet specifically designed for children as young as 7 years old. The recommended dosing is one 10-mg mini-tablet twice daily, even during symptom-free periods. Singulair (montelukast sodium) is the first of the leukotriene blockers intended for both adults and children as young as 6, and the first developed for once-daily use.

Montelukast Sodium (Singulair)

Actions

Singulair is a selective and orally active leukotriene receptor antagonist that inhibits the cysteinyl leukotriene CysLT1 receptor. It is able to block leukotriene action in the lung, resulting in less constriction of the bronchial tissue and less inflammation.

Uses

It is indicated for the prophylaxis and chronic treatment of asthma in adults and pediatric patients 6 years of age and older.

Contraindications

Montelukast Sodium is contraindicated in patients with hypersensitivity to any component of this product.

Precautions

Singulair is not indicated for use in the reversal of bronchospasm in acute asthma attacks, including status asthmaticus. Patients should be advised to have appropriate rescue medication available. Singulair should not be used as monotherapy for the treatment and management of exercise-induced bronchospasm. Patients who have exacerbations of asthma after exercise should continue to use their usual regimen of inhaled medication.

> **Caution:**
>
> *Rare cases in which an inflammatory condition associated with a type of cell called eosinophils has been detected among users of Singulair. Most of the affected patients were taking several asthma medications; Singulair has not been shown to be directly involved with the development of the inflammatory condition.*

Adverse Reactions

Reactions include asthenia, fatigue, fever, abdominal pain, dyspepsia, gastroenteritis, dizziness, headache, nasal congestion, cough, influenza, and rash.

Less common side effects include increased bleeding tendency, allergic reactions, behavior and mood related changes (agitation including aggressive behavior, bad/vivid dreams, depression, feeling anxious, hallucinations, irritability, restlessness, suicidal thoughts and actions including suicide, tremor, trouble sleeping), nose bleed, joint pain, and muscle aches.

Dosage and Route

The dosage for adults and adolescents 15 years of age and older is one 10-mg tablet daily to be taken in the evening. The dosage for pediatric patients 6 to 14 years of age is one 5-mg chewable tablet daily to be taken in the evening.

Implications for Patient Care

The medical assistant should monitor the patient for improvement and adverse reactions. Patients on Singulair should be monitored for suicidality and changes in mood or behavior. Assist the patient and his or her family to identify and eliminate or minimize factors that trigger symptoms.

Patient Teaching

Educate patients:

- to take the medications as prescribed and not to exceed the dosage.
- that the drug should be continued during acute attacks as well as during symptom-free periods.
- to report if increased use and frequency of inhalers is needed for symptom control.
- to continue other prescribed anti-asthma medications during this therapy.
- to report any unusual side effects, changes in disease, or significant drop in peak flow readings.
- to notify physician if pregnancy is suspected or planned.
- as to how to reduce environmental triggers and appropriate steps to minimize or avoid exposure. ▪

ANTICHOLINERGIC AGENTS

Inhalational anticholinergic agents inhibit cholinergic receptors in bronchial smooth muscle, resulting in decreased concentrations of cyclic guanosine monophosphate (cGMP). This action produces local bronchodilation. Intranasal local application inhibits secretions from glands lining the nasal mucosa. Atrovent (ipratropium bromide) is an anticholinergic agent prescribed for long-term treatment of bronchial spasms (wheezing) associated with chronic obstructive pulmonary disease, including chronic bronchitis and emphysema.

The usual starting dose for adults and children 12 years of age and older is two inhalations, four times a day. Additional inhalations may be taken, but the total should not exceed 12 in 24 hours. For intranasal application (nasal spray 0.03%), the dosage is two sprays (42 mcg) per nostril b.i.d. to t.i.d. for a total daily dose of 168 to 252 mcg/day. For intranasal application (nasal spray 0.06%), the dosage is two sprays (84 mcg) per nostril t.i.d. to q.i.d. for a total daily dose of 504 to 672 mcg/day.

Adverse reactions may include blurred vision, cough, dizziness, dry mouth, headache, nausea, nervousness, rash, stomach and intestinal upset, and worsening of symptoms.

GLUCOCORTICOIDS

Glucocorticoids are anti-inflammatory agents that are chemically related to the naturally occurring hormone cortisone. There are many uses for corticosteroids, but inhalational forms are used in the treatment of bronchial asthma, and in seasonal or perennial allergic conditions when other forms of treatment are not effective. Examples of inhalation via metered-dose inhaler steroids are flunisolide (Aerobid and Nasalide), and triamcinolone acetonide (Azmacort). See Table 24-7 for selected glucocorticoids.

Flonase (fluticasone propionate) and Rhinocort (budesonide) are two examples of anti-inflammatory glucocorticoid nasal medications that are used for the treatment of **allergic rhinitis** (hay fever). Flonase is a nasal spray, indicated for patients 4 years of age and older, and provides 24-hour relief of nasal allergy symptoms. The usual recommended starting dose is one 50-mcg spray in each nostril once a day, for a total dose of 100 mcg/day. Maximum dose is two sprays (200 mcg) in each nostril once a day. The most common adverse reactions are headache, pharyngitis, and epistaxis. Instructions for use are included with the medication and the patient is advised to follow the directions carefully and use only as directed.

Rhinocort is prescribed as a nasal inhaler. The usual recommended starting dose for adults and children 6 years of age and older is 256 micrograms a day, either as two sprays in each nostril twice a day, morning and evening, or as four sprays in each nostril once a day in the morning. Rhinocort is not recommended for use in children with nasal irritation not due to allergies. The most common adverse reactions are increased coughing, irritation of nasal passages, epistaxis, and sore throat. Because steroids can suppress the immune system, people taking Rhinocort may become more susceptible to infections, and their infections could be more severe. Anyone taking Rhinocort or other glucocorticoids who has not had infections such as chickenpox and measles should avoid exposure to them. If one is taking Rhinocort and is exposed, he or she should notify the physician immediately. Instructions for use are included with the medication; patients are advised to follow the directions carefully and use only as directed.

Cromolyn Sodium

Cromolyn sodium inhibits the degranulation of sensitized mast cells that occurs after exposure to specific antigens. It inhibits the release of histamine and SRS-A (the slow-reacting substance of anaphylaxis, that is, leukotrienes). Cromolyn sodium is used for the prophylactic treatment of bronchial asthma and for the prevention and treatment of the symptoms of allergic rhinitis.

Spotlight

Tuberculosis

Tuberculosis is a contagious disease caused by the bacillus *Mycobacterium tuberculosis*. It is spread from person to person by airborne transmission. An infected person releases large and small droplets through talking, coughing, sneezing, laughing, or singing. The large droplets settle, while the small droplets remain suspended in the air and can be inhaled by a susceptible person.

Tuberculosis, once called *consumption*, is not a new disease. At one time it was the number-one killer in the United States and it is still a major cause of death worldwide. One of public health's oldest enemies is back, and with a vengeance. An estimated 10 million Americans are infected with the TB bacterium. Compounding the problem are drug-resistant strains of TB that can shrug off as many as seven of the antibiotics traditionally used to treat this disease.

At the present time, TB is occurring primarily among patients with AIDS, the homeless, drug abusers, prison inmates, and immigrants. Health officials are concerned about the rapid spread of this disease and the risks it poses to the general public. Virtually anyone who comes in contact with an infected person is at risk of contracting TB. Studies show that exposure to an infected person in confined quarters such as homes and classrooms increases an individual's risk.

Symptoms

Symptoms include a chronic cough, fatigue, low-grade fever, night sweats, weakness, chills, anorexia, weight loss, hemoptysis and, in the early stages, scanty, whitish, or grayish-yellow, frothy sputum.

During the early stages of TB, the sputum is expectorated in small quantities, but later, when consolidation takes place, it becomes more copious, tenacious, and grayish-yellow. In the late stages of TB, the sputum becomes mucopurulent, musty and fetid, and containing fibers and tubercle bacilli, and blood-tinged or mixed with blood.

Diagnosis

To determine a diagnosis of tuberculosis, a careful history is taken and a complete physical examination is performed. After evaluation of the patient, the physician may order a tuberculin test (if the patient has not had a previous positive reaction), chest X-ray, a bronchoscopy, or a sputum analysis to obtain a conclusive diagnosis.

Treatment

Treatment of TB requires long-term drug therapy (6 to 9 months), often utilizing a regimen that includes a combination of antituberculosis agents. The use of multiple drugs is indicated in all but a few active cases, because any large population of *Mycobacterium tuberculosis* will have naturally occurring mutants that are resistant to each of the drugs administered. The primary drug regimen for active tuberculosis combines the drugs isoniazid (INH), rifampin (RIF), and ethambutol (EMB). Other drugs that are also used are streptomycin (SM) and pyrazinamide (PZA). Diet and rest are also important aspects of treatment for this disease. It is recommended that patients receive a liver function test before and while taking antituberculosis drugs. See Table 24-8 for selected antituberculosis agents.

The effectiveness of treatment can be evaluated by monitoring patients' sputum smear results. It takes about two weeks for the drugs to kill enough bacteria so that they cannot infect other people. It takes 6 to 9 months of continuous drug therapy for a cure. Follow-up care is essential. A sputum culture is essential to confirming a diagnosis, determining the organisms' susceptibility to drugs, and assessing response to treatment. If the TB bacteria become resistant to two of the drugs that are used to treat tuberculosis, then MDR-TB (multidrug resistant tuberculosis) is suspected and appropriate measures must be instituted promptly to treat and prevent the spread of MDR-TB.

Some people are at high risk for drug-resistant TB: people who have been recently exposed to drug-resistant TB, especially if they are immunocompromised; TB patients who failed to take medications as prescribed; TB patients who were prescribed an ineffective treatment regimen; and people previously treated for TB.

Rifapentine (Priftin) is the first new medication for tuberculosis in 25 years. The drug is important because it makes patients more likely to complete their therapy. Treatment with rifapentine is broken down into two phases: an intensive phase, and a continuation phase. In the intensive phase of treatment, rifapentine is administered at 72-hour intervals for two months. It must be administered along with at least one other

TABLE 24-8   Antituberculosis Agents

MEDICATION	USUAL DOSAGE	ADVERSE REACTIONS
FIRST-LINE DRUGS		
ethambutol HCl (Myambutal)	Oral: 15 to 25 mg/kg/day in a single dose Twice weekly: 50 mg/kg	Optic neuritis, decreased visual acuity and red-green color discrimination, skin rash
isoniazid (Nydrazid)	Oral: 300 mg daily in a single dose, or 4 to 5 mg/kg of body weight per day Twice weekly: 15 mg/kg	Hepatotoxicity, flulike syndrome, neuropathy, hypersensitivity Note: The physician may prescribe pyridoxine to prevent or decrease neuropathy.
pyrazinamide (PZA)	Oral: 15 to 30 mg/kg/day	Hepatotoxicity, hyperuricemia, arthralgia, skin rash, gastrointestinal irritation
rifabutin (Mycobutin)	Oral: 300 mg once daily	Fever, headache, flulike syndrome, gastrointestinal symptoms, brown-orange discoloration of body fluids Note: Interacts with zidovudine and protease inhibitors except indinavir
rifampin (Rifadin) (Rimactane)	Oral (Adult): 600 mg/day or 10 mg/kg/day Oral (Child): 10 to 20 mg/kg/day	Gastrointestinal disturbances, flulike symptoms, orange-tinged body fluids, fever, headache
rifampin and isoniazid (Rifamate, Rimactane/ INH Dual Pack)	Oral: two capsules once daily	Gastrointestinal disturbances, flulike symptoms, hepatotoxicity, neuropathy, hypersensitivity, headache
rifapentine (Priftin)	Oral: Intensive phase: 300 mg at 72 hour intervals for two months Continuation phase: 600 mg once a week for 4 months	Hyperuricemia, headache, dizziness, elevation of liver enzymes, neutropenia, pyuria, hematuria, reddish discoloration of body fluids including saliva, rash
isoniazid, rifampin, and pyrazinamide (Rifater)	Oral: Each tablet contains a fixed-dose combination 50 mg of isoniazid, 120 mg of rifampin, and 300 mg of pyrazinamide Daily: 99 lb: 4 tabs; 99 to 120 lb: 5 tabs; above 120 lb: 6 tabs	Same as for isoniazid, rifampin, and pyrazinamide
streptomycin sulfate	IM: 0.75 to 1 g daily, then reduced to 1 g 2 to 3 times weekly	Ototoxicity, nephrotoxicity, hypokalemia
SECOND-LINE DRUGS		
ciprofloxacin (Cipro)	Oral: 750 to 1500 mg daily	Abdominal cramps, nausea, diarrhea, rash, headache, photosensitivity, insomnia
cycloserine (Seromycin)	Oral: 15 to 20 mg/kg/day; 250 to 1000 mg daily in divided doses	Psychosis, personality changes, rash, impaired coordination, depression, increased phenytoin (Dilantin) levels

(continues)

TABLE 24-8 (continued)		
MEDICATION	**USUAL DOSAGE**	**ADVERSE REACTIONS**
ethionamide (Trecator-SC)	Oral: 15 to 20 mg/kg/day; 500 to 1000 mg daily in divided doses	Gastrointestinal disturbance, hepatotoxicity, hyperthyroidism, metallic taste and distorted sense of smell, severe acne
kanamycin, amikacin, and capreomycin	IM: 15 to 30 mg/kg/day	Renal and auditory toxicity, vestibular toxicity, hypokalemia
levofloxacin (Levaquin)	Oral: 500 mg daily	Nausea, diarrhea, abdominal cramps
oxfloxacin (Floxin)	Oral: 400 to 800 mg daily in divided doses	Abdominal cramps, nausea, diarrhea

antibiotic accepted for the treatment of tuberculosis. Streptomycin or ethambutol may also be required until the results of susceptibility testing for the specific *M. tuberculosis* isolate are known. Following the intensive phase of treatment, the dose of rifapentine is reduced to one dose per week and should continue to be administered along with an appropriate antibiotic. Susceptibility testing should be conducted at regular intervals during therapy. Patients should be educated as to the importance of compliance during the entire course of therapy, because lack of compliance has been associated with a high incidence of relapse and delayed sputum conversion. Rifapentine may cause serious hepatic damage. It should be administered to patients with liver test function abnormalities only in cases where the advantages of treatment outweigh the disadvantages of delay. Rifapentine may produce a red-orange discoloration of skin, teeth, tongue, urine, sweat, sputum, and tears. This may result in permanent staining of contact lenses. In addition, the effectiveness of oral contraceptives in women may be decreased while taking rifapentine. Women relying on oral contraceptives should consider switching to other forms of birth control while taking rifapentine. Patients who experience nausea or vomiting after administration of rifapentine should try taking the medication with food.

CDC Guidelines

The following specific actions that are used to reduce the risk of tuberculosis transmission are taken from the Centers for Disease Control and Prevention's booklet on *Guidelines for Preventing the Transmission of Tuberculosis in Health-Care Settings*:

- Screening patients for active TB and TB infection
- Providing rapid diagnostic services
- Prescribing appropriate curative and preventive therapy
- Maintaining physical measures to reduce microbial contamination of the air
- Providing isolation rooms for people with, or suspected of having, infectious TB
- Screening health care facility personnel for TB infection
- Promptly investigating and controlling outbreaks

Transmission-Based Precautions

The Centers for Disease Control and Prevention (CDC) recommends the use of transmission-based precautions to reduce the risk of airborne, droplet, and contact transmission of pathogens. These precautions are to be used in addition to standard precautions, and are intended for patients diagnosed with or suspected of specific highly transmissible diseases, such as tuberculosis. See Figures 24-2 and 24-3.

AIRBORNE PRECAUTIONS
(in addition to Standard Precautions)

VISITORS: Report to nurse before entering.

Use Airborne Precautions as recommended for patients known or suspected to be infected with infectious agents transmitted person-to-person by the airborne route (e.g., M. tuberculosis, measles, chickenpox, disseminated herpes zoster).

Patient placement

Place patients in an **AIIR** (Airborne Infection Isolation Room).
Monitor air pressure daily with visual indicators (e.g., flutter strips).

Keep door closed when not required for entry and exit.

In ambulatory settings instruct patients with a known or suspected airborne infection to wear a surgical mask and observe Respiratory Hygiene/Cough Etiquette. Once in an AIIR, the mask may be removed.

Patient transport

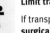

Limit transport and movement of patients to **medically-necessary purposes.**

If transport or movement outside an AIIR is necessary, instruct patients to **wear a surgical mask**, if possible, and observe Respiratory Hygiene/Cough Etiquette.

Hand Hygiene

Hand Hygiene according to Standard Precautions.

Personal Protective Equipment (PPE)

Wear a fit-tested NIOSH-approved **N95** or higher level respirator for respiratory protection when entering the room of a patient when the following diseases are suspected or confirmed: Listed on back.

APR   ©2007 Brevis Corporation www.brevis.com

FIGURE 24-2

Airborne Precautions, One Category of Transmission-Based Precautions for use i n hospital settings. *Source: Reprinted with permission from Brevis Corporation (www.brevis.com).*

■ Special Considerations: **OLDER ADULTS**

With aging, there may be an increased risk of developing tuberculosis. Two factors that may contribute to an increased incidence of tuberculosis among older adults are the following:

1. Previous exposure to the *Mycobacterium tuberculosis* bacillus as a child.
2. Actually having had an active case of tuberculosis as a younger person and the disease process was not treated sufficiently.

CONTACT PRECAUTIONS

(in addition to Standard Precautions)

STOP **VISITORS: Report to nurse before entering.**

Gloves

Don gloves upon entry into the room or cubicle.
Wear gloves whenever touching the patient's intact skin or surfaces and articles in close proximity to the patient.
Remove gloves before leaving patient room.

Hand Hygiene

Hand Hygiene according to Standard Precautions.

Gowns

Don gown upon entry into the room or cubicle.
Remove gown and observe hand hygiene before leaving the patient-care environment.

Patient Transport

Limit transport of patients to medically necessary purposes.
Ensure that infected or colonized areas of the patient's body are contained and covered.
Remove and dispose of contaminated PPE and perform hand hygiene prior to transporting patients on Contact Precautions.
Don clean PPE to handle the patient at the transport destination.

Patient–Care Equipment

Use disposable noncritical patient-care equipment or implement patient-dedicated use of such equipment.

Form No. **CPR7**   BREVIS CORP., 225 West 2855 South, SLC, UT 84115   © 2007 Brevis Corp.

FIGURE 24-3

Contact Precautions, one category of Transmission-Based Precautions, for use in hospital settings. *Source: Reprinted with permission from Brevis Corporation (www.brevis.com).*

The *Mycobacterium tuberculosis* bacillus can remain dormant in a person's body for years. With the aging of the immune system, the dormant bacillus can become active and tuberculosis can emerge again. In addition to age-related immune system changes, the presence of chronic diseases often seen in older adults can make them more susceptible to infection. Some age-related changes seen in older adults respiratory system that may make them more susceptible to infection are:

- Decline in the protective mechanisms of the respiratory mucosa.
- Decrease in the effectiveness of bronchial cilia.
- Changes in the connective tissues of the lungs and chest.

- Decline in elastic recoil of the lungs.
- Increase in the stiffness of the chest wall decreases the lung's air-moving efficiency.
- Decreased airflow delivers less oxygen to the blood and therefore to the body's tissues.

Symptoms, Diagnosis, and Treatment

The classic symptoms of tuberculosis may not be obvious in older adults. Older adults may only have weight loss and anorexia as presenting symptoms. The diagnosis and treatment are the same for older adults as they are for anyone with tuberculosis. The exception is in the monitoring of drug therapy for older adults. Adverse reactions are more likely to occur in older adults. One should be especially aware of possible toxic effects of streptomycin: deafness, dizziness, unsteadiness of gait, ringing in the ears, or severe headache. Some of the effects of isoniazid may be numbness, tingling, and weakness of the extremities. Additionally, individuals who have a previous history of drug treatment for tuberculosis may be at an increased risk of developing drug-resistant TB. Their drug regimen should be monitored very carefully.

◼▪ Special Considerations: **CHILDREN**

When exposed to the *Mycobacterium tuberculosis* bacillus, children may be at greater risk of contracting tuberculosis because of the following factors:

1. The airway diameter is smaller of children and this increases the potential for obstruction.
2. The airway mucous membranes are highly vascular and susceptible to trauma, edema, infection, and spasm.
3. The accessory muscles of respiration are not as strong in children as in adults.
4. Children with respiratory problems are more prone to infections.

Symptoms, Diagnosis, and Treatment

The classic symptoms of tuberculosis may be more difficult to identify in children than in adults. The child may appear weak, have a history of weight loss, anorexia, and a low-grade fever. Because several conditions could cause the same symptoms, a careful analysis of a child's physical state should be evaluated and a differential diagnosis should include a tuberculin test, chest X-ray, and a positive smear or sputum culture indicating the presence of acid-fast bacteria (AFB). When a positive diagnosis is determined, the child is placed on antituberculosis agents for six to nine months. The drug regimen is determined by the attending physician and the dosage is based upon kilogram of body weight. The following dosage chart is taken from the Centers for Disease Control and Prevention's publication, *TB/HIV The Connection, What Health Care Workers Should Know*:

Dosage Recommendations for the Treatment of TB in Children (12 years of age and younger)

DRUG	DAILY DOSE	TWICE-WEEKLY DOSE	THRICE-WEEKLY DOSE
ethambutol* (EMB)	15 to 25 mg/kg Max. 2.5 g	50 mg/kg	25 to 30 mg/kg
isoniazid	10 to 20 mg/kg Max. 300 mg	20 to 40 mg/kg Max. 900 mg	20 to 40 mg/kg Max. 900 mg
pyrazinamide (PZA)	15 to 30 mg/kg Max. 2 g	50 to 70 mg/kg	50 to 70 mg/kg
rifampin (Rimactane)	10 to 20 mg/kg Max. 600 mg	10 to 20 mg/kg Max. 600 mg	10 to 20 mg/kg Max. 600 mg
streptomycin (SM)	20 to 40 mg/kg Max. 1 g	25 to 30 mg/kg	25 to 30 mg/kg

*Ethambutol is generally not recommended for children whose visual acuity cannot be monitored (children under 6 years of age). However, ethambutol should be considered for all children with organisms resistant to other drugs, if susceptibility to ethambutol has been demonstrated or susceptibility is likely.

▪▪ Critical Thinking QUESTIONS AND ACTIVITIES

An estimated 10 million Americans are infected with the TB bacterium. To help protect yourself, your family, and your patients, you should know certain facts about tuberculosis. Ask yourself the following:

- How is tuberculosis spread?
- What are the symptoms of tuberculosis?
- How is tuberculosis diagnosed?
- What is the treatment regimen for tuberculosis?
- How is the effectiveness of the treatment regimen evaluated?
- What is MDR-TB?
- What people are at high risk for MDR-TB?
- What are the recommended CDC guidelines for preventing the transmission of tuberculosis in health care settings?

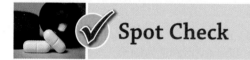 Spot Check

There are several medications that may be used to treat tuberculosis. For each of the selected drugs, give the recommended children's dosage:

DRUG	DAILY DOSE	TWICE-WEEKLY DOSE	THRICE-WEEKLY DOSE
ethambutol (EMB)			
isoniazid			
rifampin (Rimactane)			
pyrazinamide (PZA)			
streptomycin (SM)			

◼️◼️ REVIEW QUESTIONS

Directions. Select the best answer to each of the following multiple-choice questions, circling the letter of your choice.

1. Allergic rhinitis is also known as _____.

   a. rhinovirus   b. coryza   c. hay fever   d. hives

2. _____ is an inflammation of the respiratory mucous membrane caused by a rhinovirus.

   a. Urticaria   b. Coryza   c. Pruritus   d. Rhinorrhea

3. Antihistamines are effective in the treatment of _____.

   a. allergy symptoms   c. urticaria and pruritus

   b. seasonal upper respiratory disorders   d. all of these

4. Adverse reactions to antihistamines are _____.

   a. drowsiness, dryness of mouth, dizziness, epigastric distress

   b. diarrhea, constipation, hypotension

   c. anorexia, nausea, and vomiting

   d. muscle weakness, bitter taste, hypertension

5. In children, aspirin should not be used as an antipyretic because of the risk of _____.

   a. a flulike syndrome   c. Reye's syndrome

   b. neuropathy   d. hepatotoxicity

6. Allegra (fexofenadine) is a/an _____.

   a. antihistamine   c. antitussive

   b. decongestant   d. expectorant

7. Decongestants that are commonly used for symptomatic relief of nasal congestion produce the following effects: _____.

   a. dilate the nasal mucosa

   b. increase blood flow to the affected area

   c. slow the formation of mucus

   d. close nasal passages

8. Adverse reactions to pseudoephedrine HCl (Sudafed) are _____.

   a. drowsiness, rebound nasal congestion, anxiety, headache, and palpitation

   b. sneezing, dryness of the mouth, light-headedness, and headache

   c. sneezing, stinging of the mucosa, light-headedness, and headache

   d. nausea, vomiting, diarrhea, and hypotension

9. Although antitussives have no effect on the underlying coughing condition, they do _____.

   a. increase respiratory discomfort   c. reduce irritation

   b. facilitate sleep   d. b and c

10. Adverse reactions to diphenhydramine (Benylin) are _____.

    a. nausea, dizziness, and constipation

    b. drowsiness, dry mouth, and constipation

    c. nausea, constipation, lightheadedness

    d. headache, rash, drowsiness

11. Bronchodilators are used to improve pulmonary airflow in patients with chronic obstructive pulmonary disease (COPD) and asthma.

     a. True   b. False

12. Adverse reactions to epinephrine HCl are _____.

     a. nausea, vomiting, and diarrhea

     b. anxiety, headache, palpitations, tremor, and tachycardia

     c. bradycardia, hypotension, nausea, and vomiting

     d. constipation, tremor, headache, and vomiting

13. The most popular regimen for active tuberculosis combines the drugs _____.

     a. para-aminosalicylic acid, cycloserine, and rifampin

     b. streptomycin, capreomycin, and ethambutol

     c. isoniazid, rifampin, and ethambutol

     d. isoniazid, streptomycin, and para-aminosalicylic

14. Patients on Singulair should be monitored for suicidality and changes in mood.

     a. True   b. False

15. Adverse reactions to rifampin (Rifadin) are _____.

     a. nephrotoxicity, ototoxicity, hypokalemia

     b. psychoses, convulsions, tremor, seizures

     c. peripheral neuritis and hepatotoxicity

     d. gastrointestinal disturbance, headache, flulike symptoms

16. Respiratory ailments are caused by _____.

     a. pathogenic microorganisms, allergens, and environmental factors

     b. nonpathogenic organisms, allergens, and environmental factors

     c. pathogenic organisms, antibodies, and environmental factors

     d. none of these

17. The thin-walled air sacs of the lungs are called _____.

     a. alveoli   b. bronchi   c. bronchus   d. aveoli

Matching. Place the correct letter from Column II on the appropriate line of Column I:

Column I	Column II
18. _C_ allergic rhinitis	A. one of a subgroup of viruses that causes the common cold in humans
19. _G_ coryza	B. severe itching
20. _F_ histamine	C. an inflammation of the nasal mucosa that is due to the sensitivity of the nasal mucosa to an allergen
21. _B_ pruritus	D. the flow of thin watery discharge from the nose
22. _D_ rhinorrhea	E. hives
23. _A_ rhinovirus	F. a substance that is normally present in the body
24. _E_ urticaria	G. the common cold
25. _I_ Robitussin	H. antihistamine
	I. expectorant

UNIT 25
Diuretics and Medications Used for Urinary System Disorders

OBJECTIVES

Upon completing this unit, you should be able to:

- Define the terms listed in the vocabulary.
- State two vital functions of the kidneys.
- State the actions, uses, contraindications, adverse reactions, dosage and route, implications for patient care, patient teaching, and special considerations for thiazide, loop, potassium-sparing, osmotic, and carbonic anhydrase inhibitor diuretics, sulfonamides, and urinary tract antiseptics.
- Describe the symptoms, diagnosis, and treatment regimen for cystitis.
- Describe interstitial cystitis.
- Describe the effect of the aging process on the kidneys.
- Explain why it is important to assess an older adult's voiding history and medication history.
- State the signs of nephrotoxicity.
- Describe the signs and symptoms of a urinary tract infection in children.
- Explain the treatment regimen for a child with a urinary tract infection.
- Complete the critical thinking questions and activities presented in this unit.
- Complete the Spot Check on selected drugs used to treat urinary tract infections.
- State the action, usual dosage, and adverse reactions of selected drugs used for urologic disorders.
- Identify selected agents that discolor urine.
- Answer the review questions correctly.

VOCABULARY

edema (e-de′ma). Swelling. A local or generalized collection of fluid in the body tissues.

excretion (eks-kre′shun). The process of eliminating waste products from the body.

Escherichia coli (esh-er″ik′e-a ko′li). A type of bacteria that is commonly found in the alimentary canal of humans and other animals.

nephrotic syndrome. A disease of the basement membrane of the glomerulus. It causes proteinuria, hypoalbuminemia, edema, and hyperlipidemia.

Proteus mirabilis (pro′te-us mi″ra-bi′lis). A species of enteric bacilli that may cause urinary tract infections. It is found in the intestines of humans and animals.

INTRODUCTION

The urinary system is composed of two kidneys, two ureters, one bladder, and one urethra (see Figure 25-1). Within each kidney, there are a million or more functional units called *nephrons* where the filtration and reabsorption process occurs (see Figure 25-2).

Blood undergoes a process of filtration and reabsorption as it passes through the kidneys. During this process, two vital functions are performed: (1) urine is produced for excretion, and (2) the amount of water, electrolytes, and other substances in the blood is regulated.

Diseases and disorders of the urinary system may involve the kidneys, ureters, bladder, and urethra. Approximately 20 million Americans are affected by kidney and urologic diseases. Diabetes mellitus (Type 2) is the leading cause of chronic kidney failure, and uncontrolled or poorly controlled high blood pressure is the second leading cause. Glomerulonephritis, an inflammatory disease of the glomerulus of the kidney, is the third leading cause. Some of the other conditions that may affect the kidney are kidney stones, polycystic kidney disease, and cancer.

Urinary tract infections (UTIs), another common disorder of the urinary system, are more common in women than men. They are usually confined to the bladder (cystitis), and if they spread to the kidneys, they can lead to nephritis. Urinary incontinence, the loss of the ability to retain urine due to lack of sphincter control, is a health problem in older adults. An estimated 3 million older Americans suffer from this condition. Other types of bladder-control problems involve (1) overactive bladder, (2) stress incontinence, and (3) mixed symptoms. These conditions may affect men and women of all ages; it is estimated that 17 million Americans are affected by bladder problems.

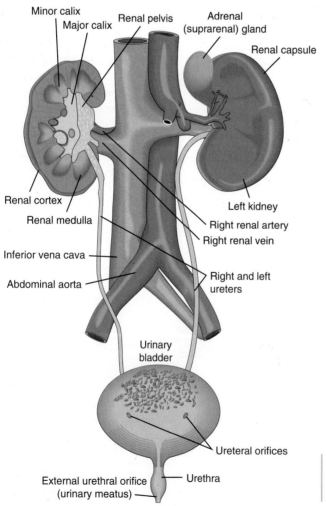

FIGURE 25-1

The organs of the urinary system

Source: Delmar/Cengage Learning

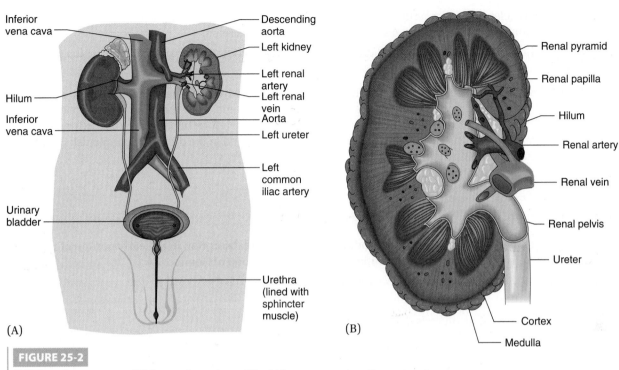

FIGURE 25-2

(A) The urinary system; (B) Internal structure of the kidney *Source: Delmar/Cengage Learning*

Kidney and urologic diseases continue to be one of the major causes of work loss among men and women. The National Kidney Foundation lists the following warning signs of kidney and urinary tract disease:

- Burning or difficulty during urination
- More frequent urination, particularly at night (nocturia)
- Passage of bloody-appearing urine (hematuria)
- Puffiness around eyes, swelling of hands and feet, especially in children
- Pain in small of back just below the ribs (not aggravated by movement)
- High blood pressure (hypertension)

Medications used to treat urinary system diseases and disorders described in this unit are diuretics, urinary tract antibacterials, urinary tract antiseptics, and miscellaneous agents.

DIURETICS

Diuretics decrease reabsorption of sodium chloride by the kidneys, thereby increasing the amount of salt and water excreted in the urine. This action reduces the amount of fluid retained in the body and prevents edema. Diuretics are classified according to site and mechanism of action.

- *Thiazide diuretics* appear to act by inhibiting sodium and chloride reabsorption in the early portion of the distal tubule. They may also block chloride reabsorption in the ascending loop of Henle.
- *Loop diuretics* act by inhibiting the reabsorption of sodium and chloride in the ascending loop of Henle.
- *Potassium-sparing diuretics* act by inhibiting the exchange of sodium for potassium in the distal tubule. They inhibit potassium excretion.
- *Osmotic diuretics* are agents that are capable of being filtered by the glomerulus, but have a limited capability of being reabsorbed into the bloodstream. Any increase in the concentration of osmotically

active particles in the glomerular filtrate is accompanied by retention of an equivalent amount of water in the tubular lumen, which increases the volume of urine excreted.

- *Carbonic anhydrase inhibitor diuretics* act to increase the excretion of bicarbonate ion, which carries out sodium, water, and potassium.

Diuretics are used in the treatment of congestive heart failure, hypertension, the nephrotic syndrome, chronic renal failure, idiopathic edema, diabetes insipidus, and glaucoma. They may also be used selectively for premenstrual syndrome. With most diuretics, potassium is excreted; therefore, bananas, prunes, raisins, oranges, orange juice, cereals, dried peas, and fresh vegetables should be included in the diet to help replenish potassium.

Selected diuretics are included in Table 25-1.

Thiazide Diuretics

Actions

Thiazide diuretics appear to act by inhibiting sodium and chloride reabsorption in the early portion of the distal tubule. They may also block chloride reabsorption in the ascending loop of Henle.

Uses

Use for edema, hypertension, diuresis.

Contraindications

Thiazide diuretics are contraindicated in patients who are known to be hypersensitive to any of the ingredients. They should not be used in anuria and/or renal decompensation.

> **Caution:**
>
> *Use with caution in patients with severe renal disease, impaired hepatic function, or progressive liver disease.*

Adverse Reactions

Reactions can include weakness, hypotension, orthostatic hypotension, pancreatitis, jaundice, diarrhea, vomiting, constipation, nausea, anorexia, aplastic anemia, agranulocytosis, leukopenia, hemolytic anemia, thrombocytopenia, electrolyte imbalance, hyperglycemia, glycosuria, hyperuricemia, muscle spasm, vertigo, dizziness, headache, restlessness, renal failure, blurred vision, xanthopsia, anaphylactic reactions, rash, urticaria, photosensitivity, and fever.

Dosage and Route

The dosage and route of administration are determined by the physician and individualized for each patient (see Table 25-1).

Implications for Patient Care

Observe patient for evidence of fluid or electrolyte imbalance. **Warning signs:** dryness of mouth, thirst, weakness, lethargy, drowsiness, restlessness, muscle pains or cramps, muscular fatigue, hypotension, oliguria, tachycardia, nausea, and vomiting. Monitor weight, intake and output ratio, blood pressure, respirations, and serum electrolytes.

TABLE 25-1   Diuretics

MEDICATION	CLASSIFICATION	USUAL DOSAGE	ADVERSE REACTIONS
acetazolamide (Diamox)	Carbonic anhydrase inhibitor	Oral: 250 to 375 mg once daily	Tingling in the extremities, loss of appetite, polyuria
amiloride	Potassium-sparing diuretic	Oral (Adult): 5 to 10 mg/day	Dizziness, headache, arrhythmias, constipation, photosensitivity, hyperkalemia
bendroflumethiazide	Thiazide diuretic	Oral: 2.5 to 5 mg/day following an initial dose of up to 20 mg	Anorexia, nausea, vomiting, dizziness
bumetanide (Bumex)	Loop diuretic	Oral (Adult): 0.5 to 2.0 mg as a single dose IM (Adult): 0.5 to 1.0 mg	Muscle cramps, dizziness, hypotension, headache, nausea, encephalopathy
chlorothiazide (Diuril)	Thiazide diuretic	Oral: 500 mg to 1 g 1 to 2 times/day	Weakness, anorexia, gastric irritation, hyperglycemia, purpura, muscle spasm
chlorthalidone (Thalitone)	Thiazide diuretic	Oral (Adult): 25 to 100 mg once daily	Dizziness, anorexia, hypotension, nausea, photosensitivity, hypokalemia, dehydration
furosemide (Lasix)	Loop diuretic	Oral (Adult): 20 to 80 mg as a single dose Oral (Child): 1 to 2 mg/kg 1 to 2 times/day	Anorexia, vertigo, purpura, hyperglycemia, anemia
glycerin/systemic (Glyrol) (Osmoglyn)	Osmotic diuretic	Oral (Adult): To lower eye pressure: 1 to 2 g/kg of body weight taken one time. Additional doses of 500 mg/kg every six hours may be taken if needed.	Headache, nausea, vomiting, diarrhea, dizziness, confusion, irregular heartbeat
hydrochlorothiazide	Thiazide diuretic	Oral (Adult): 50 mg to 100 mg 1 to 2 times/day Oral (Child): 1 mg/lb daily in 2 doses	Orthostatic hypotension, muscle spasm, pancreatitis, vertigo, aplastic anemia
indapamide	Thiazide diuretic	Oral (Adult): Hypertension: 1.25 to 5 mg daily in the morning	Dizziness, headache, arrhythmias, constipation, photosensitivity, hyperkalemia
methyclothiazide (Enduron)	Thiazide diuretic	Oral (Adult): 2.5 to 10 mg once daily Oral (Child): 0.05 to 0.2 mg/kg daily	Anorexia, nausea, vomiting, dizziness, headache, rash, leukopenia, hyperglycemia
metolazone	Thiazide-like diuretic	Oral (Adult): 0.5 to 1 mg/day	Drowsiness, nausea, hypotension, photosensitivity, hypokalemia
polythiazide	Thiazide diuretic	Oral (Adult): 1 to 4 mg daily	Anorexia, dizziness, purpura, leukopenia, hypoglycemia
spironolactone (Aldactone)	Potassium-sparing diuretic	Oral (Adult): 50 to 100 mg daily Oral (Child): 3.3 mg/kg in divided doses	Gynecomastia, cramping and diarrhea, drowsiness, rash, irregular menses

(continues)

TABLE 25-1 *(continued)*

MEDICATION	CLASSIFICATION	USUAL DOSAGE	ADVERSE REACTIONS

orsemide (Demadex)	Loop diuretic	Oral (Adult):
		Congestive heart failure:
		  10 to 20 mg once daily
		Chronic renal failure: 20 mg
		  once daily
		Hypertension: 5 mg once daily
			Dizziness, headache, ototoxicity, nausea hypotension, constipation, hypokalemia

triamterene (Dyrenium)	Potassium-sparing diuretic	Oral (Adult): 100 to 300 mg
		  daily in divided doses
		Oral (Child): 2 to 4 mg/kg
		  daily in divided doses
			Diarrhea, nausea, vomiting, weakness, headache, rash, dry mouth, anaphylaxis

Patient Teaching

Educate patients:

- to increase fluid intake to 2 to 3 liters per day unless contraindicated and to eat potassium-rich foods such as bananas, oranges, prunes, raisins, dried peas and beans, fresh vegetables, nuts, meats, and cereals.
- about warning signs of fluid or electrolyte imbalance.
- to contact the physician without delay if warning signs occur.
- that the medication should be taken in the morning to avoid nocturia. ■

Special Considerations

- Thiazide diuretics may increase blood sugar in diabetic patients. Dosage adjustment of oral hypoglycemic agents and insulin may be required.
- Use in pregnancy is not recommended.
- Alcohol, barbiturates, and narcotics may potentiate the occurrence of orthostatic hypotension.
- There may be an additive effect when taken with other antihypertensive agents.
- Electrolyte depletion may be intensified when taken with corticosteroids.
- Patients taking lithium should not take diuretics because they reduce the renal clearance of lithium and add a high risk of lithium toxicity.

Loop Diuretics

Actions

Loop diuretics act by inhibiting reabsorption of sodium and chloride in the proximal and distal tubules and in the ascending loop of Henle.

Uses

Use loop diuretics for edema, hypertension, and as adjunctive therapy in acute pulmonary embolism.

Contraindications

This medicine is contraindicated in patients who are known to be hypersensitive to any of the ingredients. They should not be used in patients with anuria, electrolyte depletion, hypovolemia, for infants, and during breast-feeding.

> ### ⚠ Caution:
>
> 1. *Lasix (furosemide) is a potent loop diuretic and, if given in excessive amounts, can lead to profound diuresis with water and electrolyte depletion. Careful medical supervision is required.*
> 2. *In patients with hepatic cirrhosis and ascites, drug therapy should be initiated in the hospital, after the basic condition is improved.*
> 3. *Ototoxicity has been reported and is usually associated with rapid injection, severe renal impairment, doses higher than recommended, and when given with other agents that cause ototoxicity.*

Adverse Reactions

Reactions include anorexia, jaundice, pancreatitis, diarrhea, cramping, constipation, nausea, vomiting, tinnitus, hearing loss, paresthesia, vertigo, dizziness, headache, blurred vision, xanthopsia, aplastic anemia, thrombocytopenia, leukopenia, purpura, photosensitivity, urticaria, rash, pruritus, orthostatic hypotension, hyperglycemia, glycosuria, muscle spasm, weakness, restlessness, thrombophlebitis, fever, and necrotizing angiitis.

Dosage and Route

The dosage and route of administration are determined by the physician and individualized for each patient (see Table 25-1).

Implications for Patient Care

Observe patients for evidence of fluid or electrolyte imbalance. Monitor weight, intake and output ratio, blood pressure, respirations, and serum electrolytes.

Patient Teaching

Educate patients:

- to increase fluid intake to 2 to 3 liters per day unless contraindicated and to eat potassium-rich foods.
- that potassium supplements may be prescribed by the physician.
- about warning signs of fluid and electrolyte imbalance.
- to contact the physician without delay if warning signs occur.
- that the medication should be taken in the morning to avoid nocturia. ▪

Special Considerations

- Loop diuretics may increase blood sugar in patients with diabetes. Dosage adjustment of oral hypoglycemic agents and insulin may be required.
- Some patients may be more sensitive to sunlight while taking loop diuretics.
- Use in pregnancy is not recommended.
- Loop diuretics may increase ototoxicity effect of aminoglycosides.
- Patients taking lithium should not take loop diuretics because they reduce the renal clearance of lithium and add a higher risk of lithium toxicity.

- There may be an additive effect when taken with other antihypertensive agents.
- Alcohol, barbiturates, and narcotics may potentiate the occurrence of orthostatic hypotension.

Potassium-Sparing Diuretics

Actions

Potassium-sparing diuretics exert their action in the distal tubule. They cause increased amounts of sodium and water to be excreted, while potassium is retained.

Uses

Use potassium-sparing diuretics in patients with edema, primary hyperaldosteronism, congestive heart failure, cirrhosis of the liver, essential hypertension, and hypokalemia.

Contraindications

These diuretics are contraindicated in patients who are known to be hypersensitive to any of the ingredients. They should not be used in patients with anuria, acute renal disease, or hyperkalemia, and during pregnancy or lactation.

> **Caution:**
>
> *Potassium supplements and foods rich in potassium should not generally be given with potassium-sparing diuretics. Hyperkalemia could occur. Also, most salt substitutes contain potassium salts, therefore cautious use should be followed.*

Adverse Reactions

Reactions can include gynecomastia, agranulocytosis, cramping, diarrhea, drowsiness, lethargy, headache, urticaria, rash, pruritus, mental confusion, drug fever, ataxia, impotence, irregular menses or amenorrhea, postmenopausal bleeding, hirsutism, gastritis, and vomiting.

Dosage and Route

The dosage and route of administration are determined by the physician and individualized for each patients (see Table 25-1).

Implications for Patient Care

Observe patient for evidence of fluid and electrolyte imbalance. Monitor cardiac function and be alert for signs of hyperkalemia: nausea, diarrhea, muscle weakness, marked ECG changes (elevated T waves, depressed P waves), atrial systole, slow irregular pulse, ventricular fibrillation, and cardiac arrest. Treatment of hyperkalemia: IV administration of 20 percent to 50 percent glucose and 0.25 to 0.5 units of regular insulin per gram of glucose. Assess weight, intake and output ratio, vital signs, serum electrolytes, and mental status.

Patient Teaching

Educate patients:

- not to take potassium supplements or eat foods rich in potassium.
- that the medication may cause drowsiness, mental confusion, gynecomastia, and menstrual irregularities.

- about the warning signs of fluid and electrolyte imbalance.
- to contact the physician without delay if warning signs occur. ■

Special Considerations

- Excessive potassium intake may cause hyperkalemia in patients taking potassium-sparing diuretics.
- When used in combination with other diuretics or antihypertensive agents, potassium-sparing diuretics potentiate their effects. Dosage of such drugs, particularly the ganglionic blocking agents, should be reduced by 50 percent.
- Severe hyperkalemia may occur when ACE inhibitors or indomethacin is administered concurrently with potassium-sparing diuretics.
- Reduces the vascular response to norepinephrine; therefore, cautious use in patients undergoing regional or general anesthesia should be the rule.
- Potassium-sparing diuretics increase the half-life of digoxin; therefore, patients receiving any form of digitalis should be monitored very carefully while taking any potassium-sparing diuretic.

Osmotic Diuretics

Actions

Osmotic diuretics are agents that are capable of being filtered by the glomerulus, but have a limited capability of being reabsorbed into the bloodstream. They act by increasing the osmolality of the plasma, glomerular filtrate, and tubular fluid, thereby increasing the excretion of water, chloride, sodium, and potassium.

Uses

Use to prevent acute renal failure during trauma or prolonged surgery; to prevent increased cerebral, cerebrospinal, or intraocular pressures during trauma, surgery, or disease; and to reduce intraocular pressure in acute glaucoma.

Contraindications

Osmotic diuretics are contraindicated in patients who are known to be hypersensitive to any of the ingredients. They should not be used in anuria, diagnosed acute renal failure, cardiac dysfunction, congestive heart failure, active intracranial hemorrhage, severe dehydration, or severe pulmonary congestion.

Adverse Reactions

Reactions can include marked diuresis, urinary retention, thirst, dizziness, headache, convulsions, nausea, vomiting, dry mouth, diarrhea, thrombophlebitis, hypotension, hypertension, tachycardia, angina-like chest pains, fever, chills, pulmonary congestion, fluid, electrolyte imbalance, dehydration, loss of hearing, blurred vision, nasal congestion, and decreased intraocular pressure.

Dosage and Route

The dosage and route of administration are determined by the physician and individualized for each patient (see Table 25-1).

Implications for Patient Care

Observe patient for evidence of fluid or electrolyte imbalance and signs of circulatory overload. Monitor weight, intake and output ratio, vital signs, and serum electrolytes. Observe IV administration sites for signs of local irritation, extravasation, or thrombophlebitis.

Patient Teaching

Educate patients:

- to increase fluid intake to 2 to 3 liters per day unless contraindicated.
- that sucking on ice chips or hard candy will help relieve thirst. ■

Special Considerations

- Parenteral mannitol crystallizes at low temperatures. Store at 59°F to 89°F, unless otherwise ordered. Do not allow it to freeze. If the medication crystallizes, warm it in a hot-water bath and shake container vigorously, then allow the solution to return to room temperature before administration.
- Do not add whole blood to IV lines used for mannitol.
- Do not mix this medication with any other drug or solution.

Carbonic Anhydrase Inhibitor Diuretics

Actions

Carbonic anhydrase inhibititor diuretics act to promote the reabsorption of sodium and bicarbonate from the proximal tubules. They block the action of the enzyme carbonic anhydrase (found in the kidneys, eyes, and other organs), thereby reversing the hydration of carbon dioxide and producing a bicarbonate diuresis that promotes the excretion of water, sodium, and potassium. These effects also decrease the formation of aqueous humor, thus reducing intraocular pressure.

Uses

For adjunctive therapy of chronic simple (open-angle) glaucoma, secondary glaucoma, and preoperatively in acute angle-closure glaucoma where delay of surgery is desired to lower intraocular pressure.

Contraindications

Carbonic anhydrase inhibitor diuretics are contraindicated in patients who are known to be hypersensitive to any of the ingredients. They should not be used in patients with hepatic insufficiency, renal failure, adrenocortical insufficiency, hyperchloremic acidosis, in conditions where serum levels of sodium and potassium are depressed, or in severe pulmonary obstruction.

Adverse Reactions

Reactions include anorexia, nausea, vomiting, drowsiness, paresthesia, ataxia, tremor, tinnitus, headache, weakness, nervousness, depression, confusion, dizziness, constipation, hepatic insufficiency, loss of weight, electrolyte imbalance, metabolic acidosis, skin eruptions, pruritus, fever, agranulocytosis, thrombocytopenia, frequency of urination, renal colic, renal calculi, and phosphaturia.

Dosage and Route

The dosage and route of administration are determined by the physician and individualized for each patient (see Table 25-1).

Implications for Patient Care

Observe patient for evidence of fluid or electrolyte imbalance. Monitor weight, intake and output ratio, vital signs, and serum electrolytes. Administer medication by mouth or IV if possible, because administration by IM injection is painful. Monitor patient for signs of metabolic acidosis.

Patient Teaching

Educate patients:

- to increase fluid intake to 2 to 3 liters per day unless contraindicated.
- to eat potassium-rich foods.
- to avoid hazardous activities if drowsiness or dizziness occurs.
- about warning signs of fluid or electrolyte imbalance.
- to contact the physician without delay if warning signs occur.
- that the medication should be taken in the morning to avoid nocturia.
- that any eye pain should be reported to the physician without delay. ■

Special Considerations

- If serum potassium is below 3.0, potassium supplements are needed.
- Use caution in patients receiving high doses of aspirin, and during pregnancy and lactation.
- Watch for signs and symptoms metabolic acidosis: headache, fatigue, hypotension, anorexia, nausea, vomiting, dysrhythmia, drowsiness, confusion, seizures, coma, and Kussmaul's respirations.

Spotlight

Urinary Tract Infections: Cystitis

Cystitis is an inflammation of the urinary bladder. The urinary bladder is a muscular, membranous sac that serves as a reservoir for urine. It is located in the anterior portion of the pelvic cavity and consists of a lower portion, the neck, which is continuous with the urethra, and an upper portion, the apex, which is connected to the umbilicus by the median umbilical ligament. The urethra is the musculomembranous tube extending from the bladder to the outside of the body. The external urinary opening is the urinary meatus. The male urethra is approximately 8 inches long and the female urethra is approximately 1.5 inches long.

Each year, in the United States, approximately 10 million patients seek treatment for urinary tract infections, with cystitis being the most common. Cystitis is most often caused by an ascending infection from the urethra and it is more common in the female because the short length of the urethra promotes the transmission of bacteria from the skin and genitals to the internal bladder. The most common type of bacteria that causes cystitis in the female is Escherichia coli (*E. coli*), the colon bacillus. This bacillus is constantly present in the alimentary canal and is normally nonpathogenic, but when it enters the urinary tract and is transmitted to the bladder, it can cause infection. Cystitis in men is usually secondary to some other type of infection such as epididymitis, prostatitis, gonorrhea, syphilis, or kidney stones.

Symptoms

Urgency
Pyuria
Chills and fever
Burning sensation and pain during urination

Frequency

Hematuria

Pain or spasm in the region of the bladder and pelvic area

Diagnosis

History of symptoms

Microscopic urinalysis

Urine culture

Dipstick

Gram stain

Treatment

Treatment of cystitis usually consists of taking an antibiotic or antibacterial agent for a specified number of times and days, depending on the type of infection and its severity. The sulfonamides and antibiotics such as penicillins, cephalosporins, tetracyclines, and aminoglycosides are generally the drugs of first choice. Always ask patients if they are allergic to any medication before the initiation of drug therapy. *Note:* If there is any question about a person's hypersensitivity to an antibiotic or sulfa drugs, an appropriate skin test should be performed before the initiation of drug therapy.

Patients should be informed about possible adverse reactions to the prescribed medication and be instructed to report any signs to their physician. Advise patients to take the medication as prescribed until all of the drug has been taken.

Interstitial Cystitis

Interstitial cystitis (IC) is a painful inflammation of the bladder wall. Approximately 450,000 people suffer from this condition and 90 percent are women. Research showed that the median age of onset was 40, with many women experiencing symptoms as early as their twenties and thirties.

Symptoms can vary from mild to severe and are similar to a urinary tract infection (cystitis). There is usually pelvic pain and pressure, and frequent urination, sometimes as often as 50 times a day. Diagnosis is difficult because the standard blood tests, urine tests, and X-rays come up negative. The cause is unknown and IC does not respond to antibiotic therapy. Women with IC often live in chronic pain. They are always tired because they have to go to the bathroom so often, and their sexual, social, and work life is affected.

For a referral to a database center, send a self-addressed, stamped, business-size envelope to the Interstitial Cystitis Association, P.O. Box 1553, Madison Square Station, New York, NY 10159.

Guidelines to Help Avoid Cystitis (Female)

- Drink plenty of fluids (8 glasses or more a day).
- To avoid contaminating the urinary meatus, females should wipe themselves from front to back.
- Females who have repeated infections (cystitis) should drink a glass of water before engaging in sexual intercourse and then urinate right after intercourse. This helps flush out any bacteria that may have entered the urethra.
- Have your sexual partner wear a condom.
- Do not use vaginal deodorants, bubble baths, colored toilet paper, and other substances that could cause irritation to the urinary meatus.
- Wear cotton underclothes and keep the genital area dry.

▪▪ Special Considerations: **OLDER ADULTS**

As aging occurs, the kidneys may lose mass as blood vessels degenerate. The loss of glomerular capillaries causes a decrease in glomerular filtration and the kidneys lose their ability to conserve water and sodium. Additionally, the tubules of the aging kidneys diminish their capacity for conserving base and ridding the body of excess hydrogen ions. Because the renal system helps to regulate acid-base balance, fluid and electrolyte imbalance may occur quickly in older adults.

During the fourth decade, the kidneys begin to decrease in size and function. By the eighth decade, the kidneys have generally shrunk 30 percent and have lost a proportionate amount of function. If stressed, kidneys respond more slowly to changes in one's internal environment. Some causes of stressful situations that may cause the kidneys to respond more slowly and contribute to fluid and electrolyte imbalance are:

- Vomiting and diarrhea
- Fever
- Diuretics
- Decreased fluid intake
- Surgery
- Renal damage from medications

When assessing urinary system disorders or diseases in the older adult, it is important to assess the patient's voiding history and medication history. Fluid intake and output should be carefully monitored, because older adults who are having urinary problems, such as dribbling urine or losing urine when coughing or sneezing, may be limiting their fluid intake in an attempt to control the symptoms. This self-imposed fluid restriction can cause dehydration, or water and electrolyte imbalance. The older adult who takes many medications (polypharmacy) may be at a higher risk of developing nephrotoxicity.

> **Note:** Signs of nephrotoxicity are oliguria and proteinuria. Because many medications are metabolized by the liver and then excreted via the kidneys, it is important that older adults be informed of these signs and have renal function tests performed on a regular basis.

▪▪ Special Considerations: **CHILDREN**

In children, the kidneys are more susceptible to trauma because children usually do not have as much fat padding as adults. Children who are 1 to 2 years old have a lower glomerular filtration and absorption rate than older children or adults. Infants are more prone to fluid volume changes that can result in excess fluid or dehydration. Additionally, infants do not concentrate urine.

Urinary tract infections are common in children. The microorganisms *Escherichia coli*, *Klebsiella*, and *Proteus* cause most urinary tract infections seen in children. *Escherichia coli* is the most common cause, contributing to 75 percent to 90 percent of the infections. Except during the neonatal period, girls are more prone to UTIs than boys. This is because of the shorter urethra of the female, and the location of the urethra near the anus.

The signs and symptoms of urinary tract infection are age related:

- **Infants**—fever, loss of weight, nausea, vomiting, increased urination, foul-smelling urine, persistent diaper rash, failure to thrive.
- **Older children**—increased urination (frequency), pain during urination, abdominal pain, hematuria.

- **Other indications** of infection—bed-wetting in a "trained children." When the kidneys are involved, fever, chills, and flank pain may be present.
- **No apparent indications**—some children do not exhibit any symptoms.

Diagnosis is based upon a urine culture and the presence of bacteria in the urine. When a urinary tract infection is diagnosed, treatment should begin immediately to prevent the possible development of pyelonephritis. Treatment of cystitis usually consists of taking an antibiotic or antibacterial agent for a specified number of times and days, depending on the type of infection and its severity. A careful assessment of the child's allergies, body weight, and body surface area are essential before the initiation of drug therapy. The dosage prescribed must be individualized for each child. Parents should be informed of possible adverse reactions to the prescribed medication and told to report any signs to the physician. Advise parents to be sure to give the medication as ordered, and to complete the drug regimen for the specified number of days.

■ Critical Thinking **QUESTIONS AND ACTIVITIES**

Your patient is a 30-year-old female who complains of urinary frequency and urgency. She states that she has pain in her pelvic area and that it burns and "hurts" when she uses the bathroom. Ask yourself:

- What do these symptoms indicate?
- What diagnostic tests might the physician order to determine the cause of the patient's symptoms?
- After the diagnosis is determined, what treatment regimen will the patient most likely be placed on?
- With regards to a medication history, what questions should be asked of this patient?
- What information should you give the patient about a prescribed medication regimen?
- What are some guidelines that you could use to explain ways this patient could possibly help avoid the cause(s) of her symptoms?

URINARY TRACT ANTIBACTERIALS

Sulfonamides are among the drugs of choice for treating acute, uncomplicated urinary tract infections, especially those caused by *Escherichia coli* and Proteus mirabilis bacterial strains. The sulfonamides may be classified according to the length of time they remain in the body. Using this criterion, these drugs can be separated into three groupings: short-, intermediate-, and long-acting sulfonamides. The short-acting sulfonamides are used in the treatment of urinary infections because they are rapidly absorbed, can be terminated quickly if adverse reactions occur, and produce high levels of the drug in urine. See Table 25-2 for selected sulfonamides and antibacterials.

Sulfonamides

Actions

Sulfonamides exert a bacteriostatic effect against a wide range of gram-positive and gram-negative microorganisms. They prevent the growth of microorganisms by inhibiting the production of dihydrofolic acid in the bacterial cells by competing with para-aminobenzoic acid (PABA).

Uses

Use sulfonamides with acute, recurrent, or chronic urinary tract infections due to susceptible organisms (*Escherichia coli, Klebsiella-enterobacter, staphylococcus, Proteus mirabilis,* and *Proteus vulgaris*). Also use in meningococcal meningitis, acute otitis media, trachoma, inclusion conjunctivitis, nocardiosis, and chancroid.

Contraindications

Sulfonamides are contraindicated in patients who are known to be hypersensitive to any of the ingredients. They should not be used in infants less than 2 months of age, or during pregnancy and breast-feeding.

TABLE 25-2 Selected Sulfonamides

MEDICATION	USUAL DOSAGE	ADVERSE REACTIONS
sulfadiazine (Microsulfon)	Oral (Adult): 2 to 4 g initially, then 0.5 to 1 g every 6 hours times 10 days Oral (Child): 75 mg/kg initially, then 150 mg/kg in 4 to 6 divided doses	Nausea, vomiting, headache, confusion, drug fever, headache, blood dyscrasias
sulfamethoxazole	Oral (Adult): 1 to 2 g initially, then 1 g two times a day Oral (Child—over 2 months): 50 to 60 mg/kg initially, then 25 to 30 mg/kg two times a day (maximum 75 mg/kg/day)	Blood dyscrasias, hemolysis, drug fever, rash, nausea, vomiting, headache
sulfisoxazole	Oral (Adult): 2 to 4 g initially, then 1 to 2 g every 4 to 6 hours Oral (Child): 75 mg/kg initially, then 150 mg/kg/day in divided doses every 4 hours (maximum, 6 g daily)	Agranulocytosis, erythema multiform, nausea, emesis, headache, drug fever, chills
MIXTURES trimethoprim and sulfamethoxazole (Bactrim) (Septra)	Oral (Adult): 2 tablets or 4 teaspoons (20 mL) of suspension every 12 hours for 10 to 14 days Oral (Child): 8 mg/kg of trimethoprim and 40 mg/kg of sulfamethoxazole daily in 2 divided doses every 12 hours for 10 days	Blood dyscrasias, nausea, vomiting, anorexia, rash, urticaria

Caution:

Sulfinomides should not be used for the treatment of group A beta-hemolytic streptococcal infections.

Adverse Reactions

Reactions include agranulocytosis, aplastic anemia, myocarditis, serum sickness, hemolytic anemia, purpura, anaphylaxis, hepatitis, pancreatitis, nausea, vomiting, abdominal pain, diarrhea, anorexia, convulsions, peripheral neuritis, ataxia, vertigo, headache, tinnitus, depression, apathy, arthralgia, myalgia, edema, fever, chills, weakness, fatigue, insomnia, and photosensitivity.

Dosage and Route

The dosage and route of administration are determined by the physician and individualized for each patient (see Table 25-2).

Implications for Patient Care

Before initiating drug therapy, make sure that patients are not allergic to sulfonamides. Monitor patients for any adverse reactions, especially for signs that may indicate serious reactions or blood dyscrasia (fever, sore throat, arthralgia, cough, shortness of breath, pallor, purpura, or jaundice). Monitor intake and output ratio and kidney function studies, and note the color, character, and pH of the patient's urine.

Patient Teaching

Educate patients:

- to drink plenty of fluids.
- to take the medication with 8 ounces of water.
- to take the medication as ordered and for the full-time period to prevent superimposed infection.
- to avoid direct sunlight, as one may be more sensitive to burns and photosensitivity while taking sulfonamides.
- not to take over-the-counter medications that contain aspirin and vitamin C unless prescribed by a physician.
- about signs of serious adverse reactions.
- to contact a physician without delay if signs of serious adverse reactions occur.
- that sulfonamides may decrease the effectiveness of oral contraceptives. Therefore, one may choose to use additional methods of birth control.
- that some sulfonamide preparations may produce orange-yellow discoloration of the urine. ■

Special Considerations

- Sulfonamides may decrease the absorption of digoxin; therefore, serum digoxin levels should be carefully monitored and dosage adjustment made as necessary.
- Sulfonamides can potentiate the blood sugar lowering activity of sulfonylurea. Blood glucose levels should be monitored and dosage adjustment made as necessary.
- Sulfonamides may increase the anticoagulant effect of warfarin agents. Coagulation time should be monitored and dosage adjustment made as necessary.
- Sulfonamides can displace methotrexate from plasma protein-binding sites, thereby increasing free methotrexate concentrations.

URINARY TRACT ANTISEPTICS

The urinary antiseptics, although used against urinary tract infections, are not usually drugs of first choice in such treatments. The sulfonamides and antibiotics such as penicillins, cephalosporins, tetracyclines, and aminoglycosides are generally the drugs of first choice that are used to treat urinary tract infections.

Urinary antiseptics are most often used in patients who are either intolerant of or unresponsive to one of the first-choice antibiotics. They are also used for the control of chronic urinary infections due to microorganisms that have developed resistance to other drugs.

Actions

Urinary antiseptics may inhibit the growth of microorganisms by bactericidal, bacteriostatic, anti-infective, or antibacterial action.

Uses

Treatment of acute and chronic upper and lower urinary tract infections, asymptomatic bacteriuria caused by susceptible strains of *Escherichia coli, Proteus mirabilis, Morganella morganii, Providencia rettgeri, Proteus vulgaris, Pseudomonas, Enterobacter,* and *Enterococci.*

Contraindications

These antiseptics are contraindicated in patients who are known to be hypersensitive to any of the ingredients. They should not be used in patients with anuria, renal insufficiency, severe dehydration, pregnancy, and lactation. Certain urinary tract antiseptics are contraindicated in children and patients with convulsive disorders, anemia, diabetes, or chronic lung disease.

Adverse Reactions

The adverse reactions of urinary antiseptics are listed according to the drug (see Table 25-3).

Dosage and Route

The dosage and route of administration are determined by the physician and individualized for each patient (see Table 25-3).

Implications for Patient Care

Observe the patient for signs of improvement or adverse reactions. Monitor intake and output ratio, vital signs, culture and sensitivity tests.

Methenamine yields formaldehyde in the presence of an acidic urine, which helps suppress the growth and multiplication of bacteria.

Ascorbic acid may be prescribed to help maintain the acidity of urine. Ascorbic acid tablets should not be crushed as they allow the formation of formaldehyde in the stomach, resulting in nausea and belching.

TABLE 25-3   Urinary Antiseptics

MEDICATION	USUAL DOSAGE	ADVERSE REACTIONS
ciprofloxacin (Cipro)	Oral (Adult): 250 to 500 mg every 12 hours	CNS stimulation, superinfection, nausea, diarrhea, vomiting, GI discomfort, headache, restlessness, rash, crystalluria
methenamine (Hiprex)	Oral (Adult): 1 g 4 times/day after meals and at bedtime Oral (Child 6 to 12): one-half the adult dose as shown above	Mild gastric irritation, rash, headache, nausea, vomiting
nalidixic acid (NegGram)	Oral (Adult): 4 g/day in 4 divided doses for 2 weeks, reduced to 2 g per day for long-term therapy Oral (Child under 12): 55 mg/kg/day in 4 divided doses	Headache, malaise, weakness, convulsions, photosensitivity, nausea, vomiting
nitrofurantoin (Furadantin) (Macrodantin)	Oral (Adult): 50 to 100 mg 4 times/day Oral (Child): 5 to 7 mg/kg/24 hours in 4 divided doses (dose reduced by half if continued past 10 days)	Nausea, vomiting, diarrhea, fever, rash, urticaria
norfloxacin (Noroxin)	Oral (Adult): 400 mg twice a day for 7 to 10 days. Take 1 hr before or 2 hrs after meals with 8 ounces of water.	Crystalluria, dizziness, nausea, headache
trimethoprim	Oral (Adult): 100 to 200 mg every 24 hours for 10 days	Rash, pruritus, GI discomfort, blood dyscrasias, drug fever, liver and renal disorders, exfoliative dermatitis

Patient Teaching

Educate patients:

- to increase fluid intake to 2 to 3 liters per day unless contraindicated.
- to report any signs of adverse reactions.
- to take medication as prescribed until all of the drug has been taken. (It is most important that patients understand this, as many times once the patients start to feel better, they may discontinue taking the drug, causing a relapse to occur.)
- about proper personal hygienic practices. ■

Special Considerations

- A culture and sensitivity test should be performed prior to the initiation of drug therapy to determine the causative type of microorganism.
- Medication must be taken in equal intervals, day and night, to maintain proper blood levels.

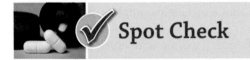 **Spot Check**

There are several medications that may be used to treat urinary tract infections. For each of the selected drugs, give the usual dosage and several adverse reactions:

DRUG	USUAL DOSAGE	ADVERSE REACTIONS
Cipro (ciprofloxacin)		
Furadantin (nitrofurantoin)		
Sulfisoxazole		
Hiprex (methenamine)		
Phenazopyridine		

MISCELLANEOUS AGENTS

Miscellaneous agents are used to treat disorders of the lower urinary tract. These agents either stimulate, inhibit, or relax smooth muscle activity and help control involuntary contractions of the bladder muscle. These actions help improve the functions of the urinary bladder, such as storage of urine and its subsequent excretion from the body. See Table 25-4 for selected agents used for urologic disorders.

TABLE 25-4 Drugs Used for Urologic Disorders

MEDICATION	CLASSIFICATION	USUAL DOSAGE	ADVERSE REACTIONS
bethanechol chloride (Duvoid) (Urecholine)	Facilitates bladder emptying	Oral (Adult): 25 mg every 6 hours	Flushing, headache, nausea, vomiting, diarrhea, sweating, salivation
dimethyl sulfoxide (Rimso-50)	Treatment of interstitial cystitis	Intravesical instillation: 50 mL of a 50% solution into the bladder	Garlic-like taste and odor
flavoxate HCl (Urispas)	Reduces dysuria, nocturia, and urinary frequency	Oral (Adult): 100 to 200 mg 3 to 4 times/day	Nausea, vomiting, dryness of the mouth, nervousness, blurred vision, vertigo
hyoscyamine sulfate (Cystospaz-M) (Levsin)	Relaxes smooth muscle bladder spasm	Oral (Adult): 1 capsule every 12 hours	Dryness of the mouth, photophobia, constipation
imipramine HCl (Tofranil)	Treatment of nocturnal enuresis in children	Oral (Child): 10 mg nightly for 1 week or as needed	Drowsiness, dryness of the mouth, constipation, nausea, blurred vision
oxybutynin chloride (Ditropan XL)	Relaxes the muscles in the bladder, thereby decreasing the occurrence of wetting accidents	Oral (Adult): one 5-mg tablet once a day	Dry mouth, constipation, sleepiness, headache, diarrhea, nausea, loss of energy, dizziness
pentosan polysulfate (Elmiron)	Exact mechanism of action is unkown; used for the relief of bladder pain or discomfort associated with interstitial cystitis	Oral (Adult): 300 mg/day taken as one 100-mg capsule 3 times a day. Should be taken with water and at least 1 hour before meals or 2 hours after meals	Diarrhea, sodium nausea, dizziness, alopecia (reversible), headache, rash, dyspepsia, abdominal pain, liver function abnormalities
phenazopyridine HCl	Analgesic, anesthetic action on the urinary tract mucosa	Oral (Adult): 200 mg 3 times a day after meals. Stains urine and fabric red-orange	Headache, rash, GI discomfort, hemolytic anemia, renal and hepatic toxicity (*Note:* phenazopyridine may cause the sclera to turn yellow; this may indicate an accumulation of the drug due to decreased renal function.)
tolterodine tartrate (Detrol)	Helps control involuntary contractions of the bladder muscle	Oral (Adult): 2-mg tablet 2 times a day. May be lowered to 1-mg tablet 2 times a day	Dry mouth, headache, constipation, indigestion, dry eyes

SELECTED AGENTS THAT DISCOLOR URINE

Agent	*Color of Urine*
Aldomet (methyldopa)	red to black
Aralen (chloroquine)	rust-yellow to brown
Azulfidine (sulfasalazine)	orange-yellow
Coumadin sodium (warfarin sodium)	orange
Desferal (deferoxamine mesylate)	red
Dilantin (phenytoin)	pink or red to red-brown
Dopar (levodopa)	darkening of urine upon standing
Dyrenium (triamterene)	pale blue fluorescence
Flagyl (metronidazole)	darkened urine
Furadantin (nitrofurantoin)	rust-yellow or brownish
Furoxone (furazolidone)	brown, orange-brown
Indocin (indomethacin)	green
Iron (IV)	blackening
Macrodantin (nitrofurantoin)	rust-yellow or brownish
Phenazopyridine HCl	red or orange
Rifadin (rifampin)	bright red-orange
Robaxin (methocarbamol)	brown to black to green upon standing
Sulfonamides	rust-yellow or brownish
Vitamin B_2 (riboflavin)	yellow

■ ■ REVIEW QUESTIONS

Directions. Select the best answer to each of the following multiple-choice questions, circling the letter of your choice:

1. A local or generalized collection of fluid in the body tissues is known as _____.
   a. excretion
   b. emia
   c. edema
   d. secretion

2. Diuretics are agents that _____.
   a. increase reabsorption of sodium chloride in the kidneys
   b. decrease reabsorption of sodium chloride in the kidneys
   c. increase the amount of fluid retained in the body
   d. decrease the amount of salt and water excreted in the urine

3. Potassium-sparing diuretics exert their action in the _____.
   a. distal tubule
   b. loop of Henle
   c. proximal tubule
   d. glomerulus

4. The leading cause of chronic kidney failure is _____.
   a. hypertension
   b. glomerulonephritis
   c. polycystic kidney disease
   d. diabetes mellitus (Type 2)

5. Adverse reactions to furosemide (Lasix) are _____.

   a. hypoglycemia, headache, rash

   b. anorexia, vertigo, purpura, hyperglycemia, anemia

   c. dry mouth, gynecomastia, diarrhea

   d. polydipsia, chills, fever

6. _____ are among the drugs of choice for treating acute, uncomplicated urinary tract infections.

   a. Urinary antiseptics   c. Sulfonamides

   b. Diuretics   d. none of these

7. The National Kidney Foundation lists warning signs of kidney and urinary tract disease. All of the following are included in this list except _____.

   a. tachycardia

   b. burning or difficulty during urination

   c. nocturia

   d. hematuria

8. Adverse reactions to ciprofloxacin (Cipro) are _____.

   a. constipation, pruritus, drug fever

   b. liver and renel disorders

   c. urticaria, convulsions, photosensitivity

   d. CNS stimulation, superinfection, nausea, diarrhea, headache.

9. Adverse reactions to chlorothiazide (Diuril) are _____.

   a. decreased blood pressure and blurred vision

   b. drowsiness and constipation

   c. weakness, anorexia, gastric irritation, and purpura

   d. nausea and vomiting

10. Two vital functions of the kidneys are _____.

    a. production of urine

    b. regulation of water, electrolytes, and other substances

    c. excretion of urine

    d. a and b

11. Individuals who take diuretics should include foods that are rich in _____ in their diet.

    a. sodium   c. chloride

    b. potassium   d. iron

12. The functional units of the kidneys are called _____.

    a. neurons   c. glomerulus

    b. nephrons   d. Bowman's capsule

13. Disorders of the urinary system may be caused by _____.

    a. infection   c. dysfunction

    b. damage   d. all of these

14. Blood undergoes a process of _____ and _____ as it passes through the kidneys.

    a. dilution and absorption   c. filtration and reabsorption

    b. filtration and absorption   d. none of these

15. Thiazide diuretics appear to act by inhibiting _____ and _____ reabsorption in the early portion of the distal tubule.

    a. potassium and chloride   c. sodium and chloride

    b. potassium and sodium   d. calcium and sodium

16. Osmotic diuretics are agents that are capable of being filtered by the _____.

    a. distal tubule   c. glomerulus

    b. loop of Henle   d. proximal tubule

17. Carbonic anhydrase inhibitor diuretics act to promote the reabsorption of _____ and _____ from the proximal tubule.

    a. potassium and chloride

    b. potassium and sodium

    c. sodium and chloride

    d. sodium and bicarbonate

18. Diuretics may be used in the treatment of _____.

    a. congestive heart failure

    b. hypertension

    c. idiopathic edema

    d. all of these

19. Foods rich in potassium include _____.

    a. bananas, prunes, raisins, oranges, and fresh vegetables

    b. milk, cheese, and other dairy products

    c. butter, breads, and nuts

    d. none of these

Matching. Place the correct letter from Column II on the appropriate line of Column I:

	Column I		*Column II*
20.	_C_ edema	A.	a species of enteric bacilli that may cause urinary tract infections
21.	_D_ excretion	B.	a disease of the basement membrane of the glomerulus
22.	_E_ *escherichia coli*	C.	swelling
23.	_b_ nephrotic syndrome	D.	the process of eliminating waste products from the body
24.	_a_ *proteus mirabilis*	E.	a type of bacteria that is commonly found in the alimentary canal of humans and other animals
25.	_g_ Lasix	F.	antibacterial
		G.	diuretic

UNIT 26
Medications Used in Treatment of Endocrine Disorders

OBJECTIVES

Upon completing this unit, you should be able to:

- Define the terms listed in the vocabulary.
- Give the location and functions of the primary endocrine glands.
- State the actions, uses, contraindications, adverse reactions, dosage and route, implications for patient care, patient teaching, and special considerations for thyroid hormones, antithyroid hormones, insulin, and oral hypoglycemic agents.
- Describe diabetes mellitus.
- Contrast the signs and symptoms of hypoglycemia and hyperglycemia.
- Describe some risk factors associated with older adults developing diabetes.
- Explain why drug therapy may present special problems for older adults.
- Explain why the management of diabetes mellitus during childhood is most difficult.
- Describe some of the factors associated with the management of diabetes in children.
- Complete the critical thinking questions and activities presented in the unit.
- List the types of insulin preparations according to rapid-acting, short-acting, intermediate-acting, and long-acting.
- State why hyperglycemic agents are used and give examples.
- Complete the Spot Check on insulin.
- Answer the review questions correctly.

VOCABULARY

acromegaly (ak"ro-meg'a-le). A condition in which there is enlargement of the extremities and certain head bones, accompanied by enlargement of the nose and lips caused by excessive growth hormone.

cretinism (kre'tin-ism). A congenital condition that is due to a deficiency in the secretion of thyroid hormones. There is arrested physical and mental development.

diabetes insipidus (di"a-be'tez in-sip'e-dus). A condition caused by inadequate secretion of vasopressin or antidiuretic hormone (ADH). Classic symptoms are polyuria and polydipsia.

diabetes mellitus (di"a-be'tez mel-i'tus). A disorder of carbohydrate metabolism. Classic symptoms are polyuria, polydipsia, and polyphagia. Also glycosuria and hyperglycemia.

dwarfism (dwar'fizm). A condition of being abnormally small caused by deficiency of growth hormone.

gigantism (ji'gan-tizm). A condition in which there is excessive development of the body or of a body part caused by overproduction of growth hormone.

myxedema (miks"e-de'ma). An acquired condition (in older children and adults) that is due to a deficiency in the secretion of thyroid hormones.

sulfonylurea (sul"fo-nil-u're-ah). A class of chemical compounds that includes oral hypoglycemia agents.

473

INTRODUCTION

The primary glands of the endocrine system are the pituitary, the thyroid, the parathyroids, the pancreas (islets of Langerhans), the adrenals, the testes, and the ovaries (see Figure 26-1). This unit covers each of these glands, with the exception of the testes and ovaries, which are discussed as parts of the reproductive system in Unit 28.

The ductless glands of the endocrine system secrete chemical substances, known as *hormones*, directly into the bloodstream. Each of the endocrine glands performs an important part in growth, development, and maintenance of normal body functions. The hormones secreted by these glands act as chemical transmitters that either stimulate or inhibit specific organs of the body. When abnormal production of hormones occurs (too little or too much), the resultant disorders can be life-threatening.

THE PITUITARY

The *pituitary* is a small gland located at the base of the brain. Sometimes called the *master gland*, the pituitary secretes hormones that are essential for the body's growth and development and the regulation of actions by other endocrine glands. Pituitary hormones are grouped according to the lobe of the gland in which they originate.

An improperly functioning pituitary gland can be caused by a genetic condition or it may be the result of injury, surgery, tumors, or radiation. Disorders of the pituitary relate to the overproduction or underproduction of certain hormones.

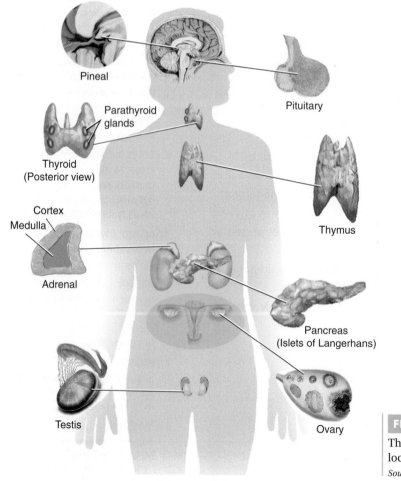

FIGURE 26-1

The endocrine glands and their locations in the body

Source: Delmar/Cengage Learning

- Hyperpituitarism occurs with the *overproduction* of hormones and can cause gigantism if the condition is present prior to puberty. If hyperpituitarism occurs after puberty, the feet, hands, and face show overgrowth and the resultant condition is known as acromegaly. The overproduction of pituitary hormones is often associated with the presence of a tumor. Treatment may involve radiation, chemotherapy, or surgery.

- Hypopituitarism occurs with the *underproduction* of hormones by the gland. An inadequate supply of pituitary hormones can cause dwarfism in developing children, as well as poor growth and function of the thyroid gland, the sex glands, and the adrenal cortex. Somatropin (Asellacrin) is administered to individuals with this condition following careful screening.

- Diabetes insipidus occurs with the underproduction or absence of the hormone *vasopressin*, also known as antidiuretic hormone (ADH). This condition should not be confused with diabetes mellitus, and is treated by the administration of natural and synthetic substances (vasopressin, Lypressin) that produce antidiuretic hormone activity.

THE THYROID

The thyroid gland is a large, bilobed gland located in the neck. Two hormones, thyroxine (T_4) and triiodothyronine (T_3), are stored and secreted by the thyroid. When released into the bloodstream, these hormones influence the metabolic rate (the rate at which foods are burned in the tissues). Iodine, which is obtained from the diet, is essential for the production of thyroid hormones.

The amount of hormone produced is also important. If the thyroid produces too much hormone, the resulting condition is known as *hyperthyroidism* and is characterized by a high basal metabolism rate. Should the gland produce too little hormone, a condition known as *hypothyroidism* results and is characterized by a low metabolic rate. The thyroid-stimulating hormone, thyrotropin (TSH), from the anterior lobe of the pituitary gland regulates the activity of the thyroid and must be present along with an adequate iodine intake for it to function properly. Cretinism in children and myxedema in adults are conditions resulting from untreated hypothyroidism. Graves' disease, characterized by bulging eyeballs and other symptoms, is the most common form of hyperthyroidism. Early detection and appropriate replacement therapy with thyroid preparations are necessary in treating hypothyroidism. Antithyroid drugs, radiation, or surgery is used in the treatment of hyperthyroidism.

See Table 26-1 for selected drugs used in thyroid disorders.

Thyroid Hormones

Actions

Thyroid hormones increase metabolic rate, cardiac output, oxygen consumption, body temperature, respiratory rate, blood volume, and carbohydrate, fat, and protein metabolism, and influence growth and development at the cellular level.

Uses

Thyroid hormones are used as supplements or replacement therapy in hypothyroidism, myxedema, and cretinism.

Contraindications

Thyroid hormones are contraindicated in patients with adrenal insufficiency, myocardial infarction, and thyrotoxicosis.

Adverse Reactions

Reactions can include sweating, alopecia, anxiety, insomnia, tremors, headache, heat intolerance, fever, tachycardia, palpitations, angina, dysrhythmia, hypertension, nausea, diarrhea, and increased or decreased appetite.

Dosage and Route

The dosage and route of administration are determined by the physician and individualized for each patient. See Table 26-1 for selected drugs used to treat hypothyroidism.

TABLE 26-1 Drugs Used in Thyroid Disorders

MEDICATION	USUAL DOSAGE	ADVERSE REACTIONS
HYPERTHYROIDISM		
methimazole (Tapazole)	Oral (Adult): Initial: 15 to 60 mg in divided doses every 6 hours, then 5 to 15 mg daily Oral (Child): 0.4 mg/kg/day in 3 doses every 8 hours initially, then 0.2 mg/kg/day	Pruritus, rash, abdominal discomfort, nausea, headache, agranulocytosis
potassium iodide solution (SSKI)	Oral: 0.3 mL 3 times daily	Brassy taste, burning in the mouth, hypersalivation, rash, productive cough, diarrhea
propranolol HCl (Inderal)	Oral: 10 to 30 mg 3 to 4 times daily	Bradycardia, bronchospasm, nausea, abdominal cramping, hypotension
propylthiouracil (PTU)	Oral (Adult): 300 mg/day divided into 3 doses at 8-hour intervals, maintenance dosage 100 to 150 mg/day	Pruritus, nausea, headache, agranulocytosis, abdominal discomfort, rash, serious liver injury
strong iodine solution (Lugol's solution)	Oral: 0.3 mL 3 times daily	Brassy taste, diarrhea, rash, hypersalivation, burning in the mouth, cough
HYPOTHYROIDISM		
levothyroxine sodium (Levothroid) (Synthroid)	Oral: 50 to 100 mcg/day, increased by increments of 50 to 100 mcg/day at 2- to 3-week intervals until the desired response is maintained	Symptoms of hyperthyroidism may occur with overdose
liothyronine sodium (Cytomel)	Oral: 25 mcg/day, increased by increments of 12.5 to 25 mcg/day at 1- to 2-week intervals until the desired response is maintained	Symptoms of hyperthyroidism may occur with overdose
liotrix (Thyrolar)	Oral: Initially 1 tablet daily (15 or 30 mg), increased by 1 tablet every 2 weeks until the desired response is maintained	Symptoms of hyperthyroidism may occur with overdose
thyroglobulin	Oral: Same as for thyroid, USP	Same as for thyroid, USP
thyroid, USP	Oral: Initially 15 to 30 mg/daily, increased by increments of 15 to 30 mg/day at 2-week intervals until the desired response is obtained. Usual maintenance dose is 60 to 120 mg in a single dose	Symptoms of hyperthyroidism may occur with overdose

Implications for Patient Care

Assess pulse before each dose. If pulse is above 100 beats per minute in adults and in excess of the normal range in children, withhold the medication and notify the physician. Monitor weight gain and/or loss, intake and output ratio, and, in the child, height and growth rate. Report any signs of hyperthyroidism (loss of weight, palpitations, diaphoresis, tachycardia, and insomnia) to the patient's physician. Administer medication at the same time each day, preferably before breakfast, to maintain drug level and help reduce the possibility of insomnia.

Patient Teaching

Educate patients:

- to take the medication as prescribed (best to take before breakfast).
- to avoid foods and over-the-counter medications that contain iodine.
- to report any signs of excitability, irritability, and anxiety to the physician.
- that if loss of hair occurs, it is generally temporary.
- that children on thyroid hormone therapy will show almost immediate personality and behavior changes.

Special Considerations

- When a patient's medication regimen includes anticoagulants, the prothrombin time should be monitored carefully, as the dosage of the anticoagulant may have to be *decreased*.
- When a patient's medication regimen includes insulin, blood glucose level should be monitored carefully, as the dosage of insulin may have to be *increased*.
- Medication is generally not taken one to several weeks before thyroid function studies.
- To prevent binding of thyroid hormones by cholestyramine, administer at least four hours apart.

Antithyroid Hormones

Actions

Antithyroid hormones inhibit the synthesis of thyroid hormones by decreasing iodine use in the manufacture of thyroglobin and iodothyronine. They do not inactivate or inhibit thyroxine or triiodothyronine.

Uses

Antithyroid hormones are used to treat hyperthyroidism, in preparation for thyroidectomy, in and thyrotoxic crisis and thyroid storm.

Contraindications

Antithyroid hormones are contraindicated in patients who are hypersensitive to any of the ingredients, and during pregnancy (third trimester) and breast-feeding.

Adverse Reactions

Reactions can include rash, urticaria, pruritus, alopecia, hyperpigmentation, irregular menses, drowsiness, headache, vertigo, fever, paresthesia, neuritis, nausea, diarrhea, vomiting, jaundice, loss of taste, myalgia, arthralgia, nocturnal muscle cramps, agranulocytosis, leukopenia, and thrombocytopenia.

Dosage and Route

The dosage and route of administration are determined by the physician and individualized for each patient. See Table 26-1 for selected drugs used to treat hyperthyroidism.

Implications for Patient Care

Assess blood pressure, pulse, temperature, intake and output ratio, and weight. Observe for signs of improvement and/or hypersensitivity, edema, bleeding, petechiae, and ecchymosis. Evaluate blood work, especially CBC, for blood dyscrasia: leukopenia, agranulocytosis, or thrombocytopenia. Unless contraindicated, encourage patients to drink plenty of fluids (3 to 4 liters/day).

Patient Teaching

Educate patients:

- to follow the prescribed medication regimen.
- that the medicine should be stored in a light-resistant container.
- to dilute liquid iodine preparation and take through a straw to minimize unpleasant taste.
- to report any signs of blood dyscrasia (redness, swelling, sore throat, mouth lesions); signs of overdose (periorbital edema, cold intolerance, mental depression); or signs of inadequate dose (tachycardia, diarrhea, fever, irritability) to the physician.
- to take their pulse daily, measure weight, and be aware of mood changes.
- to avoid foods and over-the-counter medications that contain iodine. ▪

Special Considerations

- Medication may increase effect of anticoagulants. Prothrombin time should be monitored carefully.
- Best to administer with meals to decrease gastrointestinal upset and at the same time each day to maintain proper drug level.
- Liquid preparations should be diluted and given through a straw to minimize unpleasant taste.
- Medication should be stored in a light-resistant container.

THE PARATHYROIDS

The parathyroid glands are about the size of a pinhead and can be found on either side of the thyroid gland. They secrete *parathormone* in response to lowered serum calcium levels. Parathormone (PTH) acts in several ways to increase levels of calcium and phosphorus in the body.

A deficiency of parathormone may occur as a consequence of surgery or due to a genetic defect. Symptoms of parathormone deficiency include increased neuromuscular irritability and psychiatric disorders.

THE ADRENALS

Located atop each kidney are the triangular-shaped adrenal glands, each with a tough outer cortex and an inner medulla that secretes hormones. Adrenocorticotropic hormone (ACTH) from the pituitary gland stimulates the adrenals to produce a number of important hormones that regulate fat, salt, and water metabolism. These hormones are essential to the development of male secondary sex characteristics and assist in the regulation of the sympathetic branch of the autonomic nervous system. The adrenal cortex secretes three groups of hormones: the glucocorticoids, the mineralocorticoids, and the androgens. The adrenal medulla synthesizes, stores, and secretes dopamine, epinephrine, and norepinephrine.

Primary adrenocortical insufficiency (Addison's disease) is a progressive condition associated with adrenal atrophy. Symptoms of this disease include hyperpigmentation (copper-colored skin), nausea, vomiting, weight loss, anorexia, weakness, hypotension, and a danger of dehydration. Cortisone and cortisol are the agents most often used in replacement therapy for primary adrenal insufficiency.

Prolonged administration of adrenocortical hormones will cause Cushing's syndrome. Symptoms of this syndrome include adiposity, fatigue and weakness, osteoporosis, amenorrhea, impotence, edema, excess hair growth, skin discoloration and turgidity, and purplish striae of the skin.

THE PANCREAS (ISLETS OF LANGERHANS)

The word *insulin* comes from the Latin *insula*, which means island. Therefore, it is not surprising that the source of the hormone insulin is the beta cells of the islets of Langerhans. These endocrine glands are masses of cells scattered throughout the pancreas.

Insulin is essential for the proper metabolism of carbohydrates, fats, and proteins. Normally, insulin is released following the rise in blood glucose level that accompanies the ingestion of food. As with other endocrine glands, the oversecretion or undersecretion of hormone results in specific disorders.

When too much insulin is present in the blood, an abnormally low level of blood sugar (glucose) is the result. This condition, known as *hypoglycemia*, is characterized by acute fatigue, marked irritability, and weakness. An overdose of insulin can produce a condition known as insulin shock.

When too little insulin is present in the blood, an abnormally high level of blood sugar is the result. This condition, known as *hypoglycemia*, increases the body's susceptibility to infection and produces symptoms of the disease diabetes mellitus.

Spotlight

Diabetes Mellitus

Diabetes mellitus is a complex metabolic disorder that disrupts the body's ability to produce or use insulin. Insulin is a hormone secreted by the beta cells of the islets of Langerhans. It is essential for the metabolism of carbohydrates, fats, and proteins. Insulin helps convert food into the vital energy source that is needed by the body to help make it function properly. The insulin in the body must be maintained at a certain level, usually between 70 and 100 mg/dL of blood. When the level of insulin is too high, hypoglycemia (low blood sugar) can occur. When the level of insulin is too low, hyperglycemia (high blood sugar) can occur.

Diabetes affects 23.6 million Americans, with care and treatment costing $20 billion annually. The National Institute of Diabetes and Digestive and Kidney Diseases conducted a ten-year Diabetes Control and Complications Trial on how best to control the complications of insulin-dependent diabetes mellitus (IDDM) and found that those in the intensive-control group who tested their blood sugar four or more times a day and injected insulin three or more times a day, or who used an insulin pump and followed a special diet showed reductions in complications.

The American Diabetes Association estimates that 5.9 million Americans have diabetes and do not know it. Are you at risk for diabetes? Do you have any, some, or many of the signs and symptoms of diabetes? If your answer is yes, you should see a physician and be carefully evaluated and tested for diabetes. For more information on diabetes you may call 1-800-DIABETES.

Warning Signs and Symptoms of Diabetes

- Frequent urination (polyuria)
- Excessive thirst (polydipsia)
- Extreme hunger (polyphagia)
- Unexplained weight loss
- Extreme fatigue
- Blurred vision

- Slow-healing wounds
- Tingling or numbing in your feet and/or hands
- Frequent vaginal (female) or skin infections
- Itchy skin
- Irritability
- Drowsiness

There are three major types of diabetes: Type 1, Type 2, and gestational diabetes. Type 1 diabetes used to be known as insulin-dependent diabetes mellitus or juvenile-onset diabetes. It results from the body's failure to produce insulin, the hormone that "unlocks" the cells of the body, allowing glucose to enter and fuel them. So, individuals with this type of diabetes will need to take insulin injections each day for the rest of their life. It is estimated that 5 percent to 10 percent of Americans who are diagnosed with diabetes have Type 1 diabetes.

Type 2 diabetes used to be known as noninsulin-dependent diabetes mellitus, NIDDM, or adult-onset diabetes. It results from insulin resistance combined with relative insulin deficiency. This is by far the most common type of diabetes. Approximately 90 percent to 95 percent of Americans have Type 2 diabetes. Someone with Type 2 diabetes might make healthy or even high levels of insulin, but obesity makes the body resistant to its effect. Type 2 diabetes used to be rare in children. But with the increase in obesity in children, doctors are now finding that as many as 1 out of 20 children have Type 2 diabetes. Of these children, 85 percent are obese. Obesity is the main cause of Type 2 diabetes in both adults and children. A recent study showed a 33 percent increase in the number of Americans with Type 2 diabetes over the past 8 years. The increase was 70 percent in people ages 30 to 39 years old and was linked to a sharp rise in obesity in this group.

It may be possible to prevent Type 2 diabetes. Even modest lifestyle changes can help prevent the onset of Type 2 diabetes. The key is to eat a healthy diet, exercise 30 minutes a day at least 5 days a week, and maintain a proper body weight for age and body type.

Gestational diabetes or pregnancy-induced diabetes develops in a pregnant woman. In most cases, this type of diabetes goes away after the woman's child is born. It affects about 4 percent of all pregnant women, about 135,000 cases in the United States each year.

Prediabetes is a condition that occurs when a person's blood glucose levels are higher than normal but not high enough for a diagnosis of Type 2 diabetes. It is estimated that at least 16 million Americans have prediabetes, in addition to the 17 million with diabetes. Without lifestyle changes, most people who have prediabetes will progress to Type 2 diabetes within 10 years.

Another precursor condition to developing Type 2 diabetes is called the metabolic syndrome. The underlying causes of this syndrome are overweight, obesity, physical inactivity, and genetic factors. People with the metabolic syndrome are at increased risk of coronary heart disease, other diseases related to plaque buildups in artery walls (stroke and peripheral vascular disease), and Type 2 diabetes. The metabolic syndrome is characterized by a group of metabolic risk factors in one person. They include:

- Central obesity (excessive fat tissue in and around the abdomen)
- Atherogenic dyslipidemia (blood fat disorders—mainly high triglycerides and low HDL cholesterol—that foster plaque buildups in artery walls)
- Raised blood pressure (130/85 mm Hg or higher)
- Insulin resistance or glucose intolerance (in which the body can't properly use insulin or blood sugar)
- Prothrombotic state (high fibrinogen or plasminogen activator inhibitor in the blood)
- Proinflammatory state (elevated high-sensitivity C-reactive protein in the blood)

The metabolic syndrome has become increasingly common in the United States. It is estimated that about 20 percent to 25 percent of U.S. adults have it. The syndrome is closely associated with a generalized metabolic disorder called insulin resistance, in which the body can't use insulin efficiently. This is why the metabolic syndrome is also called the insulin resistance syndrome. Some people are genetically predisposed to insulin resistance. Acquired factors, such as excess body fat and physical inactivity, can elicit insulin resistance and the metabolic syndrome in these people. Most people with insulin resistance have central obesity. The biologic mechanisms at the molecular level between insulin resistance and metabolic risk factors aren't fully understood and appear to be complex.

Understanding diabetes is the best method for controlling the disease. Through knowledge, self-regulation, discipline and following the proper medication regimen, diet, exercise program, and weight control, one may be successful in living a full life. Self-monitoring of blood glucose is an important part of managing diabetes. To teach self-monitoring to a patient you must consider the person's age, cognitive level of understanding, physical ability, and desire to learn the skill. The following are suggestions that you may use as you teach patients self-monitoring of their blood glucose level.

Show and instruct patients how to:

- use the blood glucose monitoring equipment that the physician has recommended.
- use a prepackaged sterile alcohol swab to cleanse the finger before performing a skin puncture.
- if recommended, wipe off the first drop of blood with a sterile cotton ball.
- place a drop of blood onto the test strip and how to place the strip in or on the monitor.
- read the test results.
- record the results in a daily log, with time(s) and date.
- determine the dosage of insulin based upon the physician's ordered sliding scale.
- properly dispose of used materials.

Patients should be instructed as to how many times a day to check their blood glucose level and when. Usually, this is before meals and when one "feels" different than normal. Patients should report a high blood glucose level to their physician and take insulin as instructed. When the blood glucose level is low, patients should eat some "quick sugar," ($\frac{1}{2}$ cup of orange juice, milk, or soda; several hard candies; three glucose tablets, or a combination of these).

SIGNS AND SYMPTOMS OF HYPOGLYCEMIA	SIGNS AND SYMPTOMS OF HYPERGLYCEMIA
• tremors (shaking)	• skin flushed, hot, and dry
• fast heartbeat (palpitations)	• pulse rapid and weak
• blurred vision	• drowsiness, loss of consciousness
• sweating	• low blood pressure
• hunger	• rapid, deep respirations
• irritability	• sweet, fruity odor to breath
• headache	• thirst
• weakness	• blood sugar above 200 mg/dL
• confusion	
• loss of consciousness	
• convulsions	
• blood sugar subnormal: 20 to 50 mg/dL	

Drugs and Blood Glucose Levels

Many medications can affect blood glucose levels. Patients with diabetes need to know about these medications and the physician should be informed about all drugs taken by patients with diabetes. The following are some drugs that can affect blood glucose levels.

DRUGS THAT CAN CAUSE HYPOGLYCEMIA	DRUGS THAT CAN CAUSE HYPERGLYCEMIA
• alcohol	• calcium channel blockers
• allopurinol (Lopurin, Zyloprim)	• corticosteroids
• monoamine oxidase inhibitors (MAOIs)	• diazoxide (Proglycem)
• salicylates	• isoniazid (Nydrazid)
• sulfonamides	• levothyroxine (Synthroid)
	• oral contraceptives
	• phenytoin (Dilantin)
	• rifampin (Rifadin, Rimactane)
	• thiazide diuretics

■■ Special Considerations: **OLDER ADULTS**

Diabetes mellitus may develop at any age, but generally insulin-dependent diabetes (Type 1 diabetes) appears before age 30 and noninsulin-dependent diabetes (Type 2 diabetes) develops in midlife or later. Because the onset of Type 2 diabetes is gradual and symptoms may be vague, it can go undiagnosed and untreated for years. More than 90 percent of diabetics have Type 2 diabetes and it is this type that will most likely affect older adults. Older adults may not be diagnosed with diabetes until they for go in for a regular eye exam and the ophthalmologist discovers a problem. Or perhaps older adults go in for a physical exam and the blood tests indicate an elevated blood glucose level. There are multiple risk factors associated with older adults and the development of diabetes.

Risk Factors Associated with Developing Type 2 Diabetes

- Heredity
- Decreased activity
- New stressors in life
- Age-related insulin resistance
- Obesity
- Multiple diseases
- Polypharmacy
- Age-related decreased insulin production

Treatment

The treatment regimen of medication, diet, exercise, self-monitoring, and weight control are aimed at keeping the older adult's blood glucose at an acceptable level and preventing complications from occurring. This is generally a complex process and must be individualized for each patient. Older adults may have more difficulty managing their diabetes than younger people because of physical and psychosocial limitations. In addition, drug therapy may present special problems for older adults because of multiple illnesses, polypharmacy, or poor nutrition.

Drug Therapy and Some Other Special Problems

- Certain medications may cause hypoglycemia or hyperglycemia. See Spotlight on Diabetes.
- Older adults may have reduced blood flow to the liver and kidneys, causing a slowing of drug clearance, and thereby increasing the drug concentration in their blood that could cause lactic acidosis or hypoglycemia.

- Cost of medication(s) may be more than the person can afford, causing the person not to adhere to a medication regimen.
- Impaired vision or loss of physical ability (dexterity) may interfere with the person following the treatment regimen.

Special Considerations: **CHILDREN**

Among American youth, Type 2 diabetes is an emerging epidemic associated with increasing rates of obesity and inactivity. In fact, nearly 20 years ago, only 2 percent of new cases were among children. Today, nearly 20 percent of those diagnosed with Type 2 diabetes are children ages 9 to 19. Research shows that the main culprits in the growing Type 2 diabetes epidemic among youth are alarming rates of obesity and maintenance of a sedentary lifestyle. And with nearly one-third of American youth overweight, it's no wonder this epidemic is spreading.

The major risk factors for Type 2 diabetes in children include:

- *Being overweight.* 85 percent of children diagnosed with Type 2 diabetes have a body mass index (BMI) in the 85th percentile or above for their age and sex. These children often eat a high-fat, low-fiber diet, which contributes to weight gain. Getting little or no physical activity also increases a child's risk for developing diabetes.
- *Family history.* At least 75 percent of children with Type 2 diabetes have a parent, sister, or brother with the disease.

The classic symptoms of diabetes mellitus—polyuria, polydipsia, and polyphagia—appear more rapidly in children. The child will excrete a large amount of urine (polyuria), complain of thirst (polydipsia), and be constantly hungry (polyphagia). Other symptoms seen during childhood are weakness, loss of weight, lethargy, anorexia, irritability, dry skin, vaginal yeast infections in female children, recurrent infections, and abdominal cramps.

The management of diabetes mellitus during childhood is most difficult, because diet, exercise, and medication has to be adjusted and regulated according to the various stages of growth and development of the child. Other factors that should be considered are age; cognitive level of understanding; financial, social, and cultural circumstances; and religious belief. Because children are growing and developing, special considerations must be provided for each stage of development.

- *Infants and toddlers.* During illness, infants, and toddlers are more prone to hydration problems.
- *Preschool children.* These children have irregular activity and eating patterns.
- *School-age children.* The disease may be used as a method of escape from responsibility or to gain attention.
- *Adolescence.* Onset of puberty will generally require adjustments in diet and insulin. Disease adds an additional stressor to a normally stressful growth period.

Other Factors Involved with Management

- The child expends a great deal of energy.
- Nutritional needs vary with growth and development.
- The normal stresses of childhood are increased by this disease process.
- Management of diabetes becomes a lifetime commitment.

Critical Thinking **QUESTIONS AND ACTIVITIES**

Diabetes mellitus is a complex metabolic disorder that disrupts the body's ability to produce or use insulin. In this unit, some basic facts about diabetes mellitus are presented. Your patient is a 67-year-old female who has been diagnosed with Type 2 diabetes. She states that she is having some problems managing her diabetes. Ask yourself:

- What factors are involved in the "juggling and balancing" of diabetes?
- What are some special problems that older adults may have with drug therapy?

- How can I explain to my patient that certain medications cause hypoglycemia and others cause hyperglycemia?
- How can I be sure that my patient knows the signs and symptoms of hypoglycemia and its treatment?
- How can I be sure that my patient knows the signs and symptoms of hyperglycemia and its treatment?
- What 1-800 number should I provide for my patient, so that she can find out more about diabetes?

INSULIN

Actions

Insulin stimulates carbohydrate metabolism by increasing the movement of glucose and other monosaccharides into cells. It also influences fat and carbohydrate metabolism in the liver and adipose cells. It decreases blood sugar, phosphate, and potassium, and increases blood pyruvate and lactate.

Uses

Insulin is used in insulin-dependent diabetes mellitus (Type 1 IDDM), noninsulin-dependent diabetes mellitus (Type 2 NIDDM) when other treatment regimens are not effective, and to treat ketoacidosis.

Contraindications

Insulin is essential for life, and if the patient becomes hypersensitive to one type of insulin, another type is prescribed by the physician.

Adverse Reactions

Reactions can include headache, lethargy, tremors, weakness, fatigue, delirium, sweating, tachycardia, palpitations, blurred vision, hunger, nausea, hypoglycemia, flushing, rash, urticaria, and anaphylaxis.

Dosage and Route

The dosage is individualized for each patient and depends upon the patient's blood glucose level. The route of administration is parenterally. It cannot be given orally because peptidases in the digestive juices destroy the protein molecule.

Implications for Patient Care

To provide essential care to a diabetic patient, you must be familiar with the various types of insulin preparations and their onset of action, peak action, duration of action, and appearance (see Table 26-2).

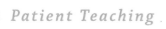 *Patient Teaching*

Patient teaching involves a wide scope of activities and the involvement of numerous health professionals. Educate patients:

- and their family about the patient's specific type of diabetes.
- about the treatment regimen (medication, diet, exercise, weight control/reduction/management, rest, stress management, and lifestyle modification).
- on how to properly test blood sugar levels, urine glucose levels, or both.

TABLE 26-2 Selected Insulin Preparations

TYPE OF INSULIN & BRAND NAMES	ONSET	PEAK	DURATION	ROLE IN BLOOD GLUCOSE MANAGEMENT
RAPID-ACTING				
Apidra	15 min	30 to 90 min	1 to 2.5 hr	Rapid-acting insulin covers insulin needs for meals eaten at the same time as the injection.
Humalog	15 to 30 min	30 min to $2\frac{1}{2}$ hr	3 to 5 hr	
Novolog	10 to 20 min	1 to 3 hr	3 to 5 hr	This type of insulin is used with longer-acting insulin.
LONG-ACTING				
Lantus	1 to $1\frac{1}{2}$ hr	No peak time; insulin is delivered at a steady level	20 to 24 hr	Long-acting insulin covers insulin needs for about 1 full day. This type of insulin is often combined, when needed, with rapid- or short-acting insulin.
PREMIXED *				
Novolin 70/30	30 min.	2 to 12 hr	Up to 24 hr	These products are generally taken twice a day before mealtime.
Novolog 70/30	10 to 20 min.	1 to 4 hr	Up to 24 hr	
Humalog mix 75/25	15 min.	30 min to $2\frac{1}{2}$ hr	16 to 20 hr	

*Premixed insulins are a combination of specific proportions of intermediate-acting and short-acting insulin in one bottle or insulin pen. (The numbers following the brand name indicate the percentage of each type of insulin.)

- on how to store and handle insulin.
- about the symptoms and treatment for hypoglycemia and hyperglycemia.
- on when to seek medical attention.
- on how to properly administer insulin. (To teach a patient or a family member how to administer insulin, you should use the information on subcutaneous injection provided in Unit 13, Administration of Parenteral Medications.) ■

Note: **Safety Information: The FDA notified health care providers and patients that insulin pens and insulin cartridges are never to be shared among patients. Sharing of insulin pens may result in transmission of hepatitis viruses, HIV, or other bloodborne pathogens. Insulin pens are not designed, and are not safe, for one pen to be used for more than one patient, even if needles are changed between patients because any blood contamination of the pen reservoir could result in transmission of already existing bloodborne pathogens from the previous user. The FDA is working with the Centers for Disease Control and Prevention, professional societies, and health care organizations to reinforce patient and health care provider education about proper and safe use of insulin pens. ●**

To teach other aspects of diabetic care, one should use an appropriate source and seek the assistance of other health professionals. It is not possible to include all the information that you need to know about diabetes and its management in this text, but the following is basic information that you should know and be able to teach patients and their family.

- Insulin is given subcutaneously, using a site rotation system.
- While using, most insulin preparations may be stored at room temperature. Other insulin should be stored in a refrigerator, and then warmed to room temperature before use. *Always check the expiration date before use. Insulin should be gently rotated in the palms of the hand to mix and it should never be shaken.*
- Patients need to know that with the initiation of insulin therapy, blurred vision may occur, and that usually vision is stabilized in one to two months. One should not change contact lens or eyeglasses without the advice of the physician.
- Patients need to know that with unusual stress, infection, or other health-related conditions, an increase in their dosage of insulin may be necessary.
- One should monitor blood glucose levels very carefully and use the correct dose of insulin to maintain proper blood glucose level during times of stress or disease.
- Patients should always wear or carry a Medic Alert ID. Patients should always have the appropriate equipment, medication (insulin), and candy or lump of sugar in their possession.
- Patients should not use over-the-counter medications without the physician's permission.
- Patients should not smoke or drink alcoholic beverages while taking insulin.
- Patients need to know that insulin is a lifetime drug, and that its proper use is essential in helping to prevent complicating conditions or diseases from occurring.

Special Considerations

- Patients need special care and consideration for the prescribed treatment regimen to be an effective lifetime mode.
- Hypoglycemia may be increased with the use of MAO inhibitors, alcohol, beta-blockers, anabolic steroids, guanethidine, salicylate, fenfluramine, tetracycline, clofibrate, and oral hypoglycemics.
- Hyperglycemia may be increased with the use of oral contraceptives, corticosteroids, estrogens, lithium, thiazides, thyroid hormones, triamterene, phenothiazines, and phenytoin.

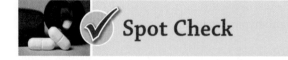 Spot Check

There are many types of insulin preparations. For each of the following types, give the onset of action, peak action, and duration of action:

TYPE OF INSULIN	ONSET	PEAK	DURATION
Humalog			
Apidra			

TYPE OF INSULIN	ONSET	PEAK	DURATION
Lantus			
Novolin 70/30			
Humalog mix 75/25			

ORAL HYPOGLYCEMIC AGENTS

Oral hypoglycemic agents may be used in conjunction with diet and exercise in the management and treatment of Type 2 diabetes. They are classified as sulfonylureas, biguanides, thiazolidinediones, alpha glucosidase inhibitors, meglitinides, and dipeptidyl peptidase-4(DPP-4) inhibitor.

- *Sulfonylureas* (Amaryl, DiaBeta, Diabinese, Glucotrol, Micronase, Orinase, Tolinase) work primarily by stimulating the pancreas to release more insulin.
- *Biguanides* (Glucophage) work by decreasing the release of glucose by the liver and by making cells more sensitive to insulin.
- *Thiazolidinediones* (Actos, Avandia) work primarily by making cells more sensitive to insulin.
- *Alpha glucosidase inhibitors* (Precose) slow the body's absorption of carbohydrates. This allows the insulin in the body to work better. The medication is taken before each meal.
- *Meglitinides* (Prandin and Starlix) prevent a rise in blood sugar levels by increasing the amount of insulin produced by the pancreas, similar to the way sulfonylurea medications work.
- *Dipeptidyl peptidase-4 (DPP-4) inhibitor* is a new class of oral hypoglycemic agent. DPP-4 is a substance in the body that blocks messages to the pancreas to make enough insulin and then the pancreas cannot signal the liver to stop making glucose. At present, Januvia (sitaliptin) is the only drug in this class. It helps the body increase the insulin made in the pancreas and decrease glucose made in the liver. It is a once-daily prescription pill (100 mg) that can be taken with or without food. It is used as an adjunct to diet and exercise to improve glycemic control in adults with Type 2 diabetes mellitus.

Sulfonylureas

Agents of the sulfonylurea class of chemical compounds are used to stimulate insulin secretion from pancreatic islet cells in Type 2 diabetes for those with some pancreatic function.

Actions

Sulfonylureas stimulate functioning beta cells in the pancreas to release insulin, thereby lowering blood glucose levels. These agents are not effective if the patient lacks functioning beta cells.

Uses

Sulfonylureas are used in noninsulin-dependent Type 2 stable adult-onset diabetes mellitus.

Contraindications

Sulfonylureas are contraindicated in patients who are hypersensitive to any of the ingredients, and in patients with juvenile or brittle diabetes, severe renal disease, and severe hepatic disease.

Adverse Reactions

Reactions include headache, weakness, paresthesia, nausea, heartburn, vomiting, abdominal pain, diarrhea, hepatotoxicity, cholestatic jaundice, leukopenia, thrombocytopenia, agranulocytosis, aplastic anemia, rash, allergic reaction, pruritus, urticaria, eczema, photosensitivity, erythema, hypoglycemia, and joint pains.

Dosage and Route

The dosage is determined by the physician and individualized for each patient. The route of administration is orally. See Table 26-3 for selected sulfonylureas.

Implications for Patient Care

Monitor the patient's blood glucose level to determine glucose balance. Observe the patient for signs of improvement and any adverse reactions.

TABLE 26-3   Sulfonylureas

MEDICATION	USUAL DOSAGE	DURATION	ADVERSE REACTIONS
acetohexamide	Oral: 250 mg to 1.5 g daily in single or divided doses	8 to 10 hours	Hypoglycemia, nausea, heartburn, epigastric fullness
chlorpropamide (Diabinese)	Oral: 100 to 500 mg once daily	72 hours	Hypoglycemia, nausea, vomiting, diarrhea, pruritus
glipizide (Glucotrol)	Oral: 5 mg initially, then increased by 2.5 to 5 mg/day until blood glucose level is satisfactory (maximum dose is 40 mg daily)	10 to 24 hours	Hypoglycemia, nausea and diarrhea, constipation and gastralgia
glyburide (DiaBeta) (Micronase)	Oral: 2.5 to 5 mg/day initially; maintenance dose ranges from 1.25 to 20 mg/daily	24 hours	Hypoglycemia, nausea, heartburn, epigastric fullness, allergic skin reactions
tolazamide	Oral: 100 to 1000 mg/day in single or divided doses	10 to 14 hours	Hypoglycemia, nausea, heartburn, epigastric fullness
tolbutamide	Oral: 1 to 2 g/day initially; maintenance dose ranges from 0.25 to 3 g/daily	6 to 12 hours	Hypoglycemia, nausea, heartburn, epigastric fullness, allergic skin reactions

Patient Teaching

Educate patients:

- and their family about the patient's specific type of diabetes.
- about the treatment regimen (medication; diet; exercise; weight control, reduction, and management; rest; stress management; and lifestyle modification).
- on how to properly test blood sugar and urine glucose levels.
- about the symptoms and treatment for hypoglycemia and hyperglycemia.
- on when to seek medical attention.
- to take the medication in the morning to prevent hypoglycemic reactions at night.
- to be alert for signs of cholestatic jaundice (dark urine, pruritus [severe itching], and yellow sclera). The physician should be notified immediately if any of these signs occur.
- to wear a Medic Alert ID.
- not to use over-the-counter medications without the physician's permission.
- not to smoke or drink alcoholic beverages while taking oral hypoglycemic agents. ■

Special Considerations

- Patient need special care and consideration for the prescribed treatment regimen to be an effective lifetime mode.
- The effect of oral hypoglycemic agents may be increased with the use of insulin, MAO inhibitors, and cimetidine.
- The effect of oral hypoglycemic agents may be decreased with the use of calcium channel blockers, corticosteroids, oral contraceptives, estrogens, thiazide diuretics, thyroid preparations, phenothiazines, phenytoin, rifampin, and isoniazid.

Biguanides

Biguanides work by decreasing the release of glucose by the liver and by making cells more sensitive to insulin.

Metformin Hydrochloride (Glucophage)

Metformin HCl (Glucophage) is an oral hypoglycemic agent in the chemical group known as biguanides. It can be used either alone or in combination with sulfonylurea agents, when glycemia control is inadequate with a sulfonylurea or the patient suffers too many adverse reactions.

Actions

Metformin HCI decreases hepatic glucose production, decreases intestinal absorption of glucose, and improves insulin sensitivity (increases peripheral glucose uptake and utilization).

Uses

Use in the management of Type 2 diabetes.

Contraindications

- Avoid using in patients with renal disease or renal dysfunction.
- It should be temporarily withheld in patients undergoing radiologic studies involving parenteral administration of iodinated contrast materials, because use of such products may result in acute alteration of renal function.

- Avoid using in patients with known hypersensitivity to metformin hydrochloride.
- Avoid using in patients with acute or chronic metabolic acidosis, including diabetic ketoacidosis, with or without coma. Diabetic ketoacidosis should be treated with insulin.
- Metformin HCI is not recommended for use during pregnancy or for use in children.

> **Warning:**
>
> *Lactic acidosis is a rare, but serious, metabolic complication that can occur due to metformin accumulation during treatment with Glucophage; when it occurs, it is fatal in approximately 50 percent of cases. Lactic acidosis is characterized by elevated blood lactate levels (>5 mmol/L), decreased blood pH, electrolyte disturbances with an increased anion gap, and an increased lactate to pyruvate ratio. When metformin is implicated as the cause of lactic acidosis, a metformin level greater than 5 microgram/mL is generally found.*

Adverse Reactions

Reactions include lactic acidosis, diarrhea, nausea, vomiting, abdominal bloating, flatulence, anorexia, unpleasant or metallic taste, rash, and dermatitis.

Dosage and Route

Dosage is individualized for each patient. The usual starting dose is 500 mg tablets, one tablet twice a day with the morning and evening meals. Dosage increases should be made in increments of one tablet every week, given in divided doses, up to a maximum of 2500 mg per day.

Implications for Patient Care

Monitor the patient's blood glucose level and urine test to determine glucose balance. Observe the patient for signs of improvement and any adverse reactions.

THIAZOLIDINEDIONES

The Food and Drug Administration has approved Avandia and Avelox (rosiglitazone maleate) and Actos (pioglitazone hydrochloride) for Type 2 diabetes. These drugs are a member of a new class of oral diabetes agents called thiazolidinediones (TZDs), which act as insulin sensitizers. In contrast to traditional Type 2 diabetes medicines, which increase insulin production in the pancreas or decrease glucose output through the liver, these drugs are believed to reduce the amount of insulin needed while improving blood sugar control.

Rosiglitazone Maleate (Avandia)

Avandia is used to treat Type 2 diabetes by helping the body use the insulin it is already making. It comes as pills that can be taken either once a day or twice a day, with or without meals, to help control blood sugar levels.

Actions

Avandia helps the body use insulin by making the cells less resistant to insulin so that the sugar can enter the cell.

Uses

It is recommended for Type 2 diabetes, and in people over 18 who do not have liver disease or severe heart disease.

Contraindications

Avandia is contraindicated in patients with known hypersensitivity or allergy to any of its components.

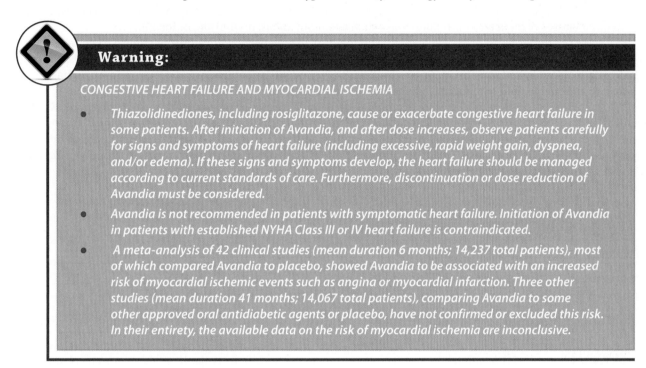

Warning:

CONGESTIVE HEART FAILURE AND MYOCARDIAL ISCHEMIA

- *Thiazolidinediones, including rosiglitazone, cause or exacerbate congestive heart failure in some patients. After initiation of Avandia, and after dose increases, observe patients carefully for signs and symptoms of heart failure (including excessive, rapid weight gain, dyspnea, and/or edema). If these signs and symptoms develop, the heart failure should be managed according to current standards of care. Furthermore, discontinuation or dose reduction of Avandia must be considered.*

- *Avandia is not recommended in patients with symptomatic heart failure. Initiation of Avandia in patients with established NYHA Class III or IV heart failure is contraindicated.*

- *A meta-analysis of 42 clinical studies (mean duration 6 months; 14,237 total patients), most of which compared Avandia to placebo, showed Avandia to be associated with an increased risk of myocardial ischemic events such as angina or myocardial infarction. Three other studies (mean duration 41 months; 14,067 total patients), comparing Avandia to some other approved oral antidiabetic agents or placebo, have not confirmed or excluded this risk. In their entirety, the available data on the risk of myocardial ischemia are inconclusive.*

Adverse Reactions

Reactons can include upper respiratory infection, headache, weight gain, edema, and anemia.

Dosage and Route

It should be taken orally, once a day in the morning or twice a day in the morning and evening.

Implications for Patient Care

Monitor the patient's blood glucose level to determine glucose balance. Observe the patient for signs of improvement and any adverse reactions.

 Patient Teaching

Educate patients:

- to call the physician immediately if they experiences nausea, vomiting, stomach pain, tiredness, lack of appetite, dark urine, or yellowing of the skin.
- that for some women with diabetes, insulin resistance may interfere with their ability to become pregnant. Because Avandia reduces insulin resistance, use of Avandia may restore their ability to become pregnant. Therefore, the patient may need to consider birth control measures.
- that although Avandia did not show signs of liver problems in studies, the physician may recommend a liver test before starting Avandia, and from time to time while the patient is using Avandia.
- that management of Type 2 diabetes includes diet control with caloric restriction, weight loss, and exercise as essential components for the proper treatment of diabetes. ■

Pioglitazone (Actos)

Actos is the latest member of the thiazolidinedione class of drugs. It is approved for use as sole therapy in diabetics who are unable to control their blood sugar with diet and exercise alone. It is also approved for use in combination with other classes of diabetes-controlling drugs, such as sulfonylureas, metformin, or insulin.

Actos (45 mg) is given orally, once daily. The majority of adverse reactions during clinical trials were mild. The most commonly reported included symptoms of upper respiratory infection, headache, sinusitis, muscle pain, tooth disorder, and sore throat. As observed with other members of this class of drugs, weight gain has been noted. Additionally, mild to moderate edema and anemia were reported in patients taking Actos.

There have been no reported cases of jaundice or liver failure associated with Actos use in the United States. However, it is recommended that patients obtain medical monitoring of liver enzyme levels prior to the start of therapy, every two months for the first year of therapy and periodically thereafter. In premenopausal anovulatory patients with insulin resistance, treatment with any thiazolidinedione may result in resumption of ovulation. These patients may be at risk of pregnancy.

ALPHA GLUCOSIDASE INHIBITORS

Alpha glucosidase inhibitors slow the body's absorption of carbohydrates. This allows the insulin in the body to work better. The medication is taken before each meal.

Acarbose (Precose)

Precose is an oral hypoglycemic agent in the chemical group known as alpha glucosidase inhibitors. It slows the body's absorption of carbohydrates. This allows the insulin in the body to work better. Precose must be taken with the first bite of food at each meal. It may be used alone or in combination with a sulfonylurea.

Actions

Acarbose blocks the enzymes that digest starches in food. This results in a slower and lower rise of blood sugar through the day.

Uses

Acarbose is used in noninsulin-dependent Type 2 diabetes.

Contraindications

Acarbose is contraindicated in patients who are hypersensitive to any of its ingredients. Use caution in patients with inflammatory bowel disease, ulcers of the colon, intestinal obstruction, or chronic intestinal disease.

Adverse Reactions

Alpha glucosidase inhibitors can cause gastrointestinal symptoms such as cramping, gas, and diarrhea. These symptoms usually pass with time as the body adjusts to the new medication. Other adverse reactions that may occur are rash, hives, or fever.

Dosage and Route

The dosage is determined by the physician and individualized for each patient. The route of administration is oral. The usual starting dose is 50 mg 3 times daily. The maximum dose is 300 mg/day.

Implications for Patient Care

Monitor the patient's blood glucose level to determine glucose balance. Observe the patient for signs of improvement and any adverse reactions.

Patient Teaching

Educate patients:

- that Precose *must* be taken with the first bite of food at each meal.
- that when Precose is given in combination with a sulfonylurea or insulin, it will cause a further lowering of blood sugar and may increase the hypoglycemic potential of these agents.
- and their family of the risk of hypoglycemia, its symptoms and treatment, and condition that predispose to its development.
- that the administration of an oral carbohydrate (CHO) such as orange juice, candy, or a lump of sugar will generally correct mild hypoglycemia.
- that because Precose prevents the breakdown of table sugar, one should have a readily available source of glucose to treat symptoms of low blood sugar when taking Precose in combination with a sulfonylurea or insulin.
- that certain drugs tend to produce hyperglycemia and may lead to loss of blood glucose control. One should ask their pharmacist for a list of these drugs.
- that management of Type 2 diabetes includes diet control with caloric restriction, weight loss, and exercise as essential components for the proper treatment of diabetes.
- that Precose has shown to change the bioavailability of digoxin when they are coadministered, which may require digoxin dose adjustment. ■

MEGLITINIDES

Prandin (repaglinide) and Starlix (nateglinide) are oral drugs used to treat Type 2 diabetes when an improved diet and exercise regime have failed to improve high blood sugar. They work by stimulating the pancreas to produce more insulin in a similar way to the sulfonylurea medications.

These drugs work quickly and the effects are of short duration. They are designed to be taken immediately before each meal and attempt to mimic the normal effects of insulin after eating. They are particularly suitable for patients who do not maintain a regular meal schedule. They are also useful for patients with potential kidney problems. Prandin or Starlix is often prescribed in combination with metformin or other diabetic medications.

The side effects of Prandin or Starlix include:

- diarrhea
- headache
- cardiac effects (slight risk only)
- low blood sugar (hypoglycemia)
- upper respiratory infections, nasal and sinus inflammation, and bronchitis
- joint and back pain
- nausea
- constipation

People who have liver problems may not be able to take meglitinides. In addition, it is unknown whether these medications are safe for use during pregnancy.

HYPERGLYCEMIC AGENTS

Hyperglycemic agents are used to cause an increase in blood glucose of diabetic patients with severe hypoglycemia (insulin shock). In patients with mild hypoglycemia, the administration of an oral carbohydrate (CHO) such as orange juice, candy, or a lump of sugar will generally correct the condition. If comatose, adults may be given 10 to 30 mL of 50 percent dextrose solution IV, and children should receive 0.5 to 1 mL/kg of 50 percent dextrose solution IV.

Glucagon, an insulin antagonist, may be used in the acute management of severe hypoglycemia. It increases blood glucose levels by increasing the breakdown of glycogen to glucose and inhibits glycogen synthesis. It is useful in hypoglycemia only if liver glycogen is available and should only be used with medical supervision. For adults, the dose is 0.5 to 1 mg IM, IV, or SC, repeated in 20 minutes when necessary. For children, the dose is 25 mcg/kg up to a maximum dose of 1 mg IM, IV, or SC, repeated in 20 minutes when necessary. It is contraindicated in individuals with hyperactivity to beef protein, pork protein, or glucagon; pheochromocytoma; or a history of insulinoma. Adverse reactions include nausea, vomiting, and an allergic reaction.

Proglycem (diazoxide) is a hyperglycemic agent that may be used in the treatment of hypoglycemia associated with hyperinsulinism or other causes. Oral diazoxide produces a prompt, dose-related increase in blood glucose levels by inhibition of pancreatic-insulin release. For adults and children, the dose is 1 mg/kg every 8 hours initially, further adjustments made on the basis of response. Usual maintenance dose is 3 to 8 mg/kg/day given in divided doses every 8 to 12 hours. For infants and newborns, the dose is 3.3 mg/kg/day divided into two or three equal doses every 8 to 12 hours. Proglycem is rapidly absorbed orally and has an onset of action within 1 hour. It has a duration of 8 hours and a half-life between 20 and 36 hours in most individuals. The adverse reactions include taste alterations, anorexia, nausea, vomiting, abdominal pain, constipation, edema, tachycardia, and allergic reaction. It is contraindicated in individuals with hypersensitivity to diazoxide, sulfonamides, or thiazides; coronary or cerebral insufficiency; acute aortic dissection; and in patients who have an inadequate cardiac reserve or compensatory hypertension.

Glucose (Glutose, Insta-Glucose) may be used to correct hypoglycemia in conscious patients. It is well absorbed following oral administration and widely distributed and rapidly utilized. For adults and children, the oral dose is 10 to 20 grams and may be repeated in 10 to 20 minutes if necessary. Glucose is available as an oral gel and in chewable tablets. It is also available as an intravenous solution for injection.

■ ■ REVIEW QUESTIONS

Directions. Select the best answer to each of the following multiple-choice questions, circling the letter of your choice:

1. An acquired condition (in older children and adults) that is due to a deficiency in the secretion of thyroid hormones is called _____.
   a. gigantism
   b. cretinism
   c. myxedema
   d. acromegaly

2. The pituitary secretes hormones that are essential for _____.
   a. body growth
   b. body development
   c. regulation of actions by other endocrine glands
   d. all of these

3. Diabetes insipidus occurs with the underproduction or absence of the hormone _____.
   a. thyroxin
   b. vasopressin
   c. parathormone
   d. adrenocorticotropic

4. Two hormones stored and secreted by the thyroid gland are _____.
   a. thyroxine
   b. triiodothyronine
   c. vasopressin
   d. a and b

5. Oral hypoglycemic agents may be used in conjunction with diet and exercise in the management and treatment of Type 2 diabetes. All of the following are included in this classification except _____.

   a. sulfonylureas and alpha glucosidase inhibitors

   b. biguanides and meglitinides

   c. thiazolidinediones

   d. insulin

6. Parathormone increases the levels of _____ and _____ in the body.

   a. sodium and chloride   c. magnesium and phosphorus

   b. calcium and phosphorus   d. calcium and sodium

7. The adrenal medulla synthesizes, stores, and secretes _____.

   a. dopamine, epinephrine, and norepinephrine

   b. glucocorticoids, mineralocorticoids, androgens

   c. parathormone

   d. thyroxine

8. _____ _____ is a complex disorder of carbohydrate metabolism.

   a. Diabetes insipidus   c. Graves' disease

   b. Diabetes mellitus   d. Addison's disease

9. Novlin 70/30 insulin's onset of action is _____.

   a. 1 to 1.5 hours   c. 4 to 8 hours

   b. 2 to 2.5 hours   d. 30 minutes

10. The duration of Humalog insulin is _____.

   a. 2 to 3 hours   c. 6 to 8 hours

   b. 3 to 5 hours   d. 10 to 12 hours

11. Hyperglycemic agents are used to cause an increase in blood glucose of diabetic patients with severe hypoglycemia (insulin shock). All of the following are included in this classification except _____.

   a. glucagon

   b. Proglycem (diazoxide)

   c. Prandin (repaglinide)

   d. glucose (Glutose, Insta-Glucose)

12. The symptoms of hypoglycemia include _____.

   a. tremors   c. irritability

   b. sweating   d. all of these

13. The symptoms of hyperglycemia include _____.

   a. hot, dry skin   c. pulse rapid and weak

   b. fruity breath odor   d. all of these

14. The ductless glands of the endocrine system secrete chemical substances known as _____ directly into the bloodstream.

   a. enzymes   c. hormones

   b. catecholamines   d. neurotransmitters

15. The _____ is sometimes called the master gland of the body.

   a. pineal   b. pituitary   c. thyroid   d. pancreas

16. All of the following are short-acting insulins except _____.

   a. Regular   b. Humulin   c. Novolin   d. Ultralente

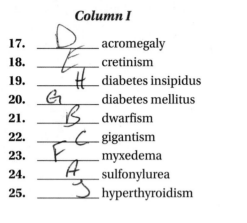

Matching. Place the correct letter from Column II on the appropriate line of Column I:

	Column I		*Column II*

17. _D_ acromegaly

18. _E_ cretinism

19. _H_ diabetes insipidus

20. _G_ diabetes mellitus

21. _B_ dwarfism

22. _C_ gigantism

23. _F_ myxedema

24. _A_ sulfonylurea

25. _J_ hyperthyroidism

A. a class of chemical compounds that includes oral hypoglycemic agents

B. a condition of being abnormally small

C. a condition in which there is excessive development of the body or a body part

D. a condition in which there is enlargement of the extremities and certain head bones

E. a congenital condition that is due to a deficiency in the secretion of thyroid hormones

F. an acquired condition that is due to a deficiency in the secretion of thyroid hormones

G. a disorder of carbohydrate metabolism that is a result of inadequate production or utilization of insulin

H. a condition caused by inadequate secretion of vasopressin

I. characterized by a low basal metabolism rate

J. characterized by a high basal metabolism rate

UNIT 27
Medications That Affect the Nervous System

OBJECTIVES

Upon completing this unit, you should be able to:

- Define the terms listed in the vocabulary.
- Describe the nervous system.
- Define pain.
- Explain the special considerations for older adults with pain.
- Give some indications of pain in neonates, infants, toddlers, and older children.
- Explain various techniques for assessing pain in children.
- Complete the critical thinking questions and activities presented in this unit.
- State the actions, uses, contraindications, warnings, adverse reactions, dosage and route, implications for patient care, patient teaching, and special considerations for narcotic analgesics, barbiturates, anti-parkinsonian drugs, and anticonvulsants.
- State the actions, usual dosage, and adverse reactions of selected analgesic-antipyretics and a narcotic antagonist (naloxone hydrochloride).
- Complete the Spot Check on selected medications used to treat pain.
- State the schedule, duration, usual sedative dose, and usual hypnotic dose of selected barbiturates.
- Give examples of benzodiazepines that are effective sedative-hypnotics drugs.
- State the schedule, usual sedative dose, and usual hypnotic dose of selected nonbarbiturate sedative-hypnotic drugs.
- Describe Alzheimer's disease (AD).
- Describe anesthetic drugs as local or general acting.
- State three uses of ophthalmic drugs.
- State the classification, usual dosage, and adverse reactions of selected drugs used to treat glaucoma.
- State four uses of mydriatic drugs.
- State the classification, usual dosage, and adverse reactions of selected mydriatic drugs.
- State the uses, usual dosage, and adverse reactions of selected drugs used in the treatment of vertigo, motion sickness, and vomiting.
- Answer the review questions correctly.

VOCABULARY

agonist (ag'on-ist). A drug that has affinity for the cellular receptors of another drug or natural substance and produces a pharmacological effect.

anhydrase (an"hi'dras). An enzyme that promotes the removal of water from a chemical compound.

aqueous humor (a'kwe-us hu'mor). The transparent liquid contained in the anterior and posterior chambers of the eye.

carbonic (kar'bon-ik). Pertaining to carbon.

carbonic anhydrase (kar'bon-ik an"hi'dras). An enzyme that catalyzes union of water and carbon dioxide to form carbonic acid. Present in red blood cells.

(*continues*)

dopamine (do'pa-men). A catecholamine synthesized in adrenergic nerve terminals, the adrenal gland, and other sites in the central nervous system. It is the immediate precursor in the synthesis of norepinephrine. It increases the force of contraction of the heart, blood pressure, and urinary output.

inhibitor (in"hib'i-tor). That which inhibits; a chemical substance that blocks enzyme activity.

sympathomimetic (sim"pa-tho-mim-et'ik). That which imitates activation or the stimulation of the sympathetic nervous system; adrenergic.

INTRODUCTION

The nervous system is comprised of the brain and spinal cord (the central nervous system or CNS), plus the network of nerves and neural tissues throughout the body (the peripheral nervous system or PNS)— (see Figure 27-1). The peripheral system connects to the brain and spinal cord by way of 12 pairs of cranial nerves and 31 pairs of spinal nerves. These two systems, functioning as a unit, regulate body functions in relationship to the environment.

Our senses of hearing, taste, equilibrium, touch, smell, and sight all rely on nerves to function properly. Pain receptors alert us to danger from inflammation or hot surfaces. Muscular activity is dependent upon proper stimulation by nerve impulses. Our ability to think, reason, feel emotions, and interact with others is directly related to our neurological processes.

Disorders that interfere with central or peripheral nervous system function are treated with a variety of drugs, some of which are discussed in this unit. Separate units cover drugs used primarily with the musculoskeletal system and for mental disorders.

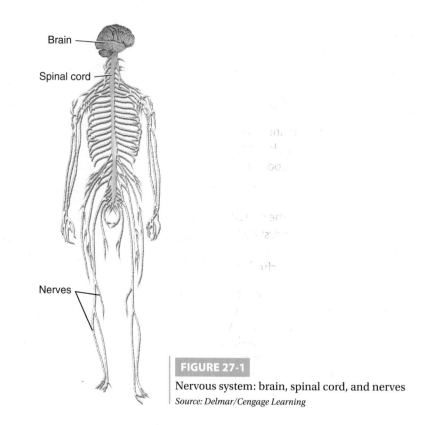

FIGURE 27-1

Nervous system: brain, spinal cord, and nerves
Source: Delmar/Cengage Learning

Spotlight

Pain

Pain is a symptom of a physical or emotional condition. The International Association for the Study of Pain defines pain as the sensory and emotional experience associated with actual or potential tissue damage.

A person's pain may be measured by its threshold and its intensity. Pain threshold is the level of stimulus that results in the perception of pain. How one responds to pain is an individual process. Some factors associated with how a person perceives pain are age, gender, and the physical, mental, social, cultural, and emotional makeup of the individual. Pain tolerance is the amount of pain a person can manage without disrupting normal functioning and without requiring pain medication. Intensity is the degree of pain felt by the individual.

In the United States, each year approximately 155 million people experience an episode of acute pain. Annually an estimated 700 million workdays are lost because of pain, with a cost of 60 billion dollars. Acute pain may be described as pain that comes on suddenly, is severe, and is a warning that something is wrong. Some signs and symptoms of acute pain are increased heart rate and respiratory rate, increased blood pressure, dilated pupils, sweating (many times profuse), nausea, vomiting, anxiety, and fear. The treatment of acute pain depends upon the cause, but generally it is treated with nonnarcotic analgesics or narcotic analgesics.

Chronic pain lasts for a long time. It is pain that persists beyond the expected time required for the healing of an injury or expected course of recovery. Some signs of chronic pain include disturbances in sleep and eating patterns, irritability, constipation, depression, fatigue, and withdrawal from social activities. Chronic pain is generally managed with analgesics, but the patient may wish to try alternative methods for relief.

Some Alternative Methods for Relief of Pain

- *Behavior modification*—relaxation training, biofeedback, and hypnosis
- *Surgery*—destroying nerves responsible for pain
- *Electrostimulation*—implanting electrodes at certain sites in the body and then stimulating them to prevent pain messages
- *Acupuncture*
- *Exercise*—aerobic exercise increases the secretion of endorphins (natural painkillers)
- *Ice*—useful for headaches, and in the first 48 hours of an injury (sprains, strains, bumps), because it reduces swelling
- *Heat*—useful for cramps and muscle aches, and after swelling of an injury has subsided

Chronic intractable pain may be caused by cancer, mental illness, neurologic disorders such as neuralgias, phantom limb pain, nerve entrapment syndromes, spinal cord damage, myofascial syndromes, or thalamic syndrome pain. New federal guidelines urge doctors to aggressively attack cancer pain, which a study showed severely afflicts one-third of Americans with spreading cancer. The guidelines issued by the Agency for Health Care Research and Quality urge doctors to start patients on mild painkillers, then work up to more potent medicines. The next step is codeine and other weak opiates, followed by morphine and similar powerful drugs.

Usual Doses and Intervals of Selected Drugs Used for Relief of Pain

DRUG	DOSE AND ROUTE	INTERVAL
acetaminophen	650 mg (Oral)	4 hour
acetylsalicylic acid	650 mg (Oral)	4 hour
codeine	15 to 60 mg (Oral)	4 hour
hydromorphone	2 mg (Oral)	4 hour
ibuprofen	400 mg (Oral)	4 to 6 hour
meperidine	50 to 150 mg (SC, IM)	3 to 4 hour
methadone	2.5 to 10 mg (SC, IM)	6 to 8 hour
morphine	10 to 20 mg (SC, IM)	4 hour
naproxen	250 to 500 mg (Oral)	12 hour

Assessment of Pain

It is important to obtain an accurate assessment of a patient's pain. Because pain is subjective, patients need to describe in detail the location, intensity, quality, onset, duration, variations, what relieves the pain and what causes or increases the pain.

- *Questions on the history of pain:* Ask patients the following questions: When did the pain start? How long does the pain last? What increases or decreases the pain? What methods are used to relieve the pain? How effective are these methods?
- *Physical signs and symptoms:* increased heart rate and respiratory rate, increased blood pressure, dilated pupils, sweating, nausea, vomiting, anxiety, fear.
- *Facial expression:* strained look, clenched teeth, tightly shut lips, tightening of the jaw muscles, furrowed brow, tears.
- *Body movements:* protective or guarding movements toward a specific area of the body, limping, clenched fist, hunched shoulders, doubling over.
- *Quality or character:* verbal description (aching, burning, prickling, sharp, cutting, throbbing, intense, pressure, mild, moderate, severe, local, deep).

Effectiveness of Treatment

Two methods that are used to monitor treatment effectiveness for pain management are questionnaires and rating scales. The McGill-Melzack Pain Questionnaire measures both sensory and affective dimensions of pain. Rating scales may use numbers, drawings, or lines. The number scale may be 0 to 5 or 0 to 10, with zero indicating no pain and the upper number signifying the most intense pain. The Wong-Baker face rating scale shows 5 faces with the numbers 0 to 5 beneath the picture; 0 indicates no pain and 5 signifies the most intense pain. This is useful for children and for patients who cannot speak English.

Standards for Pain Relief

The American Pain Society developed Standards for the Relief of Acute Pain and Cancer Pain, which are summarized as follows:

1. Acute pain and cancer pain are recognized and effectively treated. Essential to this process is the development of a clinically useful and easy-to-use scale for rating pain and its relief. Patients will be evaluated according to the scales and the results recorded as frequently as needed.

2. Information about analgesics is readily available. This includes data concerning the effectiveness of various agents in controlling pain and the availability of equianalgesic charts wherever drugs are used for pain.

3. Patients are informed on admission of the availability of methods of relieving pain, and that they must communicate the presence and persistence of pain to the health care staff.

4. Explicit policies for use of advanced analgesic technologies are defined. These advances include patient-control analgesia, epidural analgesia, and regional analgesia. Specific instructions concerning use of these techniques need to be available for the medical care staff.

5. Adherence to standards is monitored by an interdisciplinary committee. The committee is responsible for overseeing the activities related to implementing and evaluating the effectiveness of these pain standards.

■ Special Considerations: **OLDER ADULTS**

Pain is not a normal part of the aging process. Older adults may believe that their pain is just a part of "growing old" and be reluctant to report pain; therefore, pain goes untreated and unrelieved. It is true that older adults may be more vulnerable to adverse drug reactions, may have multiple disease processes, and may often take multiple medications, but older adults pain should be properly treated. Most older adults can generally take nonsteroidal anti-inflammatory drugs (NSAIDs) and analgesics for pain. There are precautions and warnings associated with these drugs, and some of the special considerations for older adults are:

- Long-term use of acetaminophen can cause end-stage renal disease and liver damage when combined with fasting. A study found that those who took 105 to 365 acetaminophen pills per year had a 40 percent increased risk of kidney failure. The risk was double in people who took more than 366 pills per year—at least one per day. Researchers also found that moderate to heavy doses of acetaminophen taken on an empty stomach can change the way the body metabolizes the analgesic. Alcohol also alters the way acetaminophen is metabolized. There is evidence that alcohol leads to liver damage if acetaminophen is taken within the recommended dose. Patients with alcoholism may be at a higher risk than nonalcoholics for liver damage because it is believed that they are more likely to exceed the recommended dose.

- Nonsteroidal anti-inflammatory drugs may cause peptic ulcer disease, bleeding and, among the frail elderly, constipation, cognitive impairment, and headaches.

- Opiates have a long serum half-life in older adults; therefore, relatively small doses may provide long-lasting pain relief. Meperidine can cause delirium and seizures. Methadone should be used with caution because it accumulates and its analgesic effect may be shorter than its serum half-life, which heightens the potential for accumulation or overdosing.

Assessment of Pain

It is important to obtain an accurate assessment of an older adult's pain. You may use the same assessment tools as used for any adult, but realize that certain normal aging processes occur that may affect the way a person perceives pain and responds to questions about pain.

Some Processes Affecting Pain Perception

- Decreasing levels of neurotransmitters or chemicals communicating in synapses between nerve cells affect short-term memory and motor coordination and control.

- Loss of cells in the brainstem changes sleep patterns. Individual variation and response to these changes are great.

- Sensory decline alters one's perception of the world. Hearing loss is common, especially at high frequencies. Smells become harder to distinguish and detect. Eyes may need corrective lenses to adjust for decreasing ability to focus. As the ciliary muscles weaken, pupil size is decreased, reducing light to the retina. The lens becomes stiff, thicker, and more opaque and begins to yellow.

▪ Special Considerations: **CHILDREN**

The mechanism for pain perception is fully developed and functioning by the time the fetus is born. Some indications of pain in the neonate are crying, eye rolling, breath holding with cyanosis, seizures, slow heart rate, and vomiting. Infants through 12 months of age show pain through body language, crying, coughing, and withdrawing the area of the body where the pain is felt. Toddlers from 1 to 3 years may indicate pain by aggressive behavior such as biting and pinching, by quiet withdrawal, and by regression. A toddler does not understand the concept of pain and is often afraid and fearful. Children who can communicate verbally can usually use words to express their pain. Hurt is a common expression said by children who are in pain. The words "Mommy, I hurt" can say it all.

Common Causes and Indications of Pain in Children

- *Earache:* pulling on the ear, crying, rubbing on the ear.
- *Stomachache:* not wanting to eat, rubbing the area, perhaps waking up in the middle of the night, crying.
- *Headache:* rubbing the head, crying, perhaps waking up in the middle of the night.

Assessment of Pain in Older Children

You may use various techniques to assess pain in older children. Some of these are:

- *Visual analog scale:* a child points to a number from 1 to 10, with 1 being no hurt and 10 being the most hurt ever felt.
- *Faces (oucher) scale:* a child tells which face represents the pain at the moment.
- *Descriptive word scale:* a child chooses the word that describes the pain (no pain, mild, moderate, quite a lot, very bad, worst).
- *Poker chip:* use four poker chips, placed horizontally in front of the child, and tell the child, "These are pieces of hurt"—one piece is a little, and four pieces are a lot. Ask the child, "How many pieces of hurt do you have right now?" Record the number (no pain equals zero chips).

▪ Critical Thinking **QUESTIONS AND ACTIVITIES**

It is important to obtain an accurate assessment of a patient's pain. Ask yourself:

- What questions must I ask the patient to obtain an accurate history of pain?
- What are the physical signs and symptoms of pain—in an adult, in a child?
- What facial expressions should I be aware of that would indicate pain?
- What body movements should I be aware of that would indicate pain?
- What are some of the verbal descriptions that a patient might use to relate the quality or character of pain?

ANALGESICS

Analgesic agents are used to relieve pain caused by disease or other conditions without causing the patient to lose consciousness. Morphine, a narcotic derivative of opium, was the forerunner of many natural and synthetic analgesics used today. Because they trace their origin back to opium, the natural and synthetic drugs derived from morphine are known as *opiates*. Other synthetic drugs, not chemically related to morphine, have been developed because they mimic the action of morphine. These drugs, called *opioids*, are also classified as narcotics because they can cause dependency. Table 27-1 lists opiate and opioid narcotic analgesics.

Narcotic Analgesics

Actions

Analgesics inhibit ascending pain pathways in the central nervous system. They increase pain threshold and alter pain perception.

Uses

Use for the relief of moderate to severe pain, as a preoperative medication, and as support of anesthesia.

Contraindications

Narcotic analgesics are contraindicated in patients with known hypersensitivity to any of the ingredients, in those with addiction; and in patients taking MAO inhibitors.

TABLE 27-1 Opiate and Opioid Analgesics

MEDICATION	CLASS/USE	USUAL DOSAGE	ADVERSE REACTIONS
codeine phosphate, codeine sulfate	ℂ analgesic	Oral, SC, IM (Adult): 15 to 60 mg 4 to 6 times/day as necessary Oral, SC, IM (Child): 0.5 mg/kg every 4 to 6 hours as necessary	Dizziness, drowsiness, palpitations, bradycardia, urinary retention, nausea, vomiting, constipation
hydromorphone HCl (Dilaudid)	ℂ analgesic	Oral, SC, IM: 2 mg every 4 to 6 hours	Respiratory depression, nausea, hypotension
levorphanol tartrate (Levo-Dromoran)	ℂ analgesic	Oral, SC: 2 to 3 mg repeated in 4 to 6 hours as necessary	As above
meperidine HCl (Demerol)	ℂ analgesic	Oral, SC, IM (Adult): 50 to 150 mg every 3 to 4 hours SC, IM (Child): 1 mg/kg every 4 hours as necessary	Dizziness, weakness, dry mouth, nausea, vomiting, respiratory depression, palpitations, bradycardia
methadone HCl (Dolophine)	ℂ analgesic	Oral, SC, IM (Adult): 2.5 to 10 mg every 3 to 4 hours, if necessary	Drowsiness, nausea, dry mouth, constipation
morphine sulfate	ℂ analgesic	Oral: 10 to 20 mg every 4 hours SC, IM: 5 to 20 mg every 4 hours SC, IM (Child): 0.05 to 0.2 mg/kg per dose	Deep sleep, respiratory depression, nausea, urinary retention, pruritus, edema, bradycardia, sweating
oxymorphone HCl	ℂ analgesic	SC, IM (Adult): 0.5 to 1.5 mg every 4 to 6 hours as needed	Nausea, vomiting, euphoria, dizziness
pentazocine HCl (Talwin)	ℂ analgesic	Oral: 50 mg every 3 to 4 hours SC, IM: 30 mg every 3 to 4 hours	Drowsiness, sweating, dry mouth, nausea, vomiting

> **Caution:**
>
> 1. *Narcotic analgesics can produce drug dependence and have the potential for being abused.*
> 2. *Narcotic analgesics must be used with great caution and in reduced dosage in patients who are concurrently taking other narcotic analgesics, general anesthetics, phenothiazines, other tranquilizers, sedative-hypnotics drugs, tricyclic antidepressants, or alcohol. Respiratory depression, hypotension, and profound sedation or coma may result.*
> 3. *Narcotic analgesics must be used with extreme caution in patients with head injury, increased intracranial pressure, asthma and other respiratory conditions, acute myocardial infarction, severe heart disease, hepatic disease, and renal disease.*
> 4. *Safe use in pregnancy prior to labor has not been established. Medication will cross the placental barrier and can produce depression of respiration and psychophysiologic functions in the newborns.*

Adverse Reactions

Reactions can include respiratory depression, circulatory depression, light-headedness, dizziness, sedation, hallucinations, nausea, vomiting, sweating, euphoria, dysphoria, weakness, headache, agitation, tremor, convulsions, dry mouth, constipation, biliary tract spasm, flushing of the face, tachycardia, bradycardia, palpitation, hypotension, syncope, urinary retention, pruritus, urticaria, rash, pain at injection site, and visual disturbances.

Dosage and Route

The dosage and route of administration are determined by the physician and individualized for each patient (see Table 27-1).

Implications for Patient Care

Observe patients for evidence of respiratory depression (respirations below 12), urinary retention (decreased output), central nervous system changes (dizziness, drowsiness, hallucinations, euphoria), allergic reactions (rash, urticaria), cardiac dysfunction (tachycardia, bradycardia, palpitation), and constipation.

 Patient Teaching

Educate patients:

- as to possible adverse reactions.
- to report any symptoms of CNS changes or allergic reactions to the physician.
- not to operate machinery or drive a motor vehicle while taking narcotics or analgesics.
- to avoid the use of alcohol and other CNS depressants that can enhance the drowsiness caused by analgesics. ■

Special Considerations

- Always assess the patient's respiratory rate before administration. Withhold medication and notify the physician if respiratory rate is 12 or below.
- Physical dependency may occur with the long-term use of narcotic analgesics. Withdrawal symptoms include nausea, vomiting, anorexia, abdominal cramps, fever, and faintness.

- Federal law requires that all controlled substances be kept separate from other drugs. They are to be stored in a substantially constructed metal box or compartment that is equipped with a double lock. A separate record book is required for information concerning the administration of controlled substances. This data system must be maintained on a daily basis and kept for a minimum of two years (three years in some states). Narcotics are counted at the end of each day, and the inventory of controlled drugs must be recorded on an audit sheet. Two individuals must sign this sheet to verify that the count is correct.

Several nonnarcotic analgesic drugs have been developed in an effort to provide alternative agents with less potential for abuse. Like the opiates, these drugs act on the central nervous system. They include butorphanol tartrate (Stadol), methotrimeprazine, and nalbuphine HCl. They produce adverse reactions similar to those listed in Table 27-1. The use of methotrimeprazine is somewhat limited by its tendency to cause orthostatic hypotension with fainting, weakness, and dizziness in a significant number of those taking the drug.

Narcotic Antagonist

Naloxone hydrochloride is a narcotic antagonist that prevents or reverses the effects of opioids including respiratory depression, sedation, and hypotension.

> **Caution:**
>
> *Narcotic antagonists should be administered cautiously to people including newborns of mothers who are known or suspected to be physically dependent on opioids.*

Dosage

Narcotic antagonists may be given intravenously, intramuscularly, and subcutaneously. For *narcotic overdose:* initial dose of 0.4 mg to 2 mg IV. Intravenous onset of action is generally apparent within 2 minutes. IV administration is performed by a physician, registered nurse, or other qualified health care professional.

Adverse Reactions

Abrupt reversal of narcotic depression may result in nausea, vomiting, sweating, tachycardia, increased blood pressure, tremulousness, seizures, and cardiac arrest.

ANALGESIC-ANTIPYRETICS

Certain medications act to relieve pain (analgesic effect) and reduce fever (antipyretic effect). Although the exact mechanism by which these drugs act is not completely understood, they appear to act peripherally by inhibition of prostaglandin synthesis at peripheral sites. Their antipyretic effect results from direct action on the heat-regulating center in the hypothalamus. In addition to their analgesic-antipyretic properties, all except acetaminophen produce significant anti-inflammatory action (see Table 27-2).

Aspirin or acetaminophen in combination with codeine phosphate or another narcotic analgesic is sometimes prescribed to provide greater relief from pain than is available from aspirin alone. Examples of such combination products include Empirin with Codeine, Percodan, Percodan-Demi, Percocet-5, Tylenol with Codeine, and Phenaphen with Codeine. Tablets and capsules containing these preparations are included in Schedule III of the Controlled Substances Act.

TABLE 27-2	Analgesic-Antipyretics		
MEDICATION	**ACTIONS**	**USUAL DOSAGE**	**ADVERSE REACTIONS**
acetaminophen (Tylenol)	analgesic-antipyretic	Oral (Adult): 325 to 650 mg at 4-hour intervals Oral (Child): 160 to 480 mg at 4- to 6-hour intervals	Nausea, vomiting, rash, urticaria, anemia, liver damage
aspirin (Bayer)	analgesic-antipyretic, anti-inflammatory, antirheumatic	Oral (Adult): 325 to 650 mg at 4- to 6-hour intervals Oral (Child): 160 to 480 mg at 4- to 6-hour intervals	Gastric irritation, easy bruising, hypersensitivity reactions such as tightness in the chest, bronchospasm, Reye's syndrome
ibuprofen (Advil) (Motrin)	anti-inflammatory, antirheumatic, analgesic-antipyretic	Oral: 200 to 800 mg 3 to 4 times per day (maximum, 2400 mg per day)	Headache, dizziness, nausea, vomiting, dyspepsia, leukopenia, flatulence
naproxen (Naprosyn)	anti-inflammatory, analgesic-antipyretic	Oral: 250 to 500 mg 2 times daily (maximum, 1000 mg/day)	Headache, blurred vision, indigestion, anorexia, agranulocytosis, pruritus

Warning:

The Food and Drug Administration has indicated new labeling for Tylenol (acetaminophen) and Motrin (ibuprofen) pain relievers. The Motrin label warns of the risk of stomach bleeding for those who drink three or more alcoholic beverages daily and take ibuprofen or other pain relievers. Tylenol's label warns that those who use acetaminophen and drink three or more alcoholic beverages daily may increase their risk of liver damage when taking in larger-than-recommended doses. Both Motrin and Tylenol labels suggest that heavy users of alcohol consult their physicians regarding use of the product.

With Motrin (ibuprofen), there is an additional warning about an allergy alert. Ibuprofen may cause a severe allergic reaction that may include hives, facial swelling, asthma (wheezing), or shock. If an allergic reaction occurs, patients are advised to stop use of the medicine and to seek medical help right away. Patients are advised not to use this product if they have ever had an allergic reaction to any other pain reliever or fever reducer.

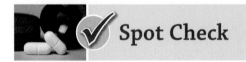

Spot Check

There are many medications that are used to help relieve pain. For each of the following drugs, give the usual dose, route, and the time interval for administration:

DRUG(S)	DOSE AND ROUTE	INTERVAL
acetaminophen (Tylenol)		

DRUG(S)	DOSE AND ROUTE	INTERVAL
codeine phosphate, codeine sulfate		
ibuprofen (Advil) (Motrin)		
meperidine (Demerol)		
methadone (Dolophine)		
morphine sulfate		
naproxen (Naprosyn)		

SEDATIVES AND HYPNOTICS

Anxiety and insomnia are conditions that often interfere with job performance and one's ability to interact with others. Sedatives and hypnotics are frequently used in the overall treatment of these disorders. These drugs depress the central nervous system by interfering with the transmission of nerve impulses. Depending upon the dosage, barbiturates, benzodiazepines, and certain other drugs can produce either a sedative or a hypnotic effect. When used as a sedative, the dosage is designed to produce a calming effect without causing sleep. Used as a hypnotic, the dosage is sufficient to cause sleep. An effective hypnotic should have fairly rapid action, produce near-normal sleep, and not give the patient a delayed effect the next day.

Barbiturates

The action of barbiturate drugs affects the entire central nervous system. Their use may produce a state ranging from mild sedation to deep sleep and anesthesia, depending upon the drug, the dosage prescribed, and the individual reaction of the patient. Large doses of barbiturates depress the respiratory vasomotor centers in the medulla and can lead to respiratory arrest and death.

Continued use of barbiturates over an extended period of time diminishes their effectiveness. Depending upon the drug, tolerance can develop as soon as a week after first administration, thereby requiring an increase in dosage to sustain the same effect. Psychological and physical dependency can result from the use of these drugs; therefore, they are subject to control under the Federal Controlled Substances Act. The adverse effects commonly associated with barbiturates include residual sedation, vertigo, nausea, and vomiting. Barbiturates used as sedatives and hypnotics are listed in Table 27-3.

Barbiturates differ widely in the duration of their action, which may range from a few seconds (ultra-short-acting) to several days (long-acting). They also differ in onset of action, which can be as little as 30 seconds or as long as 20 to 60 minutes. Short- and intermediate-acting agents are often used in the treatment of insomnia because of their rapid onset and the fact that their use rarely produces a "hangover" effect. Long-acting barbiturates (such as phenobarbital) are used as anticonvulsants in patients with epilepsy and as sedatives for a variety of anxiety and tension states.

Actions

As sedatives and hypnotics, barbiturates depress the sensory cortex, decrease motor activity, alter cerebral function, and produce drowsiness, sedation, and hypnosis. They depress activity in brain cells, primarily in the reticular activating system in the brain stem, thus interfering with the transmission of impulses to the cortex.

Uses

Use barbiturates for short-term treatment of insomnia, for sedation, as a preoperative medication, and as adjuncts to cancer chemotherapy.

Contraindications

Barbiturates are contraindicated in patients with known hypersensitivity to any of the ingredients. They should not be used in patients with a history of manifest or latent porphyria, respiratory depression, and severe liver impairment.

Caution:

1. Barbiturates may be habit-forming. Tolerance and psychological and physical dependence may occur with continued use.
2. Use caution in patients with acute and chronic pain.
3. Barbiturates can cause fetal damage when administered to a pregnant woman.
4. Alcohol and other CNS depressants may produce additive CNS depressant effects.
5. There are many precautions associated with the use of barbiturates. Please refer to a current edition of the drug reference book or go to www.fda.gov for information on precautions.

Adverse Reactions

Reactions include somnolence, agitation, confusion, hyperkinesia, ataxia, CNS depression, nightmares, nervousness, hallucinations, insomnia, anxiety, dizziness, thinking abnormality, hypoventilation, apnea, bradycardia, hypotension, syncope, nausea, vomiting, constipation, headache, angioedema, rash, exfoliative dermatitis, fever, liver damage, and megaloblastic anemia.

TABLE 27-3 Barbiturates Used as Sedatives and Hypnotics				
MEDICATION	**SCHEDULE**	**DURATION**	**USUAL SEDATIVE DOSE**	**USUAL HYPNOTIC DOSE**
pentobarbital (Nembutal)	Ⅱ	short-acting	Oral: 20 to 30 mg 2 to 4 times daily	Oral: 100 mg Rectal: 120 to 200 mg IM: 100 to 0 mg
phenobarbital	Ⅳ	long-acting	Oral: 15 to 32 mg 2 to 4 times daily	Oral: 50 to 100 mg SC, IM: 100 to 300 mg daily
secobarbital (Seconal)	Ⅱ	short-acting	Oral: 30 to 50 mg 3 times daily	Oral, IM: 100 to 200 mg

Dosage and Route

The dosage and route of administration are determined by the physician and individualized for each patient (see Table 27-3).

Implications for Patient Care

Observe patient for evidence of CNS depression and any signs of adverse reactions. Monitor vital signs, blood and hepatic tests, and therapeutic effects. Be alert for signs of drug dependency. You should be alert for the following signs of *barbiturate toxicity*, *respiratory dysfunction*, and *blood dyscrasias*:

1. *Barbiturate toxicity:* hypotension, cold and clammy skin, cyanosis of lips, insomnia, nausea, vomiting, hallucinations, delirium, and/or weakness
2. *Respiratory dysfunction:* respirations below 10/minute in adults, and pupils dilated
3. *Blood dyscrasias:* fever, rash, sore throat, bruising, jaundice, and/or epistaxis

 Patient Teaching

Educate patients:

- to take the medication as prescribed.
- to be alert for signs of adverse reactions.
- to avoid the use of alcohol and other CNS depressants.
- not to smoke, operate machinery, or drive a motor vehicle after taking the medication.
- that physical dependency may occur if medication is used for an extended period (45 to 90 days, depending on dose).
- about alternative methods of relaxation to improve sleep (exercise, reading, warm bath or shower, music, deep breathing, biofeedback, and so forth). ▪

Special Considerations

- Barbiturates are subject to control by the Federal Controlled Substances Act under Drug Enforcement Administration (DEA) Schedule II. They may be habit-forming and are often abused.
- Emergency supplies and equipment should be readily available for use when administering barbiturates to a patient in a hospital setting, long-term care facility, or other health-related facility.
- Barbiturates may decrease the effects of corticosteroids, oral anticoagulants, griseofulvin, and quinidine.
- The effects of barbiturates may be increased by alcohol, MAO inhibitors, other sedatives, and narcotics.

- Barbiturates should not be mixed with other drugs in a solution or syringe.

- Barbiturates should not be used for more than 14 days for insomnia, because they are not effective after that time and tolerance may develop.

- Barbiturates that are used for long-term therapy should not be discontinued quickly because symptoms of withdrawal can be severe and may cause death. Drugs must be tapered off over one to two weeks.

Benzodiazepines

Although benzodiazepines are best known for their use in the relief of anxiety, several drugs in this chemical classification may be used as sedative-hypnotics. These drugs generally reduce incidents of night and early morning awakening and increase the duration of total sleep time. The onset of action for these drugs is between 15 and 40 minutes and their effect has a duration of 6 to 8 hours. Examples of benzodiazepines used as sedative-hypnotics are flurazepam, lorazepam, oxazepam, temazepam, and triazolam (see Table 27-4).

Other drugs that may be used as sedative-hypnotics are chloral hydrate (one of the oldest hypnotics), zaleplon, and zolpidem (see Table 27-4).

It is recommended that any medication that is used in the treatment of *insomnia* (the inability to obtain the amount of sleep a person needs for optimal functioning and well-being) be used for short-term therapy. The medication should generally be limited to a period of 7 to 10 days.

Sedative-hypnotics have an additive central nervous system (CNS) depressant effect with other CNS depressants including alcohol, antihistamines, antidepressants, opioids, and other sedative-hypnotics.

TABLE 27-4 Nonbarbiturate Sedative-Hypnotic Drugs

MEDICATION	SCHEDULE	USUAL SEDATIVE DOSE	USUAL HYPNOTIC DOSE
chloral hydrate (Aquachloral)	C-IV	Oral, Rectal (Adult): 250 mg 3 times a day after meals Oral (Child): 8 to 25 mg/kg/24 hours divided into 2 to 3 doses	Oral, Rectal (Adult): 500 mg to 1 g before bedtime Oral (Child): 50 mg/kg to a maximum of 1 g
flurazepam HCl (Dalmane)	C-IV	No listing	Oral: 15 to 30 mg at bedtime
lorazepam (Ativan)	C-IV	No listing	Oral (Adult): 2 to 4 mg at bedtime
oxazepam (Serax)	C-IV	No listing	Oral (Adult): 15 to 30 mg at bedtime
temazepam (Restoril)	C-IV	No listing	Oral (Adult): 15 to 30 mg at bedtime Oral (Elderly): 15 mg as an initial dose
triazolam (Halcion)	C-IV	No listing	Oral (Adult): 0.25 to 0.5 mg Oral (Elderly): 0.125 to 0.25 mg
zaleplon (Sonata)	C-IV	No listing	Oral (Adult): 10 mg at bedtime
zolpidem tartrate (Ambien)	C-IV	No listing	Oral (Adult): 10 mg at bedtime

ANTI-PARKINSONIAN DRUGS

Named for British physician James Parkinson, Parkinson's disease is a neurologic disorder characterized by the development of a fine, slowly spreading tremor, muscular weakness and rigidity, and the development of disturbances in posture and equilibrium. The cause of the disease is not fully understood, but it is believed to be associated with an imbalance of the neurotransmitters *acetylcholine* and dopamine in the brain.

Anti-parkinsonian drugs are used for palliative relief from such major symptoms as bradykinesia, rigidity, tremor, and disorders of equilibrium and posture (see Figure 27-2). The drug of choice depends upon the severity of the disease at the time of diagnosis and is subject to change with the continuation of the disease. Therapy involves an attempt to replenish dopamine levels and/or inhibit the effects of the neurotransmitter acetylcholine (see Table 27-5).

Actions

The drugs exert an inhibitory effect upon the parasympathetic nervous system. They prolong the action of dopamine by blocking its uptake into presynaptic neurons in the central nervous system.

Uses

Use for treatment of all forms of parkinsonism.

Contraindications

Anti-parkinsonian drugs are contraindicated in patients with known hypersensitivity to any of the ingredients. They should not be used in patients with narrow-angle glaucoma, myasthenia gravis, gastrointestinal or genitourinary obstruction, and in children under 3 years of age.

Caution:

1. *Before initiation of drug therapy, patients should have a gonioscope evaluation and close monitoring of intraocular pressure at regular periodic intervals.*
2. *Use caution during pregnancy, lactation, and in geriatric patients.*
3. *Patients with cardiac, liver, or kidney disorders, or hypertension should be carefully monitored while on anti-parkinsonian drug.*
4. *Dopamine agonist drugs can cause drowsiness and there is a possibility of suddenly falling asleep during daily activities, which could result in an accident while operating a vehicle.*
5. *Parlodel is a synthetic derivative of natural products produced by a fungus called ergot. A rare side effect known as fibrosis (thickening or scarring of the membrane lining of body organs) has been reported.*

Adverse Reactions

Reactions include dryness of the mouth, blurring of vision, dizziness, mild nausea, nervousness, suppurative parotitis, skin rash, dilatation of the colon, paralytic ileus, delusions, hallucinations, paranoia, constipation, drowsiness, urinary hesitancy or retention, tachycardia, dilation of the pupil, increased intraocular tension, weakness, vomiting, headache, and angle-closure glaucoma.

Dosage and Route

The dosage and route of administration are determined by the physician and individualized for each patient (see Table 27-5).

Implications for Patient Care

Observe the patient for evidence of improvement and signs of adverse reactions. Monitor vital signs, intake and output ratio, gastrointestinal function, and mental status of the patient.

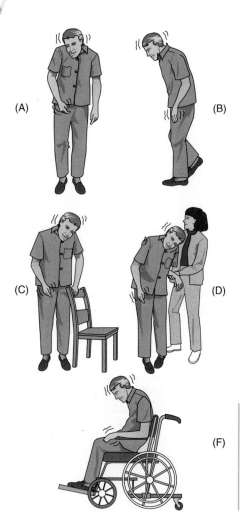

Patient Teaching

Educate patients:

- to take the medication as prescribed.
- to be alert for signs of adverse reactions.
- to avoid the use of alcohol and over-the-counter medications.
- not to operate machinery or drive a motor vehicle after taking the medication.
- not to discontinue the medication.
- that hallucinations can occur with selected anti-parkinsonian drugs such as Comtan, Requip, and Tasmar.
- that they may develop postural (orthostatic) hypotension with or without symptoms such as dizziness, nausea, syncope, and sometimes sweating with selected anti-parkinsonian drugs such as Comtan, Requip, and Tasmar.
- to the potential sedating effects associated with selected anti-parkinsonian drugs such as Comtan, Requip, and Tasmar.
- that if increased somnolence or episodes of falling asleep during activities of daily living are experienced at any time during treatment, patients should not drive or participate in potentially dangerous activities before consulting their physician. ■

TABLE 27-5 Anti-Parkinsonian Drugs

MEDICATION	DRUG ACTION	USUAL DOSAGE	ADVERSE REACTIONS
amantadine HCl (Symmetrel)	Indirectly increases dopaminergic activity	Oral: 100 mg twice daily	Dizziness, light-headedness, irritability, hypotension, edema, anorexia, nausea
benztropine mesylate (Cogentin)	Anticholinergic	Oral: 0.5 to 6 mg/day if required and tolerated	Sedation, dizziness, tachycardia, nausea, vomiting, urinary retention, dysuria
biperiden HCl (Akineton)	Anticholinergic	Oral: 2 mg 1 to 4 times daily	Dry mouth, blurred vision, constipation, dizziness
bromocriptine mesylate (Parlodel)	Dopamine receptor *agonist*	Oral: 10 to 40 mg daily in divided doses	Orthostatic hypotension, rash, shock, nausea, dizziness, epigastric pain, blurred vision
carbidopa/ levodopa (Sinemet)	Peripheral dopa decarboxylase inhibitor used in combination with L-dopa	Oral: 1 to 6 tablets 3 times daily (tablets contain 10 mg carbidopa and 100 mg levodopa)	No reactions for carbidopa For levodopa: involuntary movements, nausea, anorexia, urinary retention, dry mouth
entacapone (Comtan)	COMT inhibitor (catechol-O-methyltransferase)	Oral: 200 mg administered with a levodopa/carbidopa regimen up to a maximum of 8 times/day (1600 mg/day)	Dyskinesia, hyperkinesia hypokinesia, dizziness, anxiety, somnolence, agitation, hallucinations, nausea, vomiting, diarrhea, abdominal pain, dry mouth, dyspepsia, fatigue, asthenia, back pain, dyspnea, purpura
levodopa (Larodopa, L-dopa)	Metabolic precursor of dopamine	Oral: 0.5 to 8 g daily divided into 2 or more equal doses	Orthostatic hypotension, anorexia, nausea, abdominal distress, increased hand tremor, grinding of the teeth
ropinirole (Requip)	Dopamine agonist	Oral: 0.25 mg 3 times a day, then increased dose as needed and tolerated. The dose is usually not more than 24 mg/day	Confusion, dizziness, drowsiness, falling, light-headedness or fainting, nausea, hallucinations, swelling of legs, twitching, unusual tiredness or weakness, worsening of Parkinson's disease
trihexyphenidyl HCl (Artane)	Anticholinergic	Oral: 1 to 10 mg daily in 3 or more divided doses	Dry mouth, dizziness, nausea, blurred vision, nervousness

Special Considerations

- Medication should not be discontinued abruptly, but should be tapered off over one to two weeks. Sudden withdrawal of medication may precipitate a parkinsonian crisis characterized by anxiety, sweating, and tachycardia, and an exacerbation of tremors, rigidity, and dyskinesia.

- Administer with or after meals to help prevent gastrointestinal upset.

- Anticholinergic effects may be increased by alcohol, narcotics, barbiturates, antihistamines, MAO inhibitors, phenothiazines, or amantadine.

- Pyridoxine will reduce the therapeutic effect of levodopa; therefore, only pyridoxine-free multivitamins should be taken when taking levodopa. Larobec is a vitamin supplement made specifically for patients taking levodopa.

- When taking levodopa, adequate fluid intake and eating bulk-forming foods should be encouraged to minimize the possibility of constipation.

- When taking levodopa, the urine may turn red to black on exposure to air or alkaline substances (toilet-bowl cleansers). Patients need to be informed of this, so that they will not become alarmed.

- With selected anti-parkinsonian drugs such as Comtan, Requip, and Tasmar, patients should be advised of the potential to develop drowsiness and specifically asked about factors that may increase this risk.

ALZHEIMER'S DISEASE

Alzheimer's disease (AD) is a progressive degeneration of brain tissue that usually begins after age 60. It may also rarely affect people as young as age 30. This disease is marked by a devastating mental decline. Intellectual functions such as memory, comprehension, and speech deteriorate. Attention tends to stray, simple calculations become impossible, and ordinary daily activities grow increasingly difficult, with bewilderment and frustration worsening at night. Dramatic mood swings occur with outbursts of anger, bouts of fearfulness, and periods of deep apathy. The sufferer, increasingly disoriented, may wander off and become lost. Physical problems, such as odd gait or a loss of coordination, gradually develops. Eventually, patients may become totally noncommunicative, physically helpless, and incontinent. The disease is invariably fatal.

In Alzheimer's disease, the paths of communication between brain cells become distorted by deposits of a protein called *amyloid.* In addition, levels of acetylcholine begin to drop, causing more cell-to-cell communication problems. Eventually, the brain cells themselves are affected. They begin to shrivel and die, causing certain areas of the brain to shrink.

Alzheimer's can run its course from insidious onset to death in just a few years, or it may play out over a period of as long as 20 years; the average duration, however, is about 10 years. Among American adults, it is the fourth leading cause of death. Age and family history are the two most important risk factors for developing this disease. Alzheimer's affects an estimated 4.5 million older Americans and, as the "baby boomers" age, it may eventually affect 14 million by the year 2040. At age 65, approximately 1 percent of people are stricken, but this increases to more than 30 percent after age 85. In addition to age, there appear to be inherited factors that increase the risk of Alzheimer's disease. Current research links these genetic factors to areas on chromosomes 12 and 19. Symptoms of the disease include:

- Mood changes: depression, paranoia, agitation, anxiety, selfishness, childish behavior

- Disorientation, confusion, inattention, loss of memory for recent events, inability to retain new information.

- Increased tendency to misplace things.

- Dizziness or impaired equilibrium.

Alzheimer's disease is incurable. Certain medications seem to slow its general progress to some degree in the early stages, and others can help with mood changes, and other specific behavioral problems of the disease.

Medications that may be used to improve global functioning (including activities of daily living, behavior, and cognition) in some patients with Alzheimer's are tacrine (Cognex), donepezil hydrochloride (Aricept), rivastigmine tartrate (Exelon), and galantamine HBr (Razadyne). These drugs are classified as cholinesterase inhibitors. They work by increasing the brain's levels of acetylcholine, which helps to restore communication between brain cells.

The Food and Drug Administration has approved memantine (Namenda), the first drug to be used for the treatment of moderate to severe Alzheimer's disease. It's mechanism of action is different from that of the drugs currently available for treating this disease. It is an orally active NMDA (N-methyl-D-aspartate) receptor antagonist.

Several drugs can be prescribed for specific symptoms associated with this disease. Antipsychotic agents, such as haloperidol (Haldol) and thioridazine (Mellaril), may be prescribed for aggressive behavior and agitation. These agents alter the effect of dopamine in the central nervous system. An antidepressant such as sertraline (Zoloft) may be prescribed for depression, and a hypnotic such as zolpidem (Ambien) may be prescribed for sleep.

ANTICONVULSANTS

Epilepsy is the most common of the seizure disorders and affects approximately one percent of the population. It is characterized by recurrent abnormal electrical discharges within the brain. An epileptic convulsion may be characterized by sudden, brief episodes of altered consciousness, abnormal motor function, or sensory function interference. The disorder may be classified as *idiopathic* or *symptomatic* in origin, depending upon whether or not the cause of the condition is known. The majority of cases are idiopathic (cause is not identified), and symptoms begin during childhood or early adolescence. Tiny lesions in the brain at birth, metabolic disease, and developmental defects are possible causes. When developed in adulthood, epilepsy can usually be identified with such causes as trauma, tumors, strokes, and other disease processes affecting the brain.

Further classification has been applied to the types of seizures that are experienced by those with epilepsy. They have been divided into four main categories, some of which have subtypes:

1. *Partial seizures* (focal seizures) are those whose electrical disturbance is localized to areas of the brain near the source or focal point of the seizure.
2. *Generalized seizures* (bilateral, symmetrical) are those without local onset that involve both the right and left hemispheres of the brain.
3. *Unilateral seizures* are those in which the electrical discharge is predominately confined to one of the two hemispheres of the brain.
4. *Unclassified epileptic seizures* are those that cannot be placed into one of the other three categories because of incomplete data.

With all types of epilepsy, the objective of drug therapy is to obtain the greatest degree of control over seizures without causing intolerable side effects. Selection of the most appropriate drug for a patient with epilepsy depends upon proper diagnosis and classification. The appropriate dosage must be individualized and is related to the size, age, and condition of the patient; how the patient responds to treatment; and whether or not the patient is taking other medications.

Actions

Anticonvulsants inhibits the spread of seizure activity in the motor cortex.

Uses

Anticonvulsants are indicated for the control of tonic-clonic and psychomotor (grand mal and temporal lobe) seizures and prevention and treatment of seizures occurring during or following neurosurgery.

Contraindications

Anticonvulsants are contraindicated in patients with known hypersensitivity to any of the ingredients. They should not be used in patients with psychiatric disease and during pregnancy and breast-feeding.

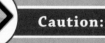

Caution:

1. *Abrupt withdrawal of medication in patients with epilepsy may precipitate status epilepticus.*
2. *There may be a relationship between anticonvulsants and the development of lymphadenopathy.*
3. *Acute alcohol intake may increase serum levels of anticonvulsant drugs, while chronic alcohol use may decrease serum levels.*

Adverse Reactions

Reactions include nystagmus, ataxia, slurred speech, mental confusion, dizziness, insomnia, transient nervousness, motor twitchings, headache, drug-induced dyskinesias similar to those induced by phenothiazines and other neuroleptic agents, nausea, vomiting, constipation, toxic hepatitis, liver damage, fever, measles-like rash, thrombocytopenia, leukopenia, granulocytopenia, agranulocytosis, pancytopenia, lymphadenopathy, coarsening of facial features, enlargement of the lips, and liver dysfunction.

Dosage and Route

The dosage and route of administration are determined by the physician and individualized for each patient (see Table 27-6).

TABLE 27-6   Anticonvulsants

MEDICATION	USUAL DOSAGE	ADVERSE REACTIONS
carbamazepine (Tegretol)	Oral (Adult): 200 mg twice/day, increased to a maximum of 1200 mg/day in 3 to 4 doses Oral (Child): 100 mg twice/day, increased to a maximum of 1000 mg/day in 3 to 4 doses	Dizziness, vertigo, drowsiness, edema, arrhythmias, skin rashes, nausea, vomiting, abdominal pain, aplastic anemia, blurred vision
clonazepam (Klonopin)	Oral (Adult): 1.5 mg/day divided into 3 doses, increased by 0.5 to 1 mg every 3 days until seizures are controlled Oral (Child): 0.01 to 0.03 mg/kg/day not to exceed 0.05 mg/day in 3 divided doses	Palpitations, bradycardia, hair loss, hirsutism, skin rash, sore gums, drowsiness, ataxia, dysuria
diazepam (Valium)	Oral (Adult): 2 to 10 mg 2 to 4 times daily IM (Adult): 2 to 10 mg repeated in 3 to 4 hours if necessary Oral (Child): 1 to 2.5 mg 3 to 4 times/day IM (Child): 0.2 to 1 mg every 2 to 5 minutes (maximum, 5 mg under age 5)	Drowsiness, fatigue, hypotension, ataxia, vivid dreams, tachycardia, urinary retention, blurred vision, hiccups, throat and chest pain, hepatic dysfunction including jaundice
ethosuximide (Zarontin)	Oral: 250 mg twice/day, increased by 250 mg every 4 to 7 hours until controlled Oral (Child under 6): 250 mg daily	Hiccups, ataxia, dizziness, anxiety, hyperactivity, nausea, epigastric distress, leukopenia
felbamate (Felbatol)	Oral (Adult): 1200 mg/day in 3 to 4 divided doses; gradually increase to 3600 mg/day Oral (Child): With Lennox-Gastaut syndrome: 15 mg/kg/day (maximum 45 mg/kg/day)	Vomiting, constipation, insomnia, headache, fatigue, nausea, dizziness, anorexia, fever
levetiracetam (Keppra)	Oral (Adult): Initial 500 mg b.i.d. Can increase dose by 1000 mg/day every 2 weeks up to a maximum daily dose of 300 mg	Somnolence, dizziness, ataxia, nervousness, vertigo, depression, amnesia, anxiety, hostility, paresthesia, psychotic symptoms, pharyngitis, rhinitis, sinusitis, increased cough, abdominal pain, constipation, diarrhea, dyspepsia, gastroenteritis, gingivitis, nausea, vomiting, headache, anorexia, diplopia, coordination difficulties
mephenytoin	Oral: 50 to 100 mg/day for first week, then increase weekly by same amount (maintenance dose 200 to 600 mg/day in 3 equal doses)	Drowsiness, dizziness, skin rashes, blood dyscrasias, hepatic damage

(continues)

TABLE 27-6   *(continued)*

MEDICATION	USUAL DOSAGE	ADVERSE REACTIONS
phenobarbital sodium	Oral (Adult): 50 to 100 mg Oral (Child): 16 to 50 mg 2 to 3 times daily	Nightmares, insomnia, hangover, dizziness, bradycardia, nausea, coughing, hiccups, liver damage
phenytoin, phenytoin sodium (Dilantin)	Oral (Adult): 100 mg 3 times/day, then gradual increase up to 600 mg/day Parenteral (Adult): 300 to 400 mg/daily Oral (Child): 4 to 8 mg/kg/day in 1 to 3 doses Parenteral (Child): 5 mg/kg in 1 to 2 doses	Nystagmus, diplopia, blurred or dimmed vision, drowsiness, ataxia, slurred speech, hypotension, nausea, epigastric pain, pruritus, acute renal failure, hyperglycemia, gingival hyperplasia, hirsutism
primidone (Mysoline)	Oral: 250 mg/day, increased by 250 mg weekly (maximum 2 g/day in 2 to 4 doses) Oral (Child under 8): half of adult dose	Drowsiness, sedation, vertigo, nausea, anorexia, nystagmus, swelling of eyelids, alopecia
trimethadione (Tridione)	Oral (Adult): 0.9 to 2.4 g/day in 3 to 4 equally divided doses Oral (Child): 0.3 to 0.9 g/day in 3 to 4 equally divided doses	Hemeralopia, photophobia, ataxia, exfoliative dermatitis, hiccups, nausea, gastric distress
valproic acid (Depakene)	Oral: 15 mg/kg/day, increased at 1 week intervals by 5 to 10 mg/kg/day (maximum recommended dose 60 mg/kg/day)	Breakthrough seizures, sedation, drowsiness, dizziness, ataxia, nausea, hypersalivation, hepatic failure, depression, skin rash

Implications for Patient Care

Observe patient for signs of improvement and adverse reactions. Monitor vital signs, weight, blood and liver function studies, intake and output ratio, and drug serum levels.

Patient Teaching

Educate patients:

- to take the medication as prescribed.
- to be alert for signs of adverse reactions.
- to avoid the use of alcohol and over-the-counter medications.
- not to operate machinery or drive a motor vehicle while taking medication.
- to wear a Medic Alert ID stating that they are an epileptic and on medication.
- to see their physician on a regular basis.
- about support groups and self-help/management programs that can assist in their treatment regimen.
- that some anticonvulsant agents may discolor the urine pink.
- that anticonvulsant medication should not be abruptly discontinued because seizures can occur.
- to notify their physician if they become pregnant or intend to become pregnant during therapy.
- that their medication may cause changes in behaviour (such as aggression, agitation, anger, anxiety, apathy, depression, hostility, and irritability) and that, in rare cases, they may experience psychotic symptoms and/or suicidal ideation.
- to read the patient information leaflet that appears as the last section of the labeling. ■

Teach the patient's family how to care for the patient during a seizure:

- Protect the patient from nearby hazards by moving hazards away from the patient.
- Do not move the patient or restrain the patient.
- Do not put anything in the patient's mouth.
- Do not try and hold the patient's tongue; it cannot be swallowed.
- Provide for privacy.
- Observe and record the time of the seizure, when it started and ended.
- Record if there is loss of bladder or bowel control, or loss of consciousness.
- Following the seizure, maintain an open airway, turn the patient on his or her side, loosen any tight clothing from the neck, reassure the patient and provide for a period of rest.
- Do not give liquid or food until the patient is fully conscious and has had an adequate time to recover from the seizure.
- If multiple seizures occur or one seizure lasts longer than 5 minutes, call 911 for help.

Special Considerations

- Drug therapy is individualized for each patient and it may be necessary to try several different drugs and dosages before therapeutic response is reached.
- The effects of anticonvulsants may be decreased by alcohol, antihistamines, antacids, antineoplastics, CNS depressants, rifampin, or folic acid.

ANESTHETICS

Anesthetics are drugs that interfere with the conduction of nerve impulses and are used to produce loss of sensation, muscle relaxation, and/or complete loss of consciousness. *Local anesthetics* block nerve transmission in the area to which they are applied. They produce loss of sensation and motor activity, but do not cause loss of consciousness (see Table 27-7). *General anesthetics* affect the central nervous system and produce either partial

TABLE 27-7 Local (Regional) Anesthetic Drugs

MEDICATION	ROUTE(S)	USUAL STRENGTH OF DOSAGE	ADVERSE REACTIONS
benzocaine (Solarcaine)	Topical	0.5 to 20%, ointment, lotion, cream, aerosol spray, liquid	Contact urticaria, erythemia, contact dermatitis, swelling
bupivacaine HCl (Marcaine HCl)	Injection	0.25 to 0.75% solution	Usually dose-related: apnea, hypotension, heart block
chloroprocaine HCl (Nesacaine)	Injection	1 to 3% solution	Usually dose-related: hypotension, ventricular arrhythmias, bradycardia
lidocaine HCl (Xylocaine HCl)	Topical, injection	2.5 to 5% cream, ointment, jelly 0.5 to 4% solution	Drowsiness, light-headedness, euphoria, tinnitus, blurred vision, numbness of lips
procaine HCl (Novocain)	Injection	1 to 10% solution	Nervousness, dizziness, hypotension, postspinal headache
tetracaine HCl (Pontocaine)	Topical, injection	0.5 to 2% ointment, cream 1% solution	Nervousness, blurred vision, drowsiness, nausea, vomiting, chills, hypotension, edema

or complete loss of consciousness. They also cause varying degrees of analgesia, skeletal muscle relaxation, and reduction of reflex activity.

OPHTHALMIC DRUGS

Medications are used in the eye for the treatment of glaucoma, during diagnostic examination of the eye, and in intraocular surgery. Glaucoma is an eye disease characterized by increased intraocular pressure, which, if not treated, causes atrophy of the optic nerve and blindness. The disease occurs when there is a failure to remove aqueous humor at a rate equal to its production. Drugs used to treat glaucoma either increase the outflow of aqueous humor, decrease its production, or produce both of these actions.

Drugs used to treat glaucoma are listed in Table 27-8.

Mydriatic Drugs

Anticholinergic agents produce dilation of the pupil (mydriasis) and interfere with the ability of the eye to focus properly (paralysis of accommodation or cycloplegia). Mydriatic drugs are used primarily as an aid in refraction, during internal examination of the eye, in intraocular surgery, and in the treatment of anterior uveitis and secondary glaucomas.

Sympathomimetic mydriatics produce mydriasis without cycloplegia. Pupil dilation is obtained as the drug causes contraction of the dilator muscle of the iris. These drugs also affect intraocular pressure by decreasing production of aqueous humor while increasing its outflow from the eyes. Mydriatic agents are listed in Table 27-9.

TABLE 27-8   Drugs Used to Treat Glaucoma

MEDICATION	CLASSIFICATION	USUAL DOSAGE	ADVERSE REACTIONS
acetazolamide (Diamox)	carbonic anhydrase inhibitor diuretic	Oral: 250 mg every 6 hours IM: 500 mg repeated in 2 to 4 hours, if necessary	Paresthesia, drowsiness, tinnitus, nausea, rash, bone marrow depression
demecarium bromide	Cholinesterase inhibitor, miotic	Topical: 1 to 2 drops of 0.125 or 0.25% solution 2 times/week up to twice daily	Stinging, burning, ciliary spasm, lacrimation, brow and eye pain, headache
echothiophate iodide (Phospholine iodide)	Cholinesterase inhibitor, miotic	Topical: 1 drop of 0.03 to 0.25% solution 1 to 2 times daily	Browache, headache, stinging, blurring of vision, iris cysts, ciliary spasm
methazolamide	Carbonic anhydrase inhibitor	Oral: 50 to 100 mg every 8 hours	Malaise, drowsiness, mild GI disturbances, vertigo
pilocarpine HCl, pilocarpine nitrate (Isopto Carpine) (Pilocar) (Ocusert Pilo) (Pilopine HS)	Miotic	Ophthalmic solution: 1 drop of 0.25% to 10% solution up to 6 times daily Ocular therapeutic system: One system (20 or 40 mcg/hour) each week Ophthalmic gel: Apply once daily at bedtime	Headache, eye and brow pain, dimness and blurring of vision, eye irritation
timolol maleate (Timoptic)	Beta-adrenergic receptor blocking agent	Ophthalmic solution: 1 drop of 0.25% solution in the affected eye(s) twice a day	Burning and stinging upon instillation, headache

TABLE 27-9	Mydriatic Agents		
MEDICATION	**CLASSIFICATION**	**USUAL DOSAGE**	**ADVERSE REACTIONS**
atropine sulfate (Atropisol)	Anticholinergic mydriatic	Topical: 1 to 2 drops of 0.5% to 1% solution 1 to 3 times daily	Blurred vision, photophobia, increased intraocular pressure
cyclopentolate HCl (Cyclogyl)	Anticholinergic mydriatic	Topical: 1 drop of 0.5% solution and, if needed, another drop after 5 minutes	Blurred vision, photophobia, increased intraocular pressure
dipivefrin (Propine)	Sympathomimetic, adrenergic agonist	Topical: 1 drop of 0.1% solution in eye every 12 hours	Burning, stinging upon application, photophobia
epinephrine	Sympathomimetic, adrenergic agonist	Topical: 1 to 2 drops of 0.1% solution in affected eye, 1 to 2 times/day	Lacrimation, headache, stinging sensation
phenylephrine HCl (Neo-Synephrine)	Sympathomimetic, adrenergic agonist	Topical: 1 drop of 2.5% to 10% solution 3 times/day	Stinging, browache, sensitivity to light
scopolamine HBr (Hyoscine)	Anticholinergic mydriatic	Topical: 1 to 2 drops of 0.5% to 1% solution	Follicular conjunctivitis, local irritation
tropicamide (Mydriacyl)	Anticholinergic mydriatic	Topical: 1 to 2 drops of 1% solution, repeat in 5 minutes	Photophobia, transient stinging, blurred vision

DRUGS USED IN VERTIGO, MOTION SICKNESS, AND VOMITING

Vertigo is a term used to describe an illusion of movement. Individuals experiencing vertigo may have the sensation of moving around in space, or know that they are stationary but sense that objects are in motion. Vertigo may be caused by a lesion or other process affecting the brain, the eighth cranial nerve, or the labyrinthine system of the ear. The result is a disturbance of equilibrium wherein the person experiences dizziness, light-headedness, and possibly nausea and vomiting.

Motion sickness is usually associated with travel. Sometimes called seasickness, carsickness, or airsickness, this condition affects large numbers of people and causes nausea and vomiting. About one-third of the population is highly susceptible to motion, and another third experiences symptoms when exposed to moderately rough travel conditions. Drugs are used for symptomatic relief rather than for treatment.

Vomiting is a complex reflex that may result from disease, drugs, radiation, toxins, and many other causes that serve to stimulate the vomiting center in the medulla. Because nausea and vomiting are symptoms of underlying causes, every effort should be made to identify and correct the causative condition.

Certain anticholinergic, antihistaminic, and antidopaminergic drugs have been identified as being effective in the treatment of vertigo, motion sickness, and vomiting; however, not all of the drugs in these classifications are effective in treating these disorders. Those that are effective are listed in Table 27-10.

TABLE 27-10	Drugs Used in Vertigo, Motion Sickness, and Vomiting		
MEDICATION	**USES**	**USUAL DOSAGE**	**ADVERSE REACTIONS**
chlorpromazine	Nausea, vomiting	Oral: 10 to 25 mg every 4 to 6 hours as needed IM: 25 to 50 mg every 3 to 4 hours as needed Rectal: One 100-mg suppository every 6 to 8 hours	Sedation, depressed cough reflex, bizarre dreams, orthostatic hypotension, constipation, blurred vision, nasal congestion, respiratory depression

(continues)

TABLE 27-10 (*continued*)

MEDICATION	USES	USUAL DOSAGE	ADVERSE REACTIONS
dimenhydrinate (Dramamine)	Motion sickness, nausea, vomiting, vertigo	Oral: 50 to 100 mg every 4 to 6 hours IM: 50 mg	Drowsiness, headache, dizziness, insomnia, hypotension, blurred vision, dry mouth
diphenhydramine HCl (Benadryl)	Motion sickness, vertigo	Oral, IM: 25 to 50 mg 3 to 4 times daily at 4 to 6-hour intervals	Drowsiness, dizziness, headache, fatigue, euphoria, dry mouth, blurred vision, dysuria
meclizine HCl (Antivert)	Nausea, vomiting, motion sickness, vertigo	Oral: 25 to 100 mg daily in divided doses	Drowsiness, blurred vision, dry mouth, fatigue
promethazine HCl (Phenergan)	Motion sickness, nausea, vomiting	Oral, IM, Rectal suppository: 12.5 to 25 mg and again at 4- to 6-hour intervals as needed	Sedation, confusion, dizziness, tremors, anorexia, dry mouth, leukopenia, blurred vision, photosensitivity
scopolamine (Transderm-scop)	Motion sickness, nausea, vomiting	Topical: transdermal delivery of 0.5 mg over 3 days. Apply to dry skin behind one of the ears	Fatigue, drowsiness, dry mouth, urinary retention, depressed respiration
trimethobenzamide HCl (Tigan)	Nausea, vomiting	Oral: 250 mg 3 to4 times daily Rectal: 200 mg 3 to 4 times daily IM: 200 mg 3 to 4 times daily	Allergic skin eruptions, hypotension, blurred vision, headache, drowsiness, diarrhea, acute hepatitis, muscle cramps

REVIEW QUESTIONS

Directions. Select the best answer to each of the following multiple-choice questions, circling the letter of your choice:

1. _____ agents are used to relieve pain.
   a. Antipyretic
   b. Analgesic
   c. Anti-inflammatory
   d. Hypnotic

2. The natural and synthetic drugs derived from morphine are known as _____.
   a. opiates
   b. opioids
   c. opium
   d. opsin

3. Tylenol acts as _____.
   a. an anti-inflammatory agent
   b. an analgesic/antipyretic
   c. an antirheumatic agent
   d. analgesic/anti-inflammatory

4. An effective hypnotic should _____.
   a. have fairly rapid action
   b. produce near-normal sleep
   c. not give the patient a delayed effect the next day
   d. all of these

5. Psychological and physical dependency can result from the use of _____.
   a. analgesics
   b. barbiturates
   c. antipyretics
   d. anticonvulsants

6. Residual sedation, vertigo, nausea, and vomiting are commonly associated adverse effects of _____.

   a. analgesics
   c. antipyretics
   b. barbiturates
   d. anticonvulsants

7. Benzodiazepines that are recognized as effective sedative-hypnotics are _____.

   a. Dalmane, Restoril, and Halcion

   b. flurazepam HCl, temazepam, and triazolam

   c. Noctec and Placidyl

   d. a and b

8. Anti-parkinsonian drugs are used for the palliative relief of _____.

   a. tachykinesia, rigidity, tremor, and disorders of equilibrium

   b. bradykinesia, rigidity, tremor, and disorders of equilibrium

   c. bradycardia, rigidity, tremor, and disorders of equilibrium

   d. none of these

9. _____ are drugs that interfere with the conduction of nerve impulses and are used to produce loss of sensation, muscle relaxation, and/or complete loss of consciousness.

   a. Barbiturates   b. Hypnotics   c. Anesthetics   d. Analgesics

10. _____ is a term used to describe an illusion of movement.

    a. Vertigo
    c. Vomiting
    b. Motion sickness
    d. Dizziness

11. Ophthalmic drugs are used _____.

    a. in the treatment of glaucoma

    b. during diagnostic examination of the eye

    c. in intraocular surgery

    d. all of these

12. Adverse reactions of Diamox include _____.

    a. dry mouth, thirst

    b. blurred vision, urinary retention

    c. congestive heart failure

    d. paresthesia, drowsiness, tinnitus, nausea

13. Mydriatic drugs are used primarily _____.

    a. as an aid in refraction

    b. during internal examination of the eye

    c. in intraocular surgery and in the treatment of anterior uveitis and secondary glaucomas

    d. all of these

14. Adverse reactions of Neo-Synephrine include _____.

    a. stinging
    c. sensitivity to light
    b. browache
    d. all of these

15. All of the following classifications of drugs are used to treat vertigo, motion sickness, and vomiting except _____.

    a. anticholinergic
    c. antidopaminergic
    b. antihistaminic
    d. antipyretic

16. Drowsiness, blurred vision, dry mouth, and fatigue are adverse reactions of _____.

    a. Tigan
    c. Marezine
    b. Dramamine
    d. Antivert

Matching. Place the correct letter from Column II on the appropriate line of Column I:

Column I	Column II
17. __C__ agonist	A. that which inhibits; a chemical substance that stops enzyme activity
18. __F__ analgesic	B. that which imitates the sympathetic nervous system; adrenergic
19. __I__ anhydrase	C. a drug that has affinity for the cellular receptors of another drug or natural substance and produces a physiological effect
20. __G__ aqueous humor	D. an enzyme that catalyzes union of water and carbon dioxide to form carbonic acid
21. __H__ carbonic	E. a catecholamine synthesized by the adrenal gland
22. __D__ carbonic anhydrase	F. agents used to relieve pain
23. __E__ dopamine	G. the transparent liquid contained in the anterior and posterior chambers of the eye
24. __A__ inhibitor	H. pertaining to carbon
25. __B__ sympathomimetic	I. an enzyme that promotes the removal of water from a chemical compound
	J. that which stimulates enzyme activity

UNIT 28
Medications That Affect the Reproductive System

OBJECTIVES

Upon completing this unit, you should be able to:

- Define the terms listed in the vocabulary.
- State the actions, uses, contraindications, warnings, adverse reactions, dosage and route, implications for patient care, patient teaching, and special considerations for estrogens.
- State the actions, uses, contraindications, adverse reactions, dosage and route, implications for patient care, patient teaching, and special considerations for progesterones.
- Give the benefits and risks of hormone replacement therapy.
- List several alternative treatment options for hormone replacement therapy.
- Describe how oral contraceptives, when used as directed, prevent the occurrence of pregnancy.
- List the adverse reactions of oral contraceptives.
- List the conditions in which taking an oral contraceptive could be dangerous.
- State the actions, uses, contraindications, adverse reactions, dosage and route, implications for patient care, patient teaching, and special considerations for testosterones.
- Describe erectile dysfunction.
- State the action, uses, contraindications, cautions, adverse reactions, dosage and route, and patient teaching for Viagra (sildenafil citrate).
- Describe the drugs that may be used during labor and delivery.
- State the uses, usual dosage, and adverse reactions of selected uterine stimulants.
- Give the signs and symptoms of specific sexually transmitted diseases (STDs).
- Complete the critical thinking questions and activities presented in this unit.

- Complete the Spot Check on sexually transmitted diseases.
- Answer the review questions correctly.

VOCABULARY

amenorrhea (a-men″o-re′a). Without or lack of the monthly menstrual flow.

cryptorchidism (kript-or′kid-izm). Failure of the testicles to descend into the scrotum.

hirsutism (hur′sut-izm). A condition characterized by excessive growth of hair, especially in women.

hypogonadism (hi″po-go′nad-izm). A condition of defective secretion of the gonads.

menopause (men′o-pawz). Climacteric. The time when there is a naturally occurring pause or stoppage of the monthly menstrual flow.

osteoporosis (os″te-o-por-o′sis). A softening of bones or increased porosity of bones, seen most often in aging women.

524

INTRODUCTION

The ovaries in the female (see Figure 28-1) and the testes in the male (see Figure 28-2) are the primary organs of sexual reproduction. With the onset of puberty (ages 9 to 16 in females, 13 to 15 in males), the pituitary gland secretes increased amounts of two gonad-stimulating hormones that cause the reproductive organs to mature and begin the production of ova and sperm. Known as *follicle-stimulating hormone* (FSH) and *luteinizing hormone* (LH), these secretions continue to exert control over the functions of the reproductive organs after maturation.

The functions of the ovaries are (1) production of ova, and (2) secretion of the female sex hormones estrogen and progesterone. The functions of the testes are (1) production of sperm, and (2) secretion of the male sex hormone testosterone. The female sex hormones are instrumental in the development of secondary sex characteristics in the female. These characteristics are sexual drive, body hair growth, breast development, feminine body features, ovulation, and menstruation (see Figure 28-3). Testosterone is essential in the development of secondary sex characteristics in the male. These characteristics are sexual desire, deepening of voice, body hair growth, masculine body features, development of sex organs, and muscle and tissue building (see Figure 28-4).

FEMALE HORMONES

One needs to be familiar with the interrelated processes of the menstrual cycle to fully appreciate the role played by the female hormones. The onset of the menstrual cycle coincides with puberty, ends during menopause, and in human females occurs monthly on an average of every 28 days.

The menstrual cycle can be divided into four distinct phases. During the *proliferation phase*, the ovarian (graafian) follicle undergoes maturation, secretes estrogen, and thickening and vascularization of the endometrium occurs. This phase ends when the ovarian follicle ruptures, expelling the ovum into the fallopian tube. Estrogen, due to the source of its secretion, is sometimes referred to as the *follicular hormone*. The next phase in the cycle is the *luteal* or *secretory phase*, which is characterized by continued thickening and vascularization of the endometrium and the secretion of progesterone by the corpus luteum, a small yellow body within the ruptured ovarian follicle. Because it is produced by the corpus luteum, progesterone is called the *luteal hormone*. At this point, the thick, spongy uterine lining is engorged with blood. If conception has not occurred, the cycle

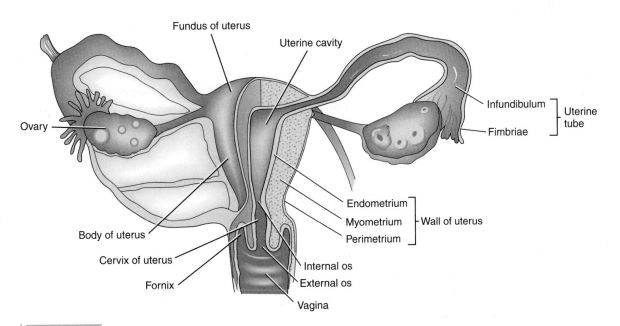

FIGURE 28-1

The position of the ovaries, uterine tubes, uterus, and vagina of the female reproductive system

Source: Delmar/Cengage Learning

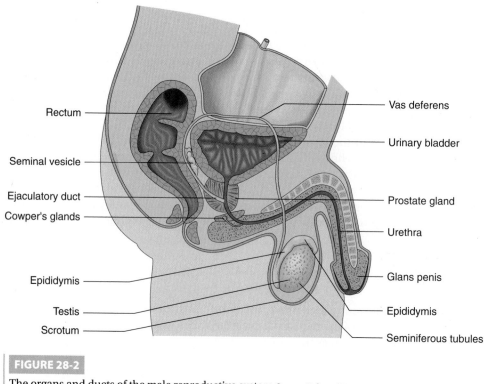

FIGURE 28-2

The organs and ducts of the male reproductive system *Source: Delmar/Cengage Learning*

enters the *premenstrual phase*, characterized by constriction of the coiled arteries within the uterine lining, shrinkage of the endometrium, and a decrease in hormonal secretion by the corpus luteum. This phase ends with the start of the menstrual flow. The fourth phase is known as *menstruation*. This is a period of uterine bleeding, lasting four to five days, containing endometrial cells, blood, and glandular secretions. After menstruation, the endometrium of the uterus is again thin and the cycle begins anew.

Estrogen

Estrogen preparations are used for a variety of conditions. They may be used in the treatment of amenorrhea, dysfunctional bleeding, and hirsutism, and in palliative therapy for breast cancer in women and prostatic cancer in men. They may also be used to relieve the uncomfortable symptoms of menopause.

Actions

Estrogens promote growth, development, and maintenance of the female reproductive system and secondary sex characteristics. They also effect the release of pituitary gonadotropins.

Uses

Estrogen is used for menopause, atrophic vaginitis, atrophic urethritis, osteoporosis, hypogonadism, castration, primary ovarian failure, breast cancer, and androgen-dependent carcinoma of the prostate.

Contraindications

Estrogen is contraindicated in patients with known hypersensitivity to any of its ingredients, known or suspected pregnancy, breast cancer, estrogen-dependent neoplasia, undiagnosed abnormal genital bleeding, thrombophlebitis, and thromboembolic disorders.

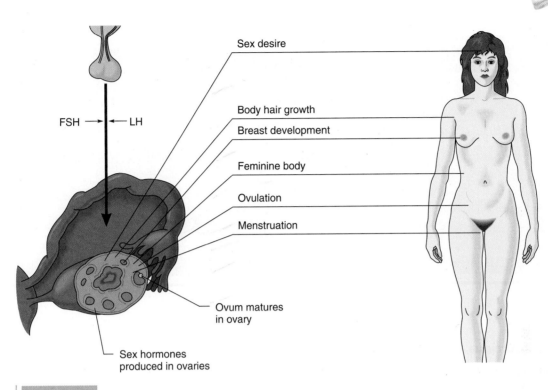

FIGURE 28-3

Secondary sex characteristics of the female *Source: Delmar/Cengage Learning*

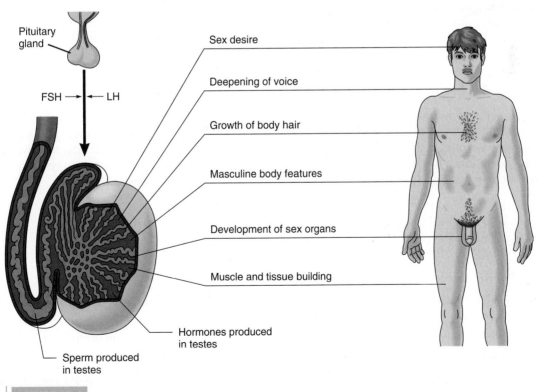

FIGURE 28-4

Secondary sex characteristics of the male *Source: Delmar/Cengage Learning*

> **⚠ Caution:**
>
> 1. *Patients who take higher doses of estrogens for a long period of time (five years or more) may have an increased risk of breast cancer.*
> 2. *There is a 2.5-fold increase in the risk of developing gallbladder disease in women receiving postmenopausal estrogens.*
> 3. *Large doses of estrogen (5 mg/day) may increase the risk of myocardial infarction in men. This dose is comparable to the dose used to treat cancer of the prostate and breast.*
> 4. *If higher doses of estrogen are used, there may be an increase in the risk of developing hypertension.*
> 5. *In patients with breast cancer and bone metastases, the administration of estrogen may lead to severe hypercalcemia. If this occurs, the drug should be stopped and appropriate action taken.*

Adverse Reactions

Reactions include breakthrough bleeding, spotting, breast tenderness and enlargement, nausea, vomiting, abdominal cramps, bloating, cholestatic jaundice, chloasma or melasma, erythema, loss of scalp hair, hirsutism, headache, migraine, dizziness, mental depression, edema, hypertension, intolerance to contact lenses, vaginal candidiasis, changes in weight, and hypercalcemia.

Dosage and Route

The dosage and route of administration are determined by the physician and individualized for each patient (see Table 28-1).

Implications for Patient Care

Observe for signs of improvement and adverse reactions. Weigh the patient daily, and if weight increases by 5 pounds within a week, notify physician. Assess blood pressure every four hours and notify physician if a consistent increase is noted in the systolic or diastolic readings. Monitor intake and output ratio and liver function studies. Be aware that a diabetic patient may have an increase in urine glucose and that the physician should be notified if such occurs. Encourage the patient to see the physician on a regular basis.

Patient Teaching

Educate patients:

- to read the package insert (leaflet) that comes with the prescription, and to call the physician if there are any questions.
- to weigh themselves daily, at the same time of day and with the same amount of clothing.
- to notify the physician if there is a 5-pound or more weight gain within a week.
- to be aware of possible adverse reactions and report any of the following to the physician without delay: abnormal vaginal bleeding, pains in the calves or chest, sudden shortness of breath, severe headache, dizziness, faintness, changes in vision, breast lumps, jaundice, pain, or swelling or tenderness in the abdomen.
- to check with the physician before taking calcium supplements.

TABLE 28-1 Estrogens

MEDICATION	USUAL DOSAGE
conjugated estrogens, USP (Premarin)	Oral: 0.3 to 1.25 mg daily Vaginal: 2 to 4 g daily
esterified estrogens (Menest)	Oral: 0.3 to 1.25 mg daily (cyclic regimen)
estradiol (Estrace)	Oral: 1 to 2 mg daily
estradiol cypionate in oil (Depo-Estradiol)	IM: 1 to 5 mg every 3 to 4 weeks
estradiol hemihydrate (Vagifem)	Vaginal tablet: Treatment of atrophic vaginitis Initial: 1 tablet, inserted vaginally, once daily for 2 weeks Maintenance: 1 tablet, inserted vaginally, twice weekly
estradiol transdermal system (Alora, Estraderm) (Climara) (Vivelle)	50 to 100 mcg/24-hour patch applied twice daily 50 to 100 mcg/24-hour patch applied weekly 25 mg/24-hour patch applied every 7 days 37.5 to 100 mcg patch applied twice weekly
estradiol valerate (Delestrogen)	Oral: 0.5 to 2 mg daily or in a cycle IM: 10 to 20 mg monthly
estropipate (Ogen)	Oral: One Ogen 0.625 tab to 2.5 mg per day Vaginal: 2 to 4 g of cream daily

- about breast self-examination.
- to see the physician on a regular basis. ■

Special Considerations

- Estrogens may decrease the action of anticoagulants and oral hypoglycemics.
- Estrogens may increase the action of corticosteroids.
- Anticonvulsants, barbiturates, phenylbutazone, and rifampin may decrease the action of estrogen.

Progesterone

Progesterone is produced by the ovaries and, to a lesser extent, by the adrenal cortex. The primary source of this hormone is the corpus luteum, which forms monthly in the ruptured ovarian follicle. Progesterone prepares the uterus for the implantation of the fertilized ovum. It also suppresses ovulation during pregnancy and stimulates the breast to secrete milk following delivery. Natural progesterone, taken orally, is quickly inactivated by the liver; therefore, chemical modification of the progesterone molecule or the use of a synthetic preparation is necessary to provide a sustained effect. Synthetic preparations are called progestins (see Table 28-2).

Progesterone is used to prevent uterine bleeding, and is combined with estrogen for treatment of amenorrhea. It is also ordered in cases of infertility and threatened or habitual miscarriage.

Actions

Progesterone is responsible for changes in the uterine endometrium during the second half of the menstrual cycle, development of maternal placenta after implantation, and development of mammary glands.

Uses

Use for secondary amenorrhea, abnormal uterine bleeding, infertility, and threatened or habitual miscarriage.

TABLE 28-2   Progestins

MEDICATION	USUAL DOSAGE
medroxyprogesterone acetate (Provera)	2.5 mg, 5 mg, 10 mg
megestrol acetate (Megace)	20 mg, 40 mg, 160 mg
natural progesterone (Prometrium)	100 mg
norethindrone acetate (Aygestin) (Micronor) (Nor-QD)	5 mg 0.35 mg 0.35 mg
norgestrel	0.075 mg

Contraindications

Progesterone is contraindicated in patients with known hypersensitivity to any of its ingredients, and in patients with thrombophlebitis, thromboembolic disorders, cerebral apoplexy, liver disease, breast cancer, reproductive organ cancer(s), undiagnosed vaginal bleeding, and missed abortion. Use during pregnancy and breast-feeding is not recommended.

Adverse Reactions

Reactions include breast tenderness, galactorrhea, urticaria, pruritus, edema, rash, acne, alopecia, hirsutism, thrombophlebitis, pulmonary embolism, breakthrough bleeding, spotting, amenorrhea, changes in weight, changes in cervical erosion and cervical secretions, cholestatic jaundice, anaphylaxis, mental depression, insomnia, nausea, and somnolence.

Dosage and Route

The dosage and route of administration are determined by the physician and individualized for each patient (see Table 28-2).

Implications for Patient Care

Observe for signs of improvement and adverse reactions. Weigh the patient daily and if weight increases by 5 pounds within a week, notify physician. Assess blood pressure every four hours and notify physician if a consistent increase is noted in the systolic or diastolic readings. Monitor intake and output ratio and liver function studies.

Patient Teaching

Educate patients:

- to weigh themselves daily, at the same time of day and with the same amount of clothing.
- to notify the physician if there is a weight gain of 5 pounds or more within a week.
- to be aware of possible adverse reactions and report any of the following to the physician without delay: abnormal vaginal bleeding, pains in the calves or chest, jaundice, dark urine, clay-colored stools, dyspnea, and blurred vision.

* about breast self-examination.
* to see the physician on a regular basis. ▓

Special Considerations

* Progestins may cause fluid retention. Use with caution in patients with epilepsy, migraine, asthma, cardiac disease, and renal dysfunction.
* Patients with mental depression should be carefully observed while using progestins. Discontinue drug if depressive state becomes severe.
* Diabetic patients should be carefully monitored while taking progestins. A decrease in glucose tolerance may occur.

HORMONE REPLACEMENT THERAPY

Hormone replacement therapy (HRT) is a medication regimen of providing a woman who has gone through menopause (natural or surgically) with hormones that her body has stopped producing.

At about 50 years of age, women begin experiencing bodily changes that are directly related to hormonal production. The ovaries cease to produce estrogen and progesterone. With decreased production of these female hormones, women enter the phase of life known as menopause. Menopause marks the permanent cessation of menstrual activity. It is also referred to as the climacteric. Natural menopause will occur in 25 percent of women by age 47, in 50 percent by age 50, in 75 percent by age 52, and 95 percent by age 55. Menopause may also be surgically produced when a woman has had an oophorectomy.

The symptoms of menopause vary from being hardly noticeable to being severe. They may include irregular periods, hot flashes, vaginal dryness, insomnia, joint pain, headache, emotional instability, irritability, and depression. Breast tissue may lose its firmness, and pubic and axillary hair becomes sparse. Without estrogen, the uterus becomes smaller, the vagina shortens, and vaginal tissues become drier. There may be loss of bone mass leading to osteoporosis.

Hormone replacement therapy may involve estrogen preparations and/or a combination of estrogen and progestin. Estrogen replacement therapy (ERT) is employed when a woman has had a hysterectomy and does not have a uterus. A combination of estrogen and progestin are employed when a woman has a uterus.

Benefits of Hormone Replacement Therapy

Estrogen remains the most effective short-term treatment for relief of menopausal symptoms such as hot flashes, night sweats, and vaginal dryness. Long-term postmenopausal hormone therapy is no longer routinely recommended. Women who take estrogen for short-term relief of menopausal symptoms may gain some protection against the following conditions:

* **Osteoporosis.** Studies show that hormone therapy may help prevent bone loss that occurs after menopause, which decreases the risk of osteoporosis-related hip fractures.
* **Colorectal cancer.** Studies show that hormone therapy may decrease the risk of colorectal cancer.
* **Heart disease.** Some data suggest that estrogen may decrease risk of heart disease when taken early in the postmenopausal years. For women who undergo menopause naturally, estrogen is typically prescribed as part of a combination therapy of estrogen and progestin. This is because estrogen without progestin can increase the risk of uterine cancer. Women who undergo menopause as the result of a hysterectomy can take estrogen alone.

Risks of Hormone Replacement Therapy

Today, there's plenty of confusion about hormone replacement therapy, which is now commonly called hormone therapy. It has been found that hormone therapy is not the magical cure for aging that it was once believed to be, but it's still the most effective treatment for unpleasant menopausal symptoms.

The following are some of the risk involved with hormone therapy.

- Taking estrogen increases a person's risk for blood clots. Generally, this risk is higher if one uses birth control pills, which contain high doses of estrogen. The risk is even higher if one smokes and takes estrogen. The risk is not as high when estrogen transdermal patches are used.

- Women who take estrogen therapy for a long period of time have a small increase in risk for breast cancer. Most guidelines currently consider hormone therapy safe for breast cancer risk when taken for up to five years.

- The risk for endometrial cancer is more than five times higher in women who take estrogen therapy alone, compared with those who do not. However, taking progesterone with estrogen seems to protect against this cancer.

- Estrogen may increase the risk of heart disease in older women. However, it may still be somewhat protective in preventing heart disease when given under certain circumstances. Estrogen is probably the safest for women under 60 years of age.

- Deep venous thrombosis (DVT) and pulmonary embolus (PE) are more common in women who take oral estrogen.

- Women who take estrogen have an increased risk for stroke.

- Several studies have shown that women who take estrogen/progestin therapy have an increased risk for developing gallstones.

Alternative Treatment Options

Before using any type of replacement therapy, patients should consult with their physician. There are risks associated with taking herbs or "natural" supplements.

The following are some alternative treatment options offered as a form of replacement therapy for menopause.

- *Natural bioidentical hormones.* These hormones are found in nature. The most common sources of these hormones are soybeans and wild yams. Soy contains phytoestrogens which are similar to estrogen and isoflavones. Isoflavones are a type of phytoestrogen, compounds that have weak estrogenic activity. There are many types of phytoestrogens and not all are in edible plants. Isoflavones are found in chickpeas and legumes. The legume soy has the most concentrated amount. Progesterone is obtained by extracting *diosgenin* from wild yams. The roots and other underground parts of wild yams used in herbal remedies are different from yams and sweet potatoes sold as food. Diosgenin is a steroid sapogenin that is isolated from various plants. Diosgenin is the starting material for the synthesis of a number of hormonal products such as DHEA (dehydroepiandrosterone). There is *no scientific evidence* showing that the wild yam has any effect on the symptoms of menopause.

- *Exercise.* Try aerobic, weight-bearing, or stretching exercises at least 30 minutes to an hour, four to five times a week.

- *Diet.* Eat a diet high in fruits and vegetables and low in saturated fats. Include four to six servings of soy products, foods such as soybeans, tofu, soymilk, and roasted soy nuts daily. Blueberries and cherries also contain bioflavonoids that are a source of phytoestrogens. Flaxseeds and flaxseed oil are lignans, also phytoestrogens, and can help relieve hot flashes and vaginal dryness. These lignans also can have a stabilizing effect on hormone-related mood swings. It is also recommend that one reduce the intake of caffeine, alcohol, hot beverages, and spicy foods.

- *Vaginal products.* As a lubricant for intercourse and moisturized for vaginal dryness, one may use over-the-counter creams that do not contain estrogen.

- *Herbal treatments.* If so desired, see an herbalist for herbal products rich in phytoestrogens. Supplements containing soy and black cohosh provide a natural support to hormonal balance.

- *Dietary supplements.* Take a multivitamin and mineral complex that contains 400 micrograms of folic acid. Also take 1200 milligrams of calcium daily and an antioxidant.

- *Do not smoke.*

- *Reduce weight* as needed.

Spotlight

Birth Control

According to the Association of Reproductive Health Professional's survey, four out of five American women ages 18 to 50 are sexually active. Of these, nine out of ten were interested in becoming more educated about various methods of birth control.

In the United States, there are numerous methods that may be used for birth control. Among them are birth control pills, condoms, a diaphragm, foams, jellies, natural planning, an IUD (intrauterine device), a cervical cap, a contraceptive sponge, a vasectomy, and female sterilization. Other methods of birth control that have been approved by the Food and Drug Administration include the Deop-Provera contraceptive injection, the female condom (Reality), NuvaRing, the birth control patch (Ortho Evra), and the cervical cap.

The NuvaRing

The NuvaRing is a small flexible contraceptive ring, about the size of a silver dollar. It contains the same hormones as many birth control pills. It is inserted manually into the vagina, where it is left for three weeks. There, a continuous, low dose of hormones is released. Then the ring is removed for one week; this is the week one will have a period. When used correctly, NuvaRing is 98 to 99 percent effective in preventing pregnancy. Women who should not consider the NuvaRing include those with a history of blood clots, heart attack, stroke, diabetes, or high cholesterol, as well as those with breast cancer, and who are pregnant or think they might be.

The most common side effects reported are:

- vaginal infections
- whitish vaginal discharge
- headache
- weight gain
- nausea
- breast tenderness

The Birth Control Patch

The birth control patch (Ortho Evra) is a tiny skin patch with the same hormones as in many birth control pills. Women can wear this patch on the buttocks, abdomen, upper torso (except for the breast), or the outer part of the upper arm. One should not place the patch on skin that is red, irritated, or cut, or skin where makeup, creams, or powders are applied. A new patch is worn for one week and then replaced on the same day of the week for three consecutive weeks. The fourth week is a "patch-free week." This is when one should have a period. The Ortho Evra contraceptive patch is 99 percent effective when used correctly. Women who should not get the Ortho Evra patch include those with blood clots, history of heart attack or stroke, those over 35 who smoke cigarettes, those with breast cancer, and those who are pregnant or think they might be.

The most common side effects reported are:

- breast tenderness
- headache
- rash or redness at the site of the patch
- nausea
- menstrual cramps

Depo-Provera

Depo-Provera is a contraceptive injection (medroxyprogesterone acetate); when administered at the recommended dose to women every 3 months, it inhibits the secretion of gonadotropins which, in turn, prevents follicular maturation and ovulation and results in endometrial thinning. These actions produce its contraceptive effect, which is 99 percent effective. Depo-Provera is given as an intramuscular injection in the dorsogluteal area or in the deltoid muscle.

Before the initiation of this type of contraception, patients should have a complete medical history and physical examination performed. The physician should inform patients of precautions, warnings, adverse reactions, and possible side effects. Because Depo-Provera is a long-acting birth control method, it takes some time after the last injection for its effect to wear off.

The Female Condom (Reality)

The female condom (Reality) affords women some protection against sexually transmitted diseases, including AIDS, as well as pregnancy. It had a 26 percent failure rate in preventing pregnancy in tests, and the FDA stresses that male latex condoms are better safeguards against pregnancy and disease.

Reality is a prelubricated polyurethane sheath that has flexible polyurethane rings on each end, one of which is inserted into the vagina like a diaphragm. One of its two flexible rings holds the device in place, fitting over the cervix, and the other ring forms the external edge and remains outside the vagina. It shields the entire vaginal and urethral area from the shaft and base of the penis. It provides women with an opportunity to protect themselves when their sexual partner refuses to use a male condom.

"Case In Point"

According to a national survey of men that was published in an issue of Family Planning Perspectives, nearly all men ages 20 to 39 in the United States are sexually experienced:

- Twenty-three percent have had 20 or more partners in their lifetimes, yet only 25 percent say they used a condom in the past four weeks.
- Single men (45 percent) are twice as likely as married men (18 percent) to use a condom.
- Twenty-seven percent of men say they are embarrassed to buy condoms.

ORAL CONTRACEPTIVES

Women who desire to prevent the occurrence of pregnancy may take oral contraceptive pills that are nearly 100 percent effective when used as directed. These pills contain mixtures of estrogen and progestin in various levels of strength. The estrogen in the pill inhibits ovulation by suppressing the normal secretion of follicle-stimulating hormone (FSH) and luteinizing hormone (LH) from the anterior pituitary gland. The progestin inhibits pituitary secretion of LH, causes changes in the cervical mucus that renders it unfavorable to penetration by sperm, and alters the nature of the endometrium.

Most oral contraceptives are taken daily for 20 to 21 days, beginning with the fifth day after menstrual bleeding starts. This cycle is then followed by a week without medication to allow bleeding to occur. An exception to this regimen is a pill that contains only progestin. Called a *minipill*, this product is taken daily and continuously. It acts by interfering with sperm and ovum transport and by adversely affecting the suitability of the endometrium for ovum implant. Progestin-only minipills have been associated with menstrual irregularities (breakthrough bleeding) and are slightly less effective than the combination products.

Combination products may contain estrogen and progestin in varying formulations; some have more estrogen, others more progestin. They are available in regular or low-dose strength, again based on the amounts of the two hormones in the product.

Adverse reactions to oral contraceptives are related to their hormone content. Those with high estrogen content tend to cause estrogen-related reactions (nausea, weight gain, edema, swelling of the breasts), and those with high progestin content cause progestin-related effects (headache, acne, fatigue). As a rule, those preparations containing the lowest hormone content, but which provide consistently effective contraceptive action, are likely to be preferred because of a lower incidence of adverse reaction.

Oral contraceptives may be grouped according to the amount of hormone that is available at a given time during the 20- to 21-day cycle of administration. *Monophasic* preparations provide a fixed concentration of hormones throughout the entire cycle. With *biphasic* preparations, estrogen is available in fixed amounts for the duration of the cycle, but the progestin content is varied. Low levels of progestin are provided during the first half of the cycle and high amounts are included during the last half when endometrial secretions are desired. *Triphasic* preparations vary both the estrogen and progestin dosages within the cycle in an effort to mimic the normal hormonal fluctuations found in women of childbearing age.

Mircette (ethinyl estradiol/desogestrel) is an oral contraceptive that contains estrogen and progesterone at varying levels throughout the cycle. It comes in a 28-day pill pack containing 26 active white and yellow pills (with hormones) and two inactive green pills (without hormones).

The regimen begins with 21 days of 20 mcg ethinyl estradiol and 150 mcg desogestrel. The last seven days in the cycle start with two days of placebo pills, followed by five days of 10 mcg ethinyl estradiol pills. Mircette has a low dose of estrogen, to help reduce estrogen-related side effects, and is more than 99 percent effective in preventing pregnancy when taken correctly. In patient studies, breakthrough bleeding occurred in only 3.5 percent of total cycles in women using Mircette, and breakthrough spotting occurred in only 8.9 percent of cycles.

Patient literature accompanying oral contraceptive preparations usually cautions those who either have or once had any of the following conditions not to take an oral contraceptive:

1. Clots in the legs or lungs
2. Angina pectoris
3. Known or suspected cancer of the breast or sex organs
4. Unusual vaginal bleeding that has not yet been diagnosed
5. Heart attack or stroke
6. Known or suspected pregnancy

Such literature will also include the following statement on cigarette smoking and the use of oral contraceptives:

Caution:

Cigarette smoking increases the risk of serious adverse effects on the heart and blood vessels from oral contraceptive use. This risk increases with age and with heavy smoking (15 or more cigarettes per day) and is quite marked in women over 35 years of age. Women who use oral contraceptives should not smoke.

The choice of an oral contraceptive depends upon a number of factors, including sensitivities to hormones, how the preparation might interact with other drugs being taken, and other considerations. Table 28-3 lists selected oral contraceptive preparations currently in use.

TABLE 28-3	Selected Oral Contraceptives		
MONOPHASIC PREPARATIONS	**BIPHASIC PREPARATIONS**	**TRIPHASIC PREPARATIONS**	**PROGESTERONE ONLY**
Alesse	Nelova 10/11	Ortho-Novum 7/7/7	Micronor
Brevicon	Ortho-Novum 10/11	Tri-Norinyl	Demulen
Nor-QD		Triphasil - 28	
Lo/Ovral - 28			
Modicon			
Nordette - 28			
Norinyl 1 + 35			
Ovcon-50			

MALE HORMONES

Adequate secretions of androgenic hormones are necessary to maintain normal male sex characteristics, the male libido, and sexual potency. *Testosterone*, the most important androgen, is secreted primarily by the Leydig cells located in the interstitial spaces of the testes. With the advent of puberty (ages 13 to 15), boys experience a dramatic increase in the amount of testosterone secreted. The increased levels of this hormone stimulate the development of male secondary sex characteristics, initiate the production of sperm, and enhance the functional capacity of the penis and the accessory sex organs in the male. Normal men produce 2.5 to 10 mg of testosterone per day. After the age of 40, there is a gradual decline in the amount of testosterone produced, and by age 80, output is approximately 20 percent of that produced during peak years.

Testosterone is rapidly inactivated by the liver; therefore, longer-lasting testosterone derivatives and synthetic forms of the hormone are available for oral and parenteral administration. These agents are used for replacement therapy in androgen deficiency, for the treatment of hypogonadism and cryptorchidism, and for palliative treatment of certain metastatic breast carcinomas in women. See Table 28-4 for selected androgens.

Actions

Testosterone is responsible for growth, development, and maintenance of the male reproductive system and secondary sex characteristics.

Uses

Use as replacement therapy in primary hypogonadism, in hypogonadotropic hypogonadism, and to stimulate puberty in carefully selected males, and in impotence. It may be used in women with advanced inoperable metastatic breast cancer who are one to five years postmenopausal.

Contraindications

These hormones are contraindicated in patients with known hypersensitivity to any of its ingredients, during pregnancy and lactation, in men with cancer of the breast or known or suspected cancer of the prostate, and in patients with pituitary insufficiency, a history of myocardial infarction, hypercalcemia, prostatic hyperplasia, hepatic dysfunction, nephrosis, and infants and young children. There are many warnings associated with testosterone preparations. Please refer to a current drug book reference for information on warnings or visit www.Drug@FDA.gov.

TABLE 28-4 Androgens

MEDICATION	USUAL DOSAGE
methyltestosterone	Oral: 10 to 40 mg/day for replacement therapy Buccal: 5 to 20 mg/day
testosterone (AndroGel)	IM: 10 to 25 mg 2 to 3 times/week for androgen deficiency Topical gel: Apply once daily to the shoulders, upper arms, and/or abdomen for replacement therapy
testosterone cypionate in oil (Depo-Testosterone)	IM: 50 to 400 mg every 2 to 4 weeks for replacement
testosterone enanthate in oil (Delatestryl)	IM: 50 to 400 mg ever 2 to 4 weeks for replacement
testosterone propionate in oil	IM: 10 to 25 mg 2 to 3 times per week for replacement
testosterone transdermal systems (ANDRODERM® ⓒ)	Controlled delivery for once-daily application to the scrotum

Caution:

Use cautiously in geriatric patients, and those with diabetes, hypertension, coronary artery disease, renal disease, hypercholesterolemia, or gynecomastia, and in males who are prepubertal.

Adverse Reactions

In males, reactions include gynecomastia; excessive frequency and duration of penile erection; oligospermia; hirsutism; male pattern of baldness; acne; retention of sodium, chloride, water, potassium, calcium, and inorganic phosphates; nausea; cholestatic jaundice; alterations in liver function tests; hepatocellular neoplasms; peliosis hepatis (liver and spleen may become engorged with blood-filled cysts); suppression of clotting factors II, V, VII, and X; increased or decreased libido; headache; anxiety; depression; generalized paresthesia; increased serum cholesterol; and, rarely, anaphylactoid reactions. *In females*, reactions include amenorrhea, menstrual irregularities, inhibition of gonadotropin secretion, and virilization (deepening of the voice, clitoral enlargement, increased growth of facial and body hair, and male-type baldness).

Dosage and Route

The dosage and route of administration are determined by the physician and individualized for each patient (see Table 28-4).

Implications for Patient Care

Observe for signs of improvement and adverse reactions. Weigh the patient daily, and if weight increases by 5 pounds within a week, notify the physician. Assess blood pressure every four hours and notify the physician if a consistent increase is noted in the systolic and/or diastolic readings. Monitor intake and output ratio and liver function studies. Monitor electrolytes: sodium, chloride, calcium, potassium, and blood cholesterol level. When used in males to stimulate puberty, assess growth pattern.

Patient Teaching

Educate patients:

- to weigh themselves daily, at the same time of day and with the same amount of clothing.
- to notify the physician if 5 pounds or more are gained within a week.
- to be aware of possible adverse reactions and report any of the following to the physician: nausea, vomiting, jaundice, and edema in all patients; frequent or persistent erections of the penis in males; signs of premature epiphyseal closure in adolescent males (they should have bone development checked every six months); and hoarseness, acne, changes in menstrual periods, growth of hair on face or body in females.
- that buccal tablets should be placed under the tongue or in the space between the cheek and gum to change the site of placement with each dose (rotate among the four locations in the mouth); and that the tablet should be completely dissolved before the patient engages in eating, drinking, or using any tobacco product.
- that oral tablets should be taken with food to minimize possible gastrointestinal distress.

Special Considerations

- In diabetic patients, the effects of testosterone may decrease blood glucose and insulin requirements.
- Testosterone may decrease the anticoagulant requirements of patients receiving oral anticoagulants. These patients require close monitoring when testosterone therapy is begun and again when it is stopped.
- Anabolic steroids (testosterone) may be abused by individuals who seek to increase muscle mass, strength, and overall athletic ability. This form of use is illegal and signs of abuse may include flulike symptoms, gastrointestinal distress, headaches, muscle aches, dizziness, bruises, needle marks, increased bleeding (nosebleeds, petechiae, gums, conjunctiva), and enlarged spleen, liver, prostate, or edema, as well as increased facial hair, menstrual irregularities, and enlarged clitoris in females.

ERECTILE DYSFUNCTION

According to the National Institutes of Health (NIH), erectile dysfunction (impotence) affects as many as 20 million men in the United States. It was once thought to be an unavoidable result of aging, but now, erectile dysfunction is understood to be caused by a variety of factors. *Erectile dysfunction* (ED) is defined as the inability to achieve or maintain an erection sufficient for sexual intercourse. It occurs when not enough blood is supplied to the penis, when the smooth muscle in the penis fails to relax, or when the penis does not retain the blood that flows into it. According to studies by the NIH, 5 percent of men have some degree of erectile dysfunction at age 40 and approximately 15 to 25 percent at age 65 or older. Although the likelihood of erectile dysfunction increases with age, it is not an inevitable part of aging. About 80 percent of erectile dysfunction has a physical cause.

Some physical causes of erectile dysfunction are:

- *Vascular diseases.* Arteriosclerosis, hypertension, high cholesterol, and other medical conditions can obstruct blood flow.
- *Diabetes.* Nerve function and blood flow to the penis can be affected by diabetes.
- *Prescription drugs.* Certain antihypertensive, cardiac medications, antihistamines, psychiatric medications, and other prescription drugs can cause erectile dysfunction.
- *Substance abuse.* Excessive smoking, alcohol, and illegal drugs constrict blood vessels and can cause erectile dysfunction.
- *Neurologic diseases.* Multiple sclerosis, Parkinson's disease, and other diseases can interrupt nerve impulses to the penis.

- *Surgery.* Prostate, colon, bladder, and other types of pelvic surgery may damage nerves and blood vessels.
- *Spinal injury.* Interruptions of nerve impulses from the spinal cord to the penis can cause erectile dysfunction.
- *Other.* Hormonal imbalance, kidney failure, dialysis, and reduced testosterone levels can cause erectile dysfunction.

There are numerous drugs that can be prescribed for erectile dysfunction. Three of these drugs are Viagra (sildenafil citrate), Cialis (tadalafil), and Levitra (vardenafil). Viagra, the little blue pill, was the first drug approved by the FDA and then, recently, the other two drugs were approved. Levitra may last a few hours longer than Viagra, and Cialis uses the same blood vessel—dilating mechanism as the other two drugs, but it provides a 36-hour opportunity for amour. It is not recommended that any of these drugs be the first line of treatment for erectile dysfunction. The following information is on Viagra, but can also apply to Cialis and Levitra.

sildenafil citrate (Viagra)

Viagra is an oral medication that may be prescribed for erectile dysfunction.

Actions

Viagra increases the body's ability to achieve and maintain an erection during sexual stimulation. It does not protect one from getting sexually transmitted diseases, including HIV.

Uses

Viagra is used to treat erectile dysfunction (impotence) in men.

Contraindications

Viagra was shown to potentiate the hypotensive effects of nitrates, and therefore its administration to patients who are using organic nitrates, either regularly or intermittently, in any form, is contraindicated. It is also contraindicated in patients with a known hypersensitivity to any component of its ingredients.

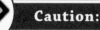

Caution:

There is a potential for cardiac risk of sexual activity in patients with preexisting cardiovascular disease. Therefore, treatments for erectile dysfunction, including Viagra, should not be generally used in men for whom sexual activity is inadvisable because of their underlying cardiovascular status.

Adverse Reactions

Reactions can include headache, flushing, dyspepsia, nasal congestion, urinary tract infection, diarrhea, dizziness, rash, abnormal vision (color tinge to vision and increased sensitivity to light or blurred vision), and prolonged erection (priapism). Serious cardiovascular events such as myocardial infarction, sudden cardiac death, ventricular arrhythmia, cerebrovascular hemorrhage, transient ischemic attack, and hypertension have been reported postmarketing in association with the use of Viagra. Most, but not all, of these patients had preexisting cardiovascular risk factors.

Dosage and Route

For most patients, the recommended dose is a 50-mg tablet taken orally, as needed, approximately 1 hour before sexual activity. However, Viagra may be taken anywhere from 4 hours to 0.5 hour before sexual activity. Based on effectiveness and toleration, the dose may be increased to a maximum recommended dose of 100 mg or decreased to 25 mg. The maximum recommended dosing frequency is once per day.

Patient Teaching

Educate patients:

- to have a complete medical history and exam to determine the cause of impotence before taking Viagra.
- that men who have medical conditions that may cause a sustained erection such as sickle-cell anemia, leukemia, or multiple myeloma or who have an abnormally shaped penis may not be able to take Viagra.
- to inform the doctor about all medications that they are taking, as there are several medications that interact with Viagra, such as cimetidine, erythromycin, ritonavir, and nitrates
- that if they experiences symptoms (chest pain, dizziness, nausea) upon initiation of sexual activity to refrain from further activity and contact a physician.
- that if an erection persists longer than 4 hours, to seek immediate medical assistance.
- that the use of Viagra offers no protection against sexually transmitted diseases. ■

DRUGS USED DURING LABOR AND DELIVERY

Drugs that selectively stimulate contraction of the myometrium are known as *oxytocic agents* because they act on smooth muscle much like the hormone *oxytocin*, which is secreted by the posterior pituitary gland. They may be used in obstetrics to induce labor at term. They are also used to control postpartum hemorrhage and to induce therapeutic abortion. Three types of oxytocic drugs are in general use; they are synthetic oxytocin, the ergot derivatives, and the prostaglandins. These drugs are also known as *uterine stimulants* (see Table 28-5).

When labor begins before term, *uterine relaxants* may be administered to delay labor until the fetus has gained sufficient maturity so as to be likely to survive. Agents used for this purpose are generally administered in cases where spontaneous labor begins after 20 weeks of gestation.

TABLE 28-5 Uterine Stimulants

MEDICATION	USE	USUAL DOSAGE	ADVERSE REACTION
carboprost tromethamine	Used to induce abortion in weeks 13 to 20	IM: 250 mcg initially, then repeated at 1.5- to 3.5-hour intervals as indicated by uterine response	Nausea, diarrhea, vomiting, temperature increase more than 2°F, flushing, cough, pain, hiccups, chills
dinoprost tromethamine	Used to terminate pregnancy in weeks 16 to 20	Intra-amniotic instillation: 40 mg or 8 mL (5 mg/mL)	Headache, dizziness, syncope, bradycardia, renal retention, bronchoconstriction, cough
dinoprostone (Prostin E$_2$ Alpha)	Used to terminate pregnancy in weeks 12 to 20	Intravaginal: 1 suppository (20 mg) inserted high into vagina; then another every 3 to 5 hours until abortion	Same as above
methylergonovine maleate (Methergine)	Used for routine management after delivery of placenta	Oral: 0.2 mg 3 to 4 times/day in puerperium for 1 week IM: 1 mL every 2 to 4 hours as necessary after delivery of placenta	Anorexia, dizziness, headache, nervousness, insomnia, blood pressure and pulse changes, tachycardia, visual disturbances, abdominal pain

▪▪ Special Considerations: **OLDER ADULTS**

A national survey of 1,604 men and women ranging in age from 65 to 97, was conducted and reported in *PARADE* magazine. The following is a summary of portions of this survey.

The Survey's Key Findings:

- Men and women remain interested in and sexually active into their 60s, 70s, and beyond.
- Approximately 40 percent of the respondents, whose average age was 74, were sexually active.
- At all ages, more men than women say sex is important.
- Sex is not the priority for older adults. When asked what matters most in an intimate relationship, nine in ten said companionship was most important.
- Approximately half of the respondents were satisfied with their quality of sexual activity.
- More seniors than younger adults found it difficult to talk about sex with a partner.
- The most common reasons reported for a decline in sexual satisfaction in later life were health or medical problems.
- Medications often are the culprit in sexual difficulties among older adults. Two-thirds of the respondents (66 percent) reported taking medication. Half of the men and a fifth of the women on medications say that the drugs have affected their sex lives. The most common sexual side effects are lower sex drive (lack of interest) and impotence (inability to maintain an erection).

▪▪ Special Considerations: **CHILDREN**

It is reported that one in five people with gonorrhea is under 20 years of age. Sexually transmitted diseases—syphilis, gonorrhea, chlamydia, genital herpes, hepatitis B, genital warts, and HIV (human immunodeficiency virus)—are not just contracted by adults. These diseases are being seen in children ranging from 10 to 19 years of age. It is noted that young people are becoming sexually active at very early ages, therefore sex education courses should begin early. A person can have intercourse only once and contract a sexually transmitted disease (STD). STDs can be passed on to sex partners and, if left untreated, can cause such medical problems as sterility, arthritis, pelvic inflammatory disease, and many other diseases and conditions. Most STDs can be treated through the proper antibiotic therapy, except for those caused by viruses (hepatitis B, genital herpes, HIV). There is only one sure way to avoid STDs and that is through abstaining from sexual activity.

Signs and Symptoms of Gonorrhea, Herpes Simplex II, Hepatitis B, and HIV

GONORRHEA	HERPES SIMPLEX II	HEPATITIS B	HIV
Genital discharge	Painful blisters	Abdominal discomfort	Swelling in lymph glands
Genital swelling	Flulike feeling	Flulike feeling	Weight loss
Burning sensation during urination	Loss of appetite	Loss of appetite	Night sweats
Lower abdominal pain	Burning sensation during urination	Yellowing of skin and eyes	Persistent cough
		Itchy skin	
		Dark urine and light stools	

Diagnosis

Tests for the various diseases range from blood samples to genital exams and cultures. People as young as 12 may be tested at state health departments without parental consent.

CDC's National STDs and AIDS hotline 1-800-342-AIDS

■■ Critical Thinking **QUESTIONS AND ACTIVITIES**

A 14-year-old boy has noticed a discharge from his penis, a burning sensation when he urinates, and an uncomfortable feeling in his lower abdominal area. Ask yourself:

- What disease does this boy possibly have?
- What should this boy do to find out what he has?
- What is the treatment for this disease?
- How is this disease contracted?
- What could happen if this disease was left untreated?

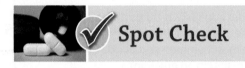 Spot Check

There are many sexually transmitted diseases that one should be informed about. For the following selected diseases, give the signs and symptoms:

DISEASE	SIGNS AND SYMPTOMS
Gonorrhea	
Hepatitis B	
Herpes Simplex II	
HIV	

REVIEW QUESTIONS

Directions. Select the best answer to each of the following multiple-choice questions, circling the letter of your choice:

1. A softening of bones or increased porosity of bones seen most often in aging women is called _____.
   a. osteoporosis
   b. menopause
   c. hirsutism
   d. amenorrhea

2. Estrogen preparations may be used for _____.
   a. amenorrhea
   b. dysfunctional bleeding
   c. hirsutism
   d. all of these

3. Women who should not consider the NuvaRing include all of the following except those with a _____.
   a. history of blood clots
   b. history of not smoking
   c. history of heart attack, stroke, high cholesterol
   d. history of diabetes

4. Adverse reactions to estrogens are _____.
   a. nausea
   b. fullness of the breasts
   c. edema
   d. all of these

5. Progesterone preparations may be used for _____.
   a. prevention of uterine bleeding
   b. infertility
   c. threatened or habitual miscarriage
   d. all of these

6. The most common side effects of Ortho Evra include all of the following except _____.
   a. breast tenderness
   b. headache
   c. nausea
   d. diarrhea

7. _____ oral contraceptive preparations provide a fixed concentration of hormones throughout the entire cycle.
   a. Biphasic
   b. Monophasic
   c. Triphasic
   d. none of these

8. An example of a triphasic oral contraceptive is _____.
   a. Modicon
   b. Ortho-Novum 10/11
   c. Ortho-Novum 7/7/7
   d. Micronor

9. Testosterone preparations may be used for _____.
   a. replacement therapy
   b. hypogonadism
   c. cryptorchidism
   d. all of these

10. There is a potential for cardiac risk of sexual activity in patients with preexisting cardiovascular disease. Therefore, treatments for erectile dysfunction, including Viagra (sildenafil citrate), should not be generally used in men for whom sexual activity is inadvisable because of their underlying cardiovascular status.
    a. True
    b. False

11. Drugs that selectively stimulate contraction of the myometrium are known as _____.
    a. relaxants
    b. oxytocic agents
    c. androgens
    d. estrogens

12. A drug used to prevent postpartum and postabortal hemorrhage is _____.
    a. Ergotate maleate
    b. Ethanol
    c. Yutopar
    d. Prostin

13. The _____ in the female and the _____ in the male are the primary organs of sexual reproduction.

   a. uterus, scrotum   c. ovaries, testes

   b. vagina, penis   d. breast, penis

14. The _____ secrete(s) increased amounts of two gonad-stimulating hormones that cause the reproductive organs to mature and begin the production of ova and sperm.

   a. ovaries   c. pineal gland

   b. pituitary gland   d. testes

15. The functions of the ovaries are _____.

   a. the production of ova

   b. secretion of estrogen and progesterone

   c. secretion of luteinizing hormone

   d. a and b

16. The functions of the testes are _____.

   a. production of semen   c. secretion of testosterone

   b. production of sperm   d. b and c

17. Estrogen, due to the source of its secretion, is sometimes referred to as a _____.

   a. luteinizing hormone   c. premenstrual hormone

   b. follicular hormone   d. all of these

18. _____ prepares the uterus for the implantation of the fertilized ovum.

   a. Estrogen   c. Testosterone

   b. Progesterone   d. Cortisone

Matching. Place the correct letter from Column II on the appropriate line of Column I:

Column I	*Column II*
19. _____ amenorrhea	A. a condition of defective secretion of the gonads
20. _____ cryptorchidism	B. a softening of bone seen most often in aging women
21. _____ hirsutism	C. literally means cessation of the monthly menstrual activity
22. _____ menopause	D. without or lack of the monthly menstrual flow
23. _____ osteoporosis	E. a condition of undescended testicles into the scrotum
24. _____ hypogonadism	F. a condition characterized by excessive growth of hair, especially in women
25. _____ testosterone	G. the least important androgen
	H. the most important androgen

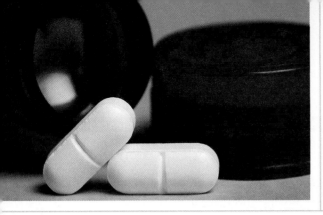

Color Photo Quick Reference Guide

This color photo quick reference guide provides rapid identification of 98 most commonly prescribed drugs. Actual-sized tablets and capsules, with their strength, are organized alphabetically by generic name and include appropriate trade name and manufacturer.

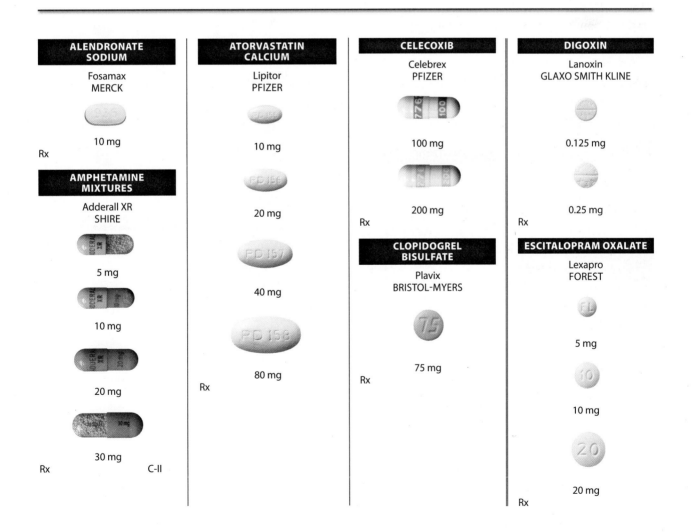

ALENDRONATE SODIUM
Fosamax
MERCK
10 mg
Rx

AMPHETAMINE MIXTURES
Adderall XR
SHIRE
5 mg
10 mg
20 mg
30 mg
Rx   C-II

ATORVASTATIN CALCIUM
Lipitor
PFIZER
10 mg
20 mg
40 mg
80 mg
Rx

CELECOXIB
Celebrex
PFIZER
100 mg
200 mg
Rx

CLOPIDOGREL BISULFATE
Plavix
BRISTOL-MYERS
75 mg
Rx

DIGOXIN
Lanoxin
GLAXO SMITH KLINE
0.125 mg
0.25 mg
Rx

ESCITALOPRAM OXALATE
Lexapro
FOREST
5 mg
10 mg
20 mg
Rx

ESOMEPRAZOLE MAGNESIUM

Nexium
ASTRA/ZENECA

20 mg

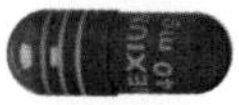

40 mg

Rx

ESTROGENS, CONJUGATED ORAL

Premarin
WYETH

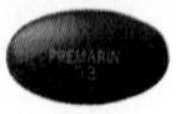

0.3 mg

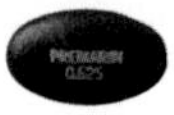

0.625 mg

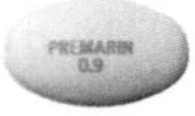

0.9 mg

Rx

ESZOPICLONE

Lunesta
SEPRACOR

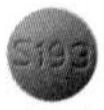

3 mg

Rx   C-IV

EZETIMIBE AND SIMVASTATIN

Vytorin
SCHERING-PLOUGH

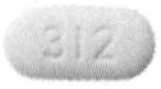

10/20 mg

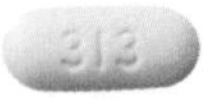

10/40 mg

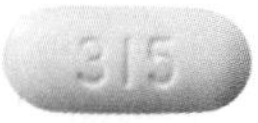

10/80 mg

Rx

FUROSEMIDE

Lasix
SANOFI

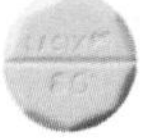

80 mg

Rx

IBANDRONATE SODIUM

Boniva
ROCHE

150 mg

Rx

IRBESARTAN

Avapro
BRISTOL-MYERS

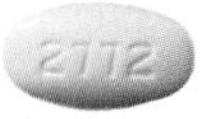

150 mg

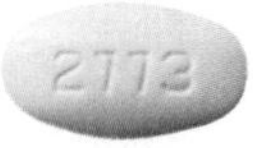

300 mg

Rx

LAMOTRIGINE

Lamictal
GLAXO SMITH KLINE

5 mg

25 mg

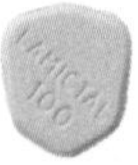

100 mg

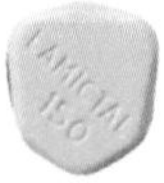

150 mg

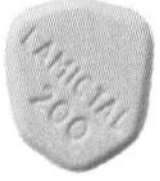

200 mg

Rx

LANSOPRAZOLE

Prevacid
TAP

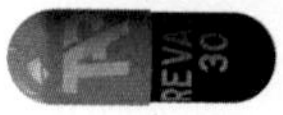

30 mg

Rx

LEVETIRACETAM

Keppra
UCB

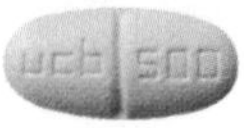

500 mg

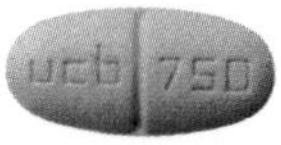

750 mg

Rx

LEVOFLOXACIN

Levaquin
OTHO-MCNEIL

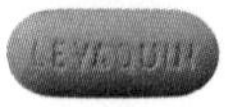

250 mg

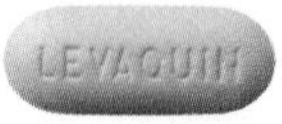

500 mg

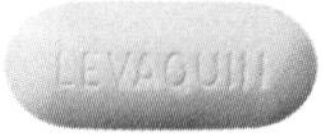

750 mg

Rx

LEVOTHYROXINE SODIUM

Synthroid
ABBOTT

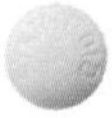

50 micrograms

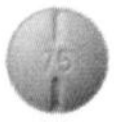

75 micrograms

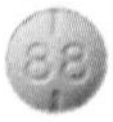

88 micrograms

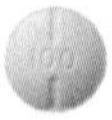

100 micrograms

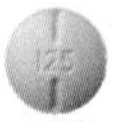

125 micrograms

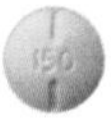

150 micrograms

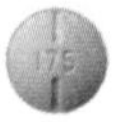

175 micrograms

Rx

LOSARTAN POTASSIUM

Cozaar
E.I. DU PONT DE NEMOURS

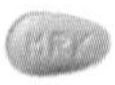

25 mg

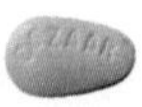

50 mg

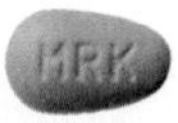

100 mg

Rx

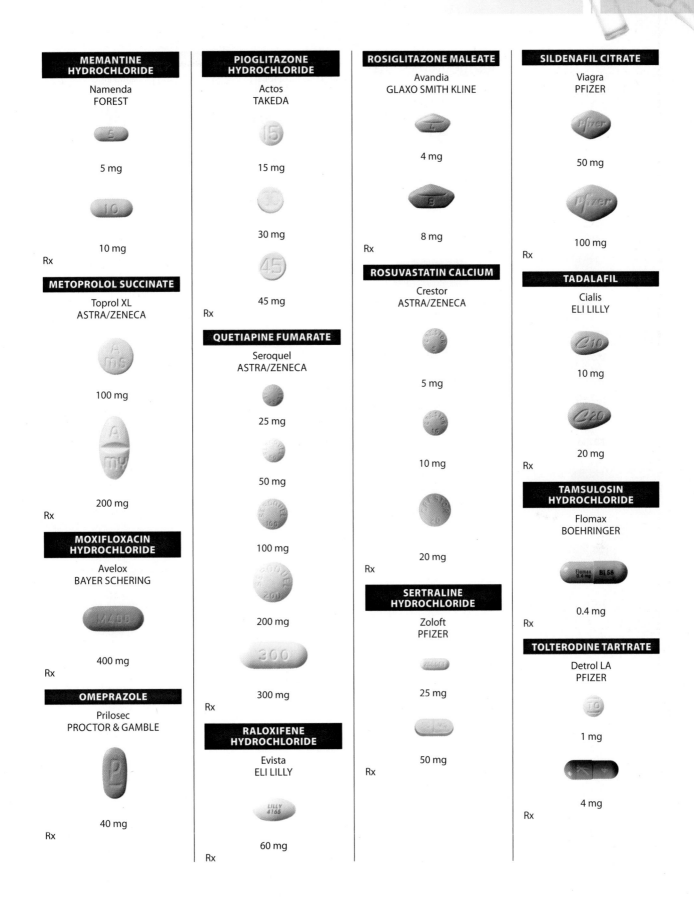

MEMANTINE HYDROCHLORIDE

Namenda
FOREST

5 mg

10 mg

Rx

METOPROLOL SUCCINATE

Toprol XL
ASTRA/ZENECA

100 mg

200 mg

Rx

MOXIFLOXACIN HYDROCHLORIDE

Avelox
BAYER SCHERING

400 mg

Rx

OMEPRAZOLE

Prilosec
PROCTOR & GAMBLE

40 mg

Rx

PIOGLITAZONE HYDROCHLORIDE

Actos
TAKEDA

15 mg

30 mg

45 mg

Rx

QUETIAPINE FUMARATE

Seroquel
ASTRA/ZENECA

25 mg

50 mg

100 mg

200 mg

300 mg

Rx

RALOXIFENE HYDROCHLORIDE

Evista
ELI LILLY

60 mg

Rx

ROSIGLITAZONE MALEATE

Avandia
GLAXO SMITH KLINE

4 mg

8 mg

Rx

ROSUVASTATIN CALCIUM

Crestor
ASTRA/ZENECA

5 mg

10 mg

20 mg

Rx

SERTRALINE HYDROCHLORIDE

Zoloft
PFIZER

25 mg

50 mg

Rx

SILDENAFIL CITRATE

Viagra
PFIZER

50 mg

100 mg

Rx

TADALAFIL

Cialis
ELI LILLY

10 mg

20 mg

Rx

TAMSULOSIN HYDROCHLORIDE

Flomax
BOEHRINGER

0.4 mg

Rx

TOLTERODINE TARTRATE

Detrol LA
PFIZER

1 mg

4 mg

Rx

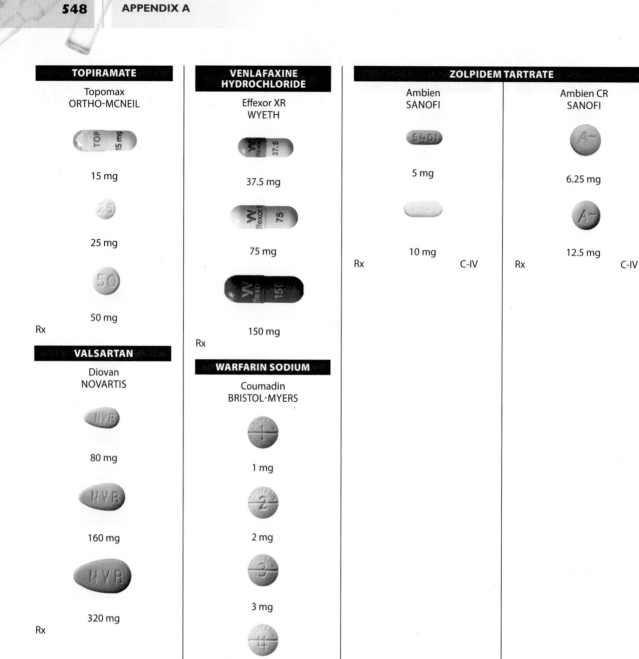

TOPIRAMATE

Topomax
ORTHO-MCNEIL

15 mg

25 mg

50 mg

Rx

VALSARTAN

Diovan
NOVARTIS

80 mg

160 mg

320 mg

Rx

VENLAFAXINE HYDROCHLORIDE

Effexor XR
WYETH

37.5 mg

75 mg

150 mg

Rx

WARFARIN SODIUM

Coumadin
BRISTOL-MYERS

1 mg

2 mg

3 mg

4 mg

5 mg

Rx

ZOLPIDEM TARTRATE

Ambien
SANOFI

5 mg

10 mg

Rx   C-IV

Ambien CR
SANOFI

6.25 mg

12.5 mg

Rx   C-IV

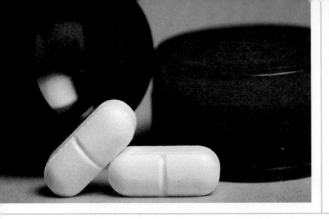

Appendix B
Helpful References

Reading Decimals

Powers of 10

Metric System Fundamental Units

Common Metric Equivalents

Household Abbreviations and Equivalents

Common Household Measures

Relationship of Household Measures

Celsius and Fahrenheit Relationship of Differences

READING DECIMALS

Reading Decimals	
0.1	Read as one-tenth
0.01	Read as one-hundredth
0.001	Read as one-thousandth
0.0001	Read as one ten-thousandth
0.00001	Read as one hundred-thousandth
0.000001	Read as one-millionth

POWERS OF 10

Power	Number	Name or Value
1st	10	ten
2nd	100	hundred
3rd	1,000	thousand
4th	10,000	ten thousand
5th	100,000	hundred thousand
6th	1,000,000	million
7th	10,000,000	ten million
8th	100,000,000	hundred million
9th	1,000,000,000	billion
10th	10,000,000,000	ten billion

METRIC SYSTEM FUNDAMENTAL UNITS

Meter (m)	=	Length
1 millimeter (mm)	=	0.001 of a meter
1 centimeter (cm)	=	0.01 of a meter
1 decimeter (dm)	=	0.1 of a meter
1 meter (m)	=	1 meter
1 dekameter (dam)	=	10 meters
1 hectometer (hm)	=	100 meters
1 kilometer (km)	=	1000 meters

Liter (L)	=	Volume
1 milliliter (mL)	=	0.001 of a liter
1 centiliter (cL)	=	0.01 of a liter
1 deciliter (dL)	=	0.1 of a liter
1 liter (L)	=	1 liter
1 dekaliter (daL)	=	10 liters
1 hectoliter (hL)	=	100 liters
1 kiloliter (kL)	=	1000 liters

Gram (g)	=	Mass and/or Weight
1 microgram (mcg, μg)	=	0.000001 gram
1 milligram (mg)	=	0.001 of a gram
1 centigram (cg)	=	0.01 of a gram
1 decigram (dg)	=	0.1 of a gram
1 gram (g)	=	1 gram
1 dekagram (dag)	=	10 grams
1 hectogram (hg)	=	100 grams
1 kilogram (kg)	=	1000 grams

COMMON METRIC EQUIVALENTS

Length	Volume	
$2\frac{1}{2}$ centimeters (cm) = 1 inch (in)	1000 milliliters (mL) or 1000 cubic centimeters (cc)	= 1 liter

Weight		
1000 micrograms (mcg)	=	1 milligram (mg)
1000 milligrams (mg)	=	1 gram (g)
1000 grams (g)	=	1 kilogram (kg)
1 kilogram	=	2.2 pounds (lb)

HOUSEHOLD ABBREVIATIONS AND EQUIVALENTS

Abbreviations		Household Equivalents				
drop (drops)	gtt	60 gtt	=	1 t or tsp		
teaspoon	t or tsp	3 t or tsp	=	1 T		
tablespoon	T or tbsp	180 gtt	=	1 T	=	$\frac{1}{2}$ oz
teacup	tcp	2 T	=	1 oz	=	6 t or tsp
cup	C	1 oz	=	30 cc or 30 mL		
pint	pt	6 oz	=	1 tcp		
quart	qt	8 oz	=	1 C or 1 glass		
gallon	gal	2 C	=	1 pt	=	16 oz
ounce	oz	2 pt	=	1 qt	=	32 oz
		4 C	=	1 qt	=	32 oz
		4 qt	=	1 gal	=	128 oz

COMMON HOUSEHOLD MEASURES

Common Household Measures

Drop (gtt) = approximate liquid measure depending on kind of liquid measured and the size of the opening from which it is dropped.

60 drops	1 teaspoon (t or tsp)	8 ounces	1 glass or cup
1 dash	Less than $\frac{1}{8}$ teaspoon	16 tablespoons	
3 teaspoons	1 tablespoon (T or tbsp)	or 8 ounces	1 measuring cup (c)
2 tablespoons	1 ounce (oz)	2 cups	1 pint (pt)
4 ounces	1 juice glass	2 pints	1 quart (qt)
6 ounces	1 teacup	4 quarts	1 gallon (gal)

RELATIONSHIP OF HOUSEHOLD MEASURES

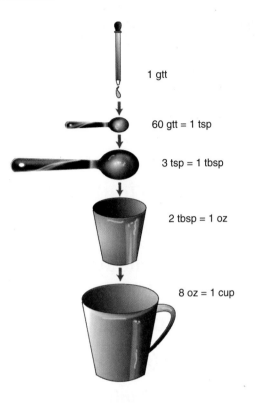

1 gtt

60 gtt = 1 tsp

3 tsp = 1 tbsp

2 tbsp = 1 oz

8 oz = 1 cup

CELSIUS AND FAHRENHEIT RELATIONSHIP OF DIFFERENCES

Relationship of Differences

	Celsius		Fahrenheit	
Boiling Point	100°		212°	Boiling Point
Freezing Point	− 0°		− 32°	Freezing Point
	100°		180°	
Relationship:	Ratio	100 : 180	Fraction	$\frac{100}{180}$
	Reduced	5 : 9		$\frac{5}{9}$

The two formulas that will be described in this unit are

$$C = (F - 32) \times \frac{5}{9}$$

$$F = \frac{9 \times C}{5} + 32$$

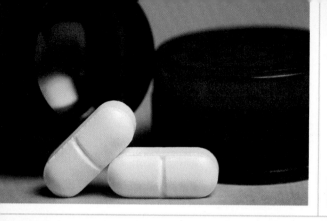

Appendix C
Performance
Checklists

☑ PERFORMANCE CHECKLIST

PROCEDURE 11-1
Administration of Oral Medications

Objective: Having been provided with a physician's order, an oral medication, and the necessary equipment and supplies, you are to correctly administer an oral medication.

Time:
Ended: _____
Started: _____
Total: _____

Directions: Write **S** or **U** to indicate a satisfactory or unsatisfactory performance.

Procedural Steps:	S or U	Comments
1. Verified the physician's order.	_____	
2. Followed the "seven rights."	_____	
3. Performed medical asepsis hand wash.	_____	
4. Worked in a well-lighted, quiet, clean area.	_____	
5. Assembled equipment and supplies.	_____	
6. Obtained the correct medication.	_____	
7. Compared the medication label with the order (first time).	_____	
8. Checked the expiration date.	_____	
9. Calculated dosage, if necessary.	_____	
10. Compared the medication label with the order (second time).	_____	
11. Correctly prepared: (a, b, or c). a. Multiple-dose solid medication b. Unit-dose medication c. Liquid medication	_____	
12. Replaced medication on shelf and compared medication label with the order (third time).	_____	
13. Transported medicine to the patient.	_____	
14. Identified the patient. Explained the procedure.	_____	
15. Assessed the patient. Took vital signs if indicated.	_____	
16. Assisted patient to a comfortable position.	_____	
17. Provided water, milk, or juice (unless contraindicated).	_____	
18. Administered the medication. Made sure that the patient took the medicine.	_____	
19. Provided for the patient's safety: Observed the patient for any adverse reactions.	_____	
20. Documented the procedure.	_____	
21. Cared for equipment and supplies according to OSHA guidelines.	_____	
22. Washed hands.	_____	

For a printable checklist, go to the Premium Website.

✓ PERFORMANCE CHECKLIST

PROCEDURE 11-2
Performing Eye Instillation

Objective: Having been provided with a physician's order, an eye medication, and the necessary equipment and supplies, you are to correctly administer an eye medication.

Time: Ended: _____
                 Started: _____
                 Total: _____

Directions: Write **S** or **U** to indicate a satisfactory or unsatisfactory performance.

Procedural Steps:	S or U	Comments
1. Washed hands.	_____	
2. Assembled supplies.	_____	
3. Checked medication, including expiration date and read label three times.	_____	
4. Identified patient.	_____	
5. Explained procedure.	_____	
6. Correctly positioned the patient.	_____	
7. Instructed the patient to stare at a fixed spot during instillation of the drops. Put on gloves.	_____	
8. Prepared eye drops or ointment for administration.	_____	
9. Had the patient look up to the ceiling and exposed the lower conjunctival sac of the affected eye.	_____	
10. Placed the number of drops ordered in the center of the lower conjunctival sac or a thin line of ointment in the lower surface of the eyelid. Replaced dropper in the bottle.	_____	
11. Had the patient close the eye and roll the eyeball.	_____	
12. Blotted excess medication from eyelids.	_____	
13. Disposed of supplies.	_____	
14. Removed gloves.	_____	
15. Washed hands.	_____	
16. Documented procedure.	_____	

For a printable checklist, go to the Premium Website.

✓ PERFORMANCE CHECKLIST

PROCEDURE 11-3
Performing Ear Instillation

Objective: Having been provided with a physician's order, an ear medication, and the necessary equipment and supplies, you are to correctly administer an ear medication.

Time: Ended: _____
Started: _____
Total: _____

Directions: Write **S** or **U** to indicate a satisfactory or unsatisfactory performance.

Procedural Steps:	S or U	Comments
1. Washed hands and assembled supplies.	_____	
2. Identified patient.	_____	
3. Explained procedure.	_____	
4. Correctly positioned the patient.	_____	
5. Checked medication, including expiration date and read label three times.	_____	
6. Drew up the prescribed amount of medication. Put on gloves.	_____	
7. Gently pulled the top of the ear upward and back (adult) or downward and backward (child).	_____	
8. Instilled prescribed dose of medication into the affected ear.	_____	
9. Had the patient maintain the position for about 5 minutes.	_____	
10. If instructed by physician, inserted moistened cotton ball into external tear canal for 15 minutes.	_____	
11. Disposed of supplies.	_____	
12. Removed gloves.	_____	
13. Washed hands.	_____	
14. Documented procedure.	_____	

For a printable checklist, go to the Premium Website.

✓ **PERFORMANCE CHECKLIST**

PROCEDURE 12-1
Handling a Sterile Syringe-Needle Unit—Disposable Peel-Back Method

Objective: Having been provided with a physician's order and the necessary equipment and supplies, you are to correctly handle a sterile syringe-needle unit—disposable peel-back method.

Time:

Ended:	_____	
Started:	_____	
Total:	_____	

Directions: Write **S** or **U** to indicate a satisfactory or unsatisfactory performance.

Procedural Steps: S or U   Comments

1. Verified physician's order.   _____
2. Worked in a well-lighted, quiet,   _____
    clean area.
3. Performed medical asepsis hand wash.   _____
4. Put on gloves.   _____
5. Obtained a sterile syringe-needle unit.   _____
6. Checked the package label.   _____
7. Opened the package correctly.   _____
8. Correctly removed the unit from   _____
    the package.
9. Held the outside of the barrel with   _____
    the sheathed needle pointing upward.
10. Loosened the plunger and pushed it   _____
    back into the barrel without touching
    the plunger's stem.
11. Assured oneself that the needle is   _____
    attached to the tip of the syringe.
12. Loosened the sheath correctly.   _____
13. Removed the sheath correctly.   _____
14. Replaced the sheath without the needle   _____
    touching the interior of the sheath.
15. Removed gloves   _____
16. Washed hands.   _____

For a printable checklist, go to the Premium Website.

PERFORMANCE CHECKLIST

PROCEDURE 12-2
Loading and Unloading a Tubex Injector

Objective: Having been provided with a physician's order and the necessary equipment and supplies, you are to correctly load and unload a Tubex injector.

Time: Ended: _____
Started: _____
Total: _____

Directions: Write **S** or **U** to indicate a satisfactory or unsatisfactory performance.

Procedural Steps:	S or U	Comments
1. Verified physician's order.	_____	
2. Worked in a well-lighted, quiet, clean area.	_____	
3. Performed medical asepsis hand wash. Put on gloves.	_____	
4. Obtained a Tubex injector and sterile cartridge-needle unit.	_____	
5. Turned the ribbed collar to the "OPEN" position until it stops.	_____	
6. Held the injector with open end up, and inserted the Tubex sterile cartridge-needle unit.	_____	
7. Tightened the ribbed collar in the direction of the "CLOSE" arrow.	_____	
8. Threaded the plunger rod into the plunger of the Tubex sterile cartridge-needle unit until slight resistance was felt.	_____	
9. After use, did not recap the needle.	_____	
10. Disengaged the plunger rod.	_____	
11. Held the injector, needle down, over sharps container and loosened the ribbed collar.	_____	
12. Discarded the needle cover.	_____	
13. Removed gloves.	_____	
14. Washed hands.	_____	

For a printable checklist, go to the Premium Website.

✓ PERFORMANCE CHECKLIST

PROCEDURE 12-3
Withdrawing (Aspirating) Medication from a Vial

Objective: Having been provided with a physician's order and the necessary equipment and supplies, you are to correctly withdraw medication from a vial.

Time:

Ended:	_____	
Started:	_____	
Total:	_____	

Directions: Write **S** or **U** to indicate a satisfactory or unsatisfactory performance.

Procedural Steps:	S or U	Comments
1. Correctly read the medication order and assembled equipment. Checked the vial label against the medication order (first time).	_____	
2. Washed hands. Put on gloves.	_____	
3. Selected the correct size syringe-needle unit.	_____	
4. Checked the vial label against the medication order (second time).	_____	
5. Removed the cap from the vial. Cleaned the rubber stopper.	_____	
6. Correctly removed the needle cover.	_____	
7. Correctly injected air into the vial.	_____	
8. Withdrew the correct amount of medication from the vial into the syringe.	_____	
9. Checked the syringe for air bubbles. Correctly removed a large air bubble.	_____	
10. Removed the needle from the vial. Correctly replaced the needle cover.	_____	
11. Checked the vial label against the medication order (third time).	_____	
12. Placed the filled syringe-needle unit on a medicine tray.	_____	
13. Returned multiple-dose vial to the proper storage area or correctly disposed of unused medication from a single-dose vial.	_____	
14. Correctly discarded used syringe-needle unit immediately after use.	_____	
15. Removed gloves.	_____	
16. Washed hands.	_____	
17. Documented procedure.	_____	

For a printable checklist, go to the Premium Website.

✓ PERFORMANCE CHECKLIST

PROCEDURE 12-4
Withdrawing (Aspirating) Medication from an Ampule

Objective: Having been provided with a physician's order and the necessary equipment and supplies, you are to correctly withdraw medication from an ampule.

Time:
Ended: _____
Started: _____
Total: _____

Directions: Write **S** or **U** to indicate a satisfactory or unsatisfactory performance.

Procedural Steps:	S or U	Comments
1. Checked the physician's order.	_____	
2. Washed hands. Gathered equipment. Put on gloves.	_____	
3. Obtained ampule of medicine. Read the label and checked medicine (first time). Checked expiration date.	_____	
4. Flicked ampule downward.	_____	
5. Thoroughly disinfected the neck of the ampule. Checked label (second time).	_____	
6. Wiped neck of ampule dry with a sterile gauze. Snapped off the top of the ampule.	_____	
7. Placed opened ampule on medicine tray. Checked label (third time).	_____	
8. Aspirated the required dose of medicine into the syringe. Covered needle with sheath and transported to the patient.	_____	
9. Identified the patient.	_____	
10. Administered the medication.	_____	
11. Discarded syringe-needle unit. Discarded alcohol swabs and gauze.	_____	
12. Removed gloves.	_____	
13. Washed hands.	_____	
14. Documented the procedure.	_____	

For a printable checklist, go to the Premium Website.

✓ **PERFORMANCE CHECKLIST**

PROCEDURE 12-5
Mixing Two Medications in One Syringe-Needle Unit

Objective: Having been provided with a physician's order and the necessary equipment and supplies, you are to correctly mix two medications in one syringe-needle unit.

Time: Ended: _____
              Started: _____
              Total: _____

Directions: Write **S** or **U** to indicate a satisfactory or unsatisfactory performance.

Procedural Steps: S or U   Comments

1. Verified the physician's order.   _____
2. Worked in a well-lighted, quiet, clean area.   _____
3. Performed medical asepsis hand wash.   _____
    Put on gloves.
4. Compared the medication labels with the physician's order.   _____
5. Prepared a syringe-needle unit for use.   _____
6. Drew up an amount of air into the   _____
    syringe that was equal to the amount
    of medication that was to be withdrawn.
7. Cleansed rubber-stoppered portion of the vial.   _____
8. Placed the syringe-needle unit in   _____
    dominant hand. Removed needle sheath.
9. Picked up vial in other hand.   _____
    Inverted vial.
10. Inserted needle into the rubber-stoppered portion of the vial. _____
11. Injected equal amount of air into the vial.   _____
12. Filled the barrel with ordered amount of medication.   _____
13. Removed needle from vial.   _____
14. Replaced sheath over needle.   _____
15. Checked for air bubbles.   _____
16. Placed syringe-needle unit on medicine   _____
    tray or clean, dry surface.
17. Compared second medication label with physician's order.   _____
18. Opened sterile needle package.   _____
19. Removed needle from filled syringe.   _____
20. Placed opened needle onto filled syringe.   _____
21. Cleansed rubber-stoppered portion of the second vial.   _____
22. Placed syringe-needle unit in   _____
    dominant hand. Removed needle sheath.
23. Picked up second vial. Inverted vial.   _____
24. Inserted needle into rubber-stoppered portion of vial.   _____
25. Did not inject air into second vial.   _____
26. Filled barrel with ordered amount of medication.   _____
27. Removed needle from vial.   _____
28. Replaced sheath over needle.   _____
29. Checked for air bubbles.   _____
30. Checked to be sure of correct total doses as ordered.   _____
31. Prepared to administer medication to the patient.   _____

For a printable checklist, go to the Premium Website.

✓ PERFORMANCE CHECKLIST

PROCEDURE 12-6
Reconstituting a Powder Medication for Administration

Objective: Having been provided with a physician's order and the necessary equipment and supplies, you are to correctly reconstitute a powder medication for administration.

Time: Ended: _____
                   Started: _____
                   Total: _____

Directions: Write **S** or **U** to indicate a satisfactory or unsatisfactory performance.

Procedural Steps:	S or U	Comments
1. Performed medical asepsis hand wash. Put on gloves.	_____	
2. Prepared a syringe-needle unit for use.	_____	
3. Removed tops from diluent and powder medication containers and wiped with alcohol swabs.	_____	
4. Injected air in an equal amount to diluent being removed from the vial.	_____	
5. Withdrew the appropriate amount of diluent to be added to the powder medication.	_____	
6. Added liquid to the powder medication.	_____	
7. Removed needle-syringe unit from vial and properly discarded.	_____	
8. Rolled the vial between the palms of the hands to completely mix the powder and diluent. Labeled the multiple-dose vial with the dilution of strength of the medication prepared, the date and time, your initials, and the expiration date.	_____	
9. Used a second sterile needle-syringe unit to withdraw the desired amount of medication.	_____	
10. Removed air bubbles.	_____	
11. Prepared medicine tray with reconstituted medication.	_____	

For a printable checklist, go to the Premium Website.

PERFORMANCE CHECKLIST

PROCEDURE 13-1
Administration of Subcutaneous, Intramuscular, and/or Intradermal Injections

Objective: Having been provided with a physician's order and the necessary equipment and supplies, you are to correctly administer a subcutaneous, intramuscular, and/or intradermal injection.

Time: Ended: _____
                 Started: _____
                 Total: _____

Directions: Write **S** or **U** to indicate a satisfactory or unsatisfactory performance.

Procedural Steps:	S or U	Comments
1. Verified the physician's order.	_____	
2. Followed the "seven rights."	_____	
3. Performed medical asepsis hand wash.	_____	
4. Worked in a well-lighted, quiet, clean area.	_____	
5. Obtained the appropriate equipment.	_____	
6. Obtained the correct medication.	_____	
7. Compared medication label with medication order (first time).	_____	
8. Checked expiration date on medicine.	_____	
9. Calculated dosage, if necessary.	_____	
10. Prepared syringe-needle unit for use.	_____	
11. Withdrew medication from container.	_____	
12. Compared medicine label with the medication order (second time).	_____	
13. Placed filled syringe-needle unit on medicine tray. Checked medication label with the medication order (third time).	_____	
14. Correctly transported the medicine to the patient.	_____	
15. Identified the patient. Explained the procedure.	_____	
16. Assessed the patient. Put on gloves.	_____	
17. Prepared the patient for the injection.	_____	
18. Selected an appropriate injection site.	_____	
19. Cleansed the injection site with a sterile antiseptic swab.	_____	
20. Allowed the skin to dry.	_____	
21. Administered the injection. Immediately disposed of syringe-needle unit in a puncture-proof container.	_____	
22. Massaged injection site unless contraindicated.	_____	
23. Observed the patient for signs of difficulty.	_____	
24. Inspected the injection site for bleeding. Applied Band-Aid if necessary.	_____	
25. Properly disposed of used equipment and supplies. Removed gloves.	_____	
26. Performed medical asepsis hand wash.	_____	
27. Correctly documented the procedure.	_____	

For a printable checklist, go to the Premium Website.

PERFORMANCE CHECKLIST

PROCEDURE 13-2
Administering a Subcutaneous Injection

Objective: Having been provided with a physician's order and the necessary equipment and supplies, you are to correctly administer a subcutaneous injection.

Time: Ended: _____
                       Started: _____
                       Total: _____

Directions: Write **S** or **U** to indicate a satisfactory or unsatisfactory performance.

Procedural Steps:	S or U	Comments
1. Verified the physician's order.	_____	
2. Followed the "seven rights."	_____	
3. Performed medical asepsis hand wash.	_____	
4. Worked in a well-lighted, quiet, clean area.	_____	
5. Obtained the appropriate equipment and supplies.	_____	
6. Obtained the correct medication.	_____	
7. Compared medication label with medication order (first time).	_____	
8. Checked expiration date on medicine.	_____	
9. Calculated dosage, if necessary.	_____	
10. Prepared parenteral medication.	_____	
11. Compared medicine label with the medication order (second time).	_____	
12. Replaced medication in appropriate area. Checked medication label with the medication order (third time).	_____	
13. Correctly transported the medicine to the patient.	_____	
14. Identified the patient. Explained the procedure.	_____	
15. Assessed the patient. Put on gloves.	_____	
16. Prepared the patient for the injection.	_____	
17. Selected an appropriate injection site.	_____	
18. Cleansed the injection site with a sterile antiseptic swab. Allowed the skin to dry.	_____	
19. Removed needle guard.	_____	
20. Grasped skin to form 1-inch fold.	_____	
21. Inserted needle correctly.	_____	
22. Aspirated.	_____	
23. Injected the medicine.	_____	
24. Removed needle and syringe.	_____	
25. Covered site. Massaged if indicated.	_____	
26. Disposed of equipment.	_____	
27. Removed gloves and washed hands.	_____	
28. Provided for patient's safety.	_____	
29. Documented the procedure.	_____	

For a printable checklist, go to the Premium Website.

✔ PERFORMANCE CHECKLIST

PROCEDURE 13-3
Administering an Intramuscular Injection

Objective: Having been provided with a physician's order and the necessary equipment and supplies, you are to correctly administer an intramuscular injection.

Time: Ended: _____
Started: _____
Total: _____

Directions: Write **S** or **U** to indicate a satisfactory or unsatisfactory performance.

Procedural Steps:	S or U	Comments
1. Verified the physician's order.	_____	
2. Followed the "seven rights."	_____	
3. Performed medical asepsis hand wash.	_____	
4. Worked in a well-lighted, quiet, clean area.	_____	
5. Obtained the appropriate equipment and supplies.	_____	
6. Obtained the correct medication.	_____	
7. Compared medication label with medication order (first time).	_____	
8. Checked expiration date on medicine.	_____	
9. Calculated dosage, if necessary.	_____	
10. Prepared parenteral medication.	_____	
11. Compared medicine label with the medication order (second time).	_____	
12. Replaced medication in appropriate area. Checked medication label with the medication order (third time).	_____	
13. Correctly transported the medicine to the patient.	_____	
14. Identified the patient. Explained the procedure.	_____	
15. Assessed the patient. Put on gloves.	_____	
16. Prepared the patient for the injection.	_____	
17. Selected an appropriate injection site.	_____	
18. Cleansed the injection site with a sterile antiseptic swab. Allowed the skin to dry.	_____	
19. Removed needle guard.	_____	
20. Stretched the skin taut, pulling it tight.	_____	
21. Using a dartlike motion, inserted needle correctly.	_____	
22. Released the skin.	_____	
23. Aspirated.	_____	
24. Injected the medicine.	_____	
25. Removed needle and syringe.	_____	
26. Covered site. Massaged if indicated.	_____	
27. Disposed of equipment.	_____	
28. Removed gloves.	_____	
29. Washed hands.	_____	
30. Observed patient.	_____	
31. Provided for patient's safety.	_____	
32. Documented the procedure.	_____	

For a printable checklist, go to the Premium Website.

✓ **PERFORMANCE CHECKLIST**

PROCEDURE 13-4
Administering an Intradermal Injection

Objective: Having been provided with a physician's order and the necessary equipment and supplies, you are to correctly administer an intradermal injection.

Time: Ended: _____
                   Started: _____
                   Total: _____

Directions: Write **S** or **U** to indicate a satisfactory or unsatisfactory performance.

Procedural Steps:	S or U	Comments
1. Verified the physician's order.	_____	
2. Followed the "seven rights."	_____	
3. Performed medical asepsis hand wash.	_____	
4. Worked in a well-lighted, quiet, clean area.	_____	
5. Obtained the appropriate equipment and supplies.	_____	
6. Obtained the correct medication.	_____	
7. Compared medication label with medication order (first time).	_____	
8. Checked expiration date on medicine.	_____	
9. Calculated dosage, if necessary.	_____	
10. Prepared parenteral medication.	_____	
11. Compared medicine label with the medication order (second time).	_____	
12. Replaced medication in appropriate area. Checked medication label with the medication order (third time).	_____	
13. Correctly transported the medicine to the patient.	_____	
14. Identified the patient. Explained the procedure.	_____	
15. Assessed the patient. Put on gloves.	_____	
16. Prepared the patient for the injection.	_____	
17. Selected an appropriate injection site.	_____	
18. Cleansed the injection site with a sterile antiseptic swab. Allowed the skin to dry.	_____	
19. Removed needle guard.	_____	
20. Stretched the skin taut, pulling it tight.	_____	
21. Carefully inserted the needle correctly.	_____	
22. Injected the medicine and produced a wheal.	_____	
23. Correctly removed the needle.	_____	
24. Covered site. Did not massage. Disposed of equipment. Removed gloves.	_____	
25. Washed hands.	_____	
26. Observed patient.	_____	
27. Provided for patient's safety.	_____	
28. Documented the procedure.	_____	

For a printable checklist, go to the Premium Website.

☑ **PERFORMANCE CHECKLIST**

PROCEDURE 13-5
"Z"-Track Intramuscular Injection Technique

Objective: Having been provided with a physician's order and the necessary equipment and supplies, you are to correctly administer a "Z"-track intramuscular injection.

Time:　　　Ended:　　　＿＿＿＿＿＿
　　　　　　　Started:　　　＿＿＿＿＿＿
　　　　　　　Total:　　　　＿＿＿＿＿＿

Directions: Write **S** or **U** to indicate a satisfactory or unsatisfactory performance.

Procedural Steps:　　　　　　　　　　　　　　　　　　S or U　　　　Comments

1. Verified the physician's order.　　　　　　　　　　＿＿＿＿
2. Followed the "seven rights."　　　　　　　　　　　＿＿＿＿
3. Performed medical asepsis hand wash.　　　　　　　＿＿＿＿
4. Worked in a well-lighted, quiet, clean area.　　　　＿＿＿＿
5. Assembled equipment and supplies.　　　　　　　　＿＿＿＿
6. Obtained the correct medication.　　　　　　　　　＿＿＿＿
7. Compared the medication label with the medication order.　＿＿＿＿
8. Checked the expiration date.　　　　　　　　　　　＿＿＿＿
9. Calculated dosage, if necessary.　　　　　　　　　＿＿＿＿
10. Prepared the parenteral medication.　　　　　　　＿＿＿＿
11. Compared the medication label with the medication order (second time).　＿＿＿＿
12. Replaced medication on shelf and compared medication label (third time).　＿＿＿＿
13. Transported medicine to the patient.　　　　　　　＿＿＿＿
14. Identified the patient. Explained procedure.　　　＿＿＿＿
15. Assessed the patient. Put on gloves.　　　　　　　＿＿＿＿
16. Prepared the patient for the injection.　　　　　　＿＿＿＿
17. Selected the injection site.　　　　　　　　　　　＿＿＿＿
18. Cleansed the injection site.　　　　　　　　　　　＿＿＿＿
19. Removed the needle guard.　　　　　　　　　　　＿＿＿＿
20. Pulled the skin laterally $1\frac{1}{2}$ inch away from the injection site.　＿＿＿＿
21. Using a dartlike motion inserted needle. Maintained "Z" position.　＿＿＿＿
22. Aspirated.　　　　　　　　　　　　　　　　　　＿＿＿＿
23. Slowly injected medication.　　　　　　　　　　　＿＿＿＿
24. Waited 10 seconds.　　　　　　　　　　　　　　＿＿＿＿
25. Removed needle and syringe at the same angle of insertion.　＿＿＿＿
26. Released traction of the "Z" position.　　　　　　＿＿＿＿
27. Covered injection site. Did not massage. Disposed of equipment.　＿＿＿＿
28. Removed gloves.　　　　　　　　　　　　　　　＿＿＿＿
29. Washed hands.　　　　　　　　　　　　　　　　＿＿＿＿
30. Observed patient for signs of difficulty.　　　　　＿＿＿＿
31. Provided for patient safety.　　　　　　　　　　　＿＿＿＿
32. Documented procedure.　　　　　　　　　　　　＿＿＿＿

For a printable checklist, go to the Premium Website.

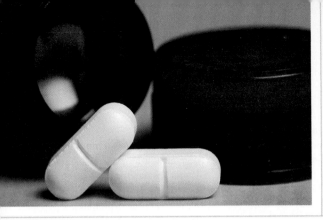

Drug Index

Page numbers followed by *f* denote figures; page numbers followed by *t* denotes tables.

Subject Index

Page numbers followed by *f* denote figures; page numbers followed by *t* denotes tables.